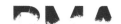

Nephrology and Fluid/ Electrolyte Physiology

Nephrology and Fluid/Electrolyte Physiology

Series Editor

Richard A. Polin, MD
William T. Speck Professor of Pediatrics
College of Physicians and Surgeons
Columbia University
Director Division of Neonatology
New York Presbyterian
Morgan Stanley Children's Hospital
New York, New York

Other Volumes in the Neonatology Questions and Controversies Series

Nephrology and Fluid/ Electrolyte Physiology

Third Edition

William Oh, MD

Professor of Pediatrics
Department of Pediatrics
Warren Altpert Medical School of Brown University
Staff Neonatologist
Department of Pediatrics
Women and Infants' Hospital
Providence, Rhode Island
Scientific Medical Director
Florida Hospital for Children
Orlando, Florida

Michel Baum, MD

Professor of Pediatrics and Internal Medicine
Department of Pediatrics
University of Texas Southwestern Medical Center
Dallas, Texas

Consulting Editor

Richard A. Polin, MD

William T. Speck Professor of Pediatrics
College of Physicians and Surgeons
Columbia University
Director Division of Neonatology
New York Presbyterian
Morgan Stanley Children's Hospital
New York, New York

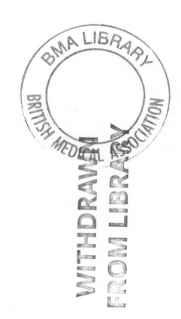

ELSEVIER

ELSEVIER

1600 John F. Kennedy Blvd.
Ste 1600
Philadelphia, PA 19103-2899

Senior Content Strategist: Sarah Barth
Content Development Specialist: Lisa M. Barnes
Publishing Services Manager: Catherine Jackson
Senior Project Manager: Daniel Fitzgerald
Designer: Paula Catalano

Contributors

Sharon P. Andreoli, MD
Byron P. and Frances D. Hollett
  Professor of Pediatrics
Division of Pediatric Nephrology and
  Hypertension
Department of Pediatrics
Indiana University Medical School
Indianapolis, Indiana
United States
  Kidney Injury in the Neonate

Timur Azhibekov, MD
Medical Director, NICU
Providence Holy Cross MC
St. Mission Hills, California
Fetal and Neonatal Institute
Division of Neonatology
Children's Hospital Los Angeles
Keck School of Medicine
University of Southern California
Los Angeles, California
United States
  *Acid-Base Homeostasis in the Fetus
  and Newborn*

Carlton Bates, MD
Nephrologist
Children's Hospital of Pittsburgh of
  University of Pittsburgh
Pittsburgh, Pennsylvania
United States
  *Renal Development and Molecular
  Pathogenesis of Renal Dysplasia*

Michel Baum, MD
Professor of Pediatrics and Internal
  Medicine
Department of Pediatrics
University of Texas Southwestern
  Medical Center
Dallas, Texas
United States
  *Prenatal Programming of
  Hypertension and Kidney and
  Cardiovascular Disease*

Stephen Baumgart, MD, FAAP
Professor, Emeritus
Department of Neonatology
Children's National Medical Center
Washington, District of Columbia
United States
  *Acute Problems of Prematurity:
  Balancing Fluid Volume and
  Electrolyte Replacements in Very
  Low Birth Weight and Extremely
  Low Birth Weight Neonates*

Marie H. Beall, MD
Los Angeles Perinatal Associates
Los Angeles, California
United States
  *Water Flux and Amniotic Fluid Volume:
  Understanding Fetal Water Flow*

Martine TP Besouw, MD, PhD
Department of Pediatric Nephrology
University of Groningen
University Medical Center Groningen
Groningen
The Netherlands
  Potassium Metabolism

Richard D. Bland, MD
Professor of Pediatrics
Stanford University
Stanford, California
United States
  *Lung Fluid Balance in Developing
  Lungs and Its Role in Neonatal
  Transition*

Detlef Bockenhauer, MD, PhD
Centre for Nephrology and Institute of
  Child Health
University College London
Great Ormond Street Hospital for
  Children
London
Great Britain
  Potassium Metabolism

Melvin Bonilla-Felix, MD
Professor and Chairman
Department of Pediatrics
University of Puerto Rico—Medical
  Sciences Campus
San Juan
Puerto Rico
  Renal Modulation: Arginine
  Vasopressin and Atrial Natriuretic
  Peptide

Debora Malta Cerqueira, PhD
Postdoctoral Fellow
Department of Pediatrics
University of Pittsburgh
Pittsburgh, Pennsylvania
United States
  Renal Development and Molecular
  Pathogenesis of Renal Dysplasia

Andrew Thomas Costarino, MD, MSCE
Professor Clinical Anesthesiology and
  Pediatrics
The Perelman School of Medicine
The University of Pennsylvania
Director Division of Cardiac Critical
  Care Medicine
Department of Anesthesiology and
  Critical Care Medicine
The Children's Hospital of Philadelphia
Philadelphia, Pennsylvania
United States
  Edema

Nilka de Jesús-González, MD, MSc
Assistant Professor
Department of Pediatrics
University of Puerto Rico—Medical
  Sciences Campus
San Juan
Puerto Rico
  Renal Modulation: Arginine
  Vasopressin and Atrial Natriuretic
  Peptide

Joseph Flynn, MD, MS
Chief
Division of Nephrology
Seattle Children's Hospital
Professor
Department of Pediatrics
University of Washington School of
  Medicine
Seattle, Washington
United States
  Neonatal Hypertension: Diagnosis
  and Management

Jyothsna Gattineni, MD
Associate Professor
Department of Pediatrics
University of Texas Southwestern
  Medical Center
Dallas, Texas
United States
  Inherited Disorders of Calcium,
  Phosphate, and Magnesium

Jean-Bernard Gouyon, MD
Professor of Pediatrics
Head of the "Centre d'Etudes Périnatales
  de l'Océan Indien-EA 7388"
University Hospital
La Reunion Island
France
  Glomerular Filtration Rate in Neonates

Jean-Pierre Guignard, MD
Honorary Professor of Pediatrics
Lausanne University Medical School
Lausanne
Switzerland
  Glomerular Filtration Rate in Neonates
  Use of Diuretics in the Newborn

Jacqueline Ho, MD
University of Pittsburgh
Pittsburgh, Pennsylvania
United States
  Renal Development and Molecular
  Pathogenesis of Renal Dysplasia

Lucky Jain, MD, MBA
Richard W. Blumberg Professor &
  Executive Vice Chairman
Department of Pediatrics
Emory University School of Medicine
Atlanta, Georgia
United States
  Lung Fluid Balance in Developing
  Lungs and Its Role in Neonatal
  Transition

Pedro A. Jose, MD, PhD
Professor
Departments of Medicine and
  Pharmacology-Physiology
Division of Renal Diseases &
  Hypertension
The George Washington University
  School of Medicine & Health
  Sciences
Washington, District of Columbia
United States
  Renal Modulation: The Renin-
  Angiotensin System

Sarah D. Keene, MD
Assistant Professor
Department of Pediatrics
Division of Neonatal/Perinatal
  Medicine
Emory University
Atlanta, Georgia
United States
  *Lung Fluid Balance in Developing
  Lungs and Its Role in Neonatal
  Transition*

Myda Khalid, MD
Assistant Professor of Clinical
  Pediatrics
Division of Pediatric Nephrology and
  Hypertension
Department of Pediatrics
James Whitcomb Riley Hospital for
  Children
Indiana University Medical Center
Indianapolis, Indiana
United States
  Kidney Injury in the Neonate

Yosef Levenbrown, DO
Division of Pediatric Critical Care
  Medicine
Nemours/Alfred I. duPont Hospital for
  Children
Wilmington, Delaware
Clinical Assistant Professor of
  Pediatrics
Sidney Kimmel Medical College of
  Thomas Jefferson University
Philadelphia, Pennsylvania
United States
  Edema

Douglas G. Matsell, MDCM
Division of Nephrology
British Columbia Children's Hospital
University of British Columbia
Vancouver, British Columbia
Canada
  *Congenital Urinary Tract
  Obstruction—Diagnosis and
  Management in the Fetus*

Ran Namgung, MD, PhD
Professor
Department of Pediatrics
Yonsei University College of Medicine
Seoul
Korea
  *Perinatal Calcium and Phosphorus
  Metabolism*

Aruna Natarajan, MD, DCH, PhD
Associate Professor (Adjunct)
Pediatrics, Pharmacology and
  Physiology
MedStar Georgetown University
  Hospital
Washington, District of Columbia
United States
  *Renal Modulation: The Renin-
  Angiotensin System*

William Oh, MD
Professor of Pediatrics
Department of Pediatrics
Warren Altpert Medical School of
  Brown University
Staff Neonatologist
Department of Pediatrics
Women and Infants' Hospital
Providence, Rhode Island
Scientific Medical Director
Florida Hospital for Children
Orlando, Florida
United States
  *Body Composition in the Fetus and
  Newborn: Effects of Intrauterine
  Growth Aberration*

Pawan Puri, PhD, DVM
Research Instructor
Department of Pediatrics
University of Pittsburgh
Pittsburgh, Pennsylvania
United States
  *Renal Development and
  Molecular Pathogenesis of Renal
  Dysplasia*

Raymond Quigley, MD
Professor
Department of Pediatrics
University of Texas Southwestern
  Medical Center
Dallas, Texas
United States
  *Renal Aspects of Sodium
  Metabolism in the Fetus and
  Neonate*

Michael G. Ross, MD, MPH
Distinguished Professor
Department of Obstetrics and
 Gynecology
Geffen School of Medicine at
 University of California, Los Angeles
Distinguished Professor
Community Health Sciences
Fielding School of Public Health at
 University of California, Los Angeles
Los Angeles, California
United States
 *Water Flux and Amniotic Fluid
 Volume: Understanding Fetal
 Water Flow*

Jeffrey Segar, MD
Stead Family Department of Pediatrics
University of Iowa Carver College of
 Medicine
University of Iowa Stead Family
 Children's Hospital
Iowa City, Iowa
United States
 *Fluid and Electrolyte Management
 of High-Risk Infants*

Istvan Seri, MD, PhD, HonD
Honorary Member
Hungarian Academy of Sciences
First Department of Pediatrics
Semmelweis University
Faculty of Medicine
Budapest
Hungary
Professor of Pediatrics (Adjunct)
Children's Hospital Los Angeles
USC Keck School of Medicine
Los Angeles, California
United States
 *Acid-Base Homeostasis in the Fetus
 and Newborn*

Reginald C. Tsang, MBBS
Emeritus Professor of Pediatrics
Cincinnati Children's Hospital Medical
 Center
Cincinnati, Ohio
United States
 *Perinatal Calcium and Phosphorus
 Metabolism*

Jeroen P.H.M. van den Wijngaard, PhD
Department of Clinical Chemistry and
 Laboratory Medicine
Leiden University Medical Center
Leiden
The Netherlands
 *Water Flux and Amniotic Fluid
 Volume: Understanding Fetal
 Water Flow*

Martin van Gemert, PhD
Department of Biomedical Engineering
 & Physics
Academic Medical Center
University of Amsterdam
Amsterdam
The Netherlands
 *Water Flux and Amniotic Fluid
 Volume: Understanding Fetal
 Water Flow*

Van Anthony M. Villar, MD, PhD
Assistant Professor
Department of Medicine
Division of Renal Diseases &
 Hypertension
The George Washington University
 School of Medicine & Health
 Sciences
Washington, District of Columbia
United States
 *Renal Modulation: The Renin-
 Angiotensin System*

Matthias Tilmann Wolf, MD
Assistant Professor
Department of Pediatric Nephrology
University of Texas Southwestern
 Medical Center Dallas
Dallas, Texas
United States
 *Inherited Disorders of Calcium,
 Phosphate, and Magnesium*

Israel Zelikovic, MD
Director
Laboratory of Developmental
 Nephrology
Faculty of Medicine
Technion
Haifa
Israel
 Hereditary Tubulopathies

Series Foreword

Richard A. Polin, MD

To study the phenomena of disease without books is to sail an uncharted sea, while to study books without patients is not to go to sea at all.

—William Osler

Physicians in training generally rely upon the spoken word and clinical experiences to bolster their medical knowledge. There is probably no better way to learn how to care for an infant than to receive teaching at the bedside. Of course, that assumes that the "clinician" doing the teaching is knowledgeable about the disease, wants to teach, and can teach effectively. For a student or intern, this style of learning is efficient because the clinical service demands preclude much time for other reading. Over the course of one's career, it becomes clear that this form of education has limitations because of the fairly limited number of disease conditions one encounters even in a lifetime of clinical rotations and the diminishing opportunities for teaching moments.

The next educational phase generally includes reading textbooks and qualitative review articles. Unfortunately, both of those sources are often outdated by the time they are published and represent one author's opinions about management. Systematic analyses (meta-analyses) can be more informative, but more often than not the conclusion of the systematic analysis is that "more studies are needed" to answer the clinical question. Furthermore, it has been estimated that if a subsequent large randomized clinical trial had not been performed, the meta-analysis would have reached an erroneous conclusion more than one-third of the time.

For practicing clinicians, clearly the best way to keep abreast of recent advances in a field is to read the medical literature on a regular basis. However, that approach is problematic given the multitude of journals, unless one reads only the two or three major pediatric journals published in the United States. That approach, however, will miss many of the outstanding articles that appear in more general medical journals (e.g., *Journal of the American Medical Association, New England Journal of Medicine, Lancet,* and the *British Medical Journal*), subspecialty journals, and the many pediatric journals published in other countries.

While there is no substitute to reading journal articles on a regular basis, the "Questions and Controversies" series of books provides an excellent alternative. This third edition of the series was developed to highlight the clinical problems of most concern to practitioners. The series has been increased from six to seven volumes and includes new sections on genetics and pharmacology. In total, there are 70 new chapters not included previously. The editors of each volume (Drs. Bancalari, Davis, Keszler, Oh, Baum, Seri, Kluckow, Ohls, Christensen. Maheshwari, Neu, Benitz, Smith, Poindexter, Cilio and Perlman) have done an extraordinary job in selecting topics of clinical importance to everyday practice. Unlike traditional review articles, the chapters not only highlight the most significant controversies, but when possible, have incorporated basic science and physiological concepts with a rigorous analysis of the current literature.

As with the first edition, I am indebted to the exceptional group of editors who chose the content and edited each of the volumes. I also wish to thank Lisa Barnes (content development specialist at Elsevier) and Judy Fletcher (global content development director at Elsevier), who provided incredible assistance in bringing this project to fruition.

Preface

It gives the editors great pleasure to present the third edition of *Nephrology and Fluid/Electrolyte Physiology*. This edition has changed considerably since the previous publication five years ago. This edition is edited by Dr. William Oh, who has been an editor of the previous two editions, and Dr. Michel Baum.

All of the chapters in this edition have been extensively updated by experts in the field. In addition, this edition of *Nephrology and Fluid/Electrolyte Physiology* contains a number of new chapters with a significant emphasis on genetics and the molecular pathogenesis of renal disease. There have been significant advances in our understanding of renal development and how genetic mutations can result in dysplastic and hyperplastic kidneys. In addition, the tools of molecular biology have provided us with an understanding of the genetic basis for many inherited fluid and electrolyte disorders. This edition has chapters devoted to the molecular basis for hereditary tubulopathies and inherited disorders of calcium, phosphate, and magnesium homeostasis. We also provide a new chapter on prenatal programming, describing how prenatal insults can result in hypertension, kidney, and cardiovascular disease. We think that this updated issue brings forth not only the clinical basis for our understanding of renal and fluid electrolyte problems but also gives the perspective of the molecular basis for many of the problems that we encounter as clinicians.

We would like to express our gratitude to the previous editors of this book, including Dr. Jean-Pierre Guignard and Dr. Stephen Baumgart, whose contributions laid the foundation for this edition. We would also like to thank all of the authors who devoted their time and expertise providing new and updated chapters for this book. Most of all, we would like to express our gratitude for the opportunity to help care for the patients and their families who inspire all of us to provide the best care possible. We hope that this book will aid in providing those who care for our patients a valuable reference for fluid and electrolyte management and a reference to understand disorders of renal, fluid, and electrolyte homeostasis.

William Oh, MD
Michel Baum, MD

Contents

SECTION D

Normal and Abnormal Renal Development and Abnormalities of Fluid and Electrolyte Homeostasis

Corresponding color figures for select images are available on Expert Consult.

Fetal and Neonatal Fluid and Electrolyte Composition

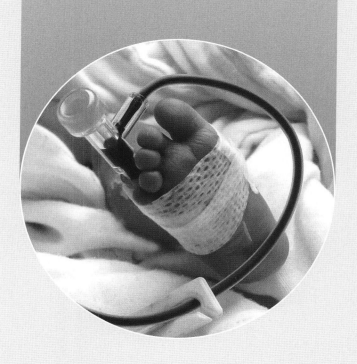

CHAPTER 1

Water Flux and Amniotic Fluid Volume: Understanding Fetal Water Flow

Marie H. Beall, MD, Jeroen P.H.M. van den Wijngaard, PhD,
Martin van Gemert, PhD, Michael G. Ross, MD, MPH

- Clinical Scenarios
- Fetal Water
- Mechanisms of Water Flow
- Aquaporins
- Conclusion

In a term human gestation, the amount of water in the fetal compartments, including the fetus, placenta, and amniotic fluid (AF), may exceed 5 L; in pathologic states, the amount may be much more because of excessive AF or fetal hydrops. Water largely flows from the maternal circulation to the fetus via the placenta, and the rate of fetal water acquisition depends on placental water permeability characteristics. Within the gestational compartment, water is circulated between the fetus and the AF. In the latter part of pregnancy, an important facet of this circulation is water flux from the AF to the fetal circulation across the amnion. Normal AF water dynamics are critical because insufficient (oligohydramnios) or excessive (polyhydramnios) amounts of AF are associated with impaired fetal outcome, even in the absence of structural fetal abnormalities. This chapter reviews data regarding the placental transfer of water and examines the circulation of water within the gestation, specifically the water flux across the amnion, as factors influencing AF volume. Finally, some controversies regarding the mechanics of these events are discussed.

Clinical Scenarios

Water flux in the placenta and chorioamnion is a matter of more than theoretical interest. Clinical experience in humans suggests that altered placental water flow may occur and can cause deleterious fetal effects in association with excessive or reduced AF volume. Similarly, primary abnormalities in fetal fluid exchange with the amniotic cavity may result in markedly abnormal AF volume.

Maternal Dehydration

Maternal dehydration has been associated with reduced fetal compartment water and oligohydramnios. As an example, the following case has been reported: a 14-year-old girl was admitted at 33 weeks' gestation with cramping and vaginal spotting. A sonogram indicated oligohydramnios and an AF index (AFI) of 2.6 cm (reference range, 5–25 cm) with normal fetal kidneys and bladder. On hospital day 2, the AFI was 0 cm. Recorded maternal fluid balance was 8 L in and 13.6 L out. Serum sodium was 153 mEq/L. Diabetes insipidus was diagnosed and treated with intranasal desmopressin acetate. With the normalization of maternal fluid and serum osmolality status, the oligohydramnios resolved rapidly. The patient ultimately delivered a healthy 2700 g male infant at 38 weeks' gestation.[1]

Reduced Maternal Plasma Oncotic Pressure

Maternal malnutrition may predispose patients to increased fetal water transfer and polyhydramnios, a result of reduced maternal plasma oncotic pressure. We recently encountered a patient who illustrated this condition: a 35-year-old gravida 4, para 3 presented at 32 to 33 weeks of gestation complaining of premature labor. On admission, the maternal hematocrit was 18.9% and hemoglobin was 5.6 g/dL with a mean corpuscular volume of 57.9 fL. Blood chemistries were normal except that the patient's serum albumin was 1.9 g/dL (reference range, 3.3–4.9 g/dL). A diagnosis of severe maternal malnutrition was made. On ultrasound examination, the AFI was 24.5 cm, and the fetal bladder was noted to be significantly enlarged, which is consistent with increased urine output. Premature labor was thought to be attributable to uterine overdistension. Subsequently, the patient delivered a 1784-g male infant with Apgar scores of 3 at 1 minute and 7 at 5 minutes. The infant was transferred to the neonatal intensive care unit for significant respiratory distress.

As described later, although the forces driving normal maternal-to-fetal water flux are uncertain, changes in the osmotic–oncotic difference between the maternal and fetal sera can affect the volume of water flowing from the mother to the fetus. In the first case of maternal dehydration, presumably because of an environment of increased maternal osmolality, less water crossed the placenta to the fetus. Similarly, maternal dehydration caused by water restriction (in a sheep model)[2] or caused by hot weather (in humans)[3] has been associated with reduced AF volumes. Conversely, reduced maternal oncotic pressure likely contributed to increased maternal-to-fetal water transfer in the second patient. Fetal renal homeostatic mechanisms then led to increased fetal urine output and increased AF volume. Similarly, studies administering DDAVP (desmopressin) to both humans[4] and sheep[5] have demonstrated that a pharmacologic reduction in maternal serum osmolality can lead to an increase in AF. As these examples illustrate, maternal-fetal water flow is a carefully balanced system that can be perturbed with clinically significant effect. The material presented below will detail the mechanisms regulating fetal–maternal–AF fluid homeostasis.

Fetal Water

Placental Water Flux

Net water flux across the placenta is relatively small. In sheep, a bulk water flow to the fetus of 0.5 mL/min[6] is sufficient for fetal needs at term. By contrast, tracer studies suggest that the total water exchanged (i.e., diffusionary flow) between the ovine fetus and the mother is dramatically larger, up to 70 mL/min.[7] Most of this diffusionary flow is bidirectional, resulting in no net accumulation of water. Although the mechanisms regulating the maternal–fetal flux of water are speculative, the permeability of the placenta to water changes with gestation,[8] suggesting that placental water permeability may be a factor in regulating the water available to the fetus.

Although fetal water may derive from sources other than transplacental flux, these other sources appear to be of minor importance. Water could, theoretically, pass from the maternal circulation to the AF across the fetal membranes (i.e., transmembrane flow), although this flow rate is thought to be small,[9] partly because the AF is hypotonic compared with maternal serum. The driving force (AF to maternal direction) resulting from osmotic and oncotic gradients between hypotonic, low-protein AF and isotonic maternal serum is far greater than that induced by maternal vascular versus AF hydrostatic pressure (maternal to AF direction). Any direct water flux between maternal serum and AF should therefore be from the fetus to the mother. In addition, a small amount of water is produced as a byproduct of fetal metabolic processes. Because these alternative routes contribute only a minor proportion of the fetal water, it is apparent that the fetus is dependent on placental flux for the bulk of water requirements.

Fetal Water Compartments

In gestation, water is partitioned between the fetus, placenta and membranes, and AF. Although term human fetuses may vary considerably in size, an average fetus contains 3000 mL of water, of which about 350 mL is in the vascular compartment. In addition, the placenta contains another 500 mL of water. As the amount of water in infants averages 75% of body weight, the volume of fetal and placental water is proportionate to the fetal weight. AF volume is less correlated with fetal weight, though reduced AF volume is associated with growth-restricted fetuses and increased AF volume is associated with macrosomic fetuses. The AF is a fetal water depot,[10] and in normal human gestations at term, the AF volume may vary from 500 mL to more than 1200 mL.[11] In pathologic states, the AF volume may vary more widely. Next, we present what is known regarding the formation of AF, the circulation of AF water, and the mechanisms controlling this circulation.

Amniotic Fluid Volume and Composition

During the first trimester, AF is isotonic with maternal plasma[12] but contains minimal protein. It is thought that the fluid arises either from a transudate of fetal plasma through nonkeratinized fetal skin or maternal plasma across the uterine decidua or placental surface.[13] With advancing gestation, AF osmolality and sodium concentration decrease, a result of the mixture of a larger volume of dilute fetal urine with a smaller volume of isotonic fetal lung liquid production. In comparison with the first half of pregnancy, AF osmolality decreases by 20 to 30 mOsm/kg H_2O with advancing gestation to levels approximately 85% to 90% of maternal serum osmolality[14] in humans, although there is no osmolality decrease in the AF near term in rats.[15] AF urea, creatinine, and uric acid increase during the second half of pregnancy, a consequence of increased renal excretion, resulting in AF concentrations of these urinary byproducts two to three times higher than those of fetal plasma.[14]

Concordant with the changes in AF content, AF volume changes dramatically during human pregnancy (Fig. 1.1). The average AF volume increases progressively from 20 mL at 10 weeks to 630 mL at 22 weeks, and to 770 mL at 28 weeks' gestation.[16] Between 29 and 37 weeks' gestation, there is little change in volume. Beyond 39 weeks, AF volume decreases sharply, averaging 515 mL at 41 weeks. When the pregnancy becomes postdate, there is a 33% decline in AF volume per week,[17–19] consistent with the increased incidence of oligohydramnios in postterm gestations.

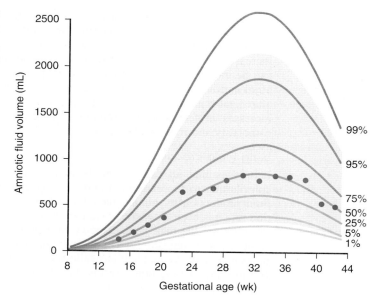

Fig. 1.1 Normal range of amniotic fluid volume in human gestation. (From Brace RA, Wolf EJ. Normal amniotic fluid volume changes throughout pregnancy. *Am J Obstet Gynecol.* 1989;161(2):382-388, used with permission.)

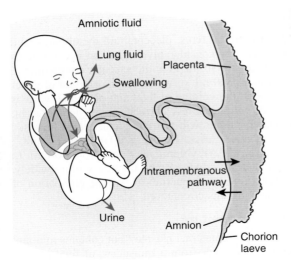

Fig. 1.2 Water circulation between the fetus and amniotic fluid (AF). The major sources of AF water are fetal urine and lung liquid; the routes of absorption are through fetal swallowing and intramembranous flow (see text).

Fetal Water Circulation

AF is produced and resorbed in a dynamic process with large volumes of water circulated between the AF and fetal compartments (Fig. 1.2). During the latter half of gestation, the primary sources of AF include fetal urine excretion and fluid secreted by the fetal lung. The primary pathways for water exit from the AF include removal by fetal swallowing and the intramembranous (IM) absorption of water into fetal vasculature. Although some data on these processes in the human fetus are available, the bulk of the information about fetal AF circulation derives from animal models, especially sheep.

Urine Production

In humans, fetal urine production changes with increasing gestation. The amount of urine produced by the human fetus has been estimated by the use of ultrasound assessment of fetal bladder volume,[20] although the accuracy of these measurements has been called into question. Exact human fetal urine production rates across gestation are not established but appear to be in the range of 25% of body weight per day or nearly 1000 mL/day near term.[20,21]

In near-term ovine fetuses, 500 to 1200 mL/day of urine is distributed to the AF and allantoic cavities.[22,23] During the last third of gestation, the fetal glomerular filtration rate (GFR) increases in parallel to fetal weight, with a similar but variable increase in the reabsorption of sodium, chloride, and free water.[24] Fetal urine output can be modulated, as numerous endocrine factors, including arginine vasopressin, atrial natriuretic factor, aldosterone, and prostaglandins, have been demonstrated to alter fetal renal blood flow, GFR, or urine flow rates.[25,26] Importantly, physiologic increases in fetal plasma arginine vasopressin significantly increase fetal urine osmolality and reduce urine flow rates.[27,28]

Lung Fluid Production

It appears that all mammalian fetuses normally secrete fluid from their lungs, contributing to the expansion and development of the lung. The absolute rate of fluid production by human fetal lungs has not been estimated; the fluid production rate has been extensively studied in the ovine fetus only. During the last third of gestation, the fetal lamb secretes an average of 100 mL/day per kilogram fetal weight. Under physiologic conditions, approximately half of the fluid exiting the lungs enters the AF and half is swallowed.[29] Therefore, an average of approximately 165 mL/day of lung liquid enters the AF near term. Fetal lung fluid production is affected by physiologic and endocrine factors, but nearly all stimuli tested have been demonstrated to reduce fetal lung liquid production, with no evidence of stimulated production and nominal changes in fluid composition. Increased arginine vasopressin,[30] catecholamines,[31] and cortisol,[32] even acute intravascular volume expansion,[33] decrease lung fluid production. Given this lack of evidence of bidirectional regulation, it appears that, unlike the kidneys, the fetal lungs may not play an important role in the maintenance of AF volume homeostasis though they do provide fluid to the amniotic cavity. Current opinion is that fetal lung fluid secretion is likely most important in providing pulmonary expansion, which promotes airway and alveolar development.

Fetal Swallowing

Studies of near-term pregnancies suggest that the human fetus swallows an average of 210 to 760 mL/day[34] of AF, which is considerably less than the volume of urine produced each day. However, fetal swallowing may be reduced beginning a few days before delivery,[35] so the rate of human fetal swallowing is probably underestimated. Little other data on human fetal swallowed volumes are available, although investigators have quantified human fetal gastric emptying as a surrogate measure of volume swallowed.[35a] In fetal sheep, there is a steady increase in the volume of fluid swallowed over the last third of gestation. In contrast to a relatively constant daily urine production/kg body weight, the daily volume swallowed increases from approximately 130 mL/kg per day at 0.75 term to more than 400 mL/kg per day near term.[36] A series of studies have measured ovine fetal swallowing activity with esophageal electromyograms and swallowed volume using a flow probe placed around the fetal esophagus.[37] These studies demonstrate that fetal swallowing increases in response to dipsogenic (e.g., central or systemic hypertonicity[38] or central angiotensin II[39]) or orexigenic (central neuropeptide Y[40]) stimulation and decreases with acute arterial hypotension[41] or hypoxia.[29,42] Thus, near-term fetal swallowed volume is subject to periodic alterations as mechanisms for "thirst" and "appetite" develop functionality, although decreases in swallowed volume appear to be more reflective of deteriorating fetal condition.

Intramembranous Flow

The amount of fluid swallowed by the fetus does not equal the amount of fluid produced by both the kidneys and the lungs in either human or ovine gestation. As the volume of AF does not greatly increase during the last half of pregnancy, another route of fluid absorption is needed. This route is the IM pathway.

The IM pathway refers to the route of absorption between the fetal circulation and the amniotic cavity directly across the amnion. Although the contribution of the IM pathway to the overall regulation and maintenance of AF volume and composition has yet to be completely understood, results from in vivo and in vitro studies of ovine membrane permeability suggest that the permeability of the fetal chorioamnion is important for determining AF composition and volume.[43–45] This IM flow, recirculating AF water to the fetal vascular compartment, is thought to be driven by the significant osmotic gradient between the hypotonic AF and isotonic fetal plasma.[46] In addition, electrolytes (e.g., Na^+) may diffuse down a concentration gradient from fetal plasma into the AF, and intraamniotic peptides (e.g., arginine vasopressin[47,48]) and other electrolytes (e.g., Cl^-) may be recirculated to the fetal plasma.

Although it has never been directly measured in humans, indirect evidence supports the presence of IM flow. Studies of intraamniotic ^{51}Cr injection demonstrated the appearance of the tracer in the circulation of fetuses with impaired swallowing.[49] Additionally, alterations in IM flow may contribute to AF clinical abnormalities because membrane ultrastructure changes are noted with polyhydramnios or oligohydramnios.[50]

Experimental estimates of the net IM flow averages 200 to 250 mL/day in fetal sheep and likely balances the flow of urine and lung liquid with fetal swallowing under homeostatic conditions. Filtration coefficients have been calculated,[51] although IM flow rates under control conditions have not been directly measured. Mathematical models of human AF dynamics also suggest significant IM water and electrolyte fluxes,[52,53] but *trans*membranous flow (AF to maternal) is extremely small compared with IM flow.[54,55]

This detailed understanding of fetal fluid production and resorption provides little explanation as to how AF volume homeostasis is maintained throughout gestation and does not account for gestational alterations in AF volume or postterm or acute-onset oligohydramnios. As an example, the acute reduction in fetal swallowing in response to hypotension or hypoxia seen in the ovine model would not produce the reduced AF volume noted in stressed human fetuses. For this reason, recent research has addressed the regulation of water flow in the placenta and fetal membranes. We will discuss the possible mechanisms for the regulation of fetal water flow, beginning with a review of the general principles of membrane water flow.

Mechanisms of Water Flow

Biologic membranes exist, in part, to regulate water flux. Flow may occur through cells (i.e., transcellular) or between cells (i.e., paracellular), and the type of flow affects the composition of the fluid crossing the membrane. In addition, transcellular flow may occur across the lipid bilayer or through membrane channels or pores (i.e., aquaporins [AQPs]); the latter route is more efficient because the water permeability of the lipid membrane is low. Because the AQPs allow the passage of water only (and sometimes other small nonpolar molecules), transcellular flow is predominantly free water. Paracellular flow occurs through relatively wide spaces between cells and consists of both water and solutes in the proportions present in the extracellular space; large molecules may be excluded. Although water molecules can randomly cross the membrane by diffusion without net water flow, net flow occurs only in response to concentration (osmotic) or pressure (hydrostatic) differences.

Osmotic and hydrostatic forces are created when there is a difference in osmotic or hydrostatic pressure on either side of the membrane. Osmotic differences arise when there is a difference in solute concentration across the membrane. For this difference to be maintained, the membrane permeability of the solute must be low (i.e., a high reflection coefficient). Commonly, osmotic differences are maintained by charged ions such as sodium, or large molecules such as proteins (also called oncotic pressure). These solutes do not cross the cell membrane readily. Osmotic differences can be *created* locally by the active transport of sodium across the membrane with water following because of the osmotic force created by the sodium imbalance. It should be noted that although the transport of sodium is active, water flux is always a passive, nonenergy-dependent process. Hydrostatic differences occur when the pressure of fluid is greater on one side of the membrane. The most obvious example is the difference between the inside of a blood vessel and the interstitial space. Hydrostatic differences may also be created locally by controlling the relative direction of two flows. Even with equal initial pressures, a hydrostatic difference will exist if venous outflow is matched with arterial inflow (countercurrent flow). The actual movement of water in response to these gradients may be more complex as a result of additional physical properties, including unstirred layer effects and solvent drag.

Net membrane water flux is a function of the membrane properties and the osmotic and hydrostatic forces. Formally, this is expressed as the Starling equation:

$$Jv = LpS(\Delta P - \sigma RT(c_1 - c_2))$$

where Jv is the volume flux; LpS is a description of membrane properties (hydraulic conductance times the surface area for diffusion); ΔP is the hydrostatic pressure difference; and $-\sigma RT(c_1 - c_2)$ is the osmotic pressure difference, with T being the temperature in degrees Kelvin, R the gas constant in Nm/Kmol, σ the reflection coefficient (a measure of the permeability of the membrane to the solute), and c_1 and c_2 the solute concentrations on the two sides of the membrane. Experimental studies most often report the membrane water permeability (a characteristic of the individual membrane). Permeability is proportionate to flux (amount of flow per second per cm^2 of membrane) divided by the concentration difference on different sides of the membrane (amount per cubic cm). Membrane water permeabilities are reported as the permeability associated with flux of water in a given direction and under a given type of force, or as the diffusional permeability. Because one membrane may have different osmotic versus hydrostatic versus diffusional permeabilities,[56] an understanding of the forces driving membrane water flow is critical for understanding flow regulatory mechanisms. This area remains controversial, but the anatomy of placenta and membranes suggests possible mechanisms for promoting water flux in one direction.

Mechanism of Placental Water Flow

Placental Anatomy[57,58]

The placenta is a complex organ, and the anatomic variation in the placentas of various species is substantial. Rodents have often been used for the study of placental water flux because primates and rodents share a hemochorial placental structure. In hemochorial placentas, the maternal blood is contained in sinuses in direct contact with one or more layers of fetal epithelium. In humans, this epithelium is the syncytiotrophoblast, a layer of contiguous cells with few or no intercellular spaces. Beneath the syncytium, there are layers of connective tissue and fetal blood vessel endothelium. (In early pregnancy, human placentas have a layer of cytotrophoblast underlying the syncytium; however, by the third trimester, this layer is not continuous and is therefore not a limiting factor for placental permeability.) The human placenta is therefore monochorial. Guinea pig placentas are also monochorial; the fetal vessels are covered with connective tissue that is in turn covered with a single layer of syncytium.[59] In mice, the layer immediately opposed to the maternal blood is a cytotrophoblast layer, covering two layers of syncytium. Because of the presence of three layers in much of the placenta, the mouse placenta is labeled trichorial. Similar to the case in humans, the mouse cytotrophoblast does not appear to be continuous, suggesting that the cytotrophoblast layer does not limit membrane permeability. The rat placenta is similar to that of the mouse.

The syncytium is therefore a common structure in all of these placental forms and a likely site of regulation of membrane permeability. In support of this hypothesis, membrane vesicles derived from human syncytial brush border were used to evaluate the permeability of the placenta. At 37°C, the osmotic permeability of apical vesicles was $1.9 \pm 0.06 \times 10^{-3}$ cm/s; the permeability of basal membrane (fetal side) vesicles was higher at $3.1 \pm 0.20 \times 10^{-3}$ cm/s.[60] The difference between the basal and apical sides of the syncytiotrophoblasts was taken to indicate that the apical (maternal) side of the trophoblast was the rate-limiting structure for water flow through the placenta. In all placentas, the fetal blood is contained in vessels, suggesting that fetal capillary endothelium may also serve as a barrier to flow between maternal and fetal circulations. However, experimental evidence suggests that the capillary endothelium is a less significant barrier to small polar molecules than the syncytium.[58]

Although sheep have been extensively used in studies of fetal physiology and placental permeability, their placentas differ from those of humans in important respects. The sheep placenta is classified as epitheliochorial, meaning that the maternal and fetal circulations are contained within blood vessels with maternal and fetal epithelial layers interposed between them. In general, compared with the hemochorial placenta, the epitheliochorial placenta would be expected to demonstrate decreased water permeability based on the increase in membrane layers. In addition, the forces driving water permeability may differ between the two placental types because the presence of maternal vessels in the sheep placenta increases the likelihood that a hydrostatic pressure difference could be maintained favoring water flux from maternal to fetal circulations.

In rodent placentas, fetal and maternal blood circulate in opposite directions (countercurrent flow), potentially increasing the opportunity for exchange between circulations based on local concentration differences. The direction of maternal blood circulation in human placentas is from the inside to the outside of the placental lobule and therefore at cross-current to the fetal blood flow (Fig. 1.3).[61] Unlike

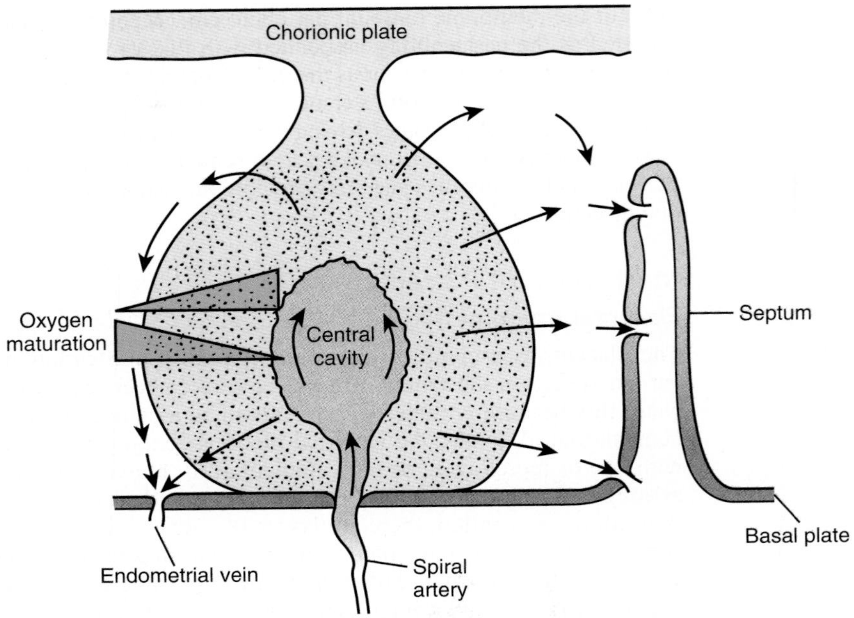

Fig. 1.3 Maternal blood flow in the human placenta. Blood flow proceeds from the spiral artery to the center of the placental lobule. Blood then crosses the lobule laterally, exiting through the endometrial vein. This creates a gradient in oxygen content from the inside to the outside of the lobule because of the changing oxygen content of the maternal blood. (From Hempstock J, Bao YP, Bar-Issac M, et al. Intralobular differences in antioxidant enzyme expression and activity reflect the pattern of maternal arterial bloodflow within the human placenta. *Placenta*. 2003;24(5):517-523, used with permission.)

in mice and rats, investigation has not revealed countercurrent blood flow in ovine placentas.[62]

The preceding is not intended to imply that there are not important differences between human and rodent placentas. The human placenta is organized into cotyledons, each with a central fetal vessel. Fetal–maternal exchange in the mouse and rat placenta occurs in the placental labyrinth. In addition, rats and mice have an "inverted yolk sac placenta," a structure with no analogy in the primate placenta. Readers are referred to Faber and Thornberg[57] and Benirschke[63] for additional details.

Controversies in Placental Flow

In the placenta, the flux of water may be driven by either hydrostatic or osmotic forces. Hydrostatic forces can be developed in the placenta by alterations in the flow in maternal and fetal circulations. Osmotic forces may be generated locally by active transport of solutes, such as sodium or by depletion of solute from the local perimembrane environment (caused by the so-called "unstirred layer" effect). The relative direction of maternal and fetal blood flows can be concurrent, countercurrent, crosscurrent, or in part combinations of these flows,[64] and differences in the direction of blood flow may be important in establishing either osmotic or hydrostatic gradients within the placenta. It has not been possible to directly study putative local pressure or osmotic differences at the level of the syncytium; therefore, theories regarding the driving forces for placental water flux are inferences from available data.

Water may be transferred from mother to fetus driven osmotically by the active transport of solutes such as sodium.[65] In rats, inert solutes, such as mannitol and inulin, are transferred *to* the maternal circulation from the fetus more readily than *from* the mother to fetus,[66] and conversely, sodium is actively transported to the fetus in excess of fetal needs. This was taken to indicate that water was being driven to the fetal side by a local osmotic effect created by the sodium flux. Water with dissolved solutes then differentially crossed from fetus to mother, probably by a paracellular route. Perfusion of the guinea pig placenta with dextran-containing solution demonstrates that the flow of water can also be influenced by colloid osmotic pressure.[67] In sheep, intact gestations have yielded estimates of osmotic placental water flow of 0.062 mL/kg min per mOsm/kg H_2O.[68] The importance of osmotically driven water flow in sheep is uncertain because the same authors found that the maternal plasma was consistently hyperosmolar to the fetal plasma. However, theoretical considerations have been used to argue that known electrolyte active transport and a modest hydrostatic pressure gradient could maintain maternal-to-fetal water flow against this osmotic gradient.[69]

Others have argued that the motive force for water flux in the placenta is hydrostatic. In perfused placentas of guinea pigs, reversal of the direction of the fetal flow reduced the rate of water transfer,[70] and increasing the fetal-side perfusion pressure increased the fetal-to-maternal water flow in both the perfused guinea pig placentas[71] and in an intact sheep model.[72] Both findings suggest that water transfer is flow dependent.

As a whole, the available data suggest that both osmotic and hydrostatic forces *can* promote placental water flux. The actual motive force in normal pregnancy is uncertain and may vary with the species, the pregnancy stage, or both. Whatever the driving force, at least some part of placental water flux involves the flow of solute-free water transcellularly, suggesting the involvement of membrane water channels in the process.

Mechanism of Intramembranous Flow

Membrane Anatomy

In sheep, an extensive network of microscopic blood vessels is located between the outer surface of the amnion and the chorion,[73] providing an extensive surface area available for IM flow. In primates, including humans, IM fluxes likely occur across the fetal surface of the placenta because the amnion and chorion are not vascularized per se. The close proximity of fetal blood vessels to the placental surface provides accessibility to the fetal circulation, explaining the absorption of AF technetium[46] and arginine vasopressin[48] into the fetal serum in subhuman fetal primates, despite esophageal ligation (eliminating the potential for swallowing). In vitro experiments with isolated layers of human amnion and chorion have also demonstrated that the membranes act as selective barriers of exchange.[74]

Studies in the ovine model suggest that the IM pathway can be regulated to restore homeostasis. Because fetal swallowing is a major route of AF fluid resorption, esophageal ligation would be expected to increase AF volume significantly. Although AF volume increased significantly 3 days after ovine fetal esophageal occlusion,[75] longer periods (9 days) of esophageal ligation reduced AF volume in preterm sheep.[76] Similarly, esophageal ligation of fetal sheep over a period of 1 month did not increase AF volume.[77] In the absence of swallowing, normalized AF volume suggests an increase in IM flow. In addition, IM flow markedly increased after the infusion of exogenous fluid to the AF cavity.[78] Collectively, these studies suggest that AF resorption pathways and likely IM flow are under dynamic feedback regulation, though the site and regulatory mechanism are unknown. That is, AF volume expansion increases IM resorption, ultimately resulting in a normalization of AF volume. Importantly, factors downregulating IM flow are less studied, and there is no functional evidence of reduced IM resorption as an adaptive response to oligohydramnios, although AQP water channel expression in the amnion may be decreased (see later). Studies have revealed that prolactin reduced the upregulation of IM flow because of osmotic challenge in the sheep model[79] and reduced diffusional permeability to water in human amnion[80] and guinea pig[81] amnion, suggesting that downregulation of IM flow is possible.

Controversies Regarding Intramembranous Flow

The specific mechanism and regulation of IM flow is key to AF homeostasis. A number of theories have been put forward to account for the observed results.

Esophageal ligation of fetal sheep resulted in the upregulation of fetal chorioamnion vascular endothelial growth factor (VEGF) gene expression.[82] It was proposed that VEGF-induced neovascularization potentiates AF water resorption. These authors also speculated that fetal urine or lung fluid (or both) may contain factors that upregulate VEGF. Their further studies demonstrated an increased water flow despite a constant membrane diffusional permeability (to technetium) in animals in which the fetal urine output had been increased by an intravenous volume load and a concurrent flow of water and solutes against a concentration gradient by the IM route.[83,84] Finally, artificial regulation of the osmolality and oncotic pressure of the AF revealed that the major force promoting IM flow in sheep was osmotic; however, there was an additional flow of about 24 mL/h, which was not osmotic dependent. Because protein was also transferred to the fetal circulation, this flow was believed to be similar to fluid flow in the lymph system.[85]

These findings, in aggregate, have been interpreted to require active bulk fluid flow across the amnion; Brace et al.[84] have proposed that this fluid transport occurs via membrane vesicles (bulk vesicular flow), as evidenced by the high prevalence of amnion intracellular vesicles seen in electron microscopy.[86] This theory is poorly accepted because vesicle water flow has not been demonstrated in any other tissue and is highly energy dependent. Most others believe that IM flow occurs through conventional paracellular and transcellular channels, driven by osmotic and hydrostatic forces. Mathematical modeling indicates that relatively small IM sodium fluxes could be associated with significant changes in AF volume, suggesting that sodium flux may be a regulator of IM flow,[53] although the observation that IM flow was independent of AF composition suggests that other forces (e.g., hydrostatic forces) may also drive IM flow.[87]

Importantly, upregulation of VEGF or sodium transfer alone cannot explain AF composition changes after fetal esophageal ligation because AF electrolyte composition indicates that water flow increases disproportionately to solute flow.[76] The passage of free water across a biologic membrane without solutes is a characteristic of transcellular flow, a process mediated by water channels in the cell membrane. Although water flow through these channels is passive, the expression and location of the channels can be modulated to regulate water flux. We will review the characteristics of AQP water channels and then comment on the evidence that AQPs may be involved in regulating gestational water flow.

Aquaporins

AQPs are cell membrane proteins approximately 30 kD in size (26–34 kD). Similarities in amino acid sequence suggest that the three-dimensional structure of all AQPs is similar. AQP proteins organize in the cell membrane as tetramers; however, each monomer forms a hydrophilic pore in its center and functions independently as a water channel (Fig. 1.4).[88] Although all AQPs function as water channels, some AQPs also allow the passage of glycerol, urea, and other small nonpolar molecules. These have also been called *aquaglyceroporins*. Multiple AQPs have been identified (≤13, depending on the mammalian species). Some are widely expressed throughout the body; others appear to be more tissue specific.

AQP function depends on cellular location. In the kidneys, several AQPs are expressed in specific areas of the collecting duct: whereas AQP3 and AQP4 are both present in the basolateral membrane of the collecting duct principal cells, AQP2 is present in the apical portion of the membrane of these same cells.[89] The presence of these different AQPs on opposite membrane sides of the same cell is important for the regulation of water transfer across the cell because altered AQP properties or AQP expression may differentially regulate water entry from the collecting duct lumen and water exit to the interstitial fluid compartment. Absence of the various renal AQPs leads to renal concentrating defects; particularly, the absence of AQP2 in humans is responsible for nephrogenic diabetes insipidus.

AQP function is also dependent on the cellular milieu. This regulation may occur through the insertion or removal of AQP into the membrane from the intracellular

Fig. 1.4 Structure of aquaporin (bovine AQP0). *Upper left* shows the structure from the extracellular side of the membrane. *Upper right* shows each monomer in a different format. *Lower figure* shows a side view of an AQP monomer, extracellular side upper. The two figures are to be viewed in crossed-eye stereo. *C* and *N*, Ends of the protein. (From Harries WE, Akhavan D, Miercke LJ, Khademi S, Stroud RM. The channel architecture of aquaporin 0 at a 2.2-A resolution. *Proc Natl Acad Sci U S A.* 2004 Sep 28;101[39]:14045-14050, used with permission. Copyright [2004] National Academy of Sciences, U.S.A.)

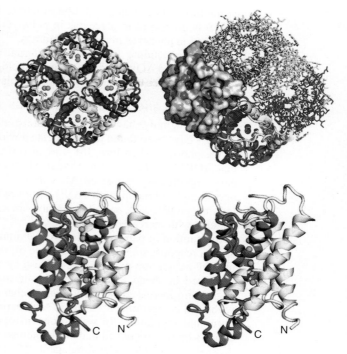

compartment. For example, in the renal tubule, AQP2 is transferred from cytoplasm vesicles to the apical cell membrane in response to arginine vasopressin[90] or forskolin.[91] AQP8 is similarly transferred from hepatocyte vesicles to the cell membrane in response to dibutyryl cyclic adenosine monophosphate (cAMP) and glucagon.[92] In longer time frames, the expression of various AQPs may be induced by external conditions. For example, AQP3 expression in cultured keratinocytes is increased when the cell culture medium is made hypertonic.[93] In summary, AQPs are important in the regulation of water flow across biologic membranes, and their expression and activity can be regulated according to the hydration status of the organism.

Aquaporins in Placentas and Membranes

Four AQPs (i.e., AQP1, 3, 8, and 9) have been widely reported in the placenta and fetal membranes of a variety of species, and alterations in the expression of these AQPs have been related to changes in AF volume. Reports also describe the finding of AQP4[94] and AQP5[95] in human placenta or membranes, but no information is available relating these AQPs to AF volume changes, and they will not be further considered here. AQP1 mRNA and protein have been demonstrated in ovine,[96] mouse,[97] and human[98] placentas associated with the placental vessels. Ovine placental AQP1 expression levels are highest early in pregnancy, with a decline thereafter, although there is an increase in expression near term.[99] AQP1 protein expression has been demonstrated in the fetal chorioamnion at term in human gestations[100] associated with amnion epithelium and cytotrophoblast of the chorion.[97] AQP3 message and protein has been demonstrated in the placentas and fetal chorioamnion of humans[100,101] and mice,[97] and in sheep placentas,[96,99] and mRNA has been found in rat placentas.[102] In humans, AQP3 protein is expressed on the apical membranes of the syncytiotrophoblast[101] on amnion epithelium and cytotrophoblast of the chorion.[103] AQP3 has also been demonstrated on the trophoblasts of mice.[97] AQP8 mRNA has been detected in mouse,[104] sheep,[99] and human placentas and in human fetal chorioamnion.[105] AQP9 protein and mRNA have been demonstrated in human placentas.[101]

Evidence suggests that AQPs may be involved in the regulation of placental water flow. In mice, AF volume is positively correlated with placental AQP3 mRNA expression.[97] In humans with abnormalities of AF volume, message for AQP3 and AQP9 is decreased in placentas in polyhydramnios,[106,107] and message for AQP3 is increased in placentas in oligohydramnios.[108] This has been interpreted as a compensatory change tending to increase maternal-to-fetal water flow. Data on placental AQP1[108,109] and AQP8[107,110] in human pathology have been inconsistent, making these AQPs less likely to be key regulators of placental water flow.

Aquaporin and Intramembranous Water Flow

AQP1, 3, 8, and 9 have all been demonstrated in human amniochorion, and AQP1, 3, and 9 have been found to be associated with amnion epithelium and cytotrophoblast of the chorion. Therefore, IM flow also may be through AQPs. There is evidence that AQP1 is necessary for normal AF homeostasis. Mice lacking the AQP1 gene have significantly increased AF volume,[111] and in normal mice, AF volume was negatively correlated with AQP1 expression.[97] In conditions with pathologic AF volume, AQP1, 3, 8, and 9 expression are increased in human amnion derived from patients with increased AF volumes,[57,106,107,110–113] and AQP1 and AQP3 are decreased in the amnion of patients with oligohydramnios.[108,109] These changes were postulated to be a response to, rather than a cause of, the AF volume abnormalities. Alterations in AQP expression may also be a cause of AF volume abnormalities; AQP1 protein increased in sheep fetal chorioallantoic membranes in response to fetal hypoxia, suggesting increased IM flow as a mechanism for the oligohydramnios associated with fetal compromise.[114] Finally, AQP expression in the chorioamnion is subject to hormonal regulation. In work done in our laboratory, AQP3, AQP8, and AQP9 expression is upregulated in cultured human amnion cells after incubation with cAMP or forskolin, a cAMP-elevating agent.[115,116] These data together support the hypothesis that AQPs, specifically AQP1, are important mediators of water flow out of the gestational sac across the amnion.

In summary, we propose the following model for human fetal water flow. Water crosses from the maternal to fetal circulation in the placenta, perhaps under the influence of local osmotic differences created by the active transport of sodium. Transplacental water flow, at least in the maternal-to-fetal direction, is through AQP water channels. Therefore, membrane permeability in the placenta is subject to regulation by upregulating or downregulating the number of AQP channels in the membrane. There is no evidence of acute changes in placental water permeability, but changes in permeability have been described over time; these could be attributable to changes in the expression of AQPs with advancing gestation. AQP3 is expressed on the apical membrane of the syncytiotrophoblasts; the membrane barrier is thought to be rate limiting for placental water flux, and its expression increases with gestation. AQP3 is therefore a candidate for the regulation of placental water flow.

In the gestational compartment, water circulates between the fetus and the AF. The available evidence suggests that the IM component of this flow is mediated by AQPs, specifically by AQP1. IM flow can be altered over gestation and in response to acute events (e.g., increased AF volume). These alterations in IM flow are likely affected by alterations in the membrane expression of AQP1. Normally, AQP1 expression in the amnion decreases with gestation associated with increasing AF volume, but expression can be increased by various humeral factors, polyhydramnios, or fetal acidosis. The osmotic water permeability of AQP1(−/−) trophoblast cells was significantly lower than that in AQP1(+/+) trophoblast cells, in response to both hypotonic and hypertonic challenges, reinforcing the important role of AQP1-mediated plasma membrane water permeability in maternal-fetal fluid balance.[117] Recent studies indicate increased expression of AQP9 in trophoblast from patients with gestational diabetes, which may contribute to increased AF volume in these pregnancies.[118]

Conclusion

The circulation of water between mother and fetus and within the fetal compartment is complex, and the mechanisms regulating water flow remain poorly understood. Water flow across the placenta must increase with increasing fetal water needs and must be relatively insensitive to transient changes in maternal status. Water circulation within the gestation must sustain fetal growth and plasma volume while also allowing for appropriate amounts of AF for fetal growth and development.

Experimental data suggest that placental water flow is affected by both hydrostatic and osmotic forces and that both transcellular and paracellular water flow occurs. IM water flow is more likely to be osmotically driven, although there are other contributing forces as well. The observation that water crosses the membrane in excess of solutes suggests a role for AQP water channels in placental and IM water flow. Experimental data have confirmed the expression of AQPs in the placenta and fetal membranes, as well as modulation of this expression by a variety of factors. AQP3 is an exciting prospect for the regulation of placental water flow given its cellular location and association with AF volume. AQP1 has been implicated in the mechanism of IM flow using a variety of experimental models. The availability of agents known to regulate the expression of AQPs suggests the possibility of treatments for AF volume abnormalities based on the stimulation or suppression of the appropriate water channel.

REFERENCES

1. Hanson RS, Powrie RO, Larson L. Diabetes insipidus in pregnancy: a treatable cause of oligohydramnios. *Obstet Gynecol.* 1997;89(5 Pt 2):816–817.
2. Schreyer P, Sherman DJ, Ervin MG, et al. Maternal dehydration: impact on ovine amniotic fluid volume and composition. *J Dev Physiol.* 1990;13(5):283–287.
3. Sciscione AC, Costigan KA, Johnson TR. Increase in ambient temperature may explain decrease in amniotic fluid index. *Am J Perinatol.* 1997;14(5):249–251.
4. Ross MG, Cedars L, Nijland MJ, Ogundipe A. Treatment of oligohydramnios with maternal 1-deamino-[8-D-arginine] vasopressin-induced plasma hypoosmolality. *Am J Obstet Gynecol.* 1996;174(5):1608–1613.
5. Ross MG, Nijland MJ, Kullama LK. 1-Deamino-[8-D-arginine] vasopressin-induced maternal plasma hypoosmolality increases ovine amniotic fluid volume. *Am J Obstet Gynecol.* 1996;174(4):1118–1125.
6. Lumbers ER, Smith FG, Stevens AD. Measurement of net transplacental transfer of fluid to the fetal sheep. *J Physiol.* 1985;364:289–299.
7. Faichney GJ, Fawcett AA, Boston RC. Water exchange between the pregnant ewe, the foetus and its amniotic and allantoic fluids. *J Comp Physiol [B].* 2004;174(6):503–510.
8. Jansson T, Powell TL, Illsley NP. Gestational development of water and non-electrolyte permeability of human syncytiotrophoblast plasma membranes. *Placenta.* 1999;20(2–3):155–160.
9. Brace RA. Progress toward understanding the regulation of amniotic fluid volume: water and solute fluxes in and through the fetal membranes. *Placenta.* 1995;16(1):1–18.
10. Moore TR. Amniotic fluid dynamics reflect fetal and maternal health and disease. *Obstet Gynecol.* 2010;116(3):759–765.
11. Goodwin JW, Godden JO, Chance GW. *Perinatal Medicine: The Basic Science Underlying Clinical Practice.* Baltimore, MD: Williams & Wilkins; 1976.
12. Campbell J, Wathen N, Macintosh M, et al. Biochemical composition of amniotic fluid and extraembryonic coelomic fluid in the first trimester of pregnancy. *Br J Obstet Gynaecol.* 1992;99(7):563–565.
13. Faber JJ, Gault CF, Green TJ, et al. Chloride and the generation of amniotic fluid in the early embryo. *J Exp Zool.* 1973;183(3):343–352.
14. Gillibrand PN. Changes in the electrolytes, urea and osmolality of the amniotic fluid with advancing pregnancy. *J Obstet Gynaecol Br Commonw.* 1969;76(10):898–905.
15. Desai M, Ladella S, Ross MG. Reversal of pregnancy-mediated plasma hypotonicity in the near-term rat. *J Matern Fetal Neonatal Med.* 2003;13(3):197–202.
16. Brace RA, Wolf EJ. Normal amniotic fluid volume changes throughout pregnancy. *Am J Obstet Gynecol.* 1989;161(2):382–388.
17. Gadd RL. The volume of the liquor amnii in normal and abnormal pregnancies. *J Obstet Gynaecol Br Commonw.* 1966;73(1):11–22.
18. Beischer NA, Brown JB, Townsend L. Studies in prolonged pregnancy. 3. Amniocentesis in prolonged pregnancy. *Am J Obstet Gynecol.* 1969;103(4):496–503.
19. Queenan JT, Von Gal HV, Kubarych SF. Amniography for clinical evaluation of erythroblastosis fetalis. *Am J Obstet Gynecol.* 1968;102(2):264–274.
20. Rabinowitz R, Peters MT, Vyas S, et al. Measurement of fetal urine production in normal pregnancy by real-time ultrasonography. *Am J Obstet Gynecol.* 1989;161(5):1264–1266.
21. Fagerquist M, Fagerquist U, Oden A, Blomberg SG. Fetal urine production and accuracy when estimating fetal urinary bladder volume. *Ultrasound Obstet Gynecol.* 2001;17(2):132–139.
22. Ross MG, Ervin MG, Rappaport VJ, et al. Ovine fetal urine contribution to amniotic and allantoic compartments. *Biol Neonate.* 1988;53(2):98–104.
23. Wlodek ME, Challis JR, Patrick J. Urethral and urachal urine output to the amniotic and allantoic sacs in fetal sheep. *J Dev Physiol.* 1988;10(4):309–319.

24. Robillard JE, Matson JR, Sessions C, Smith FG Jr. Developmental aspects of renal tubular reabsorption of water in the lamb fetus. *Pediatr Res*. 1979;13(10):1172–1176.
25. Robillard JE, Weitzman RE. Developmental aspects of the fetal renal response to exogenous arginine vasopressin. *Am J Physiol*. 1980;238(5):F407–F414.
26. Lingwood B, Hardy KJ, Coghlan JP, Wintour EM. Effect of aldosterone on urine composition in the chronically cannulated ovine foetus. *J Endocrinol*. 1978;76(3):553–554.
27. Lingwood B, Hardy KJ, Horacek I, et al. The effects of antidiuretic hormone on urine flow and composition in the chronically-cannulated ovine fetus. *Q J Exp Physiol Cogn Med Sci*. 1978;63(4):315–330.
28. Ervin MG, Ross MG, Leake RD, Fisher DA. V1- and V2-receptor contributions to ovine fetal renal and cardiovascular responses to vasopressin. *Am J Physiol*. 1992;262(4 Pt 2):R636–R643.
29. Brace RA, Wlodek ME, Cock ML, Harding R. Swallowing of lung liquid and amniotic fluid by the ovine fetus under normoxic and hypoxic conditions. *Am J Obstet Gynecol*. 1994;171(3):764–770.
30. Ross MG, Ervin G, Leake RD, et al. Fetal lung liquid regulation by neuropeptides. *Am J Obstet Gynecol*. 1984;150(4):421–425.
31. Lawson EE, Brown ER, Torday JS, et al. The effect of epinephrine on tracheal fluid flow and surfactant efflux in fetal sheep. *Am Rev Respir Dis*. 1978;118(6):1023–1026.
32. Dodic M, Wintour EM. Effects of prolonged (48 h) infusion of cortisol on blood pressure, renal function and fetal fluids in the immature ovine foetus. *Clin Exp Pharmacol Physiol*. 1994;21(12):971–980.
33. Sherman DJ, Ross MG, Ervin MG, et al. Ovine fetal lung fluid response to intravenous saline solution infusion: fetal atrial natriuretic factor effect. *Am J Obstet Gynecol*. 1988;159(6):1347–1352.
34. Pritchard JA. Fetal swallowing and amniotic fluid volume. *Obstet Gynecol*. 1966;28(5):606–610.
35. Bradley RM, Mistretta CM. Swallowing in fetal sheep. *Science*. 1973;179(77):1016–1017.
35a. Sase M, Miwa I, Sumie M, et al. Gastric emptying cycles in the human fetus. *Am J Obstet Gynecol*. 2005;193(3 Pt 2):1000–1004.
36. Nijland MJ, Day L, Ross MG. Ovine fetal swallowing: expression of preterm neurobehavioral rhythms. *J Matern Fetal Med*. 2001;10(4):251–257.
37. Sherman DJ, Ross MG, Day L, Ervin MG. Fetal swallowing: correlation of electromyography and esophageal fluid flow. *Am J Physiol*. 1990;258(6 Pt 2):R1386–R1394.
38. Xu Z, Nijland MJ, Ross MG. Plasma osmolality dipsogenic thresholds and c-fos expression in the near-term ovine fetus. *Pediatr Res*. 2001;49(5):678–685.
39. El-Haddad MA, Ismail Y, Gayle D, Ross MG. Central angiotensin II AT1 receptors mediate fetal swallowing and pressor responses in the near term ovine fetus. *Am J Physiol Regul Integr Comp Physiol*. 2004;288(4):R1014–R1020.
40. El-Haddad MA, Ismail Y, Guerra C, et al. Neuropeptide Y administered into cerebral ventricles stimulates sucrose ingestion in the near-term ovine fetus. *Am J Obstet Gynecol*. 2003;189(4):949–952.
41. El-Haddad MA, Ismail Y, Guerra C, et al. Effect of oral sucrose on ingestive behavior in the near-term ovine fetus. *Am J Obstet Gynecol*. 2002;187(4):898–901.
42. Sherman DJ, Ross MG, Day L, et al. Swallowing: response to graded maternal hypoxemia. *J Appl Physiol*. 1991;71(5):1856–1861.
43. Lingwood BE, Wintour EM. Amniotic fluid volume and in vivo permeability of ovine fetal membranes. *Obstet Gynecol*. 1984;64(3):368–372.
44. Gilbert WM, Newman PS, Eby-Wilkens E, Brace RA. Technetium Tc 99m rapidly crosses the ovine placenta and intramembranous pathway. *Am J Obstet Gynecol*. 1996;175(6):1557–1562.
45. Lingwood BE, Wintour EM. Permeability of ovine amnion and amniochorion to urea and water. *Obstet Gynecol*. 1983;61(2):227–232.
46. Gilbert WM, Brace RA. The missing link in amniotic fluid volume regulation: intramembranous absorption. *Obstet Gynecol*. 1989;74(5):748–754.
47. Ervin MG, Ross MG, Leake RD, Fisher DA. Fetal recirculation of amniotic fluid arginine vasopressin. *Am J Physiol*. 1986;250(3 Pt 1):E253–E258.
48. Gilbert WM, Cheung CY, Brace RA. Rapid intramembranous absorption into the fetal circulation of arginine vasopressin injected intraamniotically. *Am J Obstet Gynecol*. 1991;164(4):1013–1018.
49. Queenan JT, Allen FH Jr, Fuchs F, et al. Studies on the method of intrauterine transfusion. I. Question of erythrocyte absorption from amniotic fluid. *Am J Obstet Gynecol*. 1965;92:1009–1013.
50. Hebertson RM, Hammond ME, Bryson MJ. Amniotic epithelial ultrastructure in normal, polyhydramnic, and oligohydramnic pregnancies. *Obstet Gynecol*. 1986;68(1):74–79.
51. Gilbert WM, Brace RA. Novel determination of filtration coefficient of ovine placenta and intramembranous pathway. *Am J Physiol*. 1990;259(6 Pt 2):R1281–R1288.
52. Mann SE, Nijland MJ, Ross MG. Mathematic modeling of human amniotic fluid dynamics. *Am J Obstet Gynecol*. 1996;175(4 Pt 1):937–944.
53. Curran MA, Nijland MJ, Mann SE, Ross MG. Human amniotic fluid mathematical model: determination and effect of intramembranous sodium flux. *Am J Obstet Gynecol*. 1998;178(3):484–490.
54. Anderson DF, Faber JJ, Parks CM. Extraplacental transfer of water in the sheep. *J Physiol*. 1988;406:75–84.
55. Anderson DF, Borst NJ, Boyd RD, Faber JJ. Filtration of water from mother to conceptus via paths independent of fetal placental circulation in sheep. *J Physiol*. 1990;431:1–10.
56. Capurro C, Escobar E, Ibarra C, et al. Water permeability in different epithelial barriers. *Biol Cell*. 1989;66(1–2):145–148.
57. Faber JJ, Thornberg KL. *Placental Physiology: Structure and Function of Fetomaternal Exchange*. New York, NY: Raven; 1983.
58. Stulc J. Placental transfer of inorganic ions and water. *Physiol Rev*. 1997;77(3):805–836.

59. Georgiades P, Ferguson-Smith AC, Burton GJ. Comparative developmental anatomy of the murine and human definitive placentae. *Placenta*. 2002;23(1):3–19.

60. Jansson T, Illsley NP. Osmotic water permeabilities of human placental microvillous and basal membranes. *J Membr Biol*. 1993;132(2):147–155.

61. Hempstock J, Bao YP, Bar-Issac M, et al. Intralobular differences in antioxidant enzyme expression and activity reflect the pattern of maternal arterial bloodflow within the human placenta. *Placenta*. 2003;24(5):517–523.

62. Makowski EL, Meschia G, Droegemueller W, Battaglia FC. Distribution of uterine blood flow in the pregnant sheep. *Am J Obstet Gynecol*. 1968;101(3):409–412.

63. Benirschke K. Comparative placentation. Available at: http://medicine ucsd.edu/cpa/homefs.html.

64. Schroder HJ. Basics of placental structures and transfer functions. In: Brace RA, Ross MG, Robillard JE, eds. *Reproductive and Perinatal Medicine*. Vol. 11. Fetal & Neonatal Body Fluids. Ithaca, NY: Perinatology Press; 1989:187–226.

65. Stulc J, Stulcova B, Sibley CP. Evidence for active maternal-fetal transport of Na+ across the placenta of the anaesthetized rat. *J Physiol*. 1993;470:637–649.

66. Stulc J, Stulcova B. Asymmetrical transfer of inert hydrophilic solutes across rat placenta. *Am J Physiol*. 1993;265(3 Pt 2):R670–R675.

67. Schroder H, Nelson P, Power G. Fluid shift across the placenta: I. The effect of dextran T 40 in the isolated guinea-pig placenta. *Placenta*. 1982;3(4):327–338.

68. Ervin MG, Amico JA, Leake RD, et al. Arginine vasotocin-like immunoreactivity in plasma of pregnant women and newborns. *West Soc Ped Res Clin Res*. 1985;33:115A.

69. Conrad EE Jr, Faber JJ. Water and electrolyte acquisition across the placenta of the sheep. *Am J Physiol*. 1977;233(4):H475–H487.

70. Schroder H, Leichtweiss HP. Perfusion rates and the transfer of water across isolated guinea pig placenta. *Am J Physiol*. 1977;232(6):H666–H670.

71. Leichtweiss HP, Schroder H. The effect of elevated outflow pressure on flow resistance and the transfer of THO, albumin and glucose in the isolated guinea pig placenta. *Pflugers Arch*. 1977;371(3):251–256.

72. Brace RA, Moore TR. Transplacental, amniotic, urinary, and fetal fluid dynamics during very-large-volume fetal intravenous infusions. *Am J Obstet Gynecol*. 1991;164(3):907–916.

73. Brace RA, Gilbert WM, Thornburg KL. Vascularization of the ovine amnion and chorion: a morphometric characterization of the surface area of the intramembranous pathway. *Am J Obstet Gynecol*. 1992;167(6):1747–1755.

74. Battaglia FC, Hellegers AE, Meschia G, Barron DH. In vitro investigations of the human chorion as a membrane system. *Nature*. 1962;196:1061–1063.

75. Fujino Y, Agnew CL, Schreyer P. Amniotic fluid volume response to esophageal occlusion in fetal sheep. *Am J Obstet Gynecol*. 1991;165(6 Pt 1):1620–1626.

76. Matsumoto LC, Cheung CY, Brace RA. Effect of esophageal ligation on amniotic fluid volume and urinary flow rate in fetal sheep. *Am J Obstet Gynecol*. 2000;182(3):699–705.

77. Wintour EM, Barnes A, Brown EH, et al. Regulation of amniotic fluid volume and composition in the ovine fetus. *Obstet Gynecol*. 1978;52(6):689–693.

78. Faber JJ, Anderson DF. Regulatory response of intramembranous absorption of amniotic fluid to infusion of exogenous fluid in sheep. *Am J Physiol*. 1999;277(1 Pt 2):R236–R242.

79. Ross MG, Ervin MG, Leake RD. Bulk flow of amniotic fluid water in response to maternal osmotic challenge. *Am J Obstet Gynecol*. 1983;147(6):697–701.

80. Leontic EA, Tyson JE. Prolactin and fetal osmoregulation: water transport across isolated human amnion. *Am J Physiol*. 1977;232(3):R124–R127.

81. Holt WF, Perks AM. The effect of prolactin on water movement through the isolated amniotic membrane of the guinea pig. *Gen Comp Endocrinol*. 1975;26(2):153–164.

82. Matsumoto LC, Bogic L, Brace RA, Cheung CY. Fetal esophageal ligation induces expression of vascular endothelial growth factor messenger ribonucleic acid in fetal membranes. *Am J Obstet Gynecol*. 2001;184(2):175–184.

83. Daneshmand SS, Cheung CY, Brace RA. Regulation of amniotic fluid volume by intramembranous absorption in sheep: role of passive permeability and vascular endothelial growth factor. *Am J Obstet Gynecol*. 2003;188(3):786–793.

84. Brace RA, Vermin ML, Huijssoon E. Regulation of amniotic fluid volume: intramembranous solute and volume fluxes in late gestation fetal sheep. *Am J Obstet Gynecol*. 2004;191(3):837–846.

85. Faber JJ, Anderson DF. Absorption of amniotic fluid by amniochorion in sheep. *Am J Physiol Heart Circ Physiol*. 2002;282(3):H850–H854.

86. Wynn RM, French GL. Comparative ultrastructure of the mammalian amnion. *Obstet Gynecol*. 1968;31(6):759–774.

87. Anderson D, Yang Q, Hohimer A, et al. Intramembranous absorption rate is unaffected by changes in amniotic fluid composition. *Am J Physiol Renal Physiol*. 2005;288(5):F964–F968.

88. Knepper MA, Wade JB, Terris J, et al. Renal aquaporins. *Kidney Int*. 1996;49(6):1712–1717.

89. Nielsen S, Frokiaer J, Marples D, et al. Aquaporins in the kidney: from molecules to medicine. *Physiol Rev*. 2002;82(1):205–244.

90. Klussmann E, Maric K, Rosenthal W. The mechanisms of aquaporin control in the renal collecting duct. *Rev Physiol Biochem Pharmacol*. 2000;141:33–95.

91. Tajika Y, Matsuzaki T, Suzuki T, et al. Aquaporin-2 is retrieved to the apical storage compartment via early endosomes and phosphatidylinositol 3-kinase-dependent pathway. *Endocrinology*. 2004;145(9):4375–4383.

92. Gradilone SA, Garcia F, Huebert RC, et al. Glucagon induces the plasma membrane insertion of functional aquaporin-8 water channels in isolated rat hepatocytes. *Hepatology.* 2003;37(6):1435–1441.

93. Sugiyama Y, Ota Y, Hara M, Inoue S. Osmotic stress up-regulates aquaporin-3 gene expression in cultured human keratinocytes. *Biochim Biophys Acta.* 2001;1522(2):82–88.

94. De FM, Cobellis L, Torella M, et al. Down-regulation of aquaporin 4 in human placenta throughout pregnancy. *In Vivo.* 2007;21(5):813–817.

95. Liu H, Zheng Z, Wintour EM. Aquaporins and fetal fluid balance. *Placenta.* 2008;29(10):840–847.

96. Johnston H, Koukoulas I, Jeyaseelan K, et al. Ontogeny of aquaporins 1 and 3 in ovine placenta and fetal membranes. *Placenta.* 2000;21(1):88–99.

97. Beall MH, Wang S, Yang B, et al. Placental and membrane aquaporin water channels: correlation with amniotic fluid volume and composition. *Placenta.* 2007;28(5–6):421–428.

98. Liu HS, Song XF, Hao RZ. [Expression of aquaporin 1 in human placenta and fetal membranes]. *Nan Fang Yi Ke Da Xue Xue Bao.* 2008;28(3):333–336.

99. Liu H, Koukoulas I, Ross MC, et al. Quantitative comparison of placental expression of three aquaporin genes. *Placenta.* 2004;25(6):475–478.

100. Mann SE, Ricke EA, Yang BA, et al. Expression and localization of aquaporin 1 and 3 in human fetal membranes. *Am J Obstet Gynecol.* 2002;187(4):902–907.

101. Damiano A, Zotta E, Goldstein J, et al. Water channel proteins AQP3 and AQP9 are present in syncytiotrophoblast of human term placenta. *Placenta.* 2001;22(8–9):776–781.

102. Umenishi F, Verkman AS, Gropper MA. Quantitative analysis of aquaporin mRNA expression in rat tissues by RNase protection assay. *DNA Cell Biol.* 1996;15(6):475–480.

103. Wang S, Amidi F, Beall M, et al. Aquaporin 3 expression in human fetal membranes and its up-regulation by cyclic adenosine monophosphate in amnion epithelial cell culture. *J Soc Gynecol Investig.* 2006;13(3):181–185.

104. Ma T, Yang B, Verkman AS. Cloning of a novel water and urea-permeable aquaporin from mouse expressed strongly in colon, placenta, liver, and heart. *Biochem Biophys Res Commun.* 1997;240(2): 324–328.

105. Wang S, Kallichanda N, Song W, et al. Expression of aquaporin-8 in human placenta and chorioamniotic membranes: evidence of molecular mechanism for intramembranous amniotic fluid resorption. *Am J Obstet Gynecol.* 2001;185(5):1226–1231.

106. Zhu XQ, Jiang SS, Zou SW, et al. [Expression of aquaporin 3 and aquaporin 9 in placenta and fetal membrane with idiopathic polyhydramnios]. *Zhonghua Fu Chan Ke Za Zhi.* 2009;44(12):920–923.

107. Zhu X, Jiang S, Hu Y, et al. The expression of aquaporin 8 and aquaporin 9 in fetal membranes and placenta in term pregnancies complicated by idiopathic polyhydramnios. *Early Hum Dev.* 2010;86(10):657–663.

108. Zhu XQ, Jiang SS, Zhu XJ, et al. Expression of aquaporin 1 and aquaporin 3 in fetal membranes and placenta in human term pregnancies with oligohydramnios. *Placenta.* 2009;30(8):670–676.

109. Hao RZ, Liu HS, Xiong ZF. [Expression of aquaporin-1 in human oligohydramnios placenta and fetal membranes]. *Nan Fang Yi Ke Da Xue Xue Bao.* 2009;29(6):1130–1132.

110. Huang J, Qi HB. [Expression of aquaporin in human fetal membrane and placenta of idiopathic polyhydramnios]. *Zhonghua Fu Chan Ke Za Zhi.* 2009;44(1):19–22.

111. Mann SE, Ricke EA, Torres EA, Taylor RN. A novel model of polyhydramnios: amniotic fluid volume is increased in aquaporin 1 knockout mice. *Am J Obstet Gynecol.* 2005;192(6):2041–2044.

112. Mann S, Dvorak N, Taylor R. Changes in aquaporin 1 expression affect amniotic fluid volume. *Am J Obstet Gynecol.* 2004;191:S132.

113. Mann SE, Dvorak N, Gilbert H, Taylor RN. Steady-state levels of aquaporin 1 mRNA expression are increased in idiopathic polyhydramnios. *Am J Obstet Gynecol.* 2006;194(3):884–887.

114. Bos HB, Nygard KL, Gratton RJ, Richardson BS. Expression of aquaporin 1 (AQP1) in chorioallantoic membranes of near term ovine fetuses with induced hypoxia. *J Soc Gynecol Investig.* 2005;12(2 suppl):333A.

115. Wang S, Chen J, Au KT, Ross MG. Expression of aquaporin 8 and its up-regulation by cyclic adenosine monophosphate in human WISH cells. *Am J Obstet Gynecol.* 2003;188(4):997–1001.

116. Wang S, Amidi F, Beall MH, Ross MG. Differential regulation of aquaporin water channels in human amnion cell culture. *J Soc Gynecol Investig.* 2005;12(2 suppl):344A.

117. Sha XY, Liu HS, Ma TH. Osmotic water permeability diversification in primary trophoblast cultures from aquaporin 1-deficient pregnant mice. *J Obstet Gynaecol Res.* 2015;41(9):1399–1405. [Epub 2015 May 25].

118. Vilariño-García T, Pérez-Pérez A, Dietrich V, et al. Increased Expression of Aquaporin 9 in Trophoblast From Gestational Diabetic Patients. *Horm Metab Res.* 2016;48(8):535–539. [Epub 2016 Apr 15].

CHAPTER 2

Body Composition in the Fetus and Newborn: Effects of Intrauterine Growth Aberration

William Oh, MD

Body Fluid Compartments

Water is the most abundant element of body composition. It is divided into two compartments: intracellular water (ICW) and extracellular water (ECW); the latter is further divided into interstitial fluid and plasma volume (Fig. 2.1). Several methods are available for the measurements of body water in human infants. The general principle has been the use of an indicator that is infused to the subject, allowing for equilibration, and then obtaining a plasma sample to calculate the volume of interest using the principle of dilution with the following formula: $V = I \div Pl\,I$, in which V is volume of the compartment being measured, I is the amount of indicator infused, and Pl I is plasma concentration of infused indicator. Various indicators measure different body water compartments depending on their location of distribution. Table 2.1 shows the water compartments that can be measured with various indicators used.

In early gestation (24 weeks), the total body water (TBW) is very high (~86% of body weight), and most of it (60%) is in the ECW compartment. With increasing gestational age and growth, the TBW content decreases. The decline is primarily attributable to an increase in solid components of the body composition with growth as evidenced by an increase in the ICW compartment and a decline of the ECW compartment. At term, the TBW is down to 78% of body weight, with 44% being in the ECW compartment, 34% in the ICW compartment, and the rest (22%) being solid body mass. At 1 year of age the TBW is approximately 70% of body weight; most of it is in the ICW (42%), and the rest is in the ECW. Solids account for approximately 30% of body weight.[1,2] These changes also mean that a preterm infant born at 28 weeks' gestation will have a high TBW and ECW.

It should be noted that the aforementioned changes in body composition do not distinguish the variation as a result of intrauterine growth aberration and the effects of maternal nutrition and lifestyle. The aberration in intrauterine growth can be in the form of macrosomia (large for gestational age [LGA]) or intrauterine growth restriction (IUGR; also known as small for gestational age [SGA]). Their body fluid characteristics and neonatal adiposity are described later.

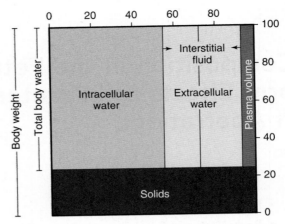

Fig. 2.1   Body water distribution in a term newborn infant.

Table 2.1   INDICATORS USED FOR BODY WATER IN HUMANS

Body Water Compartment	Indicator
Total body water	Antipyrine stable isotope of water (D_2O or $H_2^{18}O$)
Extracellular water	Bromide, sucrose, inulin
Plasma volume	Evans blue

The other body composition can be calculated by using the following formula:
Solids = Body weight − Total body water
Intracellular water = Total body water − Extracellular water
Interstitial water = Extracellular water − Plasma volume

Body Water in Fetal Growth Aberration

Large for Gestational Age

This is a heterogeneous group of infants that consists of those with accelerated fetal growth as a result of poorly controlled maternal diabetes mellitus, maternal constitutional obesity without diabetes, and genetic predisposition to enhanced fetal growth.

The data on body water in LGA infants are sparse. The only information published in the literature is that of Clapp and coworkers,[3] who used D_2O dilution technique to measure TBW and found that in seven infants of diabetic mothers (not all LGA), the value was lower than those of infants with nondiabetic mothers (73% vs. 80% body weight). It should be noted that not all of the infants of diabetic mothers were LGA; they had birth weights ranging from 1430 to 3495 g.

In the absence of good data on directly measured body water content, one may try to make an estimation of this parameter by indirect assessment of the data on body composition in these subjects.

Using dual-energy x-ray absorptiometry (DEXA), Hammami and coworkers[4] measured the body composition of 47 LGA term infants and compared the results with a group of gestational age–matched appropriate-for-gestational-age (AGA) infants. They found that the LGA infants had a higher absolute amount of body fat, lean body mass, and mineral contents. When expressed as a percentage of body weight, the LGA had higher total body fat and mineral contents but less lean body mass. They also found that the increase in total body fat was highest among LGA infants whose mothers had impaired glucose tolerance during pregnancy.

Maternal physical status, lifestyle, and dietary intake may influence the fat contents of the offspring. In a prospective study examining the association between maternal physical measurements and lifestyle, an Irish study involving a large cohort showed that increasing maternal body mass index and waist height ratio were significantly associated with increased neonatal percentage body fat. On the other hand, lifestyle such as smoking during pregnancy is significantly associated with decreased neonatal percentage body fat.[5] These findings are not new, but with a large cohort and rigorous statistical analysis, the data provide important information pointing to the importance of maternal factors affecting neonatal body composition.

Maternal dietary intake during early pregnancy can also affect neonatal body fat composition. Low glycemic index dietary intervention in pregnancy was found to have a beneficial effect on neonatal central adiposity. In addition, central adiposity was positively associated with maternal dietary fat intake and postprandial glucose, highlighting the important role of healthful diet in pregnancy in promoting normal neonatal adiposity.[6,7]

Intrauterine Growth Restriction or Small for Gestational Age

In contrast to LGA infants, there is abundant information regarding the body water and body composition of infants with IUGR.

As in LGA infants, infants with IUGR comprise a heterogeneous group resulting from maternal factors, placental pathology, or fetal causes. Maternal factors include such conditions as maternal undernutrition; maternal disease (e.g., preeclampsia, toxemia of pregnancy); or maternal exposure to adverse environmental factors such as smoking, alcohol, or substance abuse. Placental pathology includes such conditions as placental vascular disease (e.g., preeclampsia resulting in placental vascular insufficiency and placental anomalies). Fetal causes include genetic abnormalities and fetal infection. The clinical diagnosis of an SGA infant, which is also used in most body composition studies, does not differentiate between the different etiologies for impaired growth and is a categorical rather than a continuous description of growth impairment. All of these limitations complicate the interpretation of body composition measurements.

Body Water and Solids in Intrauterine Growth Restriction or Small for Gestational Age Infants

During normal intrauterine growth, TBW content decreases from 94% of body weight in the first trimester of pregnancy to 78% at term, caused by the accumulation of body solids during growth.[1,2] In the first two-thirds of gestation, body solids increase because of the accretion of protein and minerals, and there is little fat deposition. We know from postmortem chemical analyses that at 27 weeks' gestation, 86% of body weight is water, 12% is fat-free dry solids, and only 2% is fat.[8] In vivo measurements in AGA preterm infants with a birth weight less than 1500 g showed a TBW content of 83%,[9] and no fat was detectable by dual photon absorptiometry using [153]Gd magnetic resonance tomography (MRT) in preterm infants.[10] During the last trimester of gestation, the proportion of body solids increases from 14% to 24% of body weight because of the deposition of body fat, which is 2% of body weight at 27 weeks' gestation and 10% to 15% of body weight at birth.[10]

Normal intrauterine growth critically depends on the delivery of sufficient nutrients to the fetus via the placenta. When nutrient delivery was reduced by uterine artery ligation during experimental IUGR in rats, TBW was increased, reflecting the reduced deposition of body fat and protein.[11] In human IUGR neonates the TBW content of the body was also increased compared with normal intrauterine growth. In SGA preterm neonates the mean TBW content was 62 mL/kg higher than in AGA preterm neonates,[12] and in SGA term neonates, the mean TBW content was increased by 76 mL/kg[13] or by 102 mL/kg,[14] respectively. No reduction in TBW was found in only one study of a small group of SGA neonates with a wide range of gestational ages (Table 2.2).[15]

The relative increase in TBW in SGA neonates is caused by the reduction in body solids and the fat content, not by an accumulation of excess water caused by a disturbed fluid homeostasis. In preterm SGA neonates, the higher body water content reflects the reduced deposition of protein and minerals because during the first two-thirds of gestation, the fetal body consists of water and fat-free dry solids, but there is little deposition of fat. A reduction in fetal lean mass during IUGR has

Table 2.2 TOTAL BODY WATER AND EXTRACELLULAR VOLUME IN APPROPRIATE FOR GESTATIONAL AGE AND SMALL FOR GESTATIONAL AGE HUMAN NEONATES

Authors (Year)	Subjects	Patients	n	TBW (mL/kg)	Significance	Method
Cassady and Milstead (1971)	Term (37–43 weeks)	AGA	12	688 ± 16	P < .001	Indicator dilution (antipyrine)
		SGA	23	790 ± 13		
Hartnoll and coworkers (2000)	Preterm (25–30 weeks)	AGA	35	906 (833–954)	P = .019	Indicator dilution ($H_2^{18}O$)
		SGA	7	844 (637–958)		
Cheek and coworkers (1984)	Term (≥37 weeks)	AGA	7	749	Not reported	Indicator dilution (D_2O)
		SGA	6	825		
Wagen and coworkers (1986)	GA (34–40 weeks)	AGA	11	780 ± 38	NS	Indicator dilution (D_2O)
		SGA	10	776 ± 13		

Authors (Year)	Subjects	Patients	n	ECV (mL/kg)	Significance	Method
Cassady (1970)	Term (≥37 weeks)	AGA	13	376 ± 20	P = .025	Indicator dilution (bromide)
		SGA	20	419 ± 45		
Cheek and coworkers (1984)	Term (≥37 weeks)	AGA	7	361 ± 16	Not reported	Indicator dilution (bromide)
		SGA	6	395 ± 35		
Wagen and coworkers (1986)	GA (34–40 weeks)	AGA	11	355 ± 55	NS	Indicator dilution (sucrose)
		SGA	10	344 ± 35		

AGA, Appropriate for gestational age; *ECV*, extracellular volume; *GA*, gestational age; *NS*, not significant; *SGA*, small for gestational age; *TBW*, total body water.

been demonstrated by ultrasound measurements of the cross-sectional lean body area of the fetal thigh.[16]

A reduced protein and mineral deposition early in gestation is likely to disrupt organ development. In fact, preterm SGA neonates have a higher mortality rate and more chronic lung disease than gestational age–matched preterm AGA neonates,[17] and SGA preterm neonates are still smaller and lighter at 3 years of age than AGA preterm neonates.[18,19] A study by Zeitlin and coworkers[20] confirmed this association.

Different from preterm SGA neonates, the increase in body water content in term SGA neonates reflects primarily the reduced deposition of fat. The accumulation of fat is the primary cause of the physiologic reduction in TBW during normal growth throughout the third trimester of gestation. Aside from body water measurements, several lines of evidence indicate that adipose tissue is indeed reduced in SGA term neonates. Reduced abdominal wall fat thickness measured by ultrasonography in a late gestation fetus was found in IUGR.[20] The percentage of adipose tissue estimated from dual photon absorptiometry using [153]Gd MRT was 2% in SGA term neonates compared with 13% in AGA term neonates,[18] and thinner skin folds in SGA term neonates indicated a thinner subcutaneous fat layer.[21,22] A study by Lapillonne and coworkers[23] using DEXA analysis also found a reduced fat content in SGA near-term and term infants, although the difference did not reach statistical significance because of the small sample size. A prospective study using ultrasound technique of 87 pregnancies showed that fetuses with estimated fetal weight of less than 10 percentile had a significantly lower fat content in percentage when compared with those with normal fetal growth (5.1 ± 2 vs. 11.6 ± 5.6, respectively).[24]

No conclusions about the effect of altered body composition of SGA neonates on the risk for neonatal complications or long-term outcome can be drawn because studies including body composition measurements are usually small, and no clinical outcomes are reported. Yet from anthropometric studies that include large numbers of neonates, the prognostic utility of body composition estimated from anthropometry can be analyzed. Body weight less than a certain cutoff point is the parameter most often used to diagnose impaired fetal growth. In future studies of fetal growth restriction, weight deficit should be quantified and expressed on a continuous scale (e.g., as a standard deviation score) instead of using a fixed cutoff value. The more severe the weight reduction, the higher the risk of neonatal morbidity and mortality for SGA neonates regardless of the cause of the growth deficit and the higher the risk of low intellectual performance in adulthood.[25]

Another issue that complicates the interpretation of body composition changes and IUGR is the categorization of these infants as having symmetric or asymmetric IUGR. Whereas the former is often defined by clinicians as having growth restriction affecting all three morphometric parameters (weight, length, and head circumference), the latter defines the group that has growth restriction affecting the weight but not the length or head circumference. It has been shown that despite an overall small body size and lower amounts of subcutaneous fat than the reference population, symmetric SGA term newborns showed a proportionate body fat distribution and asymmetric SGA infants were thinner and had a lower percentage of central subcutaneous fat than symmetric SGA infants.[26] Although term neonates with asymmetric IUGR were more likely to demonstrate catch-up growth than preterm neonates with symmetric IUGR, preterm SGA neonates had restriction of childhood growth regardless of having symmetric or asymmetric IUGR at birth.[27] Reduced adipose tissue thickness is a more sensitive predictor for neonatal complications in SGA neonates than weight because symptomatic SGA neonates with hypoglycemia or polycythemia (or both) had a thinner subcutaneous fat layer than asymptomatic SGA neonates, but there was no difference in body weight or length between the two groups.[28]

In summary, fetal growth aberration significantly affects body composition. Accelerated fetal growth results in increase in body solids and fat with a relative decrease in body water. On the other hand, IUGR results in reduction in body fat with a relative increase in body water. Note that the body water changes in both situations are relative, without an absolute increase in actual contents.

Transitional Changes of Body Water After Birth

Although the mechanism is unknown, there is a universal contraction of ECW in infants soon after birth, associated with a weight loss of 7% to 10% of body weight by the end of the first week. The magnitude of contraction is inversely proportional to maturity. Term infants have an average of 5% to 7% weight loss during the first week (reflecting contraction of ECW),[29] but very low birth weight (VLBW)[30] and extremely low birth weight (ELBW)[31] infants may lose 10% to 15% of body weight, respectively, during that same time frame (Fig. 2.2). This study confirmed the earlier studies[32,33] showing that the magnitude of reduction of ECW is directly proportional to its content. It should be noted that these studies represented cross-sectional data and did not distinguish the type of infants with reference to growth aberration.

It is suggested that the removal of the ECW is through the renal route. The evidence for this is not direct but implied based on the concurrence of reduction in ECW, weight loss, natriuretic diuresis, and negative sodium balance.[34,35] There is also suggestion that diuresis during the first week of life is associated with an improvement in respiratory distress.

There are virtually no data available in regards to the postnatal body fluid transition in LGA infants. However, there is a significant body of literature in regards to IUGR.

Postnatal weight loss in seven SGA preterm neonates (birth weight < 5th percentile) with a mean gestational age of 35 weeks was only 5% and was accompanied by a proportionate reduction in body water and body solids.[36] This study included no information about fluid intake or diuresis and no AGA control group.

In another study comparing five SGA preterm neonates (mean gestational age, 35 weeks) with 14 weight-matched AGA neonates (mean gestational age, 31 weeks), the SGA neonates had a maximal postnatal weight loss of only 2% compared with a maximal postnatal weight loss of 8% in the AGA control infants. On days 4 to 6 of life the SGA neonates had already regained birth weight and there was no detectable change in TBW or body solids; at the same postnatal age, body weight and TBW in the AGA neonates were significantly lower than at birth. There were no

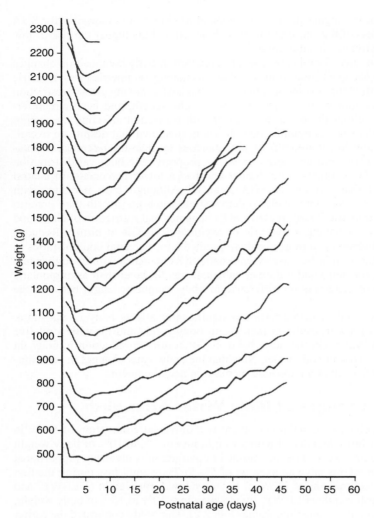

Fig. 2.2 Body weight change in low birth weight infants. Weight changes of infants at 100-g intervals are shown. (From Shaffer SG, Quimiro CL, Anderson JV, Hall RT. Postnatal weight changes in low birth weight infants. *Pediatrics.* 1987;79:702-705, with permission.)

differences in day-to-day fluid and energy intake during the first week of life in the SGA and AGA groups; however, the AGA infants had a higher urine output during this time. A possible reason for the attenuated postnatal increase in urine output in SGA preterm neonates was their altered hemodynamic adaptation. SGA preterm neonates did not show the postnatal increase in cardiac output observed in the AGA neonates.[37]

Wadhawan and coworkers[38] analyzed a large database from the National Institute of Child Health and Human Development Neonatal Research Network to compare the postnatal weight loss of SGA ($n = 1248$) versus AGA infants ($n = 8213$) and association with the risk of death or bronchopulmonary dysplasia (BPD). They found that the SGA infants had less prevalence of postnatal weight loss than the AGA infants (81.2% vs. 93.7%, respectively; $P < .001$). The association between postnatal weight loss and death or BPD was also similar between SGA and AGA groups. They suggest that clinicians who consider the association between early postnatal weight loss and risk of death or BPD should do so independent of gestation or birth weight status.

Varma and coworkers[39] analyzed a group of AGA ELBW infants ($n = 102$) and concluded that the maximal postnatal weight loss was more related to maturity than to clinical determinants. The association between postnatal weight loss and clinical morbidity clearly needs further study.

Clinical Implications of Transitional Body Water Changes in Preterm Very Low Birth Weight Infants

Fluid therapy in the immediate neonatal period in preterm and low birth weight neonates has the following objectives: It (1) allows for the physiologic postnatal contraction of the extracellular volume to occur, (2) aims at a postnatal weight loss of approximately 10% of body weight, (3) aims at a negative fluid and sodium balance on days 1 to 3 of life, and (4) minimizes transepidermal water loss.[40] These objectives can be achieved with restricted water intake and sequentially monitoring water and electrolyte balance by using the daily intake, output, weight changes, and serum electrolyte concentrations (particularly sodium) data in adjusting the appropriate amount of intake to achieve these goals. Failure to do so will result in either dehydration if inadequate amount of fluid is given or increased risk of patent ductus arteriosus (PDA), necrotizing enterocolitis (NEC), and perhaps chronic lung disease if excess fluid is given.[40-44] There is also suggestive evidence that sodium restriction during the first week of life to produce a negative sodium balance can achieve the same goals as fluid restriction.[45,46] The physiologic rationale behind the latter is that if sodium intake exceeds the requirement, the sodium retention will result in water excess producing the same result as in excess water intake with positive water balance.

Maintaining a negative water and sodium balance during the first week is the key to successful fluid and electrolyte management of VLBW infants and even more so for ELBW infants because the latter are at much higher risk for various clinical morbidities The following case presentation illustrates how a clinician can balance the fluid and electrolyte status of an ELBW infant by paying close attention to daily body weight changes in the process of prescribing the daily fluid and electrolyte.

Let us take the case of a 1.0-kg AGA infant admitted to the neonatal intensive care unit with respiratory distress who was being cared for in a hybrid-humidified incubator (Giraffe OmniBed, GE Healthcare, Pittsburgh, Pennsylvania). The latter is a new high-technology incubator that has been shown to be very effective in maintaining body temperature and fluid balance in VLBW infants.[47] The initial fluid order consisted of 70 mL/kg of 10% glucose without electrolytes. Although some clinicians may add sodium and potassium during the first 24 hours of life, most would begin sodium and potassium at 1 to 2 mEq/kg per day on the second day and increase to 3 mEq/kg per day at the end of first week. The initial fluid volume is based on the estimated insensible water loss for this infant of 50 mL/kg and an additional 20 mL/kg for estimated water required to excrete approximately 5 mOsm/kg of endogenous solute load. Recent evidence suggests beneficial effects of early initiation of amino acid.[48] Most clinicians add the protein as early as the first day of life. Soy-based fat emulsion is usually added during the second day of life to provide essential fatty acid and energy, the latter taking advantage of its high caloric density.[49]

Table 2.3 illustrates the potential scenario in body weight changes, intake, output data, and estimated insensible water loss, as well as the rationale for the prescribed fluid, electrolyte, and nutrition intake for this infant. The scenario shows that systematic data collection, interpretation, and forward calculation of intake are needed to ensure negative fluid and sodium balance in this infant during the first 72 hours. Note that the ECW contraction generally ceases at day 4 to 6 of life; thus the weight should be unchanged. By day 6 of life, the body weight should begin to increase at 20 to 30 g/kg, which reflects anabolic or the beginning of the growth phase. A useful way of ensuring the appropriate fluid balance is achieved is to plot the weight changes on a daily basis using a standard growth chart, such as the one shown in Fig. 2.3.

There is essentially no clinical trial about fluid therapy for LGA, as well as SGA, neonates. From the body water measurements, we know that despite their "wrinkled" appearance, SGA neonates are not dehydrated at birth. Rather, severely

Table 2.3 BODY WEIGHT CHANGES, INTAKE, OUTPUT, ESTIMATED INSENSIBLE WATER LOSS, AND CALCULATED INTAKE THE NEXT 24 HOURS IN A 1.0-KG INFANT AT BIRTH

Age	Weight (g)	Intake (mL/kg)	Urine (mL/kg)	Serum (Na mEq/L)	Estimated IWL	Fluid Next 24 h	Sodium (mEq/kg)
Birth	1,000	—	—	—	50	70[b]	0
24 h	970	70	20	140	80[a]	100[c]	1
48 h	950	100	48	140	72	120[d]	1
72 h	930	120	68	140	72	140	2
7 d	980[e]	140	60	140	50	140[f]	2

[a]Estimated insensible water loss = Intake − Urine output − Weight changes = 70 − 20 + 30 = 80.
[b]10% glucose.
[c]Amino acid added.
[d]Fat emulsion added.
[e]A gain of 20 g from the previous 24 hours.
[f]IWL + Urine + Stool + Weight gain = 50 + 60 + 10 + 20 = 140.
IWL, Insensible water loss.

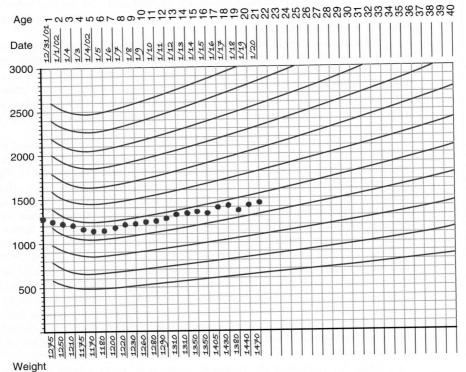

Fig. 2.3 Weight changes during the first 3 weeks of life of a very low birth weight infant.

growth-restricted neonates have an expanded extracellular volume. The only study providing data on fluid therapy in the immediate neonatal period reports an attenuated postnatal weight loss in SGA preterm infants receiving the same amount of fluid intake as weight-matched AGA preterm infants.[48] This study suggests that SGA preterm neonates do not need extra fluid intake in the immediate neonatal period, but rather a cautious approach to fluid prescription. It is probably fair to state that the description of fluid therapy above is appropriate for VLBW infants of various growth categories. However, future clinical trials to confirm this statement are desirable.

REFERENCES

1. Friis-Hansen B. Changes in body water compartments during growth. *Acta Paediatr.* 1957;46(suppl 110):1–68.
2. Friis-Hansen B. Body water compartments in children: changes during growth and related changes in body composition. *Pediatrics.* 1961;28:169–181.
3. Clapp WM, Butterfield LJ, O'Brien D. Body water compartment in premature infants with special reference to the effects of the respiratory distress syndrome and of maternal diabetes and toxemia. *Pediatrics.* 1962;29:883–889.
4. Hammami M, Walters JC, Hockman EM, et al. Disproportionate alterations in body composition of large for gestational age neonates. *J Pediatr.* 2001;138:817–821.
5. McCarthy FP, Khashan AS, Murray D, et al. Parental physical and lifestyle factors and their association with newborn body composition. *BJOG.* 2016;123:1824–1829.
6. Horan MK, McGowan CA, Gibney ER, et al. Maternal low glycemic index diet, fat intake and postprandial glucose influences neonatal adiposity—secondary analysis from the ROLO study. *Nutr J.* 2014;13:78.
7. Okubo H, Crozier SR, Harvey NC, et al. Maternal dietary glycemic index and glycemic load in early pregnancy are associated with offspring adiposity in childhood: the Southampton Women's Survey. *Am J Clin Nutr.* 2014;100:676–683.
8. Ziegler EE, O'Donnell AM, Nelson SE, Fomon SJ. Body composition of the reference fetus. *Growth.* 1976;40:329–341.
9. Bauer K, Bovermann G, Roithmaier A, et al. Body composition, nutrition, and fluid balance during the first two weeks of life in preterm neonates weighing less than 1500 grams. *J Pediatr.* 1991;118:615–620.
10. Petersen S, Gotfredsen A, Knudsen FU. Lean body mass in small for gestational age and appropriate for gestational age infants. *J Pediatr.* 1988;113:886–889.
11. Hohenauer L, Oh W. Body composition in experimental intrauterine growth retardation in the rat. *J Nutr.* 1969;99:358–361.
12. Hartnoll G, Betremieux P, Modi N. Body water content of extremely preterm infants at birth. *Arch Dis Child Fetal Neonatal Ed.* 2000;83:F56–F59.
13. Cheek DB, Wishart J, MacLennan A, Haslam R. Cell hydration in the normally grown, the premature, and the low weight for gestational age infant. *Early Hum Dev.* 1984;10:75–84.
14. Cassady G, Milstead RR. Antipyrine space studies and cell water estimates in infants of low birth weight. *Pediatr Res.* 1971;5:673–682.
15. Wagen A, Okken A, Zweens J, Zijlstra WG. Body composition at birth of growth-retarded newborn infants demonstrating catch-up growth in the first year of life. *Biol Neonate.* 1986;49:121–125.
16. Padoan A, Rigano S, Ferrazzi E, et al. Differences in fat and lean mass proportions in normal and growth restricted fetuses. *Am J Obstet Gynecol.* 2004;191:1459–1464.
17. Lal MK, Manktelow BN, Draper ES, Field DJ. Chronic lung disease of prematurity and intrauterine growth retardation: a population-based study. *Pediatrics.* 2003;111:483–487.
18. Law TL, Korte JE, Katikaneni LD, et al. Ultrasound assessment of intrauterine growth restriction: relationship to neonatal body composition. *Am J Obstet Gynecol.* 2011;205:255, e1–e6.
19. Strauss RS, Dietz WH. Growth and development of term children born with low birth weight: effects of genetic and environmental factors. *J Pediatr.* 1998;133:67–72.
20. Zeitlin J, El Ayoubi M, Jarreau PH, et al. Impact of fetal growth restriction on mortality and morbidity in a very preterm birth cohort. *J Pediatr.* 2010;157(5):733–739.
21. Gardeil F, Greene R, Stuart B, Turner MJ. Subcutaneous fat in the fetal abdomen as a predictor of growth restriction. *Obstet Gynecol.* 1999;94:209–212.
22. Brans YW, Sumners JE, Dweck HS, Cassady G. A noninvasive approach to body composition in the neonate: dynamic skinfold measurement. *Pediatr Res.* 1974;8:215–222.
23. Lapillonne A, Braillon P, Claris O, et al. Body composition in appropriate and in small for gestational age infants. *Acta Paediatr.* 1997;86:196–200.
24. Rodríguez G, Collado MP, Samper MP, Biosca M. Subcutaneous fat distribution in small for gestational age newborns. *J Perinat Med.* 2011;39:355–357.
25. Kramer MS, Olivier M, McLaen FH, et al. Impact of intrauterine growth retardation and body proportionality on fetal and neonatal outcome. *Pediatrics.* 1990;85:707–713.
26. Bergvall N, Iliadou A, Johannsson S, et al. Risks for low intellectual performance related to being born small for gestational age are modified by gestational age. *Pediatrics.* 2006;117:e460–e467.
27. Drossou V, Diamanti E, Noutsia H, et al. Accuracy of anthropometric measurements in predicting symptomatic SGA and LGA neonates. *Acta Paediatr.* 1995;84:1–5.
28. Cheek DB, Wishart J, MacLennan A, Haslam R. Cell hydration in the normally grown, the premature, and the low weight for gestational age infant. *Early Hum Dev.* 1984;10:75.
29. Shaffer SG, Quimiro CL, Anderson JV, Hall RT. Postnatal weight changes in low birth weight infants. *Pediatrics.* 1987;79:702–705.
30. Pauls J, Bauer K, Versmold H. Postnatal body weight curves for infants below 1000g birth weight receiving early enteral and parenteral nutrition. *Eur J Pediatr.* 1998;157:416–421.
31. Dancis J, O'Connell JR, Holt LE. A grid for recording the weight of preterm infants. *J Pediatr.* 1948;33:570–572.
32. Brosius KK, Ritter DA, Kenny JD. Postnatal growth curve of the infant with extremely low birth weight who was fed enterally. *Pediatrics.* 1984;74:778–782.

33. Ross BS, Cowett RM, Oh W. Renal functions of low birth weight infants during the first two months of life. *Pediatr Res.* 1977;11:1162–1164.
34. Siegel SR, Oh W. Renal function as a marker of human fetal maturation. *Acta Paediatr Scand.* 1976;65:481–485.
35. Bidiwala KS, Lorenz JM, Kleinman LI. Renal function correlates of diuresis in preterm infant. *Pediatrics.* 1988;82:50–58.
36. Wagen A, Okken A, Zweens J, Zijlstra WG. Composition of postnatal weight loss and subsequent weight gain in small for dates newborn infants. *Acta Paediatr Scand.* 1985;74:57–61.
37. Leipälä JA, Boldt T, Turpeinen U, et al. Cardiac hypertrophy and altered hemodynamic adaptation in growth-restricted preterm infants. *Pediatr Res.* 2003;53:989–993.
38. Wadhawan R, Perritt R, Laptook AR, et al. Association between early postnatal weight loss and death or broncho-pulmonary dysplasia in small and appropriate for gestational age extremely low birth weight infants. *J Perinatology.* 2007;27:359–364.
39. Varma RP, Shibli S, Fang H, et al. Clinical determinants and utility of early postnatal maximum weight loss in fluid management of extremely low birth weight infants. *Early Human Dev.* 2009;85:59–64.
40. Modi N. Management of fluid balance in the very immature neonate. *Arch Dis Child Fetal Neonatal Ed.* 2004;89:F108–F111.
41. Bell EF, Warburton D, Stonestreet BS, Oh W. High volume fluid intake predisposes premature infants to necrotizing enterocolitis. *Lancet.* 1979;2:90.
42. Bell EF, Warburton D, Stonestreet BS, Oh W. Effect of fluid administration of the development of symptomatic patent ductus arteriosus and congestive heart failure in premature infants. *N Engl J Med.* 1980;302:598–604.
43. Bell EF, Acarregui MJ. Restricted versus liberal water intake for preventing morbidity and mortality in preterm infants. *Cochrane Database Syst Rev.* 2001;(3):CD000503.
44. Bell EF, Acarregui MJ. Restricted versus liberal water intake for preventing morbidity and mortality in preterm infants. *Cochrane Database Syst Rev.* 2000;(2):CD000503.
45. Hartnoll G, Betremieux P, Modi N. Randomized controlled trial of postnatal sodium supplementation on oxygen dependency and body weight in 25–30 week gestational age infants. *Arch Dis Child.* 2000;85:F29–F32.
46. Hartnoll G, Betremieux P, Modi N. Randomized controlled trial of postnatal sodium supplementation on body composition in 25–30 week gestational age infants. *Arch Dis Child.* 2000;82(1):F24–F28.
47. Kim SM, Lee EY, Chen J, et al. Improved care and growth outcomes by using hybrid humidified incubators in very preterm infants. *Pediatrics.* 2010;125(1):e137–e145.
48. Bauer K, Cowett RM, Howard GM, et al. Effect of intrauterine growth retardation on postnatal weight change in preterm infants. *J Pediatr.* 1993;123:301–306.
49. Cassady G. Body composition in intrauterine growth retardation. *Pediatr Clin North Am.* 1970;17:79–99.

Perinatal Mineral, Electrolyte, and Acid-Base Homeostasis

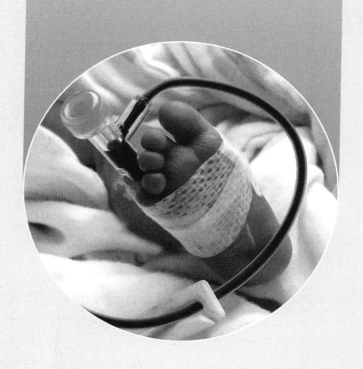

SECTION 2

Perinatal Mineral,
Electrolyte, and Acid-
Base Homeostasis

CHAPTER 3

Potassium Metabolism

Martine TP Besouw, MD, PhD, Detlef Bockenhauer, MD, PhD

- **Abnormalities in Plasma Potassium Can Reflect Changes in Internal Balance (Shift Across the Cell Membranes) or External Balance (Discrepancy Between Intake and Excretion of Potassium)**
- **Changes in Internal Balance Are Typically Acute, Whereas Disturbance of the External Balance Is More Likely to Result in Chronic Changes**
- **The Kidneys Are the Key Organs for Maintaining the External Balance by Adjusting Excretion to Intake**
- **The Distal Convoluted Tubule Is Critical for Potassium Sensing, Whereas the Aldosterone-Sensitive Nephron Is Responsible for Potassium Secretion**

Normal Metabolism

General Background

Potassium is the most abundant cation in the human body, yet only 2% of total body potassium is contained in the extracellular fluid, which is the compartment accessible to clinical assessment. Its concentration in extracellular fluid is tightly regulated between 3.5 and 5.0 mmol/L. The vast majority of potassium (98%) is located intracellularly (mainly in muscle) at concentrations between 100 and 150 mmol/L, depending on cell type (Fig. 3.1). This large difference between intracellular and extracellular potassium content is of great importance to maintain the resting membrane potential of excitable cells, such as neurons, muscle cells, and cardiac cells. In addition, redistribution between intracellular and extracellular potassium provides a first defense mechanism against hyperkalemia or hypokalemia.[1-3] The normal distribution of total body potassium is shown in Fig. 3.1.[4]

To maintain normokalemia, there needs to be a strict control between the regulation of the internal and external potassium balance. The first refers to the concentration gradient across cell membranes caused by the difference between intracellular and extracellular potassium levels, which is maintained by the influx or efflux of potassium from intracellular to extracellular spaces in different conditions. The latter refers to the regulation of total body potassium, by balancing potassium excretion with potassium intake. Although total body homeostasis mainly relies on the excretion of potassium by the kidneys, the response of the kidneys after having a meal rich in potassium is relatively slow. Therefore a transient but rapid translocation of the excess potassium from the extracellular into the intracellular space is needed to prevent potential life-threatening hyperkalemia to occur, thus showing that the internal and external potassium balance is constantly interacting with each other.[1-3]

Regulation of Internal Potassium Balance

Because of the high gradient between intracellular and extracellular potassium levels, potassium constantly leaks out of the cell via ubiquitously expressed selective potassium channels, which helps establish a voltage gradient across the membrane. This passive

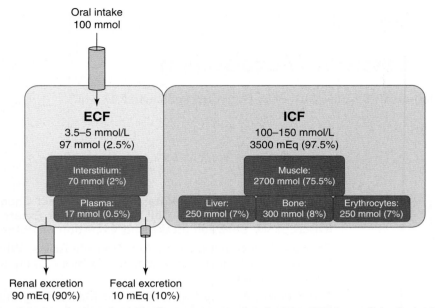

Fig. 3.1 Distribution of total body potassium in normal adults. *ECF,* Extracellular fluid; *ICF,* intracellular fluid. (From Sahni V, Gmurzcyk A, Rosa RM. Extrarenal potassium metabolism. In: Alpern RJ, Caplan MJ, Moe OW, eds. *Seldin en Giebsch's the Kidney—Physiology and Pathophysiology.* London: Elsevier Academic Press; 2013:1629-1658.)

Table 3.1 FACTORS THAT CAN INFLUENCE INTERNAL POTASSIUM BALANCE[1-3]

Factors That *Increase* Intracellular Potassium (Decreasing Serum Potassium)	Factors That *Decrease* Intracellular Potassium (Increasing Serum Potassium)
Physiologic Factors	
Insulin	
Aldosterone	
T3	
β-adrenergic stimulation	α-adrenergic stimulation
Pathologic Factors	
Alkalosis	Acidosis
Hyperosmolality	Hypoosmololality
	Hyperglycemia/uncontrolled diabetes mellitus
	Heavy exercise
	Cell lysis

potassium efflux is counteracted by active transport of potassium into the cell by Na⁺,K⁺-ATPase, which pumps two potassium ions into and three sodium ions out of the cells, at the expense of the hydrolysis of one adenosine triphosphate (ATP) molecule.[1,3] Factors that can influence this balance are shown in Table 3.1.

After ingestion of a meal, approximately 80% of the potassium that is absorbed by the gut is rapidly translocated into the intracellular space. This rapid uptake of potassium is mainly induced by increased insulin levels after the absorption of glucose and amino acids. Insulin increases the activity of the Na⁺,K⁺-ATPase in hepatocytes, muscle cells, adipose cells, and brain cells, thereby increasing their potassium uptake. This process is independent of its effect on glucose transport. Meanwhile, any rise in serum potassium levels will decrease the transmembrane potassium gradient, thereby decreasing the passive efflux of potassium out of the cells. Increased potassium intake also stimulates the secretion of aldosterone, which further stimulates potassium excretion by both the kidneys and the colon. Triiodothyronine (T3) increases Na^+,K^+-ATPase in muscle cells, increasing their potassium uptake. β-Adrenergic stimulation promotes cellular potassium uptake by liver cells, muscle cells, and cardiac cells. In contrast, α-adrenergic stimulation promotes the efflux of potassium from hepatocytes.[1–3]

Besides the abovementioned hormonal influence on internal potassium balance, extracellular potassium levels can also be affected by several pathologic conditions. These include disturbances of acid-base homeostasis, because serum pH inversely correlates with serum potassium levels.[5] In conditions causing altered serum pH, sodium and potassium are exchanged for hydrogen. Moreover, hydrogen ions impair the activity of Na^+,K^+-ATPase, thus decreasing intracellular potassium uptake. Acid-base disturbances due to metabolic conditions cause greater potassium shifts compared with respiratory conditions, as do acute changes compared with chronic acid-base derangements.[1] Changes in serum osmolality also affect extracellular potassium concentration. An increase in serum osmolality shifts water out of the cells, which inevitably leads to an increase of intracellular potassium concentration. This increased transmembrane potassium gradient promotes the passive leakage of potassium out of the cells into the extracellular fluid. In heavy exercise, intracellular ATP depletion impairs potassium uptake into muscle cells, thus increasing serum potassium levels. And lastly, in case of cell death, such as in tumor lysis syndrome, the Na^+,K^+-ATPase can no longer function and the intracellular potassium stores are released into the extracellular space.[1,2]

Regulation of External Potassium Balance

Routes of Potassium Excretion

The regulation of total body potassium is mainly controlled by renal potassium excretion, which is described in more detail later. The average daily potassium intake is approximately 1 mmol/kg per day. Although children need a positive potassium balance to grow, adults maintain a zero potassium balance.[1] Of all ingested potassium, 80% to 90% is excreted by the kidneys and 10% to 20% is lost in the stool.[1–3]

Potassium can be found in gastrointestinal secretions in various amounts. Saliva contains approximately 20 mmol/L, esophageal and gastric secretions 11 to 35 mmol/L, and pancreatic secretions 3.5 to 5.0 mmol/L. Most of this potassium is reabsorbed throughout the intestinal tract.[6] Meanwhile, the colon is the most important site for potassium excretion. Colonic cells can actively secrete potassium via the basolateral pumps Na^+,K^+-ATPase and $Na^+-K^+-2Cl^-$-cotransporter (NKCC) and the apical potassium "big" conductance (BK) channel. Colonic potassium absorption is mediated by two apical H^+-K^+-ATPases.[1] The fecal potassium content can be increased by several hormones, including aldosterone, epinephrine, and prostaglandins. Increased colonic expression of BK channels in end-stage renal disease can enhance the fecal potassium excretion to up to 30% to 80% of the ingested amount of potassium. Other pathologic conditions such as secretory diarrhea and ulcerative colitis can also be associated with increased expression or activation of BK channels, thus increasing intestinal potassium losses.[1,7] Emesis can be another route of potassium loss because it contains approximately 5 times more potassium than serum.[6] Factors that can influence gastrointestinal losses are summarized in Table 3.2.

The potassium content of sweat is generally twice as high as serum.[8] Yet, given the low volume of daily sweat production, the potassium losses via this route are usually negligible.

Regulation of Potassium Excretion: Circadian Rhythm, Feedback, and Feedforward

The regulation of the daily excretion of potassium occurs via three mechanisms. The first is characterized by a circadian rhythm, which is one of the most consistent circadian processes that occurs in humans. It enables a higher potassium excretion during daytime, when typically more potassium is ingested, thus minimizing swings in serum potassium levels. This circadian rhythm remains present when potassium intake is equally distributed throughout the day and physical activity and light exposure

Table 3.2   FACTORS THAT CAN INFLUENCE GASTROINTESTINAL POTASSIUM EXCRETION[1,7]

Factors That *Increase* Gastrointestinal Potassium Loss	Factors That *Decrease* Gastrointestinal Potassium Loss
Physiologic Factors Aldosterone Epinephrine Prostaglandins	Low dietary potassium intake
Pathologic Factors Secretory diarrhea Vomiting End-stage renal disease Ulcerative colitis	
Medications Prolonged use of laxatives[a] Intestinal potassium binders[b]	Nonsteroidal antiinflammatory drugs

[a]Mainly diphenolic laxatives (e.g., phenolphthalein and bisacodyl) and anthroquinones (e.g., senna glycosides and danthron).
[b]Polystyrene sulfonate (resonium) or sodium zirconium cyclosilicate.

are held constant. Changes in potassium intake can interfere with the amplitude of this rhythm but not with its intrinsic circadian periodicity.[1,3,9]

The second mechanism of regulation of potassium excretion is the negative feedback system, which is controlled by serum potassium levels. It relies on both the internal and external potassium balance to maintain stable serum potassium levels after a potassium load, but also after potassium depletion. Mild increases in serum potassium promote the cellular uptake of the cation (e.g., by increased insulin and aldosterone levels) and vice versa, as discussed before in the paragraph on internal potassium balance. Moreover, the urinary excretion of potassium can be regulated according to serum potassium concentration. In general, the absorption of potassium throughout the nephron is quite stable. Changes in urinary potassium content are mainly established by altering the potassium excretion by the principal cell in the late distal convoluted tubule (DCT) and collecting duct.[1-3] This is explained in more detail later.

A third mechanism of potassium regulation has been postulated in the form of a feedforward system. The exact pathways by which this system operates have not been completely elucidated, but the proposed existence of this feedforward system is based on the observation in animal studies that the kaliuretic response to a potassium load is greater with enteral intake compared with intravenous infusion.[10] This feedforward system appears to be aldosterone independent and is thought to be mediated by receptors in the gut, portal vein, and/or liver, which, via undefined pathways, lead to decreased sodium uptake in the DCT and thus enhanced delivery of sodium to the collecting duct, where it can be reabsorbed in exchange for potassium secretion.[11] This increased urinary excretion of potassium at the moment of enteral potassium intake prevents hyperkalemia when the enteral potassium load is being absorbed.[3,12]

Renal Potassium Handling

The daily urinary potassium excretion depends on glomerular potassium filtration (determined by glomerular filtration rate [GFR] and serum potassium levels) and potassium reabsorption and excretion along the different sites of the nephron (Fig. 3.2).

Potassium is freely filtered in the glomerulus. Thus, in a normal adult, approximately 755 mmol of potassium reaches the proximal tubule every day (180 L/day × average serum potassium concentration of 4.2 mmol/L). The reabsorption of potassium in the proximal tubule and loop of Henle is rather stable. According to the body's needs, the most powerful regulation of urinary potassium excretion occurs in the

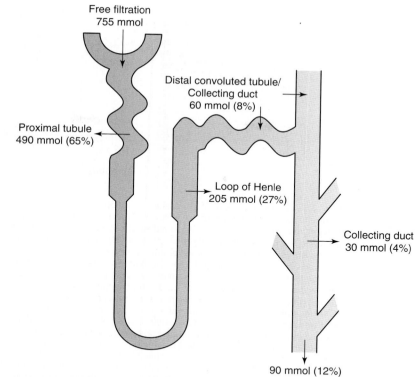

Free filtration
755 mmol

Distal convoluted tubule/
Collecting duct
60 mmol (8%)

Proximal tubule
490 mmol (65%)

Loop of Henle
205 mmol (27%)

Collecting duct
30 mmol (4%)

90 mmol (12%)

Fig. 3.2   Schematic view of renal potassium handling along the nephron. Potassium is freely filtered in the glomerulus. The majority is reabsorbed in the proximal tubule and the loop of Henle. Fine-tuning of potassium excretion is performed by the principal cells in the late distal convoluted tubule and collecting duct, by altering potassium secretion. A small amount of potassium is reabsorbed by the intercalated cells. The net excretion is around 12% of the total filtered amount of potassium. Levels given are daily amounts in healthy adults. (Satlin LM, Bockenhauer D. Physiology of the developing kidney: potassium homeostasis and its disorder. In: Avner ED, Harmon WE, Niaudet P, et al., eds. *Pediatric Nephrology*. Berlin Heidelberg: Springer-Verlag; 2016:219-246; and Hall JE. Renal regulation of potassium, calcium, phosphate, and magnesium; integration of renal mechanisms for control of blood volume and extracellular fluid volume. In: Hall JE, ed. *Textbook of Medical Physiology*. Philadelphia: Saunders Medical; 2016:389-407.)

late DCT and collecting duct. In this segment, under normal conditions, potassium will be secreted by the principal cells. The amount of potassium secreted can be increased in situations where there is a high potassium intake, to a level that can even exceed the daily amount of potassium that is filtered by the glomeruli. Besides the principal cells, in this situation the type B intercalated cells are also capable of secreting potassium. In cases of low potassium intake, potassium excretion by the principal cells is reduced and a simultaneously increase in potassium reabsorption by the type A intercalated cells in the same segment will result in a drop of net urinary potassium excretion.[1,2]

However, this response of the kidney to long-term changes in potassium intake is sluggish. In adults given a diet that is consistently rich in potassium, it takes several days until maximum urinary potassium excretion is established. In contrast, in adults who are deprived of potassium, the minimum urinary loss of potassium will still be approximately 10 mmol/day and can thus cause hypokalemia in prolonged potassium deprivation.[1] This is a well-described complication in patients who are starved after abdominal surgery and are given intravenous fluids without addition of potassium.

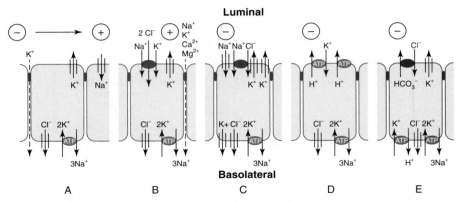

Fig. 3.3 Schematic view of potassium reabsorption and secretion on the cellular level in different parts of the nephron. (A) Proximal tubule. Potassium exits the lumen via paracellular solvent drag, caused by the reabsorption of sodium. It can subsequently enter the lumen by diffusion via potassium-specific transporters. (B) Thick ascending limb of the loop of Henle. Potassium is absorbed from the luminal fluid by Na+-K+-2Cl--cotransporter, which transports one sodium ion, one potassium ion, and two chloride ions into the cell. The favorable gradient for potassium reabsorption is maintained by rat outer medulla potassium (ROMK), that transports potassium back into the luminal fluid. The positive charge of the luminal fluid provides the driving gradient for the paracellular reabsorption of sodium, potassium, calcium, and magnesium. (C) Principal cells (late distal convoluting tubule, collecting duct). Potassium can be excreted on the basolateral side by a heterodimer of KCNJ10 and KCNJ16, which activates the NCC on the luminal side. In addition, sodium absorption via epithelial Na channel stimulates potassium excretion via ROMK, both of which are expressed on the luminal side. High tubular flow rate increases potassium excretion via luminal potassium "big" conductance (BK) channels. (D) Type A intercalated cell (late distal convoluting tubule, collecting duct). Acidification of urine is mainly performed by the luminal H+-ATPase. In hypokalemia, potassium reabsorption is mediated by the luminal H+-K+-ATPase. (E) Type B intercalated cell (late distal convoluting tubule, collecting duct). Bicarbonate is excreted while chloride is imported by the liminal transporter pendrin. In hyperkalemia, potassium can be excreted via potassium-specific channels in the luminal membrane.

Proximal Tubule

Approximately 65% of the filtered potassium is reabsorbed in the proximal tubule, which is similar to the absorption of sodium and water in this segment. This is a passive transport, occurring both by diffusion and by paracellular solvent drag. The latter is a result of active sodium transport, often coupled to the transport of other solutes like glucose or amino acids, causing paracellular hypertonicity. This local osmotic force is driving water reabsorption, with potassium being carried along in the reabsorbate. For this sodium transport to occur and also for bicarbonate to exit the cell on the basolateral side, an electrogenic gradient is needed. This gradient is provided by potassium movement across the respective membranes through potassium channels that have not yet been well defined. Because of the combined reabsorption of organic solutes and sodium in the early proximal tubule, the luminal fluid in this part will have a negative charge. In the late proximal tubule, there is a higher lumen to blood chloride concentration gradient, causing a diffusion potential in which chloride diffuses across the paracellular pathway into the blood, thus causing the luminal fluid to become positively charged. This will provide a driving force for passive paracellular potassium absorption (Fig. 3.3A).[1,13]

Thick Ascending Limb of the Loop of Henle

In this part of the nephron, approximately 20% to 25% of the total amount of filtered potassium is being absorbed by NKCC in the apical membrane. This furosemide-sensitive transporter translocates one sodium ion, one potassium ion, and two chloride ions into the cell. It is mainly driven by a low intracellular sodium concentration, which is maintained by the basolateral Na+,K+-ATPase. For NKCC to be able to transport potassium into the cell, it needs persistent availability of luminal potassium.

This is provided by the renal outer medullary potassium (ROMK) channel, which recycles the potassium back into the tubular lumen. In this way a lumen-positive transepithelial voltage is generated, which is driving the paracellular reabsorption of sodium, potassium, calcium, and magnesium (see Fig. 3.3B).[1]

Distal Nephron

Insights garnered from the rare inherited Gordon syndrome, or pseudohypoaldosteronism (PHA) type 2, have identified the DCT as critical for the regulation of potassium excretion.[14] Although potassium secretion itself is occurring in the collecting duct, it is greatly dependent on the delivery of sodium: sodium is passively transported across the luminal membrane of the principal cell along the electrochemical gradient via the epithelial Na channel (ENaC). This uptake of sodium creates lumen negativity, which enables potassium secretion via potassium channels. These include the high-conductance BK channels and the small-conductance secretory potassium (SK) channel, the latter consisting of ROMK (see Fig. 3.3C). Although potassium secretion via BK channels depends mainly on tubular flow rate, the potassium secretion via ROMK is more continuous and greatly depends on the electrochemical gradient provided by ENaC-medicated sodium reabsorption.[1] Thus, by regulating sodium delivery to the collecting duct, potassium secretion can be adjusted: with increased sodium reabsorption in the DCT, little sodium is delivered downstream and thus potassium secretion is impaired. Conversely, if sodium transport in DCT is inhibited, distal sodium delivery is increased, enabling potassium secretion. The fine-tuning of renal potassium excretion is regulated by several factors (Table 3.3). These obviously include aldosterone, which enhances sodium transport through ENaC. However, the observation that aldosterone apparently can enhance potassium secretion without sodium retention (and vice versa), created the so-called "aldosterone paradox."[15] A solution was provided by the discovery of mutations in WNK4 as a cause of Gordon syndrome.[16] This kinase regulates activity of Na-Cl-Cotransporter (NCC), the sodium transporter in the DCT, as well as paracellular chloride flux and ROMK, so that under conditions of sodium and potassium excess, sodium reabsorption can be decreased, while maintaining potassium secretion (electrically balanced by chloride efflux). Conversely, in conditions of sodium and potassium depletion, sodium reabsorption is enhanced (via NCC) without stimulating potassium secretion.

Given the critical importance of sodium reabsorption in the DCT to enable potassium secretion, it has been proposed that the basolateral potassium channel in the DCT may act as a "potassium sensor" in the kidney.[14] This channel, a heterotetramer of KCNJ10 and KCNJ16 subunits, gives rise to a 40-pS potassium channel, which recycles potassium out of the cell after it is pumped in by the basolateral Na+,K+-ATPase. In this way, it provides sufficient potassium for the pump to keep functioning and thus enables sodium reabsorption. To maintain electrochemical balance, the transport of potassium via this channel results in a simultaneous transport of chloride across the basolateral membrane, resulting in net transport of NaCl across the basolateral membrane. This causes a decrease in intracellular chloride levels, which stimulates WNK4 activity. This in turn mediates the phosphorylation and thereby activation of the luminal NCC, which imports sodium and chloride from the lumen into the cell. In case of high extracellular potassium concentrations, potassium recycling will be impaired, thereby reducing Na+,K+-ATPase and consequently NCC activity. This results in a higher sodium and water load being delivered more distally in the aldosterone-sensitive part of the distal nephron. The increased expression of ENaC, ROMK, and BK channels in the distal nephron will result in a net excretion of potassium, without changing the overall sodium absorption. In contrast, in case of low extracellular potassium, recycling is enhanced, thereby increasing Na+,K+-ATPase and NCC activity. The result is decreased sodium delivery to the aldosterone-sensitive distal nephron with consequently decreased potassium secretion (Fig. 3.4).[14]

Influencing Renal Potassium Excretion

Increased extracellular potassium levels (e.g., after dietary loading) induce a series of responses in the principal cells to increase net urinary potassium secretion besides

Table 3.3 FACTORS THAT CAN INFLUENCE RENAL POTASSIUM EXCRETION[1–3]

Factors That *Increase* Renal Potassium Excretion	Mechanism
***In Vivo* Factors**	
High extracellular potassium levels	Increased Na^+,K^+-ATPase activity leading to higher intracellular K^+ levels that favor excretion into luminal fluid; reduced NCC activity and increased aldosterone activity causing increased distal Na delivery, increased tubular flow rate, and increased expression of ENaC, ROMK, and BK channels
Volume expansion	Increased distal Na delivery and increased tubular flow rate
Aldosterone	Increased ENaC and increased Na^+,K^+-ATPase activity
Alkalosis	Increased Na reabsorption and increased K-channel activity
Chronic acidosis	Increased distal Na delivery and increased tubular flow rate
Medications	
Osmotic, loop and thiazide diuretics, CA inhibitors	Increased distal Na delivery and increased tubular flow rate
Beta-2 agonists	Increased Na^+,K^+-ATPase activity

Factors That *Decrease* Renal Potassium Excretion	Mechanism
***In Vivo* Factors**	
Low extracellular potassium levels	Decreased Na^+,K^+-ATPase activity diminishes the K^+ gradient that favors K^+ excretion into luminal fluid; increased NCC activity and decreased aldosterone activity causing decreased distal Na delivery, decreased tubular flow rate, and decreased expression of ENaC, ROMK, and BK channels
Volume depletion	Decreased distal Na delivery and decreased tubular flow rate
Acute acidosis	Decreased Na^+,K^+-ATPase and ROMK activity
Medications	
Amiloride, triamterene, trimethoprim, pentamidine	Inhibition of ENaC, decreasing electrochemical gradient
Digoxin	Decreased Na^+,K^+-ATPase activity
Beta blockers	Decreased Na^+,K^+-ATPase activity and decreased renin release
NSAIDs	Decreased renin secretion; decreased distal Na delivery and decreased tubular flow rate
Calcineurin inhibitors	Decreased Na^+,K^+-ATPase activity; decreased number of mineralocorticosteroid receptors; increased NCC activity
Heparins, azole antifungals	Blocking adrenal aldosterone synthesis
ACE inhibitors, ARBs	Blocking aldosterone secretion
Spironolactone, eplerenone	Blocking aldosterone receptor

ACE, Angiotensin converting enzyme; *ARB*, angiotensin II receptor blockers; *BK channel*, high conductance "big" potassium channel; *CA*, carbonic anhydrase; *NCC*, sodium-chloride cotransporter; *NSAIDs*, nonsteroidal antiinflammatory drugs; *ROMK*, renal outer medullary potassium channel.

the previously described changes in NCC expression. A more extensive list of factors that can influence renal potassium excretion is provided in Table 3.3. First, increased activity of Na^+,K^+-ATPase leads to an increase in the electrochemical gradient over the luminal membrane, thus favoring potassium excretion. At the same time the increased potassium levels result in aldosterone secretion. Aldosterone promotes sodium reabsorption by further increasing the activity of the basolateral Na^+,K^+-ATPase and by increasing expression of the luminal ENaC channels. This enhanced sodium reabsorption increases the electrochemical gradient over the luminal membrane, favoring potassium excretion into the luminal fluid. Furthermore, the activity of protein tyrosine kinase reduces after potassium loading. Protein tyrosine kinase causes phosphorylation of ROMK channels. Phosphorylation promotes endocytosis of the channel, thus reducing its expression in the luminal membrane and thereby inhibiting the secretion of potassium into the tubular fluid. The expression of ROMK

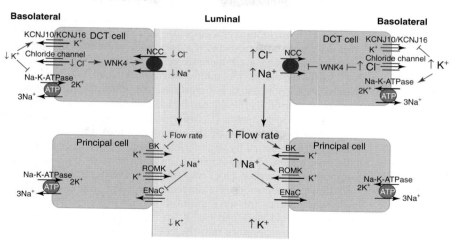

Fig. 3.4 WNK4 signaling in response to extracellular potassium levels. Signaling of WNK4 in response to hypokalemia (depicted on the left). Low extracellular potassium levels decrease Na+,K+-ATPase, while enhancing potassium recycling via the KCNJ10/KCNJ16 heterotetramer in distal convoluted tubule (*DCT*) cells. Potassium leaves the cell together with chloride, resulting in low intracellular chloride levels which in turn activate WNK4. The latter activates NCC, causing increased sodium and chloride uptake from the lumen. This results in low intraluminal sodium levels and a low tubular fluid flow rate at the site of the principal cells. The first diminishes activity of epithelial Na channel (*ENaC*) (resulting in decreased sodium reabsorption) and rat outer medulla potassium (*ROMK*) (resulting in reduced potassium excretion). The latter causes reduced expression of potassium "big" conductance (*BK*) channels, thus further reducing potassium excretion. The opposite occurs in the case of hyperkalemia (depicted on the right).

channels in the luminal membrane increases within hours after potassium loading; the expression of BK channels takes days to increase and is the result of a chronic high potassium load.[1,2]

Moreover, potassium loading results in a decreased reabsorption of sodium and water in the proximal tubule and loop of Henle. This causes increased sodium delivery to the distal nephron. As a result, sodium uptake into the principal cells via ENaC is enhanced, which creates the electrochemical driving force for potassium excretion via ROMK and BK channels, as described previously. In addition, the increased tubular flow due to increased water delivery to the distal nephron further stimulates potassium secretion. This occurs via increased ENaC activity (increasing the time that the channel is in an open state), by maintaining an electrochemical gradient favorable for potassium excretion, by immediately diluting the secreted potassium with tubular fluid that is low in potassium, and by inducing a range of biochemical signals leading to increased intracellular calcium levels which in turn result in activation of the luminal BK channels. A similar pattern of increased kaliuresis due to increased distal sodium loading and tubular flow rate is seen after extracellular fluid expansion and after the administration of carbonic anhydrase inhibitors or osmotic, loop, or thiazide diuretics. In contrast, the potassium-sparing diuretics amiloride and triamterene, as well as trimethoprim and pentamidine, inhibit ENaC, thus decreasing the electrochemical driving force for potassium excretion.[1]

An acute onset of acidosis reduces renal potassium secretion. This is caused by the fact that excess hydrogen ions inhibit the function of Na+,K+-ATPase, thereby diminishing intracellular potassium levels and thus reducing the electrochemical gradient for potassium diffusion from the intracellular space into the lumen. It also reduces the activity of ROMK in the luminal membrane, thus further inhibiting potassium efflux from the cell into the lumen. In contrast, prolonged acidosis is more complex. It promotes aldosterone release and inhibits sodium and water reabsorption in the proximal tubule. Thereby caused increased delivery of sodium to the distal nephron in combination with increased tubular flow rate will increase potassium excretion. The latter effect is stronger than the inhibitory effect of potassium ions on Na^+,K^+-ATPase, thus resulting in a net increase in urinary potassium loss. Alkalosis increases both sodium reabsorption, thereby increasing the electrochemical gradient for potassium secretion, and it increases the time that the luminal potassium channels are open, causing a net increase of potassium excretion.[1,2]

Aldosterone is the main mineralocorticosteroid, and it is a key regulator of sodium and potassium homeostasis, circulating volume status, and thereby blood pressure control. Its release can be induced either by increased extracellular potassium levels or by angiotensin II, which is produced in response to intravascular volume depletion by activation of the renin-angiotensin-aldosterone system (RAAS). The latter can be blocked by angiotensin converting enzyme (ACE) inhibitors (diminishing the conversion of angiotensin I into angiotensin II) and AII receptor blockers or angiotensin receptor blockers (ARBs) (binding to angiotensin I receptors). After binding to its receptor, the aldosterone–receptor complex translocates into the nucleus, where it induces the translation of several proteins. The net result is an increased expression of ENaC and Na^+,K^+-ATPase, both by stimulating the translocation of preexistent transporters into the cell membrane and by promoting the synthesis of new transport proteins. This can be blocked by the potassium-sparing diuretics spironolactone and eplerenone, which bind to the aldosterone receptor, thus blocking it from binding to aldosterone.[1]

Developmental Physiology

Potassium During Somatic Growth

Potassium is needed for somatic growth. Adults maintain a zero potassium balance, whereas in young children a positive potassium balance is needed. This is reflected by higher serum potassium levels in neonates. Potassium is known to be actively transported from mother to fetus during pregnancy.[1] At birth, cord potassium levels can be as high as 12.0 mmol/L in healthy newborns. This is followed by a rapid decline in the first hour of life and a more slowly decrease in serum potassium levels thereafter. These changes are due to shifts in the internal potassium balance because in the same period the potassium content of red blood cells increases.[17] In premature babies, postnatal potassium levels can be even higher and the decline is more slowly. Moreover, some children show a rise in serum potassium levels in the first 24 to 36 hours of postnatal life, which was mainly seen in babies with a birth weight less than 1500 g.[18] After the initial postnatal period, infants and young children until the age of 5 years still have slightly higher serum potassium levels compared with adults and older children to enable rapid growth in this period. After the age of 5 years, normal levels of potassium are similar to those of adults.[19] Although serum potassium levels are higher in younger children, the relative potassium content in children and adults is fairly stable. Total body potassium rapidly increases during the first trimester of pregnancy, but thereafter it remains approximately 40 to 45 mmol/kg throughout life.[20] Therefore the high potassium requirement that is seen in newborns and infants to maintain growth is mainly a reflection of their rapidly increasing cellular mass.

Changes in Internal Potassium Balance

The regulation of the internal potassium balance in newborns is influenced by the activity and expression of several potassium transporters, channels, and signal transduction pathways which are subjected to changes during development. In premature babies born before 28 weeks of gestation and with a birth weight less than 1000 g, a condition called nonoliguric hyperkalemia can be observed. This is defined by serum potassium levels greater than 7.0 mmol/L with a urine output greater than 1 mL/kg per hour in the absence of a high potassium intake. This phenomenon is attributed to decreased Na^+,K^+-ATPase activity, thus hampering the intracellular translocation of excess potassium in the intracellular space, in combination with a decreased capacity of the kidney to secrete potassium. It generally improves after 72 hours and can be prevented by prenatal maternal administration of steroids, which increases Na^+,K^+-ATPase activity.[1]

Changes in External Potassium Balance

Although the adult gut has a higher rate of potassium excretion than absorption, in the neonatal gut it is the other way around and in general there will be a net absorption of potassium. This is due to a relatively higher activity of apical K^+-ATPase, whereas there is decreased activity of the basolateral potassium transporters that are needed for potassium secretion.[21]

Newborns have a low renal excretion of potassium, even when corrected for GFR. This is despite higher aldosterone levels in premature infants and term newborns compared with healthy adults, indicating a relative aldosterone insensitivity. This cannot be explained by the density of aldosterone binding sites, receptor affinity, and the degree of nuclear binding of aldosterone, because these have been found to be unaffected by maturation in animal studies.[1]

After glomerular filtration, the potassium reabsorption in the proximal tubule of neonates has been found to be more or less similar in animal studies (50% to 60%) compared with healthy adults (65%). In contrast, the reabsorption of potassium in the thick ascending loop of the loop of Henle is lower in neonates compared with adults. Of the total filtered potassium load, approximately 35% reaches the DCT in neonates, compared with only 10% in adults. Animal studies performed in rats have shown a decreased expression of NKCC2 until day 8 of life and a decreased activity of Na^+,K^+-ATPase of only 20% of the adult activity. These data would suggest limited efficacy of loop diuretics in newborns because these inhibit the function of NKCC2. Yet in human neonates, loop diuretics have been shown to cause an adequate natriuretic response and are commonly used to increase fluid removal, arguing against impaired loop function in neonates. However, the most important differences in renal potassium excretion between neonates and adults lie in the decreased secretory capacity of principal cells. Studies on rabbits have shown no measurable potassium secretion up to the third week of life, after which secretion increases towards levels similar to adult secretion at the age of 6 weeks. This is mainly due to the absence of ROMK channels, combined with a lower activity of Na^+,K^+-ATPase. Studies again performed in rabbits have shown a progressive increase in ROMK channels only after the second week of life. Moreover, there is no effect of increased tubular flow rate on potassium secretion in newborn kidneys. Rabbit studies have shown that flow-stimulated potassium secretion only develops after 5 weeks of life, which is in line with the finding that the expression of BK channels can be first demonstrated only after 4 to 5 weeks of life. This delayed expression of BK channels fits with the clinical observation that patients with Bartter syndrome type 2 (due to mutations in ROMK) can initially present with hyperkalemia and only later develop hypokalemia, when other potassium channels can mediate potassium secretion. The potassium reabsorption in type A intercalated cells is normal in newborn animal studies, with activity of the H^+-K^+-ATPase that is equivalent to adults. Although this transporter usually only reabsorbs potassium in case of hypokalemia, the high potassium content in the luminal fluid of newborns may facilitate such increased activity.[1,22–24]

Clinical Relevance

Hyperkalemia

Pseudohyperkalemia

Elevated potassium levels *in vitro* in the absence of actual increased potassium levels in the patient is called spurious hyperkalemia or pseudohyperkalemia. It is most often caused by hemolysis of red blood cells after obtaining a whole blood sample. In small children, this can be due to small needle size, the use of a tourniquet, or squeezing of the limb from which the blood was drawn. It can also be caused by delayed processing of the sample and by tumor lysis in children with leukemia after initiation of treatment, causing lysis of the diseased white blood cells after collection. A repeat blood sample that is immediately processed (either by the laboratory or more rapidly by a blood gas analyzer) often confirms normokalemia.[1]

Disorders of Internal Potassium Balance

Disorders that promote a shift of potassium from the intracellular to the extracellular space include metabolic acidosis, diabetes mellitus, and cell lysis, the latter including hemolytic disorders, tumor lysis syndrome, and rhabdomyolysis. A more extensive list of factors and medications that can cause hyperkalemia can be found in Tables 3.1 and 3.3. In all these cases, treatment of hyperkalemia should be aimed at treating the underlying condition or withdrawal of causative agent.[1]

As described previously, very premature infants born less than 28 weeks of gestation or with a birth weight of less than 1000 g can develop nonoliguric hyperkalemia in the first 24 to 72 hours after birth, caused by the decreased movement of potassium from the extracellular into the intracellular space at the time when GFR is physiologically low. It can be treated by promoting the intracellular uptake of potassium by the administration of insulin or β-2 agonists, but the potassium will decrease anyway when the physiologic diuresis and natriuresis increase. In this phase, children can even become hypokalemic to a degree that warrants the administration of potassium supplements.[1]

Disorder of External Potassium Balance

In persons with a normal renal function, even an excessive enteral intake of potassium will not cause hyperkalemia because of rapid translocation of potassium from the extracellular to the intracellular space. When given as an intravenous bolus, the feedforward mechanism to prevent hyperkalemia is circumvented and transient higher potassium levels can occur.[1,2]

However, the most common cause of hyperkalemia is a decreased GFR. When renal function becomes impaired, the body loses its most important mechanism to maintain a stable potassium balance. Initially the potassium secretion in principal and type B intercalated cells will increase, combined with increased potassium excretion in the colon.[1,2,7] When the renal function deteriorates further, therapeutic measures will be needed to prevent hyperkalemia. These can include decreasing the dietary potassium load, correcting metabolic acidosis by administering sodium bicarbonate, and prescribing potassium binders to prevent dietary potassium from being absorbed from the gastrointestinal tract. The most commonly used potassium binders are nonspecific polymeric exchange resins (sodium or calcium polystyrene sulfonate, also called resonium). More recently sodium zirconium cyclosilicate was introduced, which is a highly sensitive potassium binder that traps potassium in exchange for sodium or hydrogen ions.[25] In acute symptomatic hyperkalemia, extracellular potassium can be lowered by shifting it into the intracellular compartment. The administration of β-2 agonists (e.g., salbutamol) and/or the combined infusion of glucose and insulin can help to temporarily reduce serum potassium, but high volumes of glucose solution need to be infused, which is often not feasible in the patient with a decreased urine output. Obviously, these are also only temporary measures because they do not promote potassium excretion. Calcium gluconate can be given as an intravenous bolus to stabilize the membrane potential of cardiomyocytes and to prevent hyperkalemia induced arrhythmia, but it does not lower serum potassium levels.

In children with severe dehydration, hyperkalemia can be caused by a combination of prerenal failure and decreased sodium delivery to the distal nephron. Treatment should be focused on volume expansion first.[1]

Although very rare, some endocrine and tubular disorders can cause hyperkalemia, often with a normal renal function. In the salt-wasting form of congenital adrenal hyperplasia and in Addison disease, the lack of aldosterone or cortisol production by the adrenals is treated by the administration of a glucocorticoid (e.g., prednisolone), a mineralocorticoid (e.g., fludrocortisone), and sodium supplements. A similar phenotype of adrenal insufficiency can be seen in patients after rapid weaning of steroid treatment that has been administered for more than 2 weeks. In type 1 PHA, there is a dysfunction of ENaC (autosomal recessive variant) or the mineralocorticoid receptor (autosomal dominant variant), in which sodium supplementation is the cornerstone of therapy. Type 2 PHA (also called familial hyperkalemia and hypertension [FHHt] or Gordon syndrome; see earlier) is caused by mutations in genes that result in a gain of function of the NCC transporter in DCT, causing hyperkalemia and hypertension, both of which respond well to thiazide diuretics. The administration of calcineurin inhibitors can provoke a clinical similar picture.[26] Type 3 PHA is a transient phenomenon which can be attributed to other pathologies, such as obstructive uropathies and pyelonephritis.[1]

To assess whether there is an adequate renal response to hyperkalemia, the transtubular potassium gradient (TTKG) can be calculated using the formula $(U_K/S_K)/(U_{Osm} \times S_{Osm})$. U and S indicate urine and serum, respectively; K and Osm indicating potassium concentration and osmolality, respectively. The TTKG serves as an indirect measure for the renal response to mineralocorticoids, this being mainly aldosterone. In hyperkalemia a TTKG less than 4 is considered to be inappropriately low because it indicates a low mineralocorticoid activity and thus a low renal potassium secretion. In contrast, a high TTKG (>13) indicates high mineralocorticoid activity and increased renal potassium secretion, thus suggesting a high potassium intake to be causing the hyperkalemia.[1,27] However, it must be stated that the main action of aldosterone is to respond to fluid shifts and that this overrides its response to a shift in potassium. Therefore, in case of hypovolemia, one would expect the TTKG to be high and, in fluid overload, one would expect the TTKG to be low, regardless of serum potassium levels.

Hypokalemia

Disorders of Internal Potassium Balance

Disorders that promote a shift of potassium from the extracellular into the intracellular space include metabolic alkalosis and the administration of insulin in patients with hyperglycemia. A more extensive list of factors and medications that can cause hypokalemia can be found in Tables 3.1 and 3.3. In these cases, treatment of hypokalemia should be focused on treating the underlying condition or withdrawal of the causative agent, whenever possible.[1]

Disorders of External Potassium Balance

Hypokalemia is often seen in patients who have fasted for a prolonged period of time (mostly after abdominal surgery) while being administered intravenous fluids without potassium. Although the kidney will try to reabsorb potassium as much as possible, there will be ongoing urinary losses of potassium even in prolonged potassium deprivation. Hypokalemia in these patients can be prevented by the addition of potassium to intravenous fluids.[1]

Gastrointestinal disorders are another well-known cause for hypokalemia (see Table 3.2). In diarrhea and vomiting a significant amount of potassium is lost in the high volumes of stool and vomit. These losses are aggravated by increased intestinal BK channel expression in secretory diarrhea, which further increases the fecal potassium loss. In ulcerative colitis an increased colonic BK channel expression is found, which promotes fecal potassium excretion. The long-term use of laxatives also promotes fecal potassium wasting. This effect is most pronounced when using diphenolic laxatives (e.g., phenolphthalein and bisacodyl) and anthroquinones (e.g., senna glycosides and danthron), which result in a cyclic adenosine monophosphate (cAMP)-mediated increase of colonic BK channel expression.[7]

Several rare hormonal and tubular disorders can cause hypokalemia. Excess of mineralocorticoids can be found in the salt-retaining form of congenital adrenal hyperplasia (in which there is increased production of aldosterone by the adrenal glands), in Cushing syndrome (in which there is increased production of cortisol by the adrenal glands), and in renovascular hypertension (in which increased renin production leads to high aldosterone levels). Proximal tubular dysfunction (also called renal Fanconi syndrome) can be congenital (e.g., cystinosis) or acquired (e.g., after administration of chemotherapy or valproate). It is defined by increased urinary loss of water and several small solutes, including sodium, potassium, phosphate, bicarbonate, glucose, and amino acids. Hypokalemia in renal Fanconi syndrome is likely due to a combination of impaired proximal reabsorption and increased distal secretion due to secondary hyperaldosteronism. Hypokalemia from secondary hyperaldosteronism is typical also for the salt-wasting disorders affecting the thick ascending limb of Henle (TAL) and the DCT. Mutations in transporters in TAL give rise to different subtypes of Bartter syndrome, characterized by hypokalemic, hypochloremic metabolic alkalosis with hypomagnesemia, and hypercalciuria causing nephrocalcinosis (type 1: NKCC2, luminal potassium sodium-potassium-chloride cotransporter; type 2: ROMK, luminal potassium transporter; type 3: ClC-Kb, basolateral chloride transporter; type 4: Barttin, activating subunit of ClC-Kb). The Bartter phenotype can be mimicked by the administration of loop diuretics, which inhibit NKCC2. In the DCT, mutations in the luminal NCC or basolateral KCNJ10 cause Gitelman and EAST (also called SeSAME) syndrome, respectively, the renal phenotype of which is characterized by hypokalemic, hypochloremic metabolic alkalosis with hypomagnesemia, and hypocalciuria. The polyuria in these conditions is less severe compared with children with renal Fanconi syndrome or Bartter syndrome. The renal phenotype can be mimicked by the administration of thiazide diuretics, which inhibit NCC. In the collecting duct, mutations in the type A intercalated cells that disturb the function of the luminal H-ATPase (autosomal recessive variants) or the intracellular anion exchanger 1 (autosomal dominant variant) cause distal renal tubular acidosis, which is characterized by metabolic acidosis with high urinary pH, hypokalemia, and hypercalciuria causing nephrocalcinosis.[1]

In all these disorders, hypokalemic alkalosis is a secondary phenomenon, mediated by increased aldosterone levels in the context of salt wasting. However, hypokalemic alkalosis can also be associated with primary increased ENaC activity, which is clinically characterized by the additional symptom of hypertension. It can be due to aldosterone excess, which can be either primary (e.g., Conn syndrome) or secondary (e.g., glucocorticoid remediable hyperaldosteronism, where aldosterone production is driven by adrenocorticotropic hormone [ACTH]), or to pathologic activation by glucocorticoids (apparent mineralocorticoid excess [AME], in which cortisol cannot be inactivated to cortisone), or to direct activation of ENaC (e.g., Liddle syndrome). Treatment typically involves ENaC blockers, such as amiloride or triamterene and/or blockers of the mineralocorticoid receptor, such as spironolactone or eplerenone, depending on the underlying etiology. In addition, if possible, treatment should focus on the underlying disease.[1] Potassium supplements are often prescribed, but especially in renal Fanconi syndrome and Bartter syndrome normokalemia is rarely achieved. The most important complications of hypokalemia include arrhythmia, muscle weakness, and paralysis. However, children with tubular disorders can be asymptomatic with chronically lower potassium levels. There is no generally accepted safe lower limit for potassium concentration, but in an expert consensus paper on Gitelman syndrome a potassium level of 3.0 mmol/L was considered a reasonable target, although this may be not achievable in all patients.[28] Of note, the administration of high amounts of potassium via the enteral route is irritating to the gastrointestinal tract and can induce vomiting and/or diarrhea, thus worsening hypokalemia. In these cases, lower doses of potassium supplements may actually improve serum potassium levels.

As is the case in hyperkalemia, the TTKG can be used to assess distal potassium secretion independent from glomerular filtration. A low TTKG of less than 4 indicates low mineralocorticoid activity and renal potassium conservation, thus suggesting a decreased intake and/or increased extrarenal (most often gastrointestinal) losses to be causing the hypokalemia.[1,27] Again it must be stated that the patient's fluid status should be taken into account when interpreting the TTKG, as explained previously. When a renal disorder is suspected to be causing hypokalemia, often the fractional excretion of potassium is calculated from paired serum and urine measurement of potassium and creatinine. The term fractional excretion is actually not physiologically appropriate because in the healthy kidney the net urinary potassium excretion depends mainly on potassium secretion by the principal cells and not on the fraction of potassium that is reabsorbed from the glomerular filtrate. However, for practical purposes, the term is still in use. It is calculated using the formula $(U_K \times S_{cr})/(S_K \times U_{cr})$. U and S indicate urine and serum, respectively, and K and cr indicate potassium and creatinine concentration, respectively. A fractional excretion of potassium greater than 15% is considered consistent with renal potassium wasting.[29]

Conclusions

- Only approximately 2% of total body potassium is in the extracellular fluid, where it is accessible to routine clinical investigations.
- Disorders of potassium can be "internal" due to a shift between the extracellular and intracellular compartment or "external" due to an imbalance between potassium intake and output.
- The secretion of potassium in the collecting duct is linked to sodium reabsorption and proton secretion, creating the distinctive biochemical pattern of hypokalemic, alkalosis with increased sodium reabsorption, and vice versa. Thus treatment of disorders of potassium often requires addressing an underlying disorder.

REFERENCES

1. Satlin LM, Bockenhauer D. Physiology of the developing kidney: potassium homeostasis and its disorder. In: Avner ED, Harmon WE, Niaudet P, et al, eds. *Pediatric Nephrology*. Berlin Heidelberg: Springer-Verlag; 2016:219–246.
2. Hall JE. Renal regulation of potassium, calcium, phosphate, and magnesium; integration of renal mechanisms for control of blood volume and extracellular fluid volume. In: Hall JE, ed. *Textbook of Medical Physiology*. Philadelphia: Saunders Medical; 2016:389–407.
3. Gumz ML, Rabinowitz L, Wingo CS. An Integrated View of Potassium Homeostasis. *N Engl J Med*. 2015;373:60–72.
4. Sahni V, Gmurzcyk A, Rosa RM. Extrarenal potassium metabolism. In: Alpern RJ, Caplan MJ, Moe OW, eds. *Seldin en Giebsch's the Kidney—Physiology and Pathophysiology*. London: Elsevier Academic Press; 2013:1629–1658.
5. Burnell JM, Scribner BH, Uyeno BT, Villamil MF. The effect in humans of extracellular pH change on the relationship between serum potassium concentration and intracellular potassium. *J Clin Invest*. 1956;35:935–939.
6. Stephens JW. Our present knowledge of potassium in physiological and pathological processes. *Can Med Assoc J*. 1952;66:19–32.
7. Sandle GI, Hunter M. Apical potassium (BK) channels and enhanced potassium secretion in human colon. *QJM*. 2010;103:85–89.
8. Schwartz IL, Thaysen JH. Excretion of sodium and potassium in human sweat. *J Clin Invest*. 1956;35:114–120.
9. Rabelink TJ, Koomans HA, Hene RJ, Dorhout Mees EJ. Early and late adjustment to potassium loading in humans. *Kidney Int*. 1990;38:942–947.
10. Oh KS, Oh YT, Kim SW, et al. Gut sensing of dietary K(+) intake increases renal K(+)excretion. *Am J Physiol Regul Integr Comp Physiol*. 2011;301:R421–R429.
11. Youn JH. Gut sensing of potassium intake and its role in potassium homeostasis. *Semin Nephrol*. 2013;33:248–256.
12. Preston RA, Afshartous D, Rodco R, et al. Evidence for a gastrointestinal-renal kaliuretic signaling axis in humans. *Kidney Int*. 2015;88:1383–1391.
13. Rector FC Jr. Sodium, bicarbonate, and chloride absorption by the proximal tubule. *Am J Physiol*. 1983;244:F461–F471.
14. Wang WH. Basolateral Kir4.1 activity in the distal convoluted tubule regulates K secretion by determining NaCl cotransporter activity. *Curr Opin Nephrol Hypertens*. 2016;25:429–435.
15. Arroyo JP, Ronzaud C, Lagnaz D, et al. Aldosterone paradox: differential regulation of ion transport in distal nephron. *Physiology (Bethesda)*. 2011;26:115–123.
16. Wilson FH, Disse-Nicodeme S, Choate KA, et al. Human hypertension caused by mutations in WNK kinases. *Science*. 2001;293:1107–1112.
17. Acharya PT, Payne WW. Blood Chemistry of Normal Full-Term Infants in the First 48 Hours of Life. *Arch Dis Child*. 1965;40:430–435.
18. Yu J, Payne WW, Ifekwunigwe A, Stevens J. Biochemical status of healthy premature infants in the first 48 hours of life. *Arch Dis Child*. 1965;40:516–525.
19. Loh TP, Metz MP. Trends and physiology of common serum biochemistries in children aged 0-18 years. *Pathology*. 2015;47:452–461.
20. Forbes GB. Chemical growth in man. *Pediatrics*. 1952;9:58–68.
21. Aizman RI, Celsi G, Grahnquist L, et al. Ontogeny of K+ transport in rat distal colon. *Am J Physiol*. 1996;271:G268–G274.
22. Schmitt R, Ellison DH, Farman N, et al. Developmental expression of sodium entry pathways in rat nephron. *Am J Physiol*. 1999;276:F367–F381.
23. Satlin LM, Palmer LG. Apical K+ conductance in maturing rabbit principal cell. *Am J Physiol*. 1997;272:F397–F404.
24. Woda CB, Miyawaki N, Ramalakshmi S, et al. Ontogeny of flow-stimulated potassium secretion in rabbit cortical collecting duct: functional and molecular aspects. *Am J Physiol Renal Physiol*. 2003;285:F629–F639.
25. Packham DK, Rasmussen HS, Lavin PT, et al. Sodium zirconium cyclosilicate in hyperkalemia. *N Engl J Med*. 2015;372:222–231.

26. Hoorn EJ, Walsh SB, McCormick JA, et al. The calcineurin inhibitor tacrolimus activates the renal sodium chloride cotransporter to cause hypertension. *Nat Med*. 2011;17:1304–1309.
27. Rodriguez-Soriano J, Ubetagoyena M, Vallo A. Transtubular potassium concentration gradient: a useful test to estimate renal aldosterone bio-activity in infants and children. *Pediatr Nephrol*. 1990;4:105–110.
28. Blanchard A, Bockenhauer D, Bolignano D, et al. Gitelman syndrome: consensus and guidance from a Kidney Disease: Improving Global Outcomes (KDIGO) Controversies Conference. *Kidney Int*. 2017;91:24–33.
29. Elisaf M, Siamopoulos KC. Fractional excretion of potassium in normal subjects and in patients with hypokalaemia. *Postgrad Med J*. 1995;71:211–212.

CHAPTER 4

Renal Aspects of Sodium Metabolism in the Fetus and Neonate

Raymond Quigley, MD

The transition from a growing fetus to a newborn infant requires many changes in fluid and electrolyte homeostasis. During gestation, the placenta controls this balance, but once the fetus is born, the kidneys will perform the task of regulating the excretion of water, electrolytes, and solutes, as well as nitrogenous waste products. This chapter will briefly review the factors that regulate the placental exchange of fluid and sodium, as well as the renal developmental changes that occur throughout the growth of the fetus and the subsequent adaptation to life outside of the womb, with a focus on the postnatal development of renal tubular transport.

Fluid Compartments

The total body water content of the adult human is approximately 60% of its weight and is broadly divided into the intracellular fluid (ICF) and extracellular fluid (ECF) compartments. The proportion of the total body water in these two main compartments changes dramatically throughout fetal life and in the first year of postnatal life.[1] In early fetal life the ECF is twice the size of the ICF, whereas in the adult the ICF is twice that of the ECF. The shift in the distribution of body water is primarily due to a decrease in the ECF after the fetus is born.

Placenta and Amniotic Fluid

During gestation, the fetus is dependent on the placenta to provide its nutrition, which includes the water and sodium necessary for amniotic fluid formation in the early part of gestation.[2] The placenta has both active and passive mechanisms for the transfer of sodium from the mother to the fetus with water following its osmotic gradient. This includes several isoforms of water channels (aquaporins [AQPs]), as well as sodium channels and sodium hydrogen exchangers (NHEs).[3–7] The driving force for the movement of sodium is provided by the sodium-potassium ATPase.[7]

The average amount of amniotic fluid in the human is approximately 40 mL at 11 weeks of gestation and increases to a maximum of approximately 920 mL at term.[8–10] During the first half of gestation, this fluid comes primarily from the placenta and has an osmolality that is isotonic to the fetus. However, as the fetal kidneys begin to produce urine, the osmolality of the amniotic fluid decreases to approximately 250 to 260 mOsm/L at term.[11]

In addition to the sodium and fluid provided to the fetus, the placenta also provides all of the nutrition necessary for fetal growth. In particular, there are specific transporters for amino acids in the placenta that are necessary for protein synthesis.[2,12,13] Because of the diversity of amino acids, there are several classes of amino acid transporters and they all appear to be present in the placenta.[13–15] The importance of these transporters is emphasized by the fact that their expression is quite diminished in models of fetal growth retardation.[16]

After the fetal kidneys begin making urine in the 10th week of gestation, the bulk of the amniotic fluid comprises urine from the fetus (Fig. 4.1).[10,17] Thus the amount of amniotic fluid in the second half of gestation is determined by the urine output. Conditions in the fetus that result in a high urine output lead to polyhydramnios, whereas conditions that limit the urine output will result in oligohydramnios.[18]

One of the kidney diseases that results in polyhydramnios is Bartter syndrome, which is a genetic defect in the thick ascending limb (TAL) of Henle (discussed later). Although most forms of Bartter syndrome are chronic and lifelong, a transient form of Bartter syndrome has been described that is caused by mutations in the gene: melanoma-associated antigen D2 (MAGED-D2) that is found on the X chromosome.[19,20] A number of patients had features of Bartter syndrome that improved with age; however, mutations were also found in a number of fetuses that were associated with polyhydramnios and fetal death. It is not clear how this gene defect affects the TAL

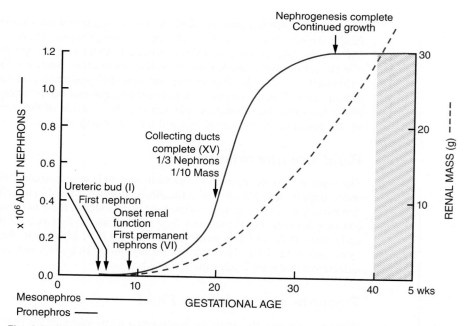

Fig. 4.1   Development of the kidneys. Renal function and urine production begins during the 10th week of gestation. (Reproduced with permission from Harrison MR, Golbus MS, Filly RA, et al. Management of the fetus with congenital hydronephrosis. *J Pediatr Surg.* 1982;17(6): 728-742.)

and why it is transient in nature.[20] These findings emphasize the role of the kidney and urine output in the formation of the amniotic fluid.

Decreased fetal renal function and urine output is associated with oligohydramnios. Severe forms of this sequence are known as Potter sequence and have characteristic facies, as well as clubfeet.[21,22] The critical issue in these patients is that the lack of amniotic fluid leads to pulmonary hypoplasia, and many of these infants die from respiratory failure.[18,23] These infants will generally not survive due to their respiratory failure.

Developmental Changes in Renal Function and Tubular Transport

As seen in Fig. 4.1, the fetal kidney begins to function around the 10th to 11th week of gestation. At term, the kidney has developed its full complement of glomeruli that it will have as an adult. However, the function of the neonatal kidney continues to undergo development in terms of its ability to filter the blood (glomerular filtration rate [GFR]) and modify the filtered fluid (tubular function).

The GFR of a term neonate is only approximately 30% of the normal adult rate when factored for body surface area.[24] The GFR increases during the first 12 to 18 months of life when the GFR is approximately the same as the adult when factored for body surface area. The glomerular ultrafiltrate is then modified by the renal tubules to eventually form the final urine. The tubules reabsorb a number of solutes, including sodium, bicarbonate, glucose, and amino acids, and also secrete a number of solutes, including potassium, acid, and ammonium. The excretion rate of the primary nitrogenous waste product, urea, is determined primarily by the filtration rate, which obligates a high rate of filtration to excrete urea and remain in nitrogen balance. This high filtration rate then obligates the renal tubules to reabsorb a large amount of sodium and fluid to remain in fluid balance.

The coordination between the GFR and tubule reabsorption rate is termed "glomerular tubular balance."[25] As will be discussed later, the neonatal tubules have much lower transport rates than the adult renal tubules. Because the developing neonate has a low GFR, the developing renal tubular reabsorption capacity is still able to meet the demand of the GFR. Thus the developing neonate is able to maintain glomerular tubular balance.[26,27]

Renal Tubular Sodium Transport

The mature adult kidneys filter approximately 150 L of blood per day so that they can excrete nitrogenous waste in the form of urea. The renal tubules then reabsorb approximately 99% of the filtered load of fluid and solutes so that the final urine volume is on the order of 1 to 2 L per day. The key regulator of the reabsorbed fluid volume is sodium transport by the renal tubules.

Although sodium reabsorption occurs via a number of different transporters throughout the nephron, all of the active transport of sodium in the renal tubules is dependent on the sodium-potassium ATPase. This enzyme is located on the basolateral membrane of the cells throughout the nephron and uses energy from adenosine triphosphate (ATP) to maintain a low intracellular sodium concentration. There is an inwardly directed electrochemical gradient for sodium to enter the cell through the luminal membrane. The entry of sodium into the cell is driven by this low intracellular sodium concentration, and the energy of this electrochemical gradient can also be linked to other solutes for transport. As will be seen, the mechanism for entry of sodium through the luminal membrane varies throughout the different segments of the nephron.

Proximal Tubule Sodium Transport

In the proximal tubule the key transporter for luminal sodium entry into the cell is the sodium-hydrogen exchanger (Fig. 4.2).[28] The primary isoform of this transporter

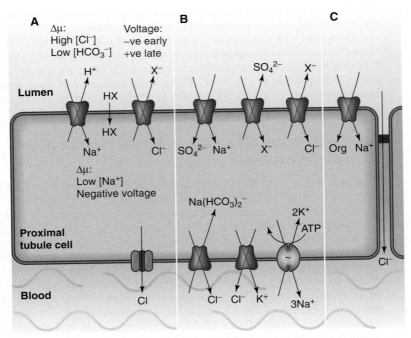

Fig. 4.2 Proximal tubule cell. The Na^+,K^+-ATPase on the basolateral membrane maintains a low intracellular sodium concentration. This sodium gradient is then used to secrete protons for the reabsorption of bicarbonate, as well as the reabsorption of organic solutes such as glucose and amino acids. X^- in the figure is an anion that is exchanged with the reabsorption of Cl^-. Thus, if X^- is OH^-, the parallel operation of a Na/H exchanger and Cl/OH exchanger will result in the reabsorption of NaCl into the cell and the secretion of H_2O into the lumen.

in the adult kidney is NHE3.[28,29] By linking the sodium entry to proton secretion, this transporter will increase the intracellular pH of the proximal tubule so there will be a gradient for sodium and bicarbonate exit through the basolateral membrane via the sodium-bicarbonate cotransporter (NBC).[30]

In the luminal fluid of the proximal tubule, the proton combines with the filtered bicarbonate to form carbonic acid that is then converted to water and carbon dioxide in the presence of carbonic anhydrase.[28] Once the water and carbon dioxide enter the cell, they are converted back to carbonic acid that ionizes into protons and bicarbonate. The proton can then be secreted again, and the bicarbonate is transported through the basolateral membrane and into the bloodstream.

Because the processes involved in the reabsorption of bicarbonate have finite rates, the entire process exhibits saturation kinetics and has a transport maximum.[31] When the filtered load of bicarbonate is below the transport maximum, all of the filtered bicarbonate will be reabsorbed. If the filtered load exceeds the transport maximum, some of the filtered bicarbonate will be excreted. Because bicarbonate is an anion, it must be excreted with a cation such as sodium or potassium. Thus bicarbonaturia can lead to volume depletion due to the sodium loss and also to hypokalemia.[32]

Other sodium-coupled transporters on the luminal membrane include the sodium-glucose cotransporters (SGLT1 and SGLT2), sodium-phosphate cotransporters (NaPi2a), and sodium–amino acid cotransporters.[33–36] (The transport of amino acids is very complex and is beyond the scope of this chapter. However, the simplistic view of the sodium–amino acid cotransporter is adequate for this discussion. Please see references 37 and 38 for further details.) These cotransporters account for only a small portion of the sodium that is reabsorbed but are responsible for reabsorbing almost the entire filtered load of glucose and amino acids. The amount of phosphate that is reabsorbed is dependent on the diet and can comprise a very wide range of the filtered load. Thus there is almost no glucose or amino acids in the final urine, but there can be considerable amounts of phosphate, depending on the dietary intake of phosphate.

Active, transcellular transport of sodium chloride occurs via the action of parallel transporters, NHE3, and the chloride-hydroxyl exchanger (see Fig. 4.2).[39,40] As discussed previously, the sodium-hydrogen exchanger raises the intracellular pH of the proximal tubule. This leads to a pH gradient that can be used to exchange intracellular base (hydroxyl ions) for luminal chloride ions. The hydrogen ion that was secreted is then combined with the hydroxyl ion to form water while the sodium and chloride exit the cell via the basolateral membrane and into the bloodstream.

The actions of these transporters for the reabsorption of bicarbonate, glucose, and amino acids in the early proximal tubule will cause the luminal fluid to have a low bicarbonate concentration and a high chloride concentration (Fig. 4.3).[41] Thus the luminal fluid in the distal portion of the proximal tubule has a very low bicarbonate

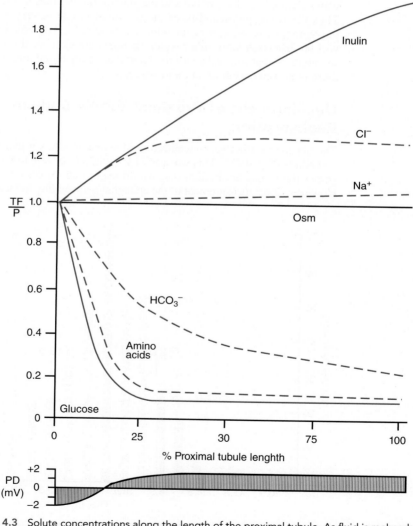

Fig. 4.3 Solute concentrations along the length of the proximal tubule. As fluid is reabsorbed, the concentration of luminal inulin/plasma inulin increases. The preferential reabsorption of bicarbonate leads to an increase in the luminal chloride concentration. (Reproduced with permission from Rector FC Jr. Sodium, bicarbonate, and chloride absorption by the proximal tubule. *Am J Physiol.* 1983;244(5):F461-F471.)

concentration, almost no glucose or amino acids, and a high concentration of chloride. The distal portion of the proximal tubule then uses the chloride concentration gradient to reabsorb salt and water by passive paracellular transport. The rate of reabsorption in this part of the nephron is dependent on the concentration gradient that was generated, as well as the paracellular permeability to chloride.[41]

The expression of the intercellular junction proteins known as claudins determines the paracellular permeability of the proximal tubule.[42] As will be discussed in the development of the proximal tubule transport, the expression of these claudins changes during development and has a direct impact on the rate of transport of sodium chloride.

Proximal Tubule Water Transport

The proximal tubule reabsorbs the bulk of the filtered load of sodium, chloride, and water in an isotonic fashion. The osmolality of the luminal fluid throughout the proximal tubule does not differ very much from the osmolality of the blood. This isotonicity is maintained because of the high expression of AQP1, the membrane water channel, in the luminal and basolateral membranes of the proximal tubule.[43,44] Thus the water permeability of the proximal tubule is very high, and the osmotic movement of water can occur with a very small solute concentration gradient. As will be discussed later, other water channels are expressed throughout the nephron segments so that salt and water transport can be separated, but in the proximal tubule, there is no separation of salt and water.

Development of Proximal Tubule Sodium Reabsorption

The plasma bicarbonate concentration of neonates is lower than that of older children and adults (Fig. 4.4).[45] This was initially thought to be due to backleak of bicarbonate across the tubule epithelium that would lead to an excess excretion of bicarbonate. However, direct measurement of the epithelial permeability to bicarbonate demonstrated

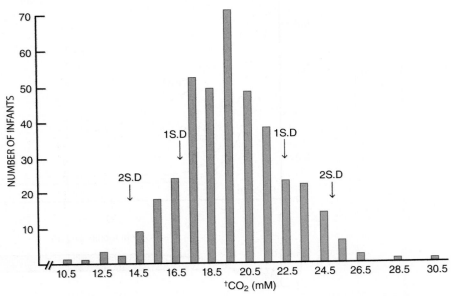

Fig. 4.4 Distribution of bicarbonate concentrations in normal newborn infants. As can be seen, the mean value of bicarbonate is lower than the normal adult value. The normal range for infants can be as low as 15 mEq/L. (Reproduced with permission from Schwartz GJ, Haycock GB, Edelmann CM, Jr., Spitzer A. Late metabolic acidosis: a reassessment of the definition. J Pediatr. 1979;95(1):102-107.)

a lower permeability in neonatal rabbit proximal tubules compared to adult rabbit proximal tubules.[46] Thus, it was clear that active transport of bicarbonate was lower in the neonatal tubule.

As the proximal tubule matures, all of the components of bicarbonate transport increase. The development of the Na^+,K^+-ATPase activity parallels that of the basolateral surface area and provides the required energy for the secondary active secretion of protons through the luminal membrane.[47] Thus the increase in the Na^+,K^+-ATPase provides the necessary energy for transporting bicarbonate, as well as other filtered solutes such as glucose, phosphate, and amino acids (Fig. 4.5).[48]

The development of the NHE is more complex. The primary isoform of the luminal sodium-proton exchanger in the adult kidney is NHE3.[28,29] Although the expression of NHE3 in neonatal rabbit proximal tubules was found to be very low, experiments demonstrated that there was sodium-hydrogen exchange activity that could not be explained by the negligible amount of NHE3 expressed.[49,50] The isoform that was subsequently found to be responsible for this exchange activity in the neonatal tubules was NHE8.[51–53] This isoform is also expressed in adult proximal tubules but is in intracellular compartments, whereas it is in the luminal membrane in the neonatal tubules. Thus there is evidence for an isoform switch for the sodium-proton exchanger throughout development.

Developmental expression of NHE3 and NHE8 is under hormonal control. A number of studies demonstrated that the expression of NHE3 is stimulated by glucocorticoids.[54,55] Treatment with glucocorticoids also will cause the luminal expression of NHE8 to decrease.[56] Thus glucocorticoids are probably one of the primary regulators of the development of transport of bicarbonate and sodium in the proximal tubule.

In addition to glucocorticoids, thyroid hormone has been shown to have a number of effects on the development of proximal tubular transport. Although thyroid hormone had some effect on the maturational increase in the expression of NHE3 and the decreased expression of NHE8, there were more significant effects on the paracellular transport of sodium chloride.[57,58] The proximal straight tubules from hypothyroid neonatal rabbits were found to have a very low chloride permeability. Proximal straight tubules from hypothyroid animals that were treated with thyroid hormone had a chloride permeability that was not different from control animals.[58] Thus the passive, paracellular transport in the proximal tubule also undergoes significant changes that appear to be affected by thyroid hormone.

The paracellular permeability properties of an epithelium are determined by the intercellular junction proteins known as claudins.[42] The claudins expressed in the neonatal proximal tubule are different from the adult tubule, which leads to the very low permeability to chloride in the neonatal proximal tubule. Claudins 6, 9, and 13 were shown to have high expression in the neonatal tubules but not in the adult tubules.[59,60] These claudins were shown in a cell culture model to have effects on chloride permeability.[61] Thus the mechanism of sodium chloride transport in the late proximal tubule has significant maturational changes that are stimulated in part by thyroid hormone.[62]

Development of Proximal Tubule Water Permeability

The active transport of sodium, chloride, and other solutes generates a small osmotic gradient across the proximal tubule. The high water permeability of this epithelium allows for high water transport rates in the presence of the low osmotic gradient. The high water permeability is due in part to the expression of AQP1 that is present in both the luminal and basolateral membranes of the tubule.

Expression of AQP1 in the proximal tubule of the neonatal rabbit kidney was found to be much lower than that of the adult proximal tubule.[63] In addition, water permeability measurements of vesicles made from proximal tubule luminal and basolateral membranes showed that the water permeability of the membranes was much lower in the neonatal tissue than the adult kidney tissue.[63,64] Thus it appeared that the water permeability of the neonatal proximal tubule should be much lower

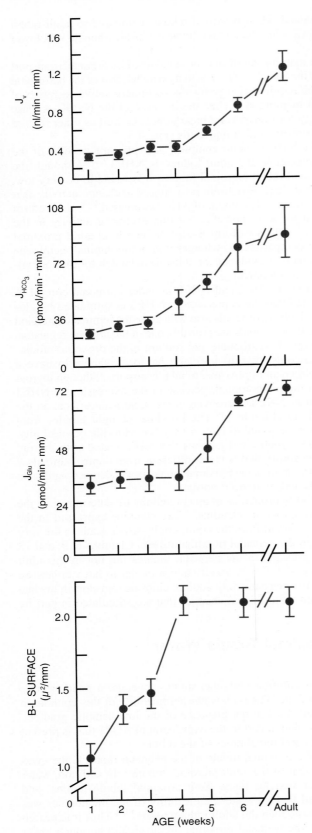

Fig. 4.5 Increase in rabbit proximal tubule transport function. The basolateral surface area increases dramatically in the first 4 weeks of life. This allows for more Na⁺,K⁺-ATPase to be present and functionally active. The increased Na⁺,K⁺-ATPase activity drives the increase in bicarbonate and glucose transport and the increase in volume reabsorption. (Reproduced with permission from Schwartz GJ, Evan AP. Development of solute transport in rabbit proximal tubule. I. HCO-3 and glucose absorption. *Am J Physiol.* 1983;245(3):F382-F390.)

B

than the adult. However, direct measurements in isolated perfused rabbit proximal tubules showed that there was no difference in the water permeability between tubules from neonatal rabbits and adult rabbits.[65] This was explained by the fact that the intracellular compartment in the neonatal tubules was much smaller than that of the adult tubules and provided less resistance to the movement of water through the epithelium.[66] Thus, although the expression of AQP1 was lower in the neonatal proximal tubule, the epithelial water permeability remained high enough so that water could be reabsorbed.[67]

Thin Descending and Thin Ascending Loops of Henle

Although transport of salt and water in the thin descending and ascending portions of the loop of Henle is primarily passive in nature, it is complex and its contribution to the medullary hypertonicity is incompletely understood.[68] The osmolality of the medullary interstitium is higher than that of the luminal fluid so that there is an osmotic gradient for water reabsorption as the thin descending limb goes further into the medulla. Some, but not all, of the thin descending limbs of Henle express AQP1, so there is high water permeability in these segments. As water is reabsorbed, solute in the lumen becomes more concentrated so that when the fluid begins to ascend to the cortex, there is a gradient for passive sodium reabsorption in the thin ascending limb of the loop of Henle. Thus the reabsorption of water and sodium in the thin portion of the loop of Henle is passive and there is no separation of salt from water.

The developing fetus has only short thin limbs of Henle. Shortly before birth, they begin to form the long loops of Henle that will eventually contribute to medullary hypertonicity. The molecular signals controlling this process have only recently been studied.[69,70] Defects in this process could contribute to the medullary hypoplasia seen in many forms of renal dysplasia.[71]

Thick Ascending Limb of Henle

The TAL of Henle actively transports sodium from the lumen to the bloodstream in a way that also causes many other ions to be reabsorbed (Fig. 4.6).[72] As in the proximal tubule, the primary active transporter is the sodium-potassium ATPase located in the basolateral membrane of the cell that maintains a very low intracellular

Fig. 4.6 Thick ascending limb cell. The Na⁺,K⁺-ATPase on the basolateral membrane provides the driving force for the entry of sodium through NKCC2. The recycling of potassium through ROMK leads to the lumen-positive electrical potential and contributes to the paracellular transport of cations. Defects in NKCC2, ROMK, the chloride channel CLC-NKB, or in Barttin lead to Bartter syndrome. *CLC-NKB,* Chloride channel; *NKCC2,* sodium-potassium-2 chloride cotransporter; *ROMK,* rat outer medullary potassium channel.

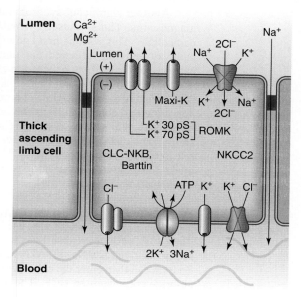

sodium concentration. The sodium-potassium-2 chloride cotransporter (NKCC2) uses this sodium concentration gradient to transport sodium, potassium, and chloride ions into the cell. This transporter is electroneutral and thus does not directly affect the luminal membrane electric potential.

Potassium enters the TAL cells through both the basolateral membrane (via the Na^+,K^+-ATPase) and the luminal membrane (via NKCC2). Both membranes have potassium channels, known as rat outer medullary potassium channel (ROMK), for the recycling of potassium ions. Because of the luminal potassium recycling, there is a lumen-positive electric potential that leads to passive paracellular reabsorption of many cations including sodium, potassium, calcium, and magnesium. Thus inhibition of transport of NKCC2 with loop diuretics such as furosemide and bumetanide results in increased excretion of not only sodium and potassium but also calcium and magnesium.

The TAL has no water channels on its luminal membrane but has AQP1 in the basolateral membrane so that the cell volume can respond to changes in interstitial osmolality.[72] In addition, the lipid composition of the luminal membrane is such that the water permeability is extremely low. As solute is actively reabsorbed from the lumen, the osmolality of the luminal fluid decreases and free water is generated. Thus the TAL is considered part of the diluting segment of the nephron.

Mutations in several of the transporters in the TAL cause Bartter syndrome, characterized by polyuria and hypokalemic alkalosis.[73–75] The first one that was identified was NKCC2, so this has been termed Bartter syndrome type 1.[76] The next defect that was identified was in ROMK, which is one of the causes of antenatal Bartter syndrome and polyhydramnios.[77] Neonates with this form of Bartter syndrome will often be hyperkalemic instead of hypokalemic because the secretion of potassium in the cortical collecting duct (CCD) will be limited due to the lack of functional potassium channels in the CCD of the neonate. As the infant matures and the maxi-K channel expression increases, they will eventually manifest the typical hypokalemic alkalosis.[78,79]

The typical patient with Bartter syndrome will have hypercalciuria and will develop nephrocalcinosis. However, in type 3 Bartter syndrome, caused by mutations in the chloride channel (CLC-NKB), there are variable amounts of calciuria due to the fact that the calcium channel is also present in the distal convoluted tubule (DCT).[80] Type 4 Bartter syndrome is caused by mutations in Barttin, an accessory protein for the chloride channel. Because Barttin is also found in the inner ear, these patients will also have sensorineural deafness.[81,82] The last form of Bartter syndrome is due to defects in the calcium-sensing receptor (CaSR), which is rare and beyond the scope of this chapter.[83]

Another significant syndrome caused by defects in the TAL is familial hypomagnesemia. This is caused by mutations in claudin 16, which was initially called paracellin.[84] This was the first known disease caused by mutations in the paracellular pathway and has furthered our understanding of the function of the paracellular pathway in the homeostasis of the electrolytes.

In the neonate the transport of sodium chloride in the TAL is only approximately 20% of that of the adult TAL.[85] This correlated with a low activity of the Na^+,K^+-ATPase that increased significantly as the animals matured.[86] This maturational increase in Na^+,K^+-ATPase activity also correlated with the increase in urinary concentrating ability, presumably due to an increase in medullary tonicity.[87] Glucocorticoids play a role in this developmental process.[88,89] Although the solute transport rate is significantly lower than the adult, the normal newborn is able to dilute its urine to excrete a water load.[90]

Distal Convoluted Tubule

The DCT continues reabsorbing sodium by an active mechanism. As in the previous segments, there is a Na^+,K^+-ATPase located on the basolateral membrane (Fig. 4.7).[91] Sodium can then enter the cell down its electrochemical gradient through the sodium-chloride cotransporter, NCC. The membranes of the DCT are similar to those of the

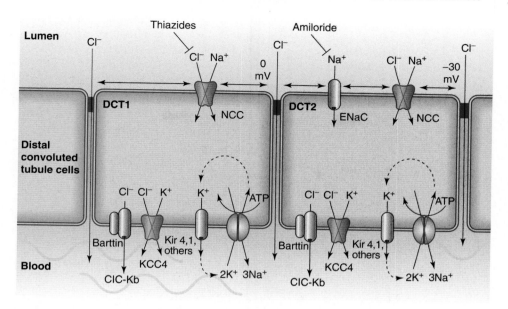

Fig. 4.7 Distal convoluted tubule cell. The Na$^+$,K$^+$-ATPase provides the driving force for sodium entry through NCC, the thiazide-sensitive sodium-chloride cotransporter. Mutations in NCC lead to Gitelman syndrome.

TAL in that they have very low water permeability. This allows the DCT to continue to remove solute from the lumen, leaving behind the water, which will continue to dilute the tubular fluid and continue to create free water.

Gitelman et al. described a group of patients who had hypokalemic alkalosis that was similar to patients with Bartter syndrome.[92,93] The key difference was that the patients they described had hypocalciuria instead of hypercalciuria that typical Bartter syndrome patients had. It was subsequently shown that these patients had a mutation in the thiazide-sensitive transporter NCC.[94] They are usually not as severely affected as Bartter syndrome patients, and many times are found incidentally when their electrolytes are measured.

Collecting Duct

The cortical and medullary collecting ducts comprise several different cell types.[95] The principal cells are involved in sodium reabsorption and potassium secretion, whereas the alpha and beta intercalated cells are involved in secretion of acid or base. We will focus on the principal cells.

As in the previous nephron segments, the collecting duct principal cells have Na$^+$,K$^+$-ATPase on the basolateral membrane for maintaining a low intracellular sodium concentration (Fig. 4.8).[95] In this segment, sodium entry occurs through the epithelial sodium channel (ENaC) instead of a cotransporter. Thus the luminal transport of sodium is electrogenic and depends on the electrochemical gradient, not just the chemical gradient.

The primary hormonal regulator of sodium reabsorption in the collecting duct is aldosterone. The collecting duct principal cells have the mineralocorticoid receptor that responds to aldosterone to increase expression of ENaC, as well as to increase Na$^+$,K$^+$-ATPase activity.[95] Because the mineralocorticoid receptor can bind cortisol and aldosterone, the enzyme 11 beta hydroxy-steroid dehydrogenase (11BHSD) is present in the principal cells and is responsible for converting cortisol to cortisone, which cannot bind to the mineralocorticoid receptor inside the CCD principal cell.[96] Defects in the recycling of ENaC, as well as the mineralocorticoid receptor or 11BHSD, have large effects on the final amount of sodium that is reabsorbed. This can then

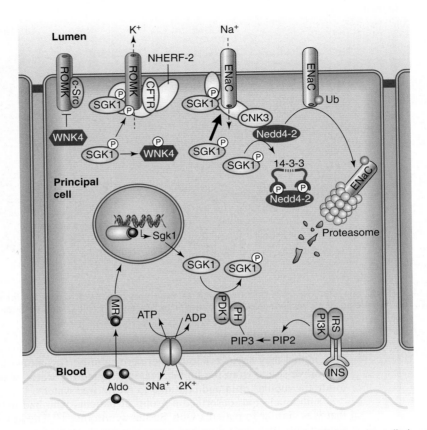

Fig. 4.8 Cortical collecting duct principal cell, sodium transport. The basolaterally located Na+,K+-ATPase maintains a low intracellular sodium concentration which allows for sodium to enter through the epithelia sodium channel. Potassium is also secreted via ROMK.

lead to hypertension if sodium is retained in excess or hypotension if too much sodium is excreted.

The first disease process involving the CCD that was described is Liddle syndrome.[97–100] These patients have a mutation in ENaC, which interferes with its intracellular recycling. Thus too many sodium channels remain in the luminal membrane of the CCD, causing excessive sodium retention. The patient becomes volume overloaded and hypertensive, causing the renin and aldosterone levels to be suppressed.

Apparent mineralocorticoid excess syndrome results from inactivation of the enzyme (11BHSD) that would usually convert cortisol to cortisone.[96] Because the serum concentrations of cortisol are much higher than aldosterone, cortisol enters the CCD principal cell and activates the mineralocorticoid receptor, acting as aldosterone, which leads to volume overload and hypertension. These patients will also have a decrease in their renin and aldosterone because cortisol is acting as a mineralocorticoid.

Glucocorticoid remediable aldosteronism is a form of hypertension caused by excessive aldosterone secretion.[101] This results from a mutation where the aldosterone synthase gene is controlled by adrenocorticotropic hormone (ACTH) instead of angiotensin II.[102,103] Thus treatment with exogenous glucocorticoids will suppress ACTH and decrease aldosterone synthase.

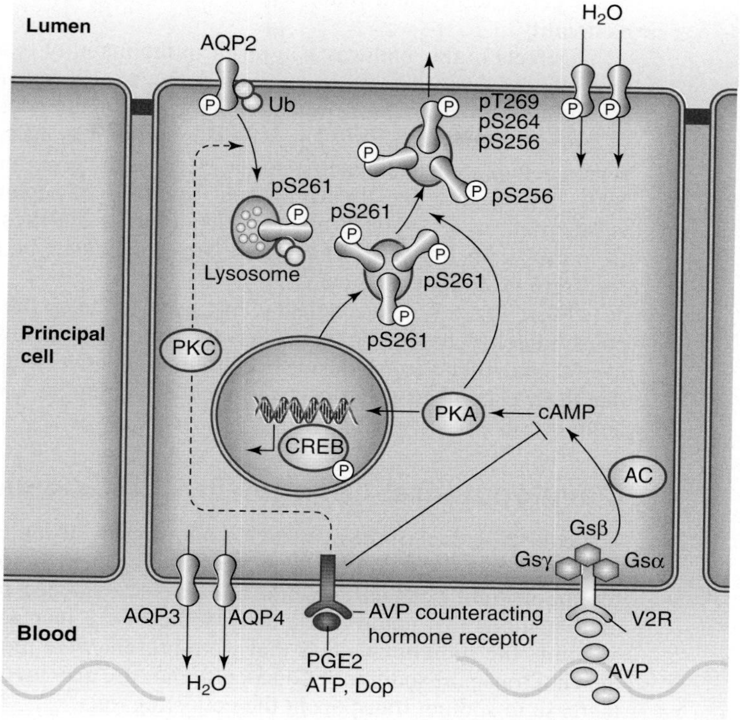

Fig. 4.9 Cortical collecting duct principal cell, water transport. AQP3 and AQP4 water channels are constitutively present in the basolateral membrane. AQP2 is inserted into the luminal membrane in response to arginine vasopressin (AVP) binding to the vasopressin receptor, V2R. Mutations in V2R cause congenital nephrogenic diabetes insipidus as well as nephrogenic syndrome of inappropriate antidiuresis. *AQP*, Aquaporins; *V2R*, V2 receptor.

Sodium wasting and hyperkalemic acidosis in the setting of high serum aldosterone concentrations is known as pseudohypoaldosteronism (PHA) type 1. Inactivating mutations of ENaC cause the autosomal recessive form of PHA type 1 that can be very severe.[104,105] Because of the sodium wasting, the patients tend to be hypotensive and can easily develop hypovolemic shock. The ENaC is also found in the lung, so these patients will often have severe respiratory distress syndrome (RDS) after birth because of difficulty in clearing the fluid from their lungs.[106–109] Another form of PHA is due to defects in the mineralocorticoid receptor and is inherited in an autosomal dominant fashion.[110] They do not have RDS because the sodium and fluid transport out of the lungs is not affected.

The collecting duct principal cells are also responsible for the final regulation of water reabsorption (Fig. 4.9).[95] The basolateral membranes of the principal cells contain AQP3 and 4, which are present in the membrane at all times. AQP2 is inserted into the apical membrane from endosomes when the tubule is stimulated by antidiuretic hormone (ADH) (also known as arginine vasopressin [AVP]). In the absence of ADH, AQP2 remains in the intracellular compartment and the water permeability of the luminal membrane of the tubule remains low. This allows for the free water that was generated in the TAL and DCT to be excreted so that hyponatremia does not develop. Under conditions of dehydration and elevated serum osmolality, ADH is released from the posterior pituitary gland and binds to the V2 receptor (V2R) on the basolateral membrane of the tubule. This initiates a cascade of events that includes stimulation of adynelate cyclase and protein kinase A and insertion of the AQP2-containing endosomes in the luminal membrane. This then increases the tubule's water permeability, and water will be reabsorbed, resulting in an increase in urine osmolality.

Defects in this pathway can result in the inability to appropriately concentrate or dilute the urine. The most common defect is nephrogenic diabetes insipidus that is caused by an inactivating mutation in the V2R and renders the tubule unresponsive to the actions of ADH.[111,112] These patients present as infants with repeated bouts of severe dehydration and hypernatremia. Because the gene for the vasopressin receptor, V2R, is located on the X chromosome, this form of nephrogenic diabetes insipidus is inherited in an X-linked manner. Nephrogenic diabetes insipidus can also result from mutations in AQP2. These are more rare and can be inherited in an autosomal recessive or dominant form.[113–115]

More recently, other defects have been found in the V2R that causes it to be constitutively activated. In these cases the patients present with chronic hyponatremia even though their serum ADH concentrations are undetectable. The clinical syndrome that these patients have has been designated "nephrogenic syndrome of inappropriate antidiuresis."[116]

Developmental Changes in CCD Sodium Transport

The collecting duct of the neonate has a lower rate of sodium transport than the adult collecting duct.[117,118] This has been shown to be due to a lower expression of mRNA for the sodium channel subunits.[119] There is evidence for some posttranslational modifications that could account for some of the increase in sodium transport. In addition, the sodium channels that were present were more likely to be closed and thus not transport sodium.[120] Glucocorticoids are also involved in the developmental increase in sodium transport in the collecting duct.[121]

Because of the lower reabsorption rate of sodium in the cortical collecting ducts in neonates, they tend to waste sodium. This leads to elevated secretion of aldosterone.[122,123] Thus, when newborns were examined in terms of the relationship between serum aldosterone and the renal handling of sodium, there is evidence for at least partial resistance of the tubules to the action of aldosterone.[124] This resistance dissipates over time as the expression of ENaC increases and the ability of the newborn kidney to reabsorb sodium.

Developmental Changes in CCD Water Transport

Neonates cannot concentrate their urine to the same degree as older children and adults.[125] This is due in part to a lower osmotic gradient that is maintained in the interstitium of the medulla. There is also evidence that the response of the neonatal collecting duct to ADH is not as robust as the adult collecting duct.

Initial experiments showed that one of the limiting factors in the response to ADH is an increase in prostaglandin secretion by the neonatal tubule.[126] When these prostaglandins were inhibited, the response of the collecting duct to produce cyclic adenosine monophosphate (cAMP) was improved. Subsequent studies also examined the role of phosphodiesterase (PDE) in the limited tubule response to ADH.[127] PDE will metabolize cAMP into AMP so that it is inactivated, thus limiting the response to ADH. Because the activity of PDE was higher in the neonatal tubules, the full response to ADH was inhibited. PDE activity was directly shown to be higher in the neonatal collecting ducts, and once PDE was blocked, the water permeability response in the neonatal tubules was the same as the adult tubules. Thus PDE is probably the most significant factor in the limited response of the neonatal collecting duct to ADH.

REFERENCES

1. Friis-Hansen B. Body water compartments in children: changes during growth and related changes in body composition. *Pediatrics*. 1961;28:169–181.
2. Lager S, Powell TL. Regulation of nutrient transport across the placenta. *J Pregnancy*. 2012;2012:179827.
3. Speake PF, Mynett KJ, Glazier JD, et al. Activity and expression of Na+/H+ exchanger isoforms in the syncytiotrophoblast of the human placenta. *Pflugers Arch*. 2005;450(2):123–130.
4. Liu H, Zheng Z, Wintour EM. Aquaporins and fetal fluid balance. *Placenta*. 2008;29(10):840–847.

5. Sha XY, Xiong ZF, Liu HS, et al. Maternal-fetal fluid balance and aquaporins: from molecule to physiology. *Acta Pharmacol Sin.* 2011;32(6):716–720.
6. Sibley CP, Glazier JD, Greenwood SL, et al. Regulation of placental transfer: the Na(+)/H(+) exchanger—a review. *Placenta.* 2002;23(suppl A):S39–S46.
7. Page KR, Ashworth CJ, McArdle HJ, et al. Sodium transport across the chorioallantoic membrane of porcine placenta involves the epithelial sodium channel (ENaC). *J Physiol.* 2003;547(Pt 3):849–857.
8. Brace RA, Wolf EJ. Normal amniotic fluid volume changes throughout pregnancy. *Am J Obstet Gynecol.* 1989;161(2):382–388.
9. Gilbert WM, Brace RA. Amniotic fluid volume and normal flows to and from the amniotic cavity. *Semin Perinatol.* 1993;17(3):150–157.
10. Magann EF, Sandlin AT, Ounpraseuth ST. Amniotic fluid and the clinical relevance of the sonographically estimated amniotic fluid volume: oligohydramnios. *J Ultrasound Med.* 2011;30(11):1573–1585.
11. Curran MA, Nijland MJ, Mann SE, Ross MG. Human amniotic fluid mathematical model: determination and effect of intramembranous sodium flux. *Am J Obstet Gynecol.* 1998;178(3):484–490.
12. Regnault TR, de Vrijer B, Battaglia FC. Transport and metabolism of amino acids in placenta. *Endocrine.* 2002;19(1):23–41.
13. Jansson T. Amino acid transporters in the human placenta. *Pediatr Res.* 2001;49(2):141–147.
14. Battaglia FC. In vivo characteristics of placental amino acid transport and metabolism in ovine pregnancy—a review. *Placenta.* 2002;23(suppl A):S3–S8.
15. Battaglia FC, Regnault TR. Placental transport and metabolism of amino acids. *Placenta.* 2001;22(2–3):145–161.
16. Cetin I. Placental transport of amino acids in normal and growth-restricted pregnancies. *Eur J Obstet Gynecol Reprod Biol.* 2003;110(suppl 1):S50–S54.
17. Harrison MR, Golbus MS, Filly RA, et al. Management of the fetus with congenital hydronephrosis. *J Pediatr Surg.* 1982;17(6):728–742.
18. Underwood MA, Gilbert WM, Sherman MP. Amniotic fluid: not just fetal urine anymore. *J Perinatol.* 2005;25(5):341–348.
19. Laghmani K, Beck BB, Yang SS, et al. Polyhydramnios, Transient Antenatal Bartter's Syndrome, and MAGED2 Mutations. *N Engl J Med.* 2016;374(19):1853–1863.
20. Quigley R, Saland JM. Transient antenatal Bartter's Syndrome and X-linked polyhydramnios: insights from the genetics of a rare condition. *Kidney Int.* 2016;90(4):721–723.
21. Potter EL. Bilateral renal agenesis. *J Pediatr.* 1946;29:68–76.
22. Potter EL. Facial characteristics of infants with bilateral renal agenesis. *Am J Obstet Gynecol.* 1946;51:885–888.
23. Bain AD, Scott JS. Renal agenesis and severe urinary tract dysplasia: a review of 50 cases, with particular reference to the associated anomalies. *Br Med J.* 1960;1(5176):841–846.
24. Rubin MI, Bruck E, Rapoport M, et al. Maturation of renal function in childhood: clearance studies. *J Clin Invest.* 1949;28(5 Pt 2):1144–1162.
25. Palmer LG, Schnermann J. Integrated control of Na transport along the nephron. *Clin J Am Soc Nephrol.* 2015;10(4):676–687.
26. Kon V, Hughes ML, Ichikawa I. Physiologic basis for the maintenance of glomerulotubular balance in young growing rats. *Kidney Int.* 1984;25(2):391–396.
27. Aperia A, Broberger O, Broberger U, et al. Glomerular tubular balance in preterm and fullterm infants. *Acta Paediatr Scand Suppl.* 1983;305:70–76.
28. Curthoys NP, Moe OW. Proximal tubule function and response to acidosis. *Clin J Am Soc Nephrol.* 2014;9(9):1627–1638.
29. Brant SR, Bernstein M, Wasmuth JJ, et al. Physical and genetic mapping of a human apical epithelial Na+/H+ exchanger (NHE3) isoform to chromosome 5p15.3. *Genomics.* 1993;15(3):668–672.
30. Romero MF, Boron WF. Electrogenic Na+/HCO3– cotransporters: cloning and physiology. *Annu Rev Physiol.* 1999;61:699–723.
31. Quigley R. Proximal renal tubular acidosis. *J Nephrol.* 2006;19(suppl 9):S41–S45.
32. Galla JH. Metabolic alkalosis. *J Am Soc Nephrol.* 2000;11(2):369–375.
33. Hummel CS, Lu C, Loo DD, et al. Glucose transport by human renal Na+/D-glucose cotransporters SGLT1 and SGLT2. *Am J Physiol Cell Physiol.* 2011;300(1):C14–C21.
34. Vallon V, Platt KA, Cunard R, et al. SGLT2 mediates glucose reabsorption in the early proximal tubule. *J Am Soc Nephrol.* 2011;22(1):104–112.
35. Biber J, Hernando N, Forster I, Murer H. Regulation of phosphate transport in proximal tubules. *Pflugers Arch.* 2009;458(1):39–52.
36. Virkki LV, Biber J, Murer H, Forster IC. Phosphate transporters: a tale of two solute carrier families. *Am J Physiol Renal Physiol.* 2007;293(3):F643–F654.
37. Broer S. Apical transporters for neutral amino acids: physiology and pathophysiology. *Physiology (Bethesda).* 2008;23:95–103.
38. Broer S. Amino acid transport across mammalian intestinal and renal epithelia. *Physiol Rev.* 2008;88(1):249–286.
39. Berry CA, Rector FC Jr. Electroneutral NaCl absorption in the proximal tubule: mechanisms of apical Na-coupled transport. *Kidney Int.* 1989;36(3):403–411.
40. Aronson PS. Ion exchangers mediating Na+, HCO3– and Cl– transport in the renal proximal tubule. *J Nephrol.* 2006;19(suppl 9):S3–S10.
41. Rector FC Jr. Sodium, bicarbonate, and chloride absorption by the proximal tubule. *Am J Physiol.* 1983;244(5):F461–F471.

42. Muto S. Physiological roles of claudins in kidney tubule paracellular transport. *Am J Physiol Renal Physiol*. 2017;312(1):F9–F24.
43. Preston GM, Carroll TP, Guggino WB, Agre P. Appearance of water channels in Xenopus oocytes expressing red cell CHIP28 protein. *Science*. 1992;256(5055):385–387.
44. Agre P, Preston GM, Smith BL, et al. Aquaporin CHIP: the archetypal molecular water channel. *Am J Physiol*. 1993;265(4 Pt 2):F463–F476.
45. Schwartz GJ, Haycock GB, Edelmann CM Jr, Spitzer A. Late metabolic acidosis: a reassessment of the definition. *J Pediatr*. 1979;95(1):102–107.
46. Quigley R, Baum M. Developmental changes in rabbit juxtamedullary proximal convoluted tubule bicarbonate permeability. *Pediatr Res*. 1990;28(6):663–666.
47. Schwartz GJ, Evan AP. Development of solute transport in rabbit proximal tubule. III. Na-K-ATPase activity. *Am J Physiol*. 1984;246(6 Pt 2):F845–F852.
48. Schwartz GJ, Evan AP. Development of solute transport in rabbit proximal tubule. I. HCO-3 and glucose absorption. *Am J Physiol*. 1983;245(3):F382–F390.
49. Baum M, Quigley R. Maturation of proximal tubular acidification. *Pediatr Nephrol*. 1993;7(6):785–791.
50. Baum M, Quigley R. Ontogeny of proximal tubule acidification. *Kidney Int*. 1995;48(6):1697–1704.
51. Goyal S, Vanden Heuvel G, Aronson PS. Renal expression of novel Na+/H+ exchanger isoform NHE8. *Am J Physiol Renal Physiol*. 2003;284(3):F467–F473.
52. Becker AM, Zhang J, Goyal S, et al. Ontogeny of NHE8 in the rat proximal tubule. *Am J Physiol Renal Physiol*. 2007;293(1):F255–F261.
53. Joseph C, Twombley K, Gattineni J, et al. Acid increases NHE8 surface expression and activity in NRK cells. *Am J Physiol Renal Physiol*. 2012;302(4):F495–F503.
54. Gupta N, Tarif SR, Seikaly M, Baum M. Role of glucocorticoids in the maturation of the rat renal Na+/H+ antiporter (NHE3). *Kidney Int*. 2001;60(1):173–181.
55. Baum M, Quigley R. Prenatal glucocorticoids stimulate neonatal juxtamedullary proximal convoluted tubule acidification. *Am J Physiol*. 1991;261(5 Pt 2):F746–F752.
56. Joseph C, Gattineni J, Dwarakanath V, Baum M. Glucocorticoids Reduce Renal NHE8 Expression. *Physiol Rep*. 2013;1(2).
57. Gattineni J, Sas D, Dagan A, et al. Effect of thyroid hormone on the postnatal renal expression of NHE8. *Am J Physiol Renal Physiol*. 2008;294(1):F198–F204.
58. Baum M, Quigley R. Thyroid hormone modulates rabbit proximal straight tubule paracellular permeability. *Am J Physiol Renal Physiol*. 2004;286(3):F477–F482.
59. Abuazza G, Becker A, Williams SS, et al. Claudins 6, 9, and 13 are developmentally expressed renal tight junction proteins. *Am J Physiol Renal Physiol*. 2006;291(6):F1132–F1141.
60. Haddad M, Lin F, Dwarakanath V, et al. Developmental changes in proximal tubule tight junction proteins. *Pediatr Res*. 2005;57(3):453–457.
61. Sas D, Hu M, Moe OW, Baum M. Effect of claudins 6 and 9 on paracellular permeability in MDCK II cells. *Am J Physiol Regul Integr Comp Physiol*. 2008;295(5):R1713–R1719.
62. Baum M. Developmental changes in proximal tubule NaCl transport. *Pediatr Nephrol*. 2008;23(2):185–194.
63. Quigley R, Harkins EW, Thomas PJ, Baum M. Maturational changes in rabbit renal brush border membrane vesicle osmotic water permeability. *J Membr Biol*. 1998;164(2):177–185.
64. Quigley R, Gupta N, Lisec A, Baum M. Maturational changes in rabbit renal basolateral membrane vesicle osmotic water permeability. *J Membr Biol*. 2000;174(1):53–58.
65. Quigley R, Baum M. Developmental changes in rabbit juxtamedullary proximal convoluted tubule water permeability. *Am J Physiol*. 1996;271(4 Pt 2):F871–F876.
66. Quigley R, Baum M. Water transport in neonatal and adult rabbit proximal tubules. *Am J Physiol Renal Physiol*. 2002;283(2):F280–F285.
67. Quigley R, Mulder J, Baum M. Ontogeny of water transport in the rabbit proximal tubule. *Pediatr Nephrol*. 2003;18(11):1089–1094.
68. Dantzler WH, Layton AT, Layton HE, Pannabecker TL. Urine-concentrating mechanism in the inner medulla: function of the thin limbs of the loops of Henle. *Clin J Am Soc Nephrol*. 2014;9(10):1781–1789.
69. Kim YM, Kim WY, Nam SA, et al. Role of Prox1 in the Transforming Ascending Thin Limb of Henle's Loop during Mouse Kidney Development. *PLoS ONE*. 2015;10(5):e0127429.
70. Cha JH, Kim YH, Jung JY, et al. Cell proliferation in the loop of henle in the developing rat kidney. *J Am Soc Nephrol*. 2001;12(7):1410–1421.
71. Song R. Yosypiv IV. Development of the kidney medulla. *Organogenesis*. 2012;8(1):10–17.
72. Mount DB. Thick ascending limb of the loop of Henle. *Clin J Am Soc Nephrol*. 2014;9(11):1974–1986.
73. Bartter FC, Pronove P, Gill JR Jr. Maccardle RC. Hyperplasia of the juxtaglomerular complex with hyperaldosteronism and hypokalemic alkalosis. A new syndrome. *Am J Med*. 1962;33:811–828.
74. Jeck N, Schlingmann KP, Reinalter SC, et al. Salt handling in the distal nephron: lessons learned from inherited human disorders. *Am J Physiol Regul Integr Comp Physiol*. 2005;288(4):R782–R795.
75. Seyberth HW. An improved terminology and classification of Bartter-like syndromes. *Nat Clin Pract Nephrol*. 2008;4(10):560–567.
76. Simon DB, Karet FE, Hamdan JM, et al. Bartter's syndrome, hypokalaemic alkalosis with hypercalciuria, is caused by mutations in the Na-K-2Cl cotransporter NKCC2. *Nat Genet*. 1996;13(2):183–188.
77. Simon DB, Karet FE, Rodriguez-Soriano J, et al. Genetic heterogeneity of Bartter's syndrome revealed by mutations in the K+ channel, ROMK. *Nat Genet*. 1996;14(2):152–156.
78. Woda CB, Miyawaki N, Ramalakshmi S, et al. Ontogeny of flow-stimulated potassium secretion in rabbit cortical collecting duct: functional and molecular aspects. *Am J Physiol Renal Physiol*. 2003;285(4):F629–F639.

79. Satlin LM. Developmental regulation of expression of renal potassium secretory channels. *Curr Opin Nephrol Hypertens*. 2004;13(4):445–450.
80. Simon DB, Bindra RS, Mansfield TA, et al. Mutations in the chloride channel gene, CLCNKB, cause Bartter's syndrome type III. *Nat Genet*. 1997;17(2):171–178.
81. Birkenhager R, Otto E, Schurmann MJ, et al. Mutation of BSND causes Bartter syndrome with sensorineural deafness and kidney failure. *Nat Genet*. 2001;29(3):310–314.
82. Jeck N, Reinalter SC, Henne T, et al. Hypokalemic salt-losing tubulopathy with chronic renal failure and sensorineural deafness. *Pediatrics*. 2001;108(1):E5.
83. Vargas-Poussou R, Huang C, Hulin P, et al. Functional characterization of a calcium-sensing receptor mutation in severe autosomal dominant hypocalcemia with a Bartter-like syndrome. *J Am Soc Nephrol*. 2002;13(9):2259–2266.
84. Simon DB, Lu Y, Choate KA, et al. Paracellin-1, a renal tight junction protein required for paracellular Mg2+ resorption. *Science*. 1999;285(5424):103–106.
85. Horster M. Loop of Henle functional differentiation: in vitro perfusion of the isolated thick ascending segment. *Pflugers Arch*. 1978;378(1):15–24.
86. Rane S, Aperia A, Eneroth P, Lundin S. Development of urinary concentrating capacity in weaning rats. *Pediatr Res*. 1985;19(5):472–475.
87. Rane S, Aperia A. Ontogeny of Na-K-ATPase activity in thick ascending limb and of concentrating capacity. *Am J Physiol*. 1985;249(5 Pt 2):F723–F728.
88. Djouadi F, Wijkhuisen A, Bastin J. Coordinate development of oxidative enzymes and Na-K-ATPase in thick ascending limb: role of corticosteroids. *Am J Physiol*. 1992;263(2 Pt 2):F237–F242.
89. Stubbe J, Madsen K, Nielsen FT, et al. Glucocorticoid impairs growth of kidney outer medulla and accelerates loop of Henle differentiation and urinary concentrating capacity in rat kidney development. *Am J Physiol Renal Physiol*. 2006;291(4):F812–F822.
90. Edelmann CM Jr, Barnett HL. Role of the kidney in water metabolism in young infants: physiologic and clinical considerations. *J Pediatr*. 1960;56:154–179.
91. Subramanya AR, Ellison DH. Distal convoluted tubule. *Clin J Am Soc Nephrol*. 2014;9(12):2147–2163.
92. Gitelman HJ, Graham JB, Welt LG. A new familial disorder characterized by hypokalemia and hypomagnesemia. *Trans Assoc Am Physicians*. 1966;79:221–235.
93. Gitelman HJ, Graham JB, Welt LG. A familial disorder characterized by hypokalemia and hypomagnesemia. *Ann N Y Acad Sci*. 1969;162(2):856–864.
94. Simon DB, Nelson-Williams C, Bia MJ, et al. Gitelman's variant of Bartter's syndrome, inherited hypokalaemic alkalosis, is caused by mutations in the thiazide-sensitive Na-Cl cotransporter. *Nat Genet*. 1996;12(1):24–30.
95. Pearce D, Soundararajan R, Trimpert C, et al. Collecting duct principal cell transport processes and their regulation. *Clin J Am Soc Nephrol*. 2015;10(1):135–146.
96. White PC, Mune T, Agarwal AK. 11 beta-Hydroxysteroid dehydrogenase and the syndrome of apparent mineralocorticoid excess. *Endocr Rev*. 1997;18(1):135–156.
97. Lifton RP, Gharavi AG, Geller DS. Molecular mechanisms of human hypertension. *Cell*. 2001;104(4):545–556.
98. Shimkets RA, Warnock DG, Bositis CM, et al. Liddle's syndrome: heritable human hypertension caused by mutations in the beta subunit of the epithelial sodium channel. *Cell*. 1994;79(3):407–414.
99. Schild L, Canessa CM, Shimkets RA, et al. A mutation in the epithelial sodium channel causing Liddle disease increases channel activity in the Xenopus laevis oocyte expression system. *Proc Natl Acad Sci USA*. 1995;92(12):5699–5703.
100. Hansson JH, Nelson-Williams C, Suzuki H, et al. Hypertension caused by a truncated epithelial sodium channel gamma subunit: genetic heterogeneity of Liddle syndrome. *Nat Genet*. 1995;11(1):76–82.
101. Sutherland DJ, Ruse JL, Laidlaw JC. Hypertension, increased aldosterone secretion and low plasma renin activity relieved by dexamethasone. *Can Med Assoc J*. 1966;95(22):1109–1119.
102. Lifton RP, Dluhy RG, Powers M, et al. A chimaeric 11 beta-hydroxylase/aldosterone synthase gene causes glucocorticoid-remediable aldosteronism and human hypertension. *Nature*. 1992;355(6357):262–265.
103. Lifton RP, Dluhy RG, Powers M, et al. Hereditary hypertension caused by chimaeric gene duplications and ectopic expression of aldosterone synthase. *Nat Genet*. 1992;2(1):66–74.
104. Chang SS, Grunder S, Hanukoglu A, et al. Mutations in subunits of the epithelial sodium channel cause salt wasting with hyperkalaemic acidosis, pseudohypoaldosteronism type 1. *Nat Genet*. 1996;12(3):248–253.
105. Strautnieks SS, Thompson RJ, Gardiner RM, Chung E. A novel splice-site mutation in the gamma subunit of the epithelial sodium channel gene in three pseudohypoaldosteronism type 1 families. *Nat Genet*. 1996;13(2):248–250.
106. Hummler E, Barker P, Beermann F, et al. Role of the epithelial sodium channel in lung liquid clearance. *Chest*. 1997;111(6 suppl):113S.
107. Hummler E, Barker P, Gatzy J, et al. Early death due to defective neonatal lung liquid clearance in alpha-ENaC-deficient mice. *Nat Genet*. 1996;12(3):325–328.
108. Barker PM, Nguyen MS, Gatzy JT, et al. Role of gammaENaC subunit in lung liquid clearance and electrolyte balance in newborn mice. Insights into perinatal adaptation and pseudohypoaldosteronism. *J Clin Invest*. 1998;102(8):1634–1640.
109. Kerem E, Bistritzer T, Hanukoglu A, et al. Pulmonary epithelial sodium-channel dysfunction and excess airway liquid in pseudohypoaldosteronism. *N Engl J Med*. 1999;341(3):156–162.

110. Geller DS, Zhang J, Zennaro MC, et al. Autosomal dominant pseudohypoaldosteronism type 1: mechanisms, evidence for neonatal lethality, and phenotypic expression in adults. *J Am Soc Nephrol.* 2006;17(5):1429–1436.
111. Morello JP, Bichet DG. Nephrogenic diabetes insipidus. *Annu Rev Physiol.* 2001;63:607–630.
112. Bichet DG. V2R mutations and nephrogenic diabetes insipidus. *Prog Mol Biol Transl Sci.* 2009;89:15–29.
113. van Os CH, Deen PM. Aquaporin-2 water channel mutations causing nephrogenic diabetes insipidus. *Proc Assoc Am Physicians.* 1998;110(5):395–400.
114. van Os CH, Deen PM. Role of aquaporins in renal water handling: physiology and pathophysiology. *Nephrol Dial Transplant.* 1998;13(7):1645–1651.
115. Savelkoul PJ, De Mattia F, Li Y, et al. p.R254Q mutation in the aquaporin-2 water channel causing dominant nephrogenic diabetes insipidus is due to a lack of arginine vasopressin-induced phosphorylation. *Hum Mutat.* 2009;30(10):E891–E903.
116. Feldman BJ, Rosenthal SM, Vargas GA, et al. Nephrogenic syndrome of inappropriate antidiuresis. *N Engl J Med.* 2005;352(18):1884–1890.
117. Vehaskari VM. Ontogeny of cortical collecting duct sodium transport. *Am J Physiol.* 1994;267(1 Pt 2):F49–F54.
118. Satlin LM, Evan AP, Gattone VH 3rd, Schwartz GJ. Postnatal maturation of the rabbit cortical collecting duct. *Pediatr Nephrol.* 1988;2(1):135–145.
119. Vehaskari VM, Hempe JM, Manning J, et al. Developmental regulation of ENaC subunit mRNA levels in rat kidney. *Am J Physiol.* 1998;274(6 Pt 1):C1661–C1666.
120. Satlin LM, Palmer LG. Apical Na+ conductance in maturing rabbit principal cell. *Am J Physiol.* 1996;270(3 Pt 2):F391–F397.
121. Nakamura K, Stokes JB, McCray PB Jr. Endogenous and exogenous glucocorticoid regulation of ENaC mRNA expression in developing kidney and lung. *Am J Physiol Cell Physiol.* 2002;283(3):C762–C772.
122. Aperia A, Broberger O, Herin P, Zetterstrom R. Sodium excretion in relation to sodium intake and aldosterone excretion in newborn pre-term and full-term infants. *Acta Paediatr Scand.* 1979;68(6):813–817.
123. Dillon MJ, Gillin ME, Ryness JM, de Swiet M. Plasma renin activity and aldosterone concentration in the human newborn. *Arch Dis Child.* 1976;51(7):537–540.
124. Martinerie L, Pussard E, Foix-L'Helias L, et al. Physiological partial aldosterone resistance in human newborns. *Pediatr Res.* 2009;66(3):323–328.
125. Bonilla-Felix M. Development of water transport in the collecting duct. *Am J Physiol Renal Physiol.* 2004;287(6):F1093–F1101.
126. Bonilla-Felix M, John-Phillip C. Prostaglandins mediate the defect in AVP-stimulated cAMP generation in immature collecting duct. *Am J Physiol.* 1994;267(1 Pt 2):F44–F48.
127. Quigley R, Chakravarty S, Baum M. Antidiuretic hormone resistance in the neonatal cortical collecting tubule is mediated in part by elevated phosphodiesterase activity. *Am J Physiol Renal Physiol.* 2004;286(2):F317–F322.

B

CHAPTER 5

Perinatal Calcium and Phosphorus Metabolism

Ran Namgung, MD, PhD, Reginald C. Tsang, MBBS

- **Body Distribution**
- **Regulation of Serum Calcium and Phosphorous Concentrations**
- **Clinical Disorders Associated With Abnormal Calcium and Phosphorus Homeostasis**

Disturbances in mineral homeostasis, common in newborns, may be caused by altered responses to normal physiologic transition from the intrauterine environment to neonatal independence. Mineral disturbances in newborns, either calcium (Ca) or phosphorus (P), may result from pathologic intrauterine conditions, fetal immaturity, birth stress, inadequate mineral intakes, or genetic defects. Diagnosis requires understanding of unique perinatal, clinical, and biochemical features of newborn mineral metabolism. This chapter reviews Ca and P metabolism during fetal and neonatal periods with emphasis on neonatal transition followed by causes, pathophysiology, and treatment of mineral disturbances.

Body Distribution of Calcium and Phosphorous

Large amounts of Ca and P are needed to allow normal mineralization of the skeleton of developing fetuses and neonates. To meet the high mineral requirements of the developing skeleton, fetuses maintain higher blood Ca and P than maternal levels through active transport of Ca and P across placenta against a concentration gradient.

Calcium

At birth, term newborns contain approximately 30 g Ca in total body, 80% of which is accrued during the last trimester of pregnancy at a maximum rate of 150 mg/kg fetal weight/day.[1] Fetal serum Ca (total and ionized) is higher than maternal serum Ca levels, primarily driven by transcellular active transport rather than passive paracellular pathways.[2]

At all ages, 99% of total body Ca is either in bone as hydroxyapatite or as noncrystalline, amorphous Ca phosphate form (predominant form in early life). One percent of total body Ca is in extracellular fluid (ECF) and soft tissues. Ca of mineral phase (at crystal surface) is in equilibrium with ECF; only about 1% is freely exchangeable with ECF.[3] Although this exchangeable pool is a small percentage of skeletal content, it approximates total Ca content in ECF and soft tissues and serves as a Ca reservoir. In children ages 3 to 16 years, total exchangeable Ca pool (TEP) size, by stable isotope technique, correlates with age independent of body weight variations. The bone Ca accretion rate (Vo^+) and Vo^+/TEP ratio are greater in children than adults, indicating increased bone flow of Ca in children compared with adults.[4]

Ca concentration in ECF is kept constant by a process that constantly feeds Ca into and withdraws Ca from this fluid compartment. Ca enters the plasma via intestinal absorption and bone resorption. In Ca balance, rates of Ca release from and uptake

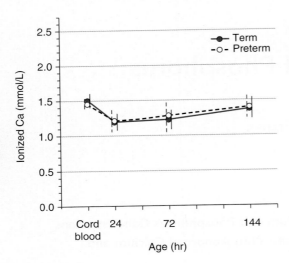

Fig. 5.1 Serum ionized calcium concentrations during the first 7 days of life in term and preterm infants. (Adapted from Wandrup J, Kroner J, Pryds O, et al. Age-related reference values for ionized calcium in the first week of life in premature and full-term neonates. *Scand J Clin Invest.* 1988;48:255-260.)

into bone are equal. In normal adults, total serum Ca ranges from 2.2 to 2.6 mmol/L (8.8–10.4 mg/dL) and is remarkably constant. Ionized Ca, although subject to changes directed by parathyroid hormone (PTH), calcitonin (CT), vitamin D, and blood pH, is also stable within individuals over prolonged periods and ranges from 1.2 to 1.3 mmol/L (4.8–5.2 mg/dL).[5]

At birth, abrupt termination of maternal-to-fetal Ca supply occurs. To maintain serum Ca homeostasis, an increase of 16% to 20% in Ca flux from bone to ECF is required unless sufficient exogenous Ca intake is achieved. In term newborns, cord blood total Ca is 2.6 mmol/L (10.2 mg/dL), and ionized Ca is 1.5 mmol/L (5.8 mg/dL). By 2 hours of age, serum total Ca declines by 5%, and by 24 to 36 hours, serum Ca reaches its nadir of total Ca of 2.3 mmol/L (9.0 mg/dL) and ionized Ca of 1.2 mmol/L (4.9 mg/dL). After a stabilization period, serum Ca slowly rises, reaching levels by 1 week of total Ca of 2.6 mmol/L (10.4 mg/dL) and ionized Ca of 1.4 mmol/L (5.5 mg/dL), similar to levels in childhood (Fig. 5.1).[6]

In preterm infants, mean cord serum ionized Ca is 1.45 mmol/L (95% confidence interval 1.29–1.61 mmol/L [5.8 (5.74–5.86) mg/dL]), which decreases during the first 24 to 36 hours of life and rises at 6 days to values exceeding original cord blood. An early decrease in ionized Ca may be associated with parathyroid glandular unresponsiveness because of prematurity or hypomagnesemia, and severe hypocalcemia may result.[7] Very low birth weight (VLBW) infants are likely to exhibit the lowest nadirs of ionized Ca; however, most are unassociated with tetany or decreased cardiac contractility (see Fig. 5.1).[8,9]

Cord serum Ca differs by season of birth (lower Ca in summer-born vs. winter-born infants) and delivery mode, but is unaffected by gender, race, or weight appropriateness for gestation.[10–12]

Phosphorus

In term newborns, total body P is approximately 16 g (0.6% of body weight). As with Ca, approximately 80% of P in term newborns is accumulated during the last pregnancy trimester at a rate of 75 mg/kg fetal weight/day, closely linked to Ca accretion, with Ca/P ratio of 1.7:1; 75% of P is for bone mineralization and 25% is in other tissues.[1] Transplacental P transport is an active sodium-dependent process against the concentration gradient.[13]

About 85% of total body P is in bone, primarily as hydroxyapatite and as more loosely complexed amorphous forms of bone crystal.[3] P plays key structural roles in bone. In contrast to Ca, P is widely distributed in nonosseous tissues, as an inorganic form, and as a component of structural macromolecules. Unlike Ca, 15% of total body P is in the ECF, largely as inorganic P ions. Soft tissue P is almost totally

P esters. P is taken up from circulation into cells via type II and type III sodium phosphate cotransporters (NPT) to facilitate cellular functions such as DNA and membrane lipid synthesis, generation of high-energy P esters (energy metabolism), and intracellular signaling. Intracellular P esters and phosphorylated intermediates are involved in important biologic processes and bone mineralization. Thus, P deficiency results in muscle weakness, impaired leukocyte function, and abnormal metabolism.[14]

Serum total P is higher in children than adults. Adult normal ranges are 1.24 to 1.86 mmol/L (3.0–4.5 mg/dL). In normal term infants, cord serum P does not differ by gender, race, season of birth, weight appropriateness for gestation, or mode of delivery.[10–12] P values in term infants range from 2.3 to 3.5 mmol/L (5.6–8.4 mg/dL) and in preterm infants from 1.7 to 3.3 mmol/L (4–8 mg/dL).[13] The relatively low initial birth values, 2.6 mmol/L (1.5–3.4) (6.2 [3.7–8.1] mg/dL), increase shortly after birth, thought to be related to increased gluconeogenesis and endogenous P release or secondary to low glomerular filtration rate (GFR) and reduced P excretion. Mean serum P increases to 3.4 mmol/L (8.1 mg/dL) by 1 week and decreases to 1.7 mmol/L (4.1 mg/dL) in childhood.[3]

Regulation of Calcium Homeostasis

After the first few days of life, serum Ca is maintained at a nearly constant level primarily through interaction of three hormones: PTH, 1,25-dihydroxyvitamin D [1,25(OH)$_2$D], and CT; these hormones direct intestinal Ca absorption, renal Ca reabsorption or excretion, and transfer of Ca stores from bone. In the fetal period, both PTH and parathyroid hormone–related peptide (PTHrP) act in regulation of fetal mineral metabolism through possible regulation of placental Ca transfer and maintaining fetal blood Ca.[3]

Placental Transport

Active Ca transport is facilitated by Ca-sensing receptor (CaSR) that "senses" extracellular Ca. Placental CaSRs regulate Ca transport from mother to fetus. Thus, the fetus develops in a "hypercalcemic state" (≈1 mg/dL higher Ca than maternal levels), and PTHrP (midregion fragment) is critical for maintaining this level.[15] Cord PTH is low, presumably suppressed by hypercalcemia in utero. The set point for fetal serum Ca is higher than the maternal set point.

Ca enters placental trophoblast at brush-border membrane (maternal–placental interface) primarily via the transient receptor potential (TRP) channel superfamily, especially the TRPV6 channel (voltage-dependent Ca^{2+} channel). The time course of TRPV6 mRNA expression in wild-type fetuses reveals a 14-fold increase during the last trimester of pregnancy, coinciding with a period of maximal Ca transfer.[16] Ca transport within trophoblast cells is facilitated by intracellular Ca-binding proteins (calbindin D9K) and actively transported into fetal circulation at the placental–fetal interface through a Ca pump, plasma membrane Ca^{2+} ATPase protein (PMCA3).[17]

Fetal PTH production is very low, especially at the end of gestation, despite a stable serum ionized Ca.[18] In mice with homozygous ablation of transcriptional factor Hox 3, fetal parathyroids are not developed, with undetectable PTH production; serum ionized Ca is significantly lower in the Hox 3 ablated fetus than in maternal serum. Measures of placental Ca transfer are not changed, suggesting that fetal PTH has no effect on transplacental Ca transfer.[19] However, PTH-ablated mice show significant abnormalities in fetal bone formation, including decreased mineralization of cartilage matrix, suggesting an additional role.[20]

In mice with lack of PTHrP, ionized Ca is significantly low in fetuses and similar to maternal levels, suggesting abolition of the maternal–fetal gradient. Transplacental Ca transfer was restored by infusions of PTHrP (1–86) or midregion fragment (67–86), but not by PTHrP (1–34) nor by PTH (1–84).[21] However, in PTHrP-ablated mice, using a different technique to assay placental Ca transfer (in situ artificially perfused placenta), surprisingly there is *increased* maternal–fetal Ca transfer, presumably related to significantly higher fetal Ca accretion, despite pronounced fetal hypocalcemia and abolition of fetomaternal Ca gradient. Thus, the influence of PTHrP on placental Ca transport is unclear, with data for facilitating and inhibiting effects.[22]

Possible factors explaining this discrepancy in these studies include technical differences in the conduct of experiments as well as modifying genes in the settings of different mouse strains. Additional studies will be required to clarify the role of PTHrP.[2]

Parathyroid Hormone

After birth, PTH is the main regulator of Ca and P homeostasis, acting in two main target tissues, kidney and bone, through the PTH/PTHrP receptor (PTHR1).[2] PTH elevates blood Ca. PTH secretion by parathyroid glands is regulated by circulating Ca ion, sensed by CaSRs in parathyroids. Increased serum Ca inhibits PTH secretion, and decreased serum Ca stimulates PTH secretion.[3] CaSRs play key roles in maintenance of a narrow range (1.2–1.3 mM/L; 4.8–5.2 mg/dL) of extracellular ionized Ca (Ca^{2+}). CaSR is expressed in target tissues for PTH, such as the kidneys, bone, and placenta, to sense alterations in Ca^{2+}, responding with changes directed at normalizing blood Ca^{2+}.[23] Genetic mutations of the *CASR* gene, on the long arm of chromosome 3, result in either activation or suppression: CaSR is "reset" so that higher or lower than normal blood Ca^{2+} is sensed by the receptor as "normal." Whereas inactivating (loss-of-function) mutations of the *CaSR* cause hypercalcemia (hyperparathyroidism), activating (gain-of-function) mutations cause a hypocalcemic syndrome of varying severity (hypoparathyroidism).[24,25]

PTH acts directly on bone, stimulating resorption, thereby releasing Ca and P into circulation. PTH acts directly on the kidneys to increase urinary P excretion and decrease urinary Ca excretion. PTH indirectly enhances intestinal Ca absorption through effects on $1,25(OH)_2D$ synthesis. Thus, the net actions of PTH increase serum Ca.

After birth, the kidneys play an important role in Ca and P homeostasis by regulating mineral loss via urine. Under normal circumstances, nearly all (98%) filtered Ca is reabsorbed in the renal tubule, but Ca excretion is modified by local and systemic factors (e.g., PTH) to regulate extracellular Ca. Urinary Ca increases over the first 2 weeks of life.[26] Both in preterm and term neonates, the kidneys respond to exogenous PTH, as measured by increased production of nephrogenous cyclic AMP (cAMP), and improve with increasing postnatal age.[27]

In normal term infants, when serum Ca decreases after birth, PTH increases appropriately (twofold to fivefold increase during 48 hours) and remains elevated for days. PTH secretion in term infants appears substantial and negatively correlates with Ca levels. Term neonates also show appropriate calcemic response when challenged with PTH. However, in extremely preterm infants, even with significant hypocalcemia as a stimulus, PTH remains low for the first 2 days. Transient hypocalcemia typically resolves within the first week and often requires no treatment.[8,9,28]

Vitamin D

Vitamin D is necessary for maintenance of normal Ca and P homeostasis. $1,25(OH)_2D$ is the major hormone affecting active intestinal Ca and P absorption. As a steroid, vitamin D binds to genomic receptors in intestinal epithelial cells and increases synthesis of Ca-binding proteins (calbindin), leading to increased Ca absorption. $1,25(OH)_2D$ acts on kidneys to conserve Ca and P. The overall result of this hormone is to increase serum Ca and P. $1,25(OH)_2D$ production by renal proximal tubule is enhanced by hypocalcemia, hypophosphatemia, PTH, and PTHrP and appears tightly regulated. $1,25(OH)_2D$ production is inhibited by elevated serum Ca and P.[3]

25-hydroxyvitamin D (25OHD) crosses the placenta, and cord 25OHD correlates significantly with maternal 25OHD; fetal vitamin D pool depends entirely on the maternal vitamin D status (i.e., maternal sun exposure and dietary D intake). $1,25(OH)_2D$ is produced by the fetal kidneys and placenta, and vitamin D receptor (VDR) is present in many fetal tissues, including the placenta.[18] The placenta synthesizes and metabolizes $1,25(OH)_2D$ through activity of 25OHD-1α hydroxylase and $1,25(OH)_2D$-24 hydroxylase, two key enzymes for vitamin D metabolism.[29,30]

However, mice deficient in 1-α-hydroxylase are grossly normal at birth and until weaning.[31] Additionally, mice with null mutation of VDR show no alteration in placental Ca transfer or fetal serum of Ca, P, or Mg despite significant maternal hypocalcemia.[32] The effect of 1,25(OH)$_2$D on placental Ca transfer, if any, could relate to expression of placental Ca transporter PMCA3 mRNA.[33]

Insufficiency of infant vitamin D arises from maternal vitamin D deficiency (sunshine deprivation with insufficient vitamin D intake), reduced production of active vitamin D metabolites caused by liver or renal disease, congenital deficiency of renal 1-α-hydroxylase, and 1,25(OH)$_2$D resistance. Deficiency of vitamin D or its metabolites causes decreased intestinal Ca absorption and renal Ca reabsorption and neonatal hypocalcemia.[34]

25-hydroxyvitamin D (25OHD), the major marker of vitamin D status, is lower in preterm than in term infants. However, conversion of 25OHD to 1,25(OH)$_2$D occurs normally in premature infants. In normal term infants, serum 1,25(OH)$_2$D is low at birth but increases to adult ranges by 24 hours, possibly reflecting a need for optimum intestinal Ca and P absorption.[35] In preterm infants, serum 1,25(OH)$_2$D at birth is comparable to that in healthy children and adults, increases significantly during the first few days, and is far above reference values between 3 and 12 weeks.[36] Cord serum 1,25(OH)$_2$D is lower in small-for-gestational-age infants compared with weight-appropriate infants, possibly reflecting decreased 1,25(OH)$_2$D production from reduced uteroplacental blood flow.[37]

Calcitonin

CT is a Ca^{2+}-lowering hormone produced by thyroid parafollicular cells and acts as a physiologic antagonist to PTH. CT secretion is under direct control of blood Ca.[38] Elevation in Ca^{2+} stimulates CaSR and lowers Ca^{2+} by enhancing CT secretion; decreased Ca^{2+} causes a decrease in CT. After being secreted, CT has a circulatory half-life of 2 to 15 minutes. CT inhibits osteoclast-mediated bone resorption (decreasing Ca and P release) and secondarily increases renal Ca and P excretion (at high doses). The net consequence of CT is decreased serum Ca and P.[38]

CT is produced in fetal thyroid; fetal and newborn CT is higher than in the mother, related to chronic fetal hypercalcemia. Recently, ablation of CT and CT gene-related peptide (CT/CGRP-null mice) produced serum Ca and placental Ca transfer identical to wild-type littermates. There was a small, nonsignificant trend toward decreased serum P, but serum Mg was reduced by almost 50%.[39] Thus, the role of CT in fetuses is unclear.

Cord serum CT decreases with increasing gestational age. Infants less than 32 weeks' gestation have nearly three times term cord serum CT.[40] After birth, serum CT further increases in both preterm and term infants, peaking at 24 to 48 hours, followed by a decline to childhood values by 1 month.[40] The physiologic importance of this increase is unclear but may relate to CT counteracting PTH bone resorptive action.

Regulation of Phosphorus Homeostasis

In contrast to regulation of Ca, the regulation of P homeostasis during the fetal and neonatal periods is less well understood. The regulation of P homeostasis involves several different hormones that act on kidney, intestine, and bone: fibroblast growth factor 23 (FGF23), PTH, and 1,25(OH)$_2$D.

Placental Transport

Similar to Ca, P is higher in fetal serum compared with maternal serum, and PTHrP appears to help prevent additional elevation. Transplacental P transport is an active sodium-dependent process against concentration gradient.[13] Inorganic P enters placental trophoblast via NaPi-IIb, a family member of sodium-dependent inorganic P transporters, critical for intestinal P transport.[41] In a mouse model that is null for NaPi-IIb, unexpected embryonic lethality was found. NaPi-IIb is expressed in the embryonic endoderm and placental labyrinthine zone (where embryonic and maternal circulations are in closest contact), consistent with a role in placental P transfer.[42] However, much remains to be learned about additional proteins involved in P transfer and about their regulation.[2]

Parathyroid Hormone

Circulating P is determined by a balance between intestinal P absorption, storage in the skeleton, and P reabsorption from the kidneys. PTH synthesis and secretion are upregulated by low serum Ca and increased serum P, and downregulated by increased serum Ca and 1,25(OH)$_2$D and by increased FGF23. The net effect of these actions is increased serum Ca and decreased serum P.[14] PTH acts on the proximal tubule, where it rapidly decreases NaPi-IIa and NaPi-IIc expression and thereby leads to phosphaturia. PTH stimulates 1,25(OH)$_2$D synthesis. Together with PTH, 1,25(OH)$_2$D furthermore acts on bone to increase the release of Ca (and P) into ECF. P regulation therefore can be either independent of, or intimately tied to, Ca regulation.[43]

1,25(OH)$_2$D expression is upregulated by PTH and downregulated by increased serum Ca, P, and FGF23. 1,25(OH)$_2$D acts through VDR/RXR dimers to stimulate intestinal P absorption, FGF23 synthesis, and secretion by osteocytes, and possibly to inhibit parathyroid PTH secretion. Its net effect is increase in serum Ca and P.[44]

Absorbed P enters the extracellular P pool in equilibrium with bone and soft tissue. In adults with a neutral P balance, P excreted by the kidneys is equal to the net P absorbed by the intestine; in growing infants, it is less than net absorbed, owing to deposition of P in soft tissues and bone. In growing infants, P preferentially goes to soft tissue with a nitrogen-to-P (weight) ratio of 15:1 and to bone with a Ca-to-P (weight) ratio of 2.15:1. The residual P constitutes renal P load, influencing plasma and urinary P. In limited P supply, bone mineral accretion may be limited, leading to significant Ca excretion associated with very low urinary P excretion.[3,45]

During P depletion, phosphaturia decreases before serum P declines through increased tubular reabsorption. Hypophosphatemic challenge results in stimulation of kidney 1,25(OH)$_2$D synthesis, enhanced mobilization of P and Ca from bone, a hypophosphatemia-induced increase in tubular maximum reabsorption for P (TmP), and decreased renal P excretion. Increased circulating 1,25(OH)$_2$D increases P and Ca absorption in the intestine and stimulates P and Ca mobilization from the bone. The increased flow of Ca from the bone and intestine inhibits PTH secretion and lowers P excretion. The net result is a return of serum P to normal without a change in serum Ca.[45] FGF23 may possibly be downregulated in low serum P and may increase NaPi-II expression, leading to decreased renal P excretion.

Defense against hyperphosphatemia consists largely of a reversal of these events. The principal humoral factor is PTH. An acute increase in serum P produces a transient decrease in serum ionized Ca and stimulation of PTH, and possibly upregulates FGF23 expression, which reduces TmP/GFR by reducing renal NaPi-II expression, leading to increased renal P excretion and readjustment in serum P and Ca.[45]

Fibroblast Growth Factor 23

FGF23, a bone derived hormone, in concert with its coreceptor Klotho, has a major role in the regulation of serum P concentration, although the mechanism by which FGF23-producing cells sense P remains to be elucidated.[46] Synthesized in bone, FGF23 is released into the circulation and acts on the proximal tubule to enhance, within hours, urinary P excretion by reducing the expression levels of NaPi-IIa and NaPi-IIc.[43] Furthermore, FGF23 decreases renal production of 1,25(OH)$_2$D and thus reduces intestinal P absorption (Fig. 5.2).[44]

FGF23 is part of the newly recognized endocrine bone–parathyroid–kidney axis modulated by PTH, 1,25(OH)$_2$D, and dietary and serum P levels.[46] Synthesis and secretion of FGF23 by osteocytes are upregulated by increased serum 1,25(OH)$_2$D and serum P and downregulated by P-regulating gene homologies to endopeptidases on the X chromosome (PHEX) and dentin matrix protein 1 (DMP1). In turn, FGF23 acts through FGF receptors, with Klotho as coreceptor, to inhibit renal P reabsorption,

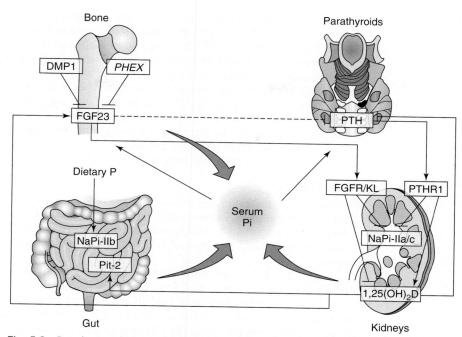

Fig. 5.2 Regulation of phosphate homeostasis. Phosphate is absorbed from the diet in the gut, stored in the skeleton, and excreted by the kidneys. 1,25-dihydroxyvitamin D [1,25(OH)$_2$D] stimulates absorption of phosphate from the diet. Fibroblast growth factor 23 (FGF23) increases renal phosphate clearance, suppresses synthesis of 1,25(OH)$_2$D, and may decrease parathyroid hormone (PTH; *dashed line*). PTH increases renal phosphate clearance and stimulates synthesis of 1,25(OH)$_2$D. *DMP1*, Dentin matrix protein 1; *FGFR/KL*, fibroblast growth factor receptor/Klotho; *NaPi*, sodium–phosphate cotransporter; *PHEX*, P-regulating gene homologies to endopeptidases on the X chromosome; *Pi*, phosphorus; *Pit-2*, Solute Carrier Family 20 (sodium-phosphate cotransporter), member 2; *PTHR1*, parathyroid hormone receptor 1. (From Bergwitz C, Jüppner H. Regulation of phosphate homeostasis by PTH, vitamin D, and FGF23. *Annu Rev Med.* 2010;61:91-104, with permission.)

1,25(OH)$_2$D synthesis, and parathyroid PTH secretion.[43,47] FGF23 synergizes with PTH to increase renal P excretion by reducing expression of renal NaPi-IIa and NaPi-IIc in the proximal tubules. Its net effect is reduction in serum P and 1,25(OH)$_2$D, which may result in hypocalcemia.

In early neonatal mineral metabolism, the role of FGF23, a novel regulator of P and vitamin D homeostasis, has not been evaluated. Recently, circulating FGF23 levels, using an intact FGF23 ELISA(iFGF23) and a C-terminal FGF23 ELISA(cFGF23), were measured in umbilical cord samples or in term infants at 5 days of life, and compared with healthy adult controls.[48] The iFGF23 (32 kDa) was low and the fragmented cFGF23 (18 kDa) was abundant in the cord blood compared with those in the healthy adults. By 5 days of life, the iFGF23 was increased to near adult concentration, and cFGF23 was twice adult values at cord blood and at 5 days of life. The iFGF23/cFGF23 ratio was very low due to the fragmentation of FGF23 during the early postpartum period, possibly indicating a considerable contribution to the P homeostasis in the healthy term infants.[48]

In healthy appropriate-for-gestational-age preterm infants (median gestational age of 31.2 weeks), iFGF23 and cFGF23 concentrations were persistently elevated at 1, 3, and 5 weeks of life and at term age, double and 10 times adult norms, respectively.[49] No infants were vitamin D deficient, and tubular reabsorption of P was normal (88% ± 8%). Persistent elevation of iFGF23 and cFGF23 was surprising. While the cFGF23 is elevated in both cord blood and at 5 days,[48] preterms maintained iFGF23 levels that were twice adult concentrations, and cFGF23 remained 10 times higher. It is not clear why cFGF23 is more markedly elevated in preterm than in term infants. Both forms of FGF23 have short half-lives of about 1 hour, and the higher concentrations of cFGF23 may reflect lack of clearance as well as rapid production of iFGF23. Of note, cFGF23 is known to inhibit iFGF23 by activating on its receptor in conjunction with alpha Klotho.[50] Considering the recent report of increased concentrations of Klotho in cord blood compared with adults, the elevated cFGF23 levels could possibly attenuate potent phosphaturic effects.[51] However, the biologic significance of the elevated FGF23 in preterm infants and in term infants at 5 days of life is unclear. Elevated FGF23 concentrations are most often associated with increased phosphaturia and are seen in a number of hereditary hypophosphatemic forms of rickets; increased levels are also described in a number of other disorders.[43,44] The role of FGF23 in early life remains to be established.

Renal Excretion

The kidneys are the major determinant of plasma P. Because intestinal P absorption is very efficient and fairly unregulated (only 30% is regulated by $1,25(OH)_2D$), renal P excretion is important in maintaining balance.[14] Serum P is maintained at close to the tubular P threshold, or TmP/GFR, via an active and saturable reabsorption process.[45]

Most filtered P is reabsorbed in the proximal tubule of the kidney through the NaPi-II. Increased P intake (e.g., from formula with a high P content) theoretically leads to rapid downregulation of NaPi-II mRNA and protein in the brush-border membrane of the proximal tubule and increased P excretion.[52] Renal P reabsorption lies under tight hormonal control by PTH and FGF23 (which inhibits P reabsorption) and, to a lesser extent, insulin and hormones of the somatotropic–pituitary axis.[43] In contrast, $1,25(OH)_2D$ synthesis, stimulated by decreased plasma P, has an indirect effect on renal P reabsorption via intestinal P absorption and bone P mobilization, resulting in increased serum P and suppression of PTH.

FGF23 principally functions as phosphaturic factor and counterregulates $1,25(OH)_2D$ production. Excess FGF23 secreted by osteocytes causes hypophosphatemia through inhibition of renal NaPi-II and suppresses $1,25(OH)_2D$ through inhibition of $25OHD-1\alpha$-hydroxylase and stimulation of 24-hydroxylase, which inactivates $1,25(OH)_2D$ in the proximal tubule. In contrast, deficiency of FGF23 results in hyperphosphatemia and elevated $1,25(OH)_2D$ production. In theory, downregulation of FGF23 could promote relative hyperphosphatemia and a relative increase in $1,25(OH)_2D$, promoting bone mineralization during early neonatal rapid growth.[46]

The kidneys contribute to positive P balance during growth by reabsorption of a relatively high fraction of filtered inorganic P (99% in newborns and 80% in adults). Growing infants, in particularly preterm infants, have high fractional reabsorption of P, reflecting their high P need. Age-related decrease in P reabsorption may relate to lower P needs with advancing age.[53]

Wide variation in serum P concentrations corresponds to few direct regulatory mechanisms. PTH, which has the greatest impact on serum P, primarily responds to changes in ionized Ca, not P. P is freely filtered at the glomerulus and presents to the renal tubules in high concentrations. The renal tubule reabsorbs P in both the proximal and distal nephrons. In states of low PTH, renal tubular cells reabsorb up to 95% to 97% of filtered P. In states of high PTH, P reabsorption in the proximal and distal tubules is inhibited, resulting in high urinary P excretion. Although markedly affected by PTH in the usual state, renal tubular cells have altered PTH responsiveness in severe P deficiency or overload. Hence, P is reabsorbed when there is severe P deficiency, even in high PTH states, and P is excreted when serum P is high despite low PTH.[54]

During early postnatal life, whereas renal P response to PTH is blunted, PTH increases tubular Ca reabsorption. Together these actions result in retention of both Ca and P in infants, which is favorable for growth. Maternal smoking during pregnancy negatively influences Ca-regulating hormones, leading to relative hypoparathyroidism in both the mother and newborn and lower PTH and 25-OHD in the smoking mother and newborn despite higher serum P.[55]

Clinical Disorders Associated With Abnormal Calcium and Phosphorus Homeostasis

Neonatal Hypocalcemia

Definition

Hypocalcemia is generally defined as serum total Ca below 2 mmol/L (8.0 mg/dL) in term and below 1.75 mmol/L (7 mg/dL) in preterm infants or ionized Ca below 0.75 to 1.1 mmol/L (3.0–4.4 mg/dL). "Early-onset" neonatal hypocalcemia typically occurs during the first few days of life, with the lowest Ca at 24 to 48 hours, and "late-onset" hypocalcemia occurs toward the end of the first week of life.

Etiology and Pathophysiology

Early-onset neonatal hypocalcemia is commonly associated with prematurity, birth asphyxia, maternal insulin-dependent diabetes, gestational anticonvulsant exposure, and maternal hyperparathyroidism. Late-onset hypocalcemia, which is less frequent, is commonly associated with relatively high P-containing diets, disturbed maternal vitamin D metabolism, intestinal malabsorption of Ca, hypomagnesemia, and hypoparathyroidism.[3,56,57]

Early-onset neonatal hypocalcemia represents exaggeration of normal serum Ca decrease during the first 24 to 48 hours of life; there is inadequate compensation for the sudden loss of placental Ca supply at birth (e.g., insufficient PTH release by immature parathyroids[8] or inadequate renal response to PTH). Preterm infants may or may not exhibit the surge in PTH secretion of term infants at birth, and restricted oral Ca intake aggravates the problem.[8,40] In asphyxiated infants, decreased Ca intake as a result of delayed feedings, increased endogenous P load, bicarbonate alkali therapy, and increased serum CT may contribute to the development of hypocalcemia. Hypocalcemia in infants of insulin-dependent diabetic mothers appears to be related to magnesium (Mg) insufficiency and consequent impaired PTH secretion. Mg is important in PTH secretion and action; chronic Mg deficiency causes impaired PTH secretion and PTH resistance at target organs.[7] Transient neonatal hypoparathyroidism occurs in infants exposed to maternal hypercalcemia in utero. Intrauterine hypercalcemia suppresses fetal parathyroids and apparently impairs PTH production response to hypocalcemia after birth.[58]

Late-onset hypocalcemia commonly results from dietary Ca and P imbalance and rarely may result from maternal hypercalcemia. Infants receiving cow's milk–derived formulas have lower serum ionized Ca and high serum P in the first week compared with breastfed infants, related to a higher absolute P amount of formula[59] or limited P excretion from low newborn GFR. P-containing enemas cause P overload and hypocalcemia.[60] Late hypocalcemia may relate to resistance of immature kidneys to PTH, leading to renal P retention and hypocalcemia; biochemical features resemble pseudohypoparathyroidism (defects in the *GNAS1* gene), but with normal nephrogenous cAMP responses to PTH.[61]

Congenital hypoparathyroidism is the most significant cause of late-onset hypocalcemia that has to be treated early. Congenital hypoparathyroidism may be a part of DiGeorge triad of hypoparathyroidism; T-cell incompetence (partial or absent thymus on chest radiograph); and conotruncal heart defects or aortic arch abnormalities, which suggest 22q11 syndrome (CARCH22 or DiGeorge sequence).[62]

Isolated hypoparathyroidism includes genetic defects that impair PTH synthesis (PTH gene defects)[63] or secretion (CASR gene defects) or parathyroid gland development (GCMB gene defects; parathyroid agenesis).[64] Gain-of-function (activating) mutations in the CASR gene-encoding CaSR are the most common cause of mild isolated hypoparathyroidism (autosomal dominant hypocalcemia), associated with inappropriately low or low-normal serum PTH and relative hypercalciuria.[23–25]

Clinical Presentation

Neonates with hypocalcemia may be asymptomatic; the less mature the infant is, the more subtle and varied the clinical manifestations will be. Main clinical signs are jitteriness, tremors, twitching, and exaggerated startle responses or seizures (generalized or focal). Frank convulsions are seen more commonly with late hypocalcemia. Infants also may be lethargic, feed poorly, vomit, and have abdominal distension. Apnea, cyanosis, tachypnea, tachycardia, vomiting, or heart failure may also be seen. The classic signs of peripheral hyperexcitability of motor nerves (carpopedal spasm and laryngospasm) are uncommon in newborns.

Diagnosis

The diagnosis of hypocalcemia is based on serum ionized or total Ca levels, history, and physical examination; serum P, Mg and glucose, and serum pH are helpful. Functional atrioventricular block from electrocardiographic prolonged QTc interval (>0.4 second) suggests hypocalcemia.[65]

When an infant is refractory to therapy or there are unusual findings, measurement of PTH, 25OHD, and 1,25(OH)$_2$D may be useful in establishing the less common causes (e.g., primary hypoparathyroidism, malabsorption, and vitamin D metabolism disorders) of hypocalcemia. Normal to moderately elevated 1,25(OH)$_2$D levels are consistent with hypoparathyroidism. Hypercalciuria (urinary Ca ≥4 mg/kg/day or urine Ca:creatinine ratio ≥0.2 [mg/mg]) associated with hypocalcemia supports low PTH states.

Prolonged hypocalcemia should prompt investigation of permanent causes, such as hypoparathyroidism. DNA analysis for causal mutations may help confirm the diagnosis in proband and relatives.[66]

Therapeutic Approaches

Treatment of symptomatic hypocalcemia is by intravenous (IV) Ca infusion with a dosage of 30 to 75 mg/kg/day of elemental Ca, titrated to clinical and biochemical response, to maintain ionized Ca in the low-normal range. Clinical hypocalcemia signs are usually reversed rapidly by correcting serum Ca, which helps confirm the diagnosis.

During seizures (serum Ca usually <1.5 mmol/L [6 mg/dL]), emergency Ca (1–2 mL/kg of Ca gluconate 10%; ≈9–18 mg/kg of elemental Ca) is given IV over 10 minutes as heart rate is measured continuously to prevent bradycardia. If this complication occurs, Ca infusion should be discontinued temporarily. Another complication of Ca infusion is potential skin tissue injury from infusate extravasation. A follow-up bolus or intermittent infusions of Ca salts are avoided because of wide serum Ca excursions.

For less urgent purposes or for follow-up after initial seizure treatment, continuous IV administration of 75 mg/kg/day of elemental Ca will maintain normocalcemia. Afterward, stepwise IV Ca reduction may help prevent rebound hypocalcemia (75 mg/kg/day for the first day, a half dose the next day, a half dose the third day, and discontinued the fourth day). Alternatively, if oral fluids are tolerated, the same dose of Ca gluconate can be given orally, divided among four to six doses per day after initial correction. Oral Ca may not be practical in sick infants because of bowel stimulation; proprietary oral Ca preparations are hypertonic (high osmolar) and are not used in infants at risk of necrotizing enterocolitis. Vitamin D metabolites are not useful for early hypocalcemia because of variable response and side effects.

With persistent hypocalcemia, serum Mg is measured because hypomagnesemic hypocalcemia cannot be corrected until hypomagnesemia is alleviated. Hypomagnesemia (serum Mg <0.6 mmol/L [1.5 mg/dL]) is treated with Mg sulfate 50% solution (500 mg or 4 mEq/mL), 0.1 to 0.2 mL/kg, IV or intramuscular (may cause local tissue necrosis) and repeated after 12 to 24 hours. Serum Mg is obtained before each dose (one or two doses may resolve transient hypomagnesemia).

Because most causes of neonatal hypocalcemia are transient, therapy duration varies with cause; commonly, as little as 2 to 3 days for early hypocalcemia is needed. Ca supplementation is usually required for long periods in hypocalcemia from malabsorption or hypoparathyroidism.

In neonates at risk, early hypocalcemia can be prevented by early oral feeding or parenteral Ca supplementation (75 mg/kg/day of elemental Ca continuously) to maintain total Ca above 2 mmol/L (8.0 mg/dL) and ionized Ca above 1 mmol/L (4.0 mg/dL). This may help prevent hypocalcemia in sick newborns with cardiovascular compromise requiring cardiotonic drugs or pressure support.

Most asymptomatic neonatal hypocalcemia resolves spontaneously with time, but hypocalcemia has potential adverse effects on the cardiovascular and central nervous systems, so treatment may be needed.[9] For asymptomatic ill infants and infants with severe hypocalcemia (serum total Ca <1.5 mmol/L [6.0 mg/dL] or ionized Ca <0.75 mmol/L [3 mg/dL]), either IV or oral therapy is usually required. In sick infants, judicious bicarbonate use and avoidance of respiratory alkalosis from excessive ventilation may reduce the risk of symptomatic hypocalcemia.

For late hypocalcemia, treatment goals are to reduce the P load and increase Ca absorption by using feedings with a Ca-to-P ratio of 4:1 or greater, such as use of low-P feedings (human milk or low-P formula) in conjunction with an oral Ca supplement.

Treatment of hypoparathyroidism is directed at maintaining plasma Ca to prevent symptoms without causing nephrocalcinosis. Hypoparathyroidism requires therapy with $1,25(OH)_2D$ (or 1 α-hydroxyvitamin D_3, a synthetic analog) and lifelong Ca supplementation. Infants with severe or persistent hypocalcemia may benefit from $1,25(OH)_2D$, IV or orally, 50 to 100 ng/kg/day in two or three divided doses. Close follow-up is required to monitor the serum Ca level. When serum Ca level is normalized, administration of $1,25(OH)_2D$ may be discontinued to prevent hypercalcemia.

Recombinant PTH (teriparatide)[67] has been tried as initial management of neonatal hypoparathyroidism. In infants with life-threatening seizures and persistent hypocalcemia despite aggressive management with high doses of $1,25(OH)_2D$ and Ca infusion, short-term use of teriparatide (5 μg subcutaneously) can raise Ca levels faster (in <4 hours) than other commonly used methods, which take 1 day or longer.[68] Theoretically, teriparatide is safer and is a more physiologic means of correcting acute hypoparathyroid hypocalcemia; however, there is a concern regarding the risk of osteosarcoma related to long-term exposure.

Neonatal Hypercalcemia

Definition

Neonatal hypercalcemia is serum total Ca greater than 2.75 mmol/L (11 mg/dL) or ionized Ca greater than 1.4 mM/L (5.6 mg/dL).

Etiology and Pathophysiology

Hypercalcemia is uncommon in term infants but relatively common in preterm infants. The most common causes are relative deficiency in P supply and hypophosphatemia from inappropriate parenteral nutrition (PN), with or without excessive Ca or human milk feeding in preterm infants (low P content relative to preterm needs).[69] Iatrogenic hypercalcemia results from excessive Ca or vitamin D for hypocalcemia or during exchange transfusion. Chronic maternal exposure to excessive vitamin D or metabolites, secondary to treatment of maternal hypocalcemic disorders, may cause hypercalcemia of the mother and neonate. Chronic diuretic therapy with thiazides during pregnancy may lead to maternal, fetal, and neonatal hypercalcemia.[70]

Other rarer causes include hyperparathyroidism (primary or secondary to maternal hypoparathyroidism) and hypercalcemia associated with subcutaneous fat necrosis, idiopathic infantile hypercalcemia, severe infantile hypophosphatasia, and a Bartter syndrome variant. Primary hyperparathyroidism is rare in neonates and children.

Elevated serum Ca in pathologic conditions with PTH or vitamin D overactivity implies increased Ca efflux into ECF from bone, intestine, or kidney. Hypophosphatemia increases circulating $1,25(OH)_2D$, which increases intestinal Ca absorption and bone resorption; Ca is not deposited in bone in the absence of P and contributes to hypercalcemia.

Homozygous inactivating mutations of CaSR produce severe hypercalcemia, termed *neonatal severe primary hyperparathyroidism* (NSPHT). Heterozygous inactivating mutations of CaSR produce a "benign" hypercalcemia, termed *familial hypocalciuric hypercalcemia* (FHH), inherited as an autosomal dominant trait with high penetrance.[24] Mutations in Ca^{+2}-sensor lead to a dual defect in parathyroid cells (causing parathyroid hyperplasia) and renal tubules (causing hypocalciuria). FHH and NSHPT are associated with mutations in the *CASR* gene at 3q13.3-21 in nearly all affected subjects[24,25]; in some families, the disorder is linked to unknown genes on the long or short arms of chromosome 19.[71]

Hypercalcemia associated with subcutaneous fat necrosis occurs in asphyxiated, large-for-gestational-age infants; possible mechanisms are increased prostaglandin E (PGE) activity, increased Ca release from fat and tissues, and unregulated production of $1,25(OH)_2D$ from macrophages infiltrating fat necrotic lesions.

Idiopathic infantile hypercalcemia (which may be part of Williams syndrome) is associated with mutations in the elastin gene on the long arm of chromosome 7; there may be a vitamin D hyperresponsive state and blunted CT response to Ca loading. Infantile hypophosphatasia is a rare autosomal recessive disorder that may be lethal in utero or shortly after birth because of inadequate bony support of the thorax and skull. Bartter variant–related hypercalcemia is associated with polyhydramnios and prematurity; in utero hypercalcemia may result in fetal hypercalciuria and polyuria, leading to early delivery; increased serum $1,25(OH)_2D$, normal serum PTH, and increased urinary PGE_2 are present.

Clinical Presentation

Clinical features of hypercalcemia depend on the underlying disorder, age, and degree of hypercalcemia. Its onset may be at birth or delayed for weeks or months. Neonates with hypercalcemia may be asymptomatic or have serious clinical signs (especially in hyperparathyroidism) requiring urgent treatment. Infants with mild increases in serum Ca (2.65–3.25 mmol/L [11–13 mg/dL]) often have no specific signs. Mild hypercalcemia may present as feeding difficulties or poor linear growth. Unrecognized hypercalcemia can result in significant morbidity or death.[72]

With moderate to severe hypercalcemia, nonspecific signs, such as anorexia, vomiting and constipation (rarely diarrhea), polyuria, and dehydration, may occur. Infants with chronic hypercalcemia may present with failure to thrive (poor growth). Severe hypercalcemia can affect the nervous system and cause lethargy, drowsiness, irritability, confusion, and seizure; in extreme cases, stupor and coma ensue. Thus, timely recognition and treatment of hypercalcemia are critical. In severely affected infants, hypertension, respiratory distress (caused by hypotonia and demineralization and deformation of the rib cage), nephrocalcinosis (from long-standing hypercalcemia), and band keratopathy of the limbus of the eye (rare) may be present. Associated features, such as elfin faces, cardiac murmur, and mental retardation (in Williams syndrome) and bluish-red skin indurations (in subcutaneous fat necrosis), may be present on physical examination.

Diagnosis

The diagnosis may be made incidentally on routine chemistry screening. The workup may include serum total Ca, ionized Ca, P, Mg, alkaline phosphatase, pH, total protein, creatinine, electrolytes, PTH, and 25OHD; urine Ca, P, tubular reabsorption of P, and cAMP with renal function evaluation; and chest and hand x-ray radiography, abdominal ultrasonography, ophthalmologic evaluation, and electrocardiography (i.e., shortened QT interval) to determine the effect of hypercalcemia.

Very elevated serum Ca (>3.75 mmol/L [15 mg/dL]) usually indicates primary hyperparathyroidism or P depletion in VLBW infants. To differentiate parathyroid from nonparathyroid conditions, measurements include serum P (low in hyperparathyroidism, FHH, and rickets of prematurity), percent renal tubular P reabsorption (<85% in hyperparathyroidism; high in rickets of prematurity associated with hypophosphatemia), and serum PTH (elevated in hyperparathyroidism). A very low urinary Ca/urinary creatinine ratio [U_{ca}/U_{cr}] in the face of hypercalcemia suggests FHH.

The diagnosis of NSPHT is based on inappropriately normal or elevated PTH along with relative hypocalciuria in severe hypercalcemia (high Ca levels, 5–6 mmol/L

[20–24 mg/dL]). Hyperparathyroidism causes erosion of bone (particularly along long bone subperiosteal margins; a "moth-eaten" appearance), which may be mistaken for rickets. In contrast to NSPHT, FHH infants usually remain asymptomatic. PTH is usually in the normal range, but inappropriately high for hypercalcemia. Urine Ca excretion is low, and nephrocalcinosis is not a problem. A family history of FHH or NSPHT in a sibling provides a strong confirmation. Care must be taken to distinguish these disorders from transient neonatal hyperparathyroidism associated with maternal hypocalcemia (e.g., in maternal pseudohypoparathyroidism or renal tubular acidosis).[73]

DNA analysis for FHH and NSPHT is available in few laboratories and requires molecular analysis of the entire *CASR* gene in a proband. Relatives of the patient's proband may be studied for genetic abnormalities and serum Ca.[66]

Bone radiographs identify demineralization, osteolytic lesions (hyperparathyroidism), or osteosclerotic lesions (occasionally with vitamin D excess).

A maternal dietary and drug history (e.g., excessive vitamin A or D, thiazides) or history of possible mineral disturbances or polyhydramnios during pregnancy should be sought. Family screening will depend on the primary diagnosis.

Additional information concerning nephrocalcinosis from hypercalcemia or soft tissue calcification (e.g., in basal ganglia) can be obtained by ultrasonography or computed tomography. If hyperparathyroidism is diagnosed (rarely), localization of a parathyroid adenoma or hyperplasia by radionuclide scintigraphy may be useful.[66]

Therapeutic Approaches

Therapy includes correction of specific underlying causes and removal of iatrogenic or external causes (e.g., surgical removal of hyperparathyroid glands, stopping excessive Ca or vitamin D intake). Treatment of neonatal hyperparathyroidism depends on the severity. For mild asymptomatic hypercalcemia in a thriving infant, conservative management is appropriate. For moderate to severe hypercalcemia, prompt investigation and more aggressive therapy are instituted; stopping excessive dietary Ca and vitamin D intake and maintenance of adequate hydration are mainstays; and renal Ca excretion is enhanced by loop-acting diuretics. Reduced dietary Ca intakes by low Ca formula and inhibition of bone resorption by antibone resorptive agent may be used.

For short-term treatment of acute hypercalcemic episodes (symptomatic or serum Ca >3.5 mmol/L [14 mg/dL]), expansion of the ECF with 10 to 20 mL/kg of 0.9% sodium chloride IV followed by IV 1 mg/kg of furosemide every 6 to 8 hours may be effective by increasing urinary Ca excretion. Fluid and electrolyte imbalance is avoided by monitoring of fluid balance and serum Ca, P, Mg, sodium, potassium, and osmolarity; reduced GFR from dehydration can worsen hypercalcemia.

For restriction of dietary intakes of Ca and vitamin D, a low-Ca, low–vitamin D_3 infant formula containing trace Ca amounts (<10 mg/100 kcal versus standard formula, 78 mg/100 kcal) and no vitamin D (also low iron) is available for short- to medium-term management (CalciloXD, Ross Laboratories, Columbus, Ohio); iron supplement is needed. As hypercalcemia resolves, usual formula or human milk (≈10 mg/oz of Ca) can be mixed with the CalciloXD to increase Ca intake, closely monitoring serum and urine Ca to prevent rickets or hypocalcemia.

Adjuvant therapies in acute hypercalcemia are CT, glucocorticoids, bisphosphonate, and dialysis. Minimal information is available in neonatal hypercalcemia. Symptomatic infants with nonparathyroid hypercalcemia may require long-term CT or bisphosphonates. Short-term salmon CT (4–8 IU/kg every 6 to 12 hours subcutaneously or intramuscularly), prednisone (1–2 mg/kg/day), or a combination may be useful. The hypocalcemic effect of CT (a potent inhibitor of bone resorption) is transient and abates after a few days, which is not ideal for chronic therapy; effects may be prolonged with concomitant glucocorticoids, although there is limited experience in neonates.

High-dose glucocorticoids reduce intestinal Ca absorption and may decrease bone resorption; methylprednisolone (1–2 mg/kg/day IV), hydrocortisone (10 mg/kg/day IV), or the equivalent is effective, but is not recommended for long-term use because of many undesirable side effects. Although effective in several types of hypercalcemia, glucocorticoids are relatively ineffective in patients with primary hyperparathyroidism.

Bisphosphonate (an antibone resorptive agent) may be useful to treat hypercalcemia that is PTH mediated and for subcutaneous fat necrosis. Infants with NSPHT and marked hypercalcemia should be managed aggressively. In the past, treatment was urgent subtotal parathyroidectomy; more recent options include IV bisphosphonates (pamidronate 0.5–2.0 mg/kg) with parathyroidectomy delayed until the patient is clinically stable.[74,75] Bisphosphonate therapy seems safe in the short term and effective in controlling hypercalcemia even in very premature infants, allowing for planned surgery when feasible.

For severe and unremitting hypercalcemia, either hemodialysis (HD) if the patient is hemodynamically stable or peritoneal dialysis (PD) with a low-Ca dialysate (1.25 mM/L) may be helpful. To avoid iatrogenic mineral depletion, for HD or PD, supplemental P or Mg is given orally or IV, or sodium phosphate is added to PD solution (<0.75 mM); in PD, crystal formation in bags should be inspected hourly and fresh solutions changed every 8 hours.

Neonatal Hypophosphatemia

Definition

Hypophosphatemia is serum P below 1.65 mmol/L (4 mg/dL). Conventionally, hypophosphatemia is often graded as mild when serum P is below 1.45 mmol/L (<3.5 mg/dL), moderate when it is below 1.0 mmol/L (<2.5 mg/dL), and severe when it is below 0.4 mmol/L (<1.0 mg/dL).

Etiology and Pathophysiology

Hypophosphatemia occurs when there is decreased P intake (decreased intestinal absorption or increased intestinal loss) or excess renal wasting from a renal tubular defect or hyperparathyroidism. P deficiency is seen in preterm infants with rickets of prematurity resulting from inadequate Ca and P intakes.[3]

The pathophysiologic consequences of P deficiency are attributable to both direct and indirect effects of hypophosphatemia. P deficiency may directly enhance bone resorption and decrease matrix formation and bone mineralization. When serum P decreases, renal P excretion decreases and renal 1,25(OH)$_2$D production increases, which in turn increases intestinal Ca absorption and mainly stimulates bone resorption, releasing P and Ca (possibly a compensatory mechanism in an attempt to maintain serum P for essential function).[76] The excess Ca results in hypercalcemia and hypercalciuria. Serum P remains low because P released from bone is used in intracellular metabolism. In VLBW infants, increased Ca absorbed from the gut or mobilized from the bone by 1,25(OH)$_2$D may not be used for bone mineralization and leads to "excess" filtered Ca being excreted in the urine.[76]

P deficiency is closely linked to metabolic bone disease in VLBW infants because P promotes bone formation and matrix production and limits bone resorption. In rats, P deficiency produces a histologic picture distinct from vitamin D deficiency.[77]

In preterm infants, a P depletion syndrome occurs in infants fed human milk,[76] with restricted enteral mineral intakes (mineral-unfortified formula), and with chronic illnesses receiving prolonged PN without mineral supplements.[78] In the latter group, biochemical signs of extreme P deficiency are prominent, with rachitic bone changes; serum 1,25(OH)$_2$D increases with increased bone resorption and turnover (increased serum bone resorption marker, cross-linked carboxyterminal telopeptide of type I collagen and osteocalcin).[79]

Pathophysiologic results of P deficiency are inadequate supplies of energy-rich P and, in particular, inhibition of glyceraldehyde-3-phosphate dehydrogenase, which occupies a key position in glycolysis. The effect of P deficiency on energy metabolism is to reduce adenosine triphosphate (ATP) and 2,3-diphosphoglycerate, leading a shift of the oxygen-hemoglobin dissociation curve to the left, with decreased peripheral oxygen uptake and transport.[80]

Prolonged starvation, malabsorption, and chronic diarrhea cause hypophosphatemia related to decreased intestinal absorption. A chronically malnourished patient is often in a catabolic state, associated with muscle breakdown and subsequent loss of intracellular P.[81] When patients subsequently receive nutrition support, they may receive a P-depleted feed, especially with PN, when large volumes of carbohydrate and amino acid solutions raise endogenous P requirements, and unbalanced amino acid solutions may induce further urinary P losses. If P replacement is insufficient, then hypophosphatemia will ensue.[82]

Diseases of vitamin D metabolism (vitamin D–dependent rickets) or renal P transport disorders (familial hypophosphatemic rickets) may lead to P deficiency in later infancy. Mutations in *FGF23* are the cause of autosomal dominant hypophosphatemic rickets[83]; and in dentin matrix protein 1 (DMP1) are a cause of autosomal recessive hypophosphatemia.[84] Mutations in the P-regulating gene *(PHEX)* occur in XLH, the most frequent form of renal P wasting.[85] In addition, low serum P may also occur in extracellular to intracellular shifts from respiratory alkalosis. In the case of cellular shifts, total body P may not be depleted.

Clinical Presentation

P deficiency is accompanied by weakness, malaise, and anorexia. Bone pain, frequently occurring in growing children with hypophosphatemic rickets, is not present in neonates with hypophosphatemia. There are no easily recognizable symptoms. Signs of hypophosphatemia are usually only seen with moderate to severe hypophosphatemia. Severe hypophosphatemia has deleterious effects on muscular, cardiac, pulmonary, hematologic, and nervous system function, including muscle weakness, poor ventricular function, and difficulty weaning from a ventilator (poor tissue oxygenation), essentially because P depletion leads to a decrease in high-energy substrate availability and respiratory muscle function (impaired diaphragm contractility).[77,86] The mechanism of muscle weakness and red blood cell dysfunction caused by hypophosphatemia may relate to the role of P in intracellular signal transduction and synthesis of ATP or creatine phosphate.[14] Other manifestations are hemolysis; impaired platelet and white blood cell function; rhabdomyolysis; and in rare cases, neurologic disorders, peripheral neuropathy, convulsions, and coma.

Physical examination of VLBW infants with P deficiency is usually benign. Clinical evidence of osteopenia or rickets is present infrequently, and pathologic fractures of the ribs or limbs are late occurrences. The clinician is, therefore, dependent on biochemical tests and radiography to detect early bone disease.

Therapeutic Approaches

Because hypophosphatemia is the most prominent feature of P deficiency in preterm infants, extra P supplement has been given; however, hypocalcemia occurs after P supplementation alone, and about 66% of supplemented P is lost in urine. In addition, these infants are Ca deficient as well as P deficient; P-induced decreases in serum Ca may lead to secondary hyperparathyroidism; large amounts of supplemental P cannot be used and are wasted in urine. Thus, both P and Ca supplements (and not P alone) are necessary to avert hypocalcemia and to allow adequate bone mineral accretion.[77] Recent recommendation of enteral Ca supplementation is 120 to 200 mg/kg/day, and the recommendation for P is 70 to 120 mg/kg/day with vitamin D 400 IU/day, which allows normophosphatemia and normocalciuria with normal vitamin D status.[1]

Provision of P and Ca in total PN solution with a Ca-to-P ratio of 1.3 to 1.7 to 1 (500–600 mg of Ca/L and 400–450 mg of P/L of PN solution) allows optimal mineral retention for preterm infants, reaching intakes of Ca of 100 mg/kg/day and P of 65 mg/kg/day.[1,87] Sodium glycerophosphate (1 mmol/L organic P) improve solubility in PN.[88] P accumulation in preterm infants is correlated with a protein content: N-to-P ratio of 17 to 1 by weight (P retained = Ca retained/2.3 + N retained/17). Adequate supply of protein is also important for normal bone formation and mineralization. Considering optimal N retention of 350 to 400 mg/kg/day and provision of

100 mg/kg/day of Ca, the P supply must reach 65 mg/kg/day corresponding to a Ca-to-P ratio close to 1.5.[87]

In hypophosphatemia with high serum Ca, supplements of 0.5 to 1.0 mM/kg/day (16–31 mg/kg/day) of elemental phosphate in divided oral doses may normalize serum P and lower serum Ca; parenteral phosphate, however, should be avoided in severe hypercalcemia (serum total Ca >3 mmol/L [12 mg/dL]) unless hypophosphatemia is severe (<1.5 mg/dL) because extraskeletal calcification theoretically may occur.[69,89]

Neonatal Hyperphosphatemia

Definition

Hyperphosphatemia is a serum level greater than 3.3 mmol/L (8 mg/dL), which reflects P overload.

Etiology and Pathophysiology

Hyperphosphatemia occurs from medication errors,[90–92] increased intestinal absorption, decreased renal excretion, and cellular release or rapid intracellular to extracellular shifts. Increased tissue P release is commonly seen in profound catabolic states.

In steady state, serum P is maintained primarily by the ability of the kidneys to excrete dietary P, with efficient renal excretion. However, if acute P load is given over several hours, transient hyperphosphatemia will ensue.[90–92] In addition to absorption of excess P, volume contraction (caused by diarrhea) and renal insufficiency (caused by volume depletion and decreased renal perfusion) may contribute to hyperphosphatemia and hypocalcemia.[93]

Hyperphosphatemia is frequently the result of increased parenteral unbalanced administration of Ca, P, and Mg or a medication error (sodium phosphate instead of Ca gluconate).[90] Increased intestinal absorption is generally caused by a large oral P intake[91] and a vitamin D overdose in preterm infants or an erroneous medical prescription (oral phosphate Joulie's solution instead of alkaline solution) in newborn infants with renal insufficiency.[92]

Life-threatening hyperphosphatemia occurs after inadvertent administration of a hypertonic Fleet enema (60 mL of pediatric formula containing 105.4 mEq of P and 130.7 mEq of Na) in newborn infants, causing hyperphosphatemia and hypocalcemia; an osmotically active high P concentration in the enema solution results in excess retention and toxicity.[93] A phosphate-containing enema (Fleet Co, Lynchburg, Virginia) is particularly dangerous in renal insufficiency or bowel dysfunction (constipation), although even without predisposing factors, a P enema can result in severe toxicity if retained.[94]

Infants receiving cow's milk–derived formulas that contain high P (67–81 mg/dL of P) who have impaired renal excretion or hypoparathyroidism may develop hyperphosphatemia. Even in normal term infants, higher serum P and lower serum ionized Ca occur in the first week, versus breastfed infants, related to higher absolute P in formula and limited P excretion from low newborn GFR.[60] The biochemical features of high serum P and low serum Ca can resemble those of pseudohypoparathyroidism[61] because there may be resistance of the immature kidneys to PTH. Persistent hyperphosphatemia occurs almost exclusively in those with acute or chronic kidney disease.

Clinical Presentation

Acute hyperphosphatemia generally does not cause signs unless the patient has hypocalcemia. In patients given high bolus doses of P orally or rectally, symptomatic acute P intoxication occurs, presenting with severe life-threatening hyperphosphatemia and hypocalcemia; carpopedal spasm[92]; vomiting; apnea; cyanosis on mechanical ventilation; hypoactivity, severe dehydration, and shock[60]; depressed level of consciousness (lethargy); shallow, difficult respirations; and generalized seizure.[93] These patients are unresponsive to multiple doses of lorazepam, but responsive only to IV Ca. Clinical signs of chronic hyperphosphatemia include ectopic mineralization of muscular and subcutaneous tissues.

Therapeutic Approaches

P intoxication is a life-threatening condition. Treatment of P-induced hypocalcemia involves increasing urinary P excretion with diuretics and hydration (isotonic solution 20 mL/kg) and administrating IV Ca in symptomatic patients (avoiding lethal cardiac instability despite concern of Ca and P deposition in the kidneys) or oral Ca as an enteral P binder (promoting fecal excretion); enteral feedings with a low-P formula or human milk; and reducing parenteral P administration.[92,93]

Ca correction is required to prevent or treat potential severe adverse effects, including cardiovascular abnormalities (prolonged QT interval, specifically ST segment), tetany, and seizures.[92] Ca chloride (IV) is generally used for acute therapy in severe cases because it contains the highest concentration of ionized Ca compared with other Ca salts. However, in patients with limited or poor venous access, IV Ca gluconate is preferred because of the potential risk of peripheral extravasation. Ca should be administered with caution and only to alleviate clinical signs related to hypocalcemic toxicity. In the presence of severe hyperphosphatemia, Ca replacement can lead to extraskeletal calcification, especially in the renal tubule.[94]

Treatment of severe life-threatening hyperphosphatemia secondary to retention of an enema may include modalities to prevent further absorption (e.g., lavage).[60] Additionally, dialysis or hemofiltration can be used to rapidly lower the P concentration in renally impaired oliguric patients. Because PD strongly depends on total dialysate turnover, continuous flow-through PD, a closed PD system using two sterile polyvinylpyrrolidone short-term urethral catheters (6 Fr in and 8 Fr out) manufactured in Brazil, has been successfully applied in neonatal enema-induced hyperphosphatemia (8-day-old newborn) after achieving hemodynamic stability with vigorous fluid resuscitation and vasoactive drugs.[60]

In children with chronic renal failure, secondary hyperparathyroidism can be suppressed using mild dietary P reduction and high-dose P binders with small vitamin D supplementation. Ca carbonate is an effective P binder with no major side effects and is a drug of choice in correcting hyperphosphatemia and hyperparathyroidism in uremic children,[95] although neonatal use of Ca carbonate has not been reported.

REFERENCES

1. Atkinson SA, Tsang RC. Calcium, magnesium, phosphorus, and vitamin D. In: Tsang RC, Uauy R, Koletzko B, Zlotkin SH, eds. *Nutrition of the Preterm Infant*. 2nd ed. Cincinnati, Ohio: Digital Education Publishing; 2005:245–276.
2. Mitchell DM, Jüppner H. Regulation of calcium homeostasis and bone metabolism in the fetus and neonate. *Curr Opin Endocrinol Diabetes Obes*. 2010;17:25–30.
3. Namgung R, Tsang RC. Neonatal calcium, phosphorus, and magnesium homeostasis. In: Polin RA, Abman HS, Rowitch DH, et al, eds. *Fetal and Neonatal Physiology*. 5th ed. Philadelphia: Elsevier; 2017:296–312.
4. Abrams SA. In utero physiology: role in nutrient delivery and fetal development for calcium, phosphorus, and vitamin D. *Am J Clin Nutr*. 2007;85(suppl):604S–607S.
5. Bowers GN Jr, Brassard C, Sena SF, et al. Measurement of ionized calcium in serum with ion-selective electrodes: a mature technology that can meet the daily service needs. *Clin Chem*. 1986;32:1437–1447.
6. Wandrup J, Kroner J, Pryds O, et al. Age-related reference values for ionized calcium in the first week of life in premature and full-term neonates. *Scand J Clin Lab Invest*. 1988;48:255–260.
7. Loughead JL, Mimouni F, Tsang RC, et al. A role for Mg in neonatal parathyroid gland function. *J Am Coll Nutr*. 1991;10:123–126.
8. Venkataraman PS, Blick KE, Fry HD, et al. Postnatal changes in calcium-regulating hormones in very-low-birth-weight infants. *Am J Dis Child*. 1985;39:913–916.
9. Venkataraman PS, Wilson DA, Sheldon RE, et al. Effect of hypocalcemia on cardiac function in very-low-birth-weight preterm neonates: studies of blood ionized calcium, echocardiography, and cardiac effect of intravenous calcium therapy. *Pediatrics*. 1985;76:543–550.
10. Namgung R, Tsang RC, Specker BL, et al. Low bone mineral content and high serum osteocalcin and 1,25-dihydroxyvitamin D in summer- versus winter-born newborn infants: an early fetal effect? *J Pediatr Gastroenterol Nutr*. 1994;19:220–227.
11. Bagnoli F, Bruchi S, Garasi G, et al. Relationship between mode of delivery and neonatal calcium homeostasis. *Eur J Pediatr*. 1990;149:800–803.
12. Namgung R, Tsang RC, Specker BL, et al. Reduced serum osteocalcin and 1,25-dihydroxyvitamin D concentrations and low bone mineral content in small for gestational age infants: evidence of decreased bone formation rates. *J Pediatr*. 1993;122:269–275.
13. Williford AL, Pare LM, Carlson GT. Bone mineral metabolism in the neonate: calcium, phosphorus, magnesium, and alkaline phosphatase. *Neonatal Netw*. 2008;27:57–63.

14. Bergwitz C, Jüppner H. Disorders of phosphate homeostasis and tissue mineralization. In: Allgrove J, Shaw NJ, eds. *Calcium and Bone Disorders in Children and Adolescents. Endocr Dev.* Vol. 16. Basel: Karger AG; 2009:133–156.

15. Kovacs CS. Calcium, phosphorus, and bone metabolism in the fetus and newborn. *Early Hum Dev.* 2015;9:623–628.

16. Suzuki Y, Kovacs CS, Takanaga H, et al. Calcium channel TRPV6 is involved in murine maternal-fetal-calcium transport. *J Bone Miner Res.* 2008;23:1249–1256.

17. Belkacemi L, Bedard I, Simoneau L, et al. Calcium channels, transporters and exchangers in placenta: a review. *Cell Calcium.* 2005;37:1–8.

18. Kovacs CS. Bone metabolism in the fetus and neonate. *Pediatr Nephrol.* 2014;29:793–803.

19. Kovacs CS, Manley NR, Moseley JM, et al. Fetal parathyroids are not required to maintain placental calcium transport. *J Clin Invest.* 2001;107(8):1007–1015.

20. Miao D, He B, Karaplis AC, et al. Parathyroid hormone is essential for normal fetal bone formation. *J Clin Invest.* 2002;109:1173–1182.

21. Kovacs CS, Lanske B, Hunzelman JL, et al. Parathyroid hormone-related peptide (PTHrP) regulates fetal-placental calcium transport through a receptor distinct from the PTH/PTHrP receptor. *Proc Natl Acad Sci USA.* 1996;93:15233–15238.

22. Bond H, Dilworth MR, Baker B, et al. Increased maternofetal calcium flux in parathyroid hormone-related protein-null mice. *J Physiol.* 2008;586:2015–2025.

23. Bai M, Quinn S, Trivedi S, et al. Expression and characterization of inactivating and activating mutations in the human Cao2+o-sensing receptor. *J Biol Chem.* 1996;271:19537–19545.

24. Egbuna OI, Brown EM. Hypercalcemic and hypocalcemic conditions due to calcium-sensing receptor mutations. *Best Pract Res Clin Rheumatol.* 2008;22:129–148.

25. Brown EM. The calcium-sensing receptor: physiology, pathophysiology and car-based therapeutics. *Subcell Biochem.* 2007;45:139–167.

26. Karlen J, Aperia A, Zetterstrom R. Renal excretion of calcium and phosphate in preterm and term infants. *J Pediatr.* 1985;106:814–819.

27. Mallet E, Basuyau JP, Brunelle P, et al. Neonatal parathyroid secretion and renal maturation in premature infants. *Biol Neonate.* 1978;33:304–308.

28. Altirkawi K, Rozycki H. Hypocalcemia is common in the first 48 h of life in ELBW infants. *J Perinat Med.* 2008;36:348–353.

29. Novakovic B, Sibson M, Ng HK, et al. Placenta-specific methylation of the vitamin D 24-hydroxylase gene: implications for feedback autoregulation of active vitamin D levels at the fetomaternal interface. *J Biol Chem.* 2009;284:14838–14848.

30. Avila E, Diaz L, Barrera D, et al. Regulation of vitamin D hydroxylase gene expression by 1,25-dihydroxyvitamin D3 and cyclic AMP in cultured human syncytiotrophoblasts. *J Steroid Biochem Mol Biol.* 2007;103:90–96.

31. Panda DK, Miao D, Tremblay ML, et al. Targeted ablation of the 25-hydroxyvitamin D 1alpha-hydroxylase enzyme: evidence for skeletal, reproductive, and immune dysfunction. *Proc Natl Acad Sci USA.* 2001;98:7498–7503.

32. Kovacs CS, Woodland ML, Fudge NJ, et al. The vitamin D receptor is not required for fetal mineral homeostasis or for the regulation of placental calcium transfer in mice. *Am J Physiol Endocrinol Metab.* 2005;289:E133–E144.

33. Martin R, Harvey NC, Crozier SR, et al. Placental calcium transporter gene expression (PMCA3) predict intrauterine bone mineral accrual. *Bone.* 2007;40:1203–1208.

34. Camadoo L, Tibott R, Isaza F. Maternal vitamin D deficiency associated with neonatal hypocalcemic convulsions. *Nutr J.* 2007;6:23–24.

35. Steichen JJ, Tsang RC, Gratton TL, et al. Vitamin D homeostasis in the perinatal period: 1,25-dihydroxyvitamin D in maternal, cord and neonatal blood. *N Engl J Med.* 1980;302:315–319.

36. Markestad T, Aksnes L, Finne PH, et al. Plasma concentrations of vitamin D metabolites in premature infants. *Pediatr Res.* 1984;18:269–272.

37. Namgung R, Tsang RC, Specker BL, et al. Reduced serum osteocalcin and 1,25-dihydroxyvitamin D concentrations and low bone mineral content in small for gestational age infants: evidence of decreased bone formation rates. *J Pediatr.* 1993;122:269–275.

38. Austin LA, Heath H 3rd. Calcitonin: physiology and pathophysiology. *N Engl J Med.* 1981;304:269–304.

39. McDonald KR, Fudge NJ, Woodrow JP, et al. Ablation of calcitonin/calcitonin gene-related peptide-alpha impairs fetal magnesium but not calcium homeostasis. *Am J Physiol Endocrinol Metab.* 2004;287:E218–E226.

40. Venkataraman PS, Tsang RC, Chen IW, et al. Pathogenesis of early neonatal hypocalcemia: studies of serum calcitonin, gastrin and plasma glucagon. *J Pediatr.* 1987;110:599–603.

41. Sabbagh Y, O'Brien SP, Song W, et al. Intestinal Npt2b plays a major role in phosphate absorption and homeostasis. *J Am Soc Nephrol.* 2009;20:2348–2358.

42. Shibasaki Y, Etoh N, Hayasaka M, et al. Targeted deletion of the type IIb Na(+)-dependent Pi-cotransporter, NaPi-IIb, results in early embryonic lethality. *Biochem Biophys Res Commun.* 2009;381:482–486.

43. Christov M, Jüppner H. Insights from genetic disorders of phosphate homeostasis. *Semin Nephrol.* 2013;3:143–157.

44. Bergwitz C, Jüppner H. Regulation of phosphate homeostasis by PTH, vitamin D, and FGF23. *Annu Rev Med.* 2010;61:91–104.

45. Favus MJ, Bushinsky DA, Lemann J Jr. Regulation of calcium, magnesium, and phosphate metabolism. In: Favus MJ, ed. *Primer on the Metabolic Bone Diseases and Disorders of Mineral Metabolism.* 7th ed. Washington DC: American Society for Bone and Mineral Research; 2009:76–83.

46. Christov M, Jüppner H. Dietary phosphate: the challenges of exploring its role in FGF23 regulation. *Kidney Int.* 2013;84:639–641.

47. Urakawa I, Yamazaki Y, Shimada T, et al. Klotho converts canonical FGF receptor into a specific receptor for FGF23. *Nature.* 2006;444:770–774.

48. Takaiwa M, Aya K, Miyai T, et al. Fibroblast growth factor 23 concentrations in healthy term infants during the early postpartum period. *Bone.* 2010;47:256–262.

49. Fatani T, Binjab A, Weiler H, et al. Persistent elevation of fibroblast growth factor 23 concentrations in healthy appropriate-for-gestational-age preterm infants. *J Pediatr Endocr Met.* 2015;28(7–8):825–832.

50. Bhattacharyya N, Chong WH, Gafni RI, et al. Fibroblast growth factor 23: state of the field and future directions. *Trends Endocrinol Metab.* 2012;23:610–618.

51. Ohata Y, Arahori H, Namba N, et al. Circulating levels of soluble alpha-Klotho are markedly elevated in human umbilical cord blood. *J Clin Endocrinol Metabol.* 2011;96:E943–S947.

52. Tenenhouse HS. Regulation of phosphorus homeostasis by the type IIa Na/phosphate cotransporter. *Annu Rev Nutr.* 2005;25:197–214.

53. Garabedian M. Regulation of phosphate homeostasis in infants, children, and adolescents, and the role of phosphatonins in this process. *Curr Opin Pediatr.* 2007;19:488–491.

54. Gertner JM. Phosphorus metabolism and its disorders in childhood. *Pediatr Ann.* 1987;16:957–965.

55. Díaz-Gómez NM, Mendoza C, González-González NL, et al. Maternal smoking and the vitamin D-parathyroid hormone system during the perinatal period. *J Pediatr.* 2007;151:618–623.

56. Cho WI, Yu HW, Chung HR, et al. Clinical and laboratory characteristics of neonatal hypocalcemia. *Ann Pediatr Endocrinol Metab.* 2015;20:86–91.

57. Do HJ, Park JS, Seo JH, et al. Neonatal late-onset hypocalcemia: is there any relationship with maternal hypovitaminosis D? *Pediatr Gastroenterol Hepatol Nutr.* 2014;17:47–51.

58. Poomthavorn P, Ongphiphadhanakul B, Mahachoklertwattana P. Transient neonatal hypoparathyroidism in two siblings unmasking maternal normocalcemic hyperparathyroidism. *Eur J Pediatr.* 2008;167:431–434.

59. Specker BL, Tsang RC, Ho ML, et al. Low serum calcium and high parathyroid hormone levels in neonates fed "humanized' cow's milk-based formula. *Am J Dis Child.* 1991;145:941–945.

60. Kostic D, Rodigues ABD, Leal A, et al. Flow-through peritoneal dialysis in neonatal enema-induced hyperphosphatemia. *Pediatr Nephrol.* 2010;25:2183–2186.

61. Lee CT, Tsai WY, Tung YC, et al. Transient pseudohypoparathyroidism as a cause of late-onset hypocalcemia in neonates and infants. *J Formos Med Assoc.* 2008;107:806–810.

62. Garcia-Garcia E, Camacho-Alonso J, Gomez-Rodriguez MJ, et al. Transient congenital hypoparathyroidism and 22q11 deletion. *J Pediatr Endocrinol Metab.* 2000;13:659–661.

63. Sunthorbthepvarakul T, Cheresigaew S, Ngowngarmratana S. A novel mutation of the signal peptide of the preproparathyroid hormone gene associated with autosomal recessive familial isolated hypoparathyroidism. *J Clin Endocrinol Metab.* 1999;84:3792–3796.

64. Ding CL, Buckingham B, Levine MA. Familial isolated hypoparathyroidism caused by a mutation in the gene for the transcription factor GCMB. *J Clin Invest.* 2001;108:1215–1220.

65. Stefanaki E, Koropuli M. Atrioventricular block in preterm infants caused by hypocalcemia: a case report and review of the literature. *Eur J Obstet Gynecol.* 2005;120:115–116.

66. Allgrove J. Disorders of calcium metabolism. *Curr Pediatr.* 2003;13:529–535.

67. Puig-Domingo M, Diaz G, Nicolau J, et al. Successful treatment of vitamin D unresponsive hypoparathyroidism with multipulse subcutaneous infusion of teriparatide. *Eur J Endocrinol.* 2008;159:653–657.

68. Newfiled RS. Recombinant PTH for initial management of neonatal hypocalcemia. *New Engl J Med.* 2007;356:1687.

69. Trindade CEP. Minerals in the nutrition of extremely low birth weight infants. *J Pediatr (Rio J).* 2005;81(suppl 1):S43–S51.

70. Mahomadi M, Bivins L, Becker KL. Effect of thiazides on serum calcium. *Clin Pharmacol Ther.* 1979;26:390–394.

71. Lloyd SE, Pannett AA, Dixon PH, et al. Localization of familial benign hypercalcemia, Oklahoma variant (FBHOk), to chromosome 19q13. *Am J Hum Genet.* 1999;64:189–195.

72. Ghirri P, Bottone U, Coccoli L, et al. Symptomatic hypercalcemia in the first months of life: calcium-regulating hormones and treatment. *J Endocrinol Invest.* 1999;22:349–353.

73. Rodriquez-Soriano J, Garcia-Fuentes M, Vallo A, et al. Hypercalcemia in neonatal distal renal tubular acidosis. *Pediatr Nephrol.* 2000;14:354–355.

74. Waller S, Kurzawinski T, Spitz L, et al. Neonatal severe hyperparathyroidism: genotype/phenotype correlation and the use of pamidronate as rescue therapy. *Eur J Pediatr.* 2004;163:589–594.

75. Fox L, Sadowsky J, Pringle KP, et al. Neonatal hyperparathyroidism and pamidronate therapy in an extremely premature infant. *Pediatrics.* 2007;120:e1350–e1354.

76. Lyon AJ, McIntosh N. Calcium and phosphorus balance in extremely low birthweight infants in the first six weeks of life. *Arch Dis Child.* 1984;59:1145.

77. Rowe JC, Carey DE. Phosphorus deficiency syndrome in very low birth weight infants. *Pediatr Clin North Am.* 1987;34:997–1017.

78. Namgung R, Joo HJ, Lee EG, et al. Radiologic (rickets) and biochemical effects of calcium and phosphorus supplementation of parenteral nutrition in very low birth weight infants. *Pediatr Res.* 1993;33:308A.

5

79. Namgung R, Park KI, Lee C, et al. High serum osteocalcin and high serum cross-linked carboxyterminal telopeptide of type I collagen in rickets of preterm infants: evidence of increased bone turnover. *Pediatr Res*. 1994;35:317A.

80. Kalan G, Derganc M, Primćić J. Phosphate metabolism in red blood cells of critically ill neonates. *Pflugers Arch*. 2000;440(suppl 5):R109–R111.

81. Kimutai D, Maleche-Obimbo E, Kamenwa R, et al. Hypo-phosphatemia in children under five years with kwashiorkor and marasmic kwashiorkor. *East Afr Med J*. 2009;86:330–336.

82. Haglin L, Burman LA, Nilsson M. High prevalence of hypophosphatemia amongst patients with infectious diseases. A retrospective study. *J Intern Med*. 1999;246:45–52.

83. White KE, Evans WE, O'Riordan JLH, et al. Autosomal dominant hypophosphatemic rickets is associated with mutations in FGF23. *Nat Genet*. 2000;26:345–348.

84. Lorenz-Depiereux B, Bastepe M, Benet-Pages A, et al. DMP1 mutations in autosomal recessive hypophosphatemia implicate a bone matrix protein in the regulation of phosphate homeostasis. *Nat Genet*. 2006;38:1248–1250.

85. The HYP Consortium. A gene (PEX) with homologies to endopeptidases is mutated in patients with X-linked hypophosphatemic rickets. *Nat Genet*. 1995;11:130–136.

86. Takeda E, Taketani Y, Sawada N, et al. The regulation and function of phosphate in the human body. *Biofactors*. 2004;21:345–355.

87. Rigo J, De Curtis M, Pieltain C, et al. Bone mineral metabolism in the micropremie. *Clin Perinatol*. 2000;27:147–170.

88. Costello I, Powell C, Williams AF. Sodium glycerophosphate in the treatment of neonatal hypophosphatemia. *Arch Dis Child Fetal Neonatal Ed*. 1995;73:F44–F45.

89. Singer FR. Medical management of nonparathyroid hypercalcemia and hypocalcemia. *Otolaryngol Clin North Am*. 1996;29:701–710.

90. Biarent D, Brumagne C, Steppe M, et al. Acute phosphate intoxication in seven infants under parenteral nutrition. *J Parenter Enteral Nutr*. 1992;16:558–560.

91. Perlman M. Fatal hyperphosphatemia after oral phosphate overdose in a premature infant. *Am J Health Syst Pharm*. 1997;54:2488–2490.

92. Dissaneewate S, Vachvanichsanong P. Severe hyperphosphatemia in a newborn with renal insufficiency because of an erroneous medical prescription. *J Renal Nutr*. 2009;19:500–502.

93. Marraffa JM, Hui A, Stork CM. Severe hyperphosphatemia and hypocalcemia following the rectal administration of a phosphate-containing Fleet® pediatric enema. *Pediatr Emerg Care*. 2004;7:453–456.

94. Biebl A, Grillenberger A, Schmitt K. Enema-induced severe hyperphosphatemia in children. *Eur J Pediatr*. 2009;168:111–112.

95. Tamanaha K, Mak RHK, Rigden SPA, et al. Long-term suppression of hyperparathyroidism by phosphate binders in uremic children. *Pediatr Nephrol*. 1987;1:145–149.

CHAPTER 6

Acid-Base Homeostasis in the Fetus and Newborn

Timur Azhibekov, MD, Istvan Seri, MD, PhD, HonD

- In Addition to the Buffering Systems, Fetal Acid-Base Homeostasis Is Regulated by Maternal Respiratory and Renal Function and the Immature Fetal Kidneys
- Fetal Acid-Base Homeostasis Affect Fetal Growth and May Have Long-Term Consequences
- Certain Aspects of Obstetrical Management of Labor and Delivery (e.g., Prenatal Steroid Administration or the Practice of Delayed Cord Clamping) and Anesthesia During Labor and Delivery Also Affect, Albeit Transiently, Fetal and Postnatal Acid-Base Homeostasis

Introduction

This chapter addresses the regulation of fetal and neonatal acid-base balance with a focus on the elimination of the acid load by the placenta, lungs, and kidneys, briefly discusses the impact of acid-base disturbance on fetal and postnatal growth, and describes the effect of selected obstetrical management approaches on fetal and neonatal acid-base balance.

Hydrogen ion concentration is tightly regulated by the intracellular and extracellular buffer systems and respiratory and renal compensatory mechanisms. The normal range of hydrogen ion concentration in the extracellular fluid is between 35 and 45 nEq/L ($3.5–4.5 \times 10^{-8}$ M), which translates to a pH range of 7.35 to 7.45 (pH = $-\log_{10}$ [H$^+$]). Under physiologic circumstances, volatile and fixed acids generated by normal metabolism are excreted and the pH remains stable.[1] Carbonic acid is the most common volatile acid produced and is readily excreted by the lungs in the form of carbon dioxide. Fixed acids, such as lactic acid, ketoacids, phosphoric acid, and sulfuric acid, are buffered principally by bicarbonate in the extracellular compartment. The bicarbonate used in this process is then regenerated by the kidneys in a series of transmembrane transport processes linked to the excretion of hydrogen ions in the form of titratable acids (phosphate and sulfate salts) and ammonium. Several aspects of the regulation of acid-base homeostasis are developmentally regulated in the fetus and neonate and thus differ from those in children and adults. These developmentally regulated differences of acid-base homeostasis and their impact on fetal and postnatal growth are reviewed in this chapter.

Regulation of Acid-Base Homeostasis

Respiratory Acidosis

Unlike in fetal respiratory acidosis, in postnatal respiratory acidosis, immediate activation of the pulmonary compensatory mechanism leads to enhanced elimination of carbon dioxide, and the resulting fall in carbon dioxide concentration increases the pH toward normal (pH = [HCO$_3^-$] ÷ pCO$_2$; where [HCO$_3^-$] = bicarbonate and pCO$_2$ = carbon dioxide tension). The *rapid activation* of the respiratory compensatory mechanism is a result of the free movement of carbon dioxide across the blood-brain barrier,[2] leading to instantaneous changes in cerebrospinal fluid (CSF) and cerebral interstitial fluid hydrogen ion concentrations. The degree of maturity of the central respiratory control system[3] and pulmonary function determines the overall effectiveness of the respiratory compensatory mechanism.

Correction of Fetal Respiratory Acidosis

Fetal respiratory acidosis develops when prolonged maternal hypoventilation occurs with maternal asthma, airway obstruction, narcotic overdosing, maternal anesthesia, severe hypokalemia, and magnesium sulfate toxicity. Fetal breathing movements increase, and the fetal kidneys exert a maturation-dependent limited response by reclaiming more bicarbonate in an attempt to restore the physiologic $20:1$ ratio of bicarbonate to carbonic acid, resulting in a return of the pH toward normal.[4] In the fetus, only the renal compensation has some limited physiologic significance when respiratory acidosis develops due to prolonged maternal hypoventilation. Rather, the placenta, coupled with maternal compensatory mechanisms, performs most of the effective compensatory functions.

Correction of Postnatal Respiratory Acidosis

In the clinical setting, acute neonatal respiratory acidosis develops most frequently in preterm infants with respiratory distress syndrome. Although stimulation of the respiratory center in the brain by the decrease in pH due to the elevated interstitial carbon dioxide concentration immediately increases respiratory rate and depth, carbon dioxide elimination by the lungs is usually limited because of immaturity and parenchymal disease. Importantly, in premature infants, increase in minute ventilation is achieved primarily by the increase in respiratory rate accompanied by only minor changes in tidal volume. On the other hand, term infants respond with increased tidal volume first.[5] Respiratory compensation can be further affected by the decreased carbon dioxide sensitivity of the premature infant[6] and the altered interaction between arterial oxygen tension (pO_2) and carbon dioxide sensitivity, particularly at the level of central receptors, during the neonatal period as compared with adults.[7]

As in the fetus, the kidneys reclaim more bicarbonate in response to respiratory acidosis. However, renal compensation is limited by the developmentally regulated immaturity of renal tubular functions, especially during the first few weeks of postnatal life.

Regulation of Acid-Base Homeostasis

Metabolic Acidosis

As in respiratory acidosis, the pulmonary gas exchange serves as the *immediate* regulator of acid-base homeostasis when *metabolic acidosis* develops. However, because plasma bicarbonate does not readily cross the blood-brain barrier, CSF bicarbonate levels change only with a delay.[8] Therefore full activation of the respiratory acid-base regulatory system occurs only hours after the development of metabolic acidosis. This is different from the previously described truly immediate activation of the respiratory acid-base regulatory system by respiratory acidosis. In the CSF, generation of bicarbonate via hydroxylation of the dissolved carbon dioxide during CSF formation is the primary source of bicarbonate.[9] On the other hand and as mentioned earlier, changes in arterial carbon dioxide tension rapidly affect carbon dioxide tension in the CSF, even in the setting of primary metabolic acidosis. Changes in CSF carbon dioxide levels also readily affect CSF bicarbonate levels.[10] In addition, the respiratory response to changes in CSF bicarbonate levels in metabolic acidosis appears to be not as robust as that triggered by changes in carbon dioxide tension.[2] Finally, the respiratory compensatory mechanism is complemented by removal of the acid load by the kidneys.

Fetoplacental Elimination of Metabolic Acid Load

Fetal respiratory and renal compensation in response to changes in fetal pH is limited by the level of maturity and the surrounding maternal environment. However, although the placentomaternal unit performs most compensatory functions,[4] the fetal kidneys have some, although limited, ability to contribute to the maintenance of fetal acid-base balance.

The most frequent cause of fetal metabolic acidosis is fetal hypoxemia owing to abnormalities of uteroplacental function or blood flow, or both. Primary maternal hypoxemia or maternal metabolic acidosis secondary to maternal diabetes mellitus, sepsis, or renal tubular abnormalities is an unusual cause of fetal metabolic acidosis.

The *pregnant woman,* at least in late gestation, maintains a somewhat more alkaline plasma environment compared with that of nonpregnant controls. This pattern of acid-base regulation in pregnant women is present during both resting and after maximal exertion and may serve as a protective mechanism from sudden decreases in fetal pH. Maintenance of the less acidic environment during pregnancy appears to be achieved through reduced plasma carbon dioxide and weak acid concentrations.[4,11]

The *placenta* plays an essential role in the maintenance of fetal acid-base balance when metabolic acidosis develops. As mentioned earlier, fetal metabolic acidosis most frequently occurs when abnormal uteroplacental function or blood flow results in fetal hypoxemia. Fetal hypoxemia then causes a shift to anaerobic metabolism and large quantities of lactic acid accumulate. As hydrogen ions are buffered by the extracellular and intracellular buffering systems of the fetus, pH drops as plasma bicarbonate decreases. Because of the unhindered diffusion of carbon dioxide through the placenta,[12] restoration of normal fetal pH initially occurs through elimination of the volatile element of the carbonic acid-bicarbonate system via the maternal lungs. However, as lactate and other fixed acids cross the placenta more slowly,[4] the onset of maternal renal compensation of fetal metabolic acidosis is delayed. In addition, if fetal oxygenation improves, the products of anaerobic metabolism are also metabolized by the fetus.

Because there is no physiologic significance to respiratory compensation of metabolic acidosis in utero, the finding that the respiratory control system in the fetus is much less sensitive to changes in pH than in the neonate[13] has little practical importance. Yet, a decrease in the fetal pH stimulates breathing movements in the fetus.[14,15]

Finally, as for the role of the *fetal kidneys* in the maintenance of acid-base balance, available evidence indicates that the fetal kidneys excrete both inorganic[16–18] and organic acids[19] and are also able to reabsorb bicarbonate.[20,21] Studies in fetal sheep have found age-dependent increases in glomerular filtration rate (GFR) and urinary titratable acid, ammonium, and net acid excretion.[16] A positive relationship also exists between changes in GFR and bicarbonate, sodium, and chloride excretions.[16,18] Yet, the adaptive capacity of the fetal kidney to changes in fetal acid-base balance is limited. In fetal sheep the hydrochloric acid infusion-induced metabolic acidosis results in increases in titratable acid, ammonium, and net acid excretion without significant changes in GFR or renal tubular bicarbonate absorption.[18] However, as mentioned earlier, under certain conditions, such as volume depletion[20] or recovery from mild hypocapnic hypoxia,[21] the fetal kidney has the ability to increase bicarbonate reabsorption. It is also important to note that the vast majority of these data have been obtained in animal models and that there is only very limited information available concerning renal acidification by the human fetus.[22] In addition, the physiologic importance of the adaptive fetal renal responses is limited compared with that in the postnatal period because the acid load excreted in the fetal urine remains within the immediate fetal environment and needs to be eliminated by the placenta or metabolized by the fetus.

Indeed, *amniotic fluid* acid-base status and electrolyte composition have been shown to affect the fetus. When the effects of amnion infusion of physiologic saline with those of lactated Ringer were compared in the fetal sheep, significant increases in fetal plasma sodium and chloride concentrations were noted only in the physiologic saline infusion group.[23] In addition, fetal arterial pH decreased in the physiologic saline group and the change in the fetal pH was directly related to the changes in plasma chloride concentrations. However, despite the significant changes in plasma sodium and chloride concentrations and pH, fetal plasma electrolyte composition and acid-base balance remained in the physiologic range, leaving these findings with little clinical significance.[23]

Postnatal Elimination of Metabolic Acid Load

The most frequent causes of increased anion gap (lactic acid) metabolic acidosis in the neonate are hypoxemia or ischemia secondary to perinatal asphyxia; vasoregulatory disturbances and/or myocardial dysfunction caused by immaturity, sepsis, or asphyxia; severe lung disease with or without pulmonary hypertension; certain types of structural heart disease; and volume depletion. Severe metabolic acidosis caused by a neonatal metabolic disorder is rare but should always be considered. Preterm neonates frequently present with a mild to moderate normal anion gap acidosis, which almost always is the consequence of the low renal bicarbonate threshold of the premature kidney.[24–27] However, the use of carbonic anhydrase inhibitors[28] and parenteral alimentation, as well as the maturation-related decreased sensitivity to aldosterone, have also been suggested to contribute to the development of normal anion gap acidosis in the neonate.[29–32]

As mentioned earlier, in metabolic acidosis caused by the accumulation of lactic acid, hydrogen ions are buffered by the intracellular and extracellular buffering systems and plasma bicarbonate concentration decreases and pH drops. Restoration of pH toward normal initially occurs through elimination of the volatile element of the carbonic acid–bicarbonate system *via the lungs*. This process may be severely compromised in the sick preterm and term neonate with parenchymal lung disease.

The principle mechanism of the *renal compensation* is the regulation of renal tubular bicarbonate and acid secretion in response to changes in extracellular pH. Although full activation of this system requires at least 2 to 3 days, changes in renal acidification may be seen as early as a few hours following the development of the acid-base disturbance. Although renal compensation is the ultimate mechanism that adjusts the hydrogen ion content of the body, this compensatory function is also affected by the immaturity of the neonatal kidneys.[27,33] Both *renal hemodynamic and tubular epithelial factors* play a role in the limited renal compensatory capacity of the newborn.

Renal blood flow (RBF) significantly increases after the immediate postnatal period, and some of the renal vasodilatory mechanisms are functionally mature as early as the 24th week of gestation.[34] Similar to RBF, GFR is also low in the immediate postnatal period and increases as a function of both gestational and postnatal age.[35–37] Indeed, the *low GFR is considered the primary hemodynamic factor* limiting the ability of the neonate to adequately handle an acid load.[27,33]

In addition, net renal acid excretion is regulated *by several tubular epithelial functions.*[38] In the proximal tubule the following major transport mechanisms regulate active acid extrusion and transepithelial bicarbonate reabsorption: the H^+-ATPase, the Na^+,K^+-ATPase–driven secondary active Na^+/H^+ antiporter in the apical membrane and the electrogenic $Na^+/3HCO_3^-$ cotransporter in the basolateral membrane, and the Na^+,K^+-ATPase–driven tertiary active Na^+-coupled organic ion transporter.[39] Because approximately 80% of the filtered bicarbonate is reabsorbed in the proximal tubule,[40] the function of these proximal tubular transporters determines the renal threshold for bicarbonate reabsorption. The bicarbonate threshold is approximately 18 mEq/L in the premature and approximately 21 mEq/L in the term infant,[24,41] and it reaches adult levels (24–26 mEq/L) only after the first postnatal year.[25,26] However, in the extremely low gestational age neonate the renal bicarbonate threshold may be as low as 14 mEq/L. Because renal carbonic anhydrase is present and active during fetal life[42] and because its activity is similar in the 26-week-old extremely immature neonate to that of the adult,[43] a developmentally regulated immaturity of the function of the previously described proximal tubular transporters is most likely responsible for the low bicarbonate threshold during early development. Indeed, both the activity and the hormonal responsiveness of the proximal tubular Na^+,K^+-ATPase are decreased in younger compared with older animals.[44] Moreover, similar to the decrease in bicarbonate reabsorption in the proximal tubule,[45] the activity of Na^+/H^+ antiporter is also decreased to approximately one-third of the adult level.[46]

In addition to immaturity, medications used in critically ill neonates may also affect proximal tubular bicarbonate reabsorption. For example, via inhibition of the proximal tubular Na^+/H^+ antiporter, dopamine may potentially decrease the low bicarbonate threshold of the neonate.[47–49] Carbonic anhydrase inhibitors also decrease proximal tubular bicarbonate reabsorption by limiting bicarbonate formation and hydrogen ion availability for the Na^+/H^+ antiporter.[50] By acting on several transport proteins along the nephron, furosemide directly increases urinary excretion of titratable acids (phosphate and sulfate salts) and ammonium.[51] On the other hand, by inhibition of the activation of aldosterone receptors, spironolactone indirectly decreases hydrogen ion excretion in the distal tubule.

Under physiologic circumstances, the thick ascending loop of Henle and the distal tubule reabsorb the remaining filtered bicarbonate via transport mechanisms similar to those of the proximal tubule. In addition, by transporting bicarbonate across the membrane,[39] the distal nephron-specific HCO_3^-/Cl^- antiporter located in the basolateral membrane contributes to the reabsorption of bicarbonate.

Hydrogen ions are excreted in the urine in the form of titratable acids (phosphate and sulfate salts) and as ammonium salts, which are formed by the combination of hydrogen with ammonia.[39] Because the major constituent of titratable acid in the urine is $H_2PO_4^-$, drugs that decrease proximal tubular phosphate reabsorption and thus increase the delivery of phosphate to the distal nephron may increase the renal acidification capacity of the neonate. Indeed, by inhibiting proximal tubular phosphate reabsorption, dopamine has been shown to increase the excretion of titratable acids in preterm infants.[52] Furthermore, net hydrogen ion secretion in the distal nephron continues after the reabsorption of virtually all bicarbonate by active extrusion of hydrogen and via the ability of the distal tubular epithelium to maintain large transepithelial concentration gradients for hydrogen and bicarbonate.[39]

Urinary excretion of titratable acid and ammonium increases as a function of gestational and postnatal age.[27,37] However, because effective urinary acidification is usually acquired by the age of 1 month, even in premature infants, postnatal distal tubular hydrogen ion secretion is inducible independent of the gestational age at birth.[53,54]

Aldosterone is one of the most important hormones influencing distal tubular acidification. By affecting the function of several different transport mechanisms, aldosterone stimulates net hydrogen ion excretion in the distal nephron.[39] Of note is that the premature neonate has a developmentally regulated relative insensitivity to aldosterone.[30,32]

In summary, the renal response to metabolic acidosis in the immediate postnatal period consists of attenuated increases in GFR, proximal tubular bicarbonate reabsorption, and distal tubular net acid secretion. However, a significant improvement in the overall renal response occurs after the first postnatal month even in the premature infant.[33,53,54]

Regulation of Acid-Base Homeostasis

Respiratory Alkalosis

Correction of Fetal Respiratory Alkalosis

Rather than causing fetal respiratory alkalosis, acute maternal hyperventilation may lead to the development fetal hypoxia and metabolic acidosis.[55] The fetal acidosis under these circumstances is thought to be the consequence of the acute decrease in placental blood flow caused by the maternal hypocapnia-induced significant uterine vasoconstriction.[56] In these cases, restoration of maternal carbon dioxide levels rapidly corrects both the abnormal uterine blood flow and the acid-base abnormality in the fetus.

The *physiologic hyperventilation* of the pregnant woman causes a compensatory decrease in her serum bicarbonate concentration to approximately 22 mM[4] without any apparent effect on the fetus (see earlier).

Correction of Postnatal Respiratory Alkalosis

Neonatal respiratory alkalosis occurs most often in the febrile nonventilated neonate or in cases with iatrogenic hyperventilation of the intubated preterm or term infant. Rarely, respiratory alkalosis may be the presenting sign of a urea cycle disorder during the first days of postnatal life because the rising ammonia level may initially stimulate the respiratory center in the brain. As for the renal compensation of respiratory alkalosis, both urinary bicarbonate reabsorption and distal tubular net acid excretion decrease and thus extracellular pH tends to return toward normal. This renal compensation plays an important although somewhat limited role in neonatal respiratory alkalosis.

Regulation of Acid-Base Homeostasis

Metabolic Alkalosis

Correction of Fetal Metabolic Alkalosis

Although metabolic alkalosis is a very rare fetal condition, it may occur in hyperemesis gravidarum. As a result of the significant and lasting hydrogen chloride losses, maternal renal compensation results in retention of bicarbonate to maintain maternal anionic balance. Because bicarbonate is transported slowly across the placenta, the development of fetal metabolic alkalosis lags behind that of the mother. On the other hand, the maternal respiratory compensation (hypoventilation with the ensuing hypercapnia) tends to restore normal pH in the fetus as carbon dioxide is rapidly transported across the placenta.

Correction of Postnatal Metabolic Alkalosis

Metabolic alkalosis most frequently develops in the preterm neonate receiving prolonged diuretic treatment for bronchopulmonary dysplasia. Although there is little evidence that chronic diuretic management results in improved medium- or long-term pulmonary outcome, many neonatologists use this treatment modality, at least intermittently. If total body chloride and potassium content is not appropriately maintained during chronic diuretic administration, severe metabolic "contraction" alkalosis may develop, which also results in poor growth. The respiratory response is a decrease in the rate and depth of breathing to increase carbon dioxide retention. This response may be interpreted as a sign of worsening pulmonary condition in the ventilated preterm neonate and may inappropriately trigger an increase in ventilatory support. Thus respiratory compensation of metabolic alkalosis may be ineffective if the intubated neonate is subjected to iatrogenic overventilation on the mechanical ventilator. As for the neonatal renal compensation for metabolic alkalosis, urinary bicarbonate reabsorption and distal tubular net acid excretion fall, resulting in a return of the extracellular pH toward normal.

Finally, metabolic alkalosis can also result from a nondiuretic administration–related loss of extracellular fluid containing disproportionally more chloride than bicarbonate. During the diuretic phase of normal postnatal adaptation, preterm and term newborns tend to retain relatively more bicarbonate than chloride.[57] The obvious benefits of allowing this physiologic extracellular volume contraction to occur clearly outweigh the clinical importance of a mild contraction alkalosis developing during postnatal adaptation. Thus no specific treatment is needed in these cases, especially because with the stabilization of the extracellular volume status and the renal function with time, acid-base balance rapidly returns to normal.

Normal Acid-Base Balance and Growth

Growth is most accelerated during fetal life. The normal fetus grows from a weight of 0.22 g at the eighth week of gestation to 3400 g at 40 weeks' completed gestation.[58] The estimated energy density of each gram of body weight gained (or lost) is 23 kJ (5.6 kcal). However, in premature infants, especially if they are critically ill and/or growth retarded, the energy density of the new tissue is estimated to be higher than 5.6 kcal/g.[59] For instance, in small-for-gestational-age infants at approximately 5 weeks after birth, the total energy expenditure is estimated to be 20% greater than in appropriate-for-gestational-age controls.[60]

Fetal growth can be negatively affected by several fetal and placentomaternal conditions. Proven fetal conditions affecting fetal growth include certain genetic conditions and infection of the fetus.[61] Placentomaternal conditions with demonstrated influence on fetal growth are primary placental insufficiency and maternal diseases, nutritional status or substance abuse leading to secondary placental insufficiency, decreased fetal nutrient availability or direct fetal toxicity, or a combination of these harmful effects on fetal well-being.[61]

Although direct evidence demonstrating an impact of chronic fetal acid-base abnormality on fetal growth is very limited, a *mild shift in the fetal acid-base status* has been suggested as the primary pathologic factor for intrauterine growth restriction caused by placental insufficiency of any etiology.[62] From 18 weeks' postconception, growth-retarded fetuses exhibit a greater degree of mild acidemia than their appropriately growing counterparts.[63] This acidemia is attributed to the reduced perfusion and mild hypoxemia the growth-retarded fetus faces as a result of the placental insufficiency. According to the above hypothesis, the small initial reduction in the pH negatively affects nitric oxide production in the fetus, and it is the decreased availability of nitric oxide that then plays a major role in the ensuing growth restriction.[62]

The following findings are in support of this hypothesis. Because locally formed nitric oxide regulates tissue perfusion and thus oxygen delivery and tissue growth itself, it has been suggested to play a pivotal role in regulation of growth in the fetus.[61,62] In addition to its effect on oxygen delivery to the tissues, nitric oxide is an anabolic factor. Indeed, it is necessary for normal growth of several tissues, including the bone and muscle, and for the action of different hormones, such as the parathyroid hormone, vitamin D, and estrogen, known to be of importance in fetal growth and development.[64,65]

Interestingly, the enzyme responsible for generating nitric oxide from L-arginine, the constitutive nitric oxide synthase (cNOS), is sensitive to changes in pH, and its activity decreases even with a mild shift in the pH toward acidosis.[66] Thus a vicious cycle may develop in growth-retarded fetuses because the initial decrease in blood flow and pH caused by placental insufficiency may lead to decreased cNOS activity and thus nitric oxide production. Decreased nitric oxide production, in turn, leads to further decreases in tissue perfusion and thus in pH, exacerbating the decrease in local nitric oxide production.[62]

In addition to being the source of locally generated nitric oxide, L-arginine also serves as the source of polyamines and L-proline. These compounds are generated by the arginase enzyme and are important when growth and tissue repair processes predominate. The function of this enzyme is also pH dependent,[67] and the proposed decrease in its activity in the growth-retarded fetus may contribute to further impairment of fetal growth.

Based on this information, it seems that elevating the pH in the fetus toward normal and supplementing L-arginine to the mother may be a plausible approach to attenuate the impact on fetal growth of the placental insufficiency–induced decreased fetal oxygen delivery. However, due to the inherent difficulties associated with attempts to effectively control fetal pH, no clinical trial has as yet attempted this combined approach.

As for the neonate, the syndrome of late metabolic acidosis of prematurity is an example how postnatal growth can be affected by alterations in the acid-base balance. This entity was first described in the 1960s, in which otherwise healthy premature infants after a few weeks developed mild to moderate anion gap acidosis and decreased growth rate. All of these infants were receiving high-protein cow's milk formulas and demonstrated increased net acid excretion compared with controls. This type of late metabolic acidosis is now rarely seen, probably because of the use of special premature formulas and the changes made to regular formulas now containing a decreased casein-to-whey ratio and lower fixed acid loads.

The diuretic administration–induced hypochloremic metabolic alkalosis is another example of the impact of acid-base balance on postnatal growth. This phenomenon is also associated with growth failure and may be a contributing factor of poor outcome in infants with bronchopulmonary dysplasia.[68] Indeed, in addition to mild chronic hypoxemia and inadequate nutrition, the decrease in cell proliferation and diminished DNA and protein synthesis in response to intracellular alkalosis may contribute to the growth failure of infants with severe bronchopulmonary dysplasia.[69] Chronic decrease in total body sodium resulting in a negative sodium balance may further hinder the growth of these infants.[70] Aggressive chloride and potassium supplementation with relatively limited sodium supplementation decreases the risk for the development of clinically significant severe contraction alkalosis associated with chronic diuretic use in these patients.

Obstetrical Management and Fetal and Neonatal Acid-Base Balance

Evidence has accumulated on the impact of certain aspects of obstetrical management of labor and delivery on fetal and neonatal acid-base homeostasis. These effects are transient, and it is unclear whether they have an independent impact on clinically relevant neonatal outcome measures.

Maternal betamethasone administration has been associated with a transient decrease in fetal movements including fetal breathing[71] and fetal heart rate variability.[71,72] Although the exact pathomechanism of these effects of antenatal betamethasone administration is unclear, animal[73] and human[74] data suggest that transient fetal acidosis following maternal steroid administration may, at least in part, explain the findings. It has been suggested that fetal acidosis is a consequence of the demonstrated fetal cardiovascular, endocrine, and metabolic effects of maternal steroid administration.[74,75] However, in growth-restricted fetuses, cardiovascular responses to maternal steroid administration differ from those of fetuses with normal growth[76,77] and may lead to significant acidosis and poor outcome.[76]

Delayed cord clamping also appears to have an impact on neonatal acid-base balance immediately after delivery, resulting in changes consistent with mixed acidosis during the first 45 seconds followed by primarily a metabolic acidosis by 90 seconds with delayed cord clamping.[78] The metabolic acidosis immediately after delivery likely occurs because the normally produced and accumulated anaerobic metabolites in nonvital organs during labor and delivery are washed out faster in the larger blood volume of neonates with delayed cord clamping, and thus they exert a smaller effect on blood pH in these infants later on.[78] Because the potential clinical relevance of fetal and immediate postnatal acidosis depends on the severity of hypoxemia and the associated acidosis, it may have importance only in the neonate with prolonged labor and difficult delivery.[79] Observations in preterm infants suggest that delaying clamping of the cord even for 30 seconds is associated with a decrease in metabolic acidosis shortly after birth.[80]

Finally, the type of anesthesia during delivery via C-section also appears to have an impact on the fetal acid-base status. Findings of a meta-analysis of 27 studies found lower cord pH and larger base deficit in newborns of mothers who received spinal anesthesia compared with those who received general and epidural anesthesia.[81] A more recent prospective observational cohort study examined the relationship between the type of anesthesia provided during C-section and fetal acid-base balance and neonatal condition upon delivery in 900 women with uncomplicated singleton pregnancies.[82] The study found that epidural anesthesia was associated with higher venous cord pH (7.30 ± 7.26–7.34) than general (7.25 ± 7.21–7.26) or spinal (7.23 ± 7.19–7.26) anesthesia and that neonatal well-being was negatively affected primarily by general anesthesia. These findings highlight the importance of taking the type of anesthesia into consideration when evaluating a neonate with metabolic acidosis in the immediate postnatal period following delivery via cesarean section.

Summary

This chapter has reviewed the available information and the gaps in our knowledge on how fetal and neonatal acid-base balance is regulated and the impact of alterations in acid-base balance on some aspects of fetal and postnatal growth, as well as how selected obstetrical management approaches affect fetal and neonatal acid-base balance. In the future, a better understanding of the role of growth factors and their interaction with the fetal acid-base status may result in improved early management of the growth-retarded fetus. This, in turn, may decrease the negative impact of growth retardation on brain and other organ development.

REFERENCES

1. Masoro EJ. An overview of hydrogen ion regulation. *Arch Intern Med.* 1982;142:1019.
2. Sorensen SC. The chemical control of ventilation. *Acta Physiol Scand.* 1971;361:1.
3. Darnall RA. The role of CO2 and central chemoreception in the control of breathing in the fetus and the neonate. *Respir Physiol Neurobiol.* 2010;173:201.
4. Blechner JN. Maternal-fetal acid-base, physiology. *Clin Obstet Gynecol.* 1993;36:3.
5. Bodegård G. Control of respiration in newborn babies. III. Developmental changes of respiratory depth and rate responses to CO2. *Acta Paediatr Scand.* 1975;64:684.
6. Abu-Shaweesh JM. Maturation of respiratory reflex responses in the fetus and neonate. *Semin Neonatol.* 2004;9:169.
7. Wolsink JG, Berkenbosch A, DeGoede J, Olievier CN. The effects of hypoxia on the ventilatory response to sudden changes in CO2 in newborn piglets. *J Physiol.* 1992;456:39.
8. Nattie EE, Romer L. CSF HCO_3^- regulation in isosmotic conditions: the role of brain PCO2 and plasma HCO_3. *Respir Physiol.* 1978;33:177.
9. Vogh BP, Maren TH. Sodium, chloride, and bicarbonate movement from plasma to cerebrospinal fluid in cats. *Am J Physiol.* 1975;228:673.
10. Javaheri S, Nardell EA, Kazemi H. Role of PCO2 as determinant of CSF [HCO-3] in metabolic acidosis. *Respir Physiol.* 1979;36:155.
11. Kemp JG, Greer FA, Wolfe LA. Acid-base regulation after maximal exercise testing in late gestation. *J Appl Physiol.* 1997;83:644.
12. Blechner JN, Meshia G, Barron DH. A study of the acid-base balance of fetal sheep and goats. *Q J Exp Physiol.* 1960;45:60.
13. Connors G, Hunse C, Carmichael L, et al. Control of fetal breathing in the human fetus between 24 and 34 weeks' gestation. *Am J Obstet Gynecol.* 1989;160:932.
14. Jansen A, Shernick V. Fetal breathing and development of control of breathing. *J Appl Physiol.* 1991;70:143L.
15. Molteni RA, Melmed MH, Sheldon RE, et al. Induction of fetal breathing by metabolic acidemia and its effect on blood flow to the respiratory muscles. *Am J Obstet Gynecol.* 1980;136:609.
16. Kesby GJ, Lumbers ER. Factors affecting renal handling of sodium, hydrogen ions, and bicarbonate in the fetus. *Am J Physiol.* 1986;251:F226.
17. Hill KJ, Lumbers ER. Renal function in adult and fetal sheep. *J Dev Physiol.* 1988;10:149.
18. Kesby GJ, Lumbers ER. The effects of metabolic acidosis on renal function of fetal sheep. *J Physiol.* 1988;396:65.
19. Elbourne I, Lumbers ER, Hill KJ. The secretion of organic acids and bases by the ovine fetal kidney. *Exp Physiol.* 1990;75:211.
20. Robillard JE, Sessions C, Burmeister L, Smith FG. Influence of fetal extracellular volume contraction on renal reabsorption of bicarbonate in fetal lambs. *Pediatr Res.* 1977;11:649.
21. Gibson KJ, McMullen JR, Lumbers ER. Renal acid-base and sodium handling in hypoxia and subsequent mild metabolic acidosis in fetal sheep. *Clin Exp Pharmacol Physiol.* 2000;27:67.
22. Blechner JN, Stenger VG, Eitzman DV, Prystowsky H. Effects of maternal metabolic acidosis on the human fetus and newborn infant. *Am J Obstet Gynecol.* 1967;9:46.
23. Shields LE, Moore TR, Brace RA. Fetal electrolyte and acid-base responses to amnioinfusion: lactated Ringer's versus normal saline in the ovine fetus. *J Soc Gynecol Investig.* 1995;2:602.
24. Svenningsen NW. Renal acid-base titration studies in infants with and without metabolic acidosis in the postneonatal period. *Pediatr Res.* 1974;8:659.
25. Edelmann CM, Soriano JR, Boichis H, et al. Renal bicarbonate reabsorption and hydrogen ion excretion in normal infants. *J Clin Invest.* 1967;46:1309.
26. Avner ED. Normal neonates and the maturational development of homeostatic mechanisms. In: Ichikawa I, ed. *Pediatric Textbook of Fluids and Electrolytes.* Baltimore: Williams & Wilkins; 1990:107–118.

27. Jones DP, Chesney RW. Development of tubular function. *Clin Perinatol*. 1992;19:33.
28. Tam B, Chhay A, Yen L, et al. Acetazolamide for the management of chronic metabolic alkalosis in neonates and infants. *Am J Ther*. 2014;21:477.
29. Trivedi A, Sinn JKH. Early versus late administration of amino acids in preterm infants receiving parenteral nutrition. *Cochrane Database Syst Rev*. 2013;(7):CD008771.
30. Sulyok E, Nemeth M, Tenyi I, et al. Relationship between maturity, electrolyte balance and the function of the renin-angiotensin-aldosterone system in newborn infants. *Biol Neonate*. 1979;35:60.
31. Brewer ED. Disorders of acid-base balance. *Pediatr Clin North Am*. 1990;37:429.
32. Stephenson G, Hammet M, Hadaway G, Funder JW. Ontogeny of renal mineralocorticoid receptors and urinary electrolyte responses in the rat. *Am J Physiol*. 1984;247:F665.
33. Guignard JP, John EG. Renal function in the tiny premature infant. *Clin Permatol*. 1986;13:377.
34. Seri I, Abbasi S, Wood DC, Gerdes JS. Regional hemodynamic effects of dopamine in the sick preterm infant. *J Pediatr*. 1998;133:728.
35. Fawer CL, Torrado A, Guignard J. Maturation of renal function in full-term and premature neonates. *Helv Paediatr Acta*. 1979;34:11.
36. Guignard JP, Torrado A, Da Cunha O, Gautier E. Glomerular filtration rate in the first three weeks of life. *J Pediatr*. 1975;87:268.
37. Arant BS. Developmental patterns of renal functional maturation compared in the human neonate. *J Pediatr*. 1978;92:705.
38. Baum M, Gattineni J, Satlin LM. Postnatal renal development. In: Alpern RJ, Moe OW, Caplan M, eds. *Seldin and Giebisch's The Kidney*. 5th ed. Academic Press; 2013:911–931.
39. Hamm LL, Alpern RJ, Preisig PA. Cellular mechanisms of renal tubular acidification. In: Alpern RJ, Moe OW, Caplan M, eds. *Seldin and Giebisch's The Kidney*. 5th ed. Academic Press; 2013:1917–1978.
40. Quigley R, Baum M. Neonatal acid base balance and disturbances. *Semin Perinatol*. 2004;28:97.
41. Schwartz GJ, Haycock GB, Edelmann CM, Spitzer A. Late metabolic acidosis: a reassessment of the definition. *J Pediatr*. 1979;95:102.
42. Robillard JP, Sessions C, Smith FG. In vivo demonstration of renal carbonic anhydrase activity in the fetal lamb. *Biol Neonate*. 1978;34:253.
43. Lonnerholm C, Wistrand PJ. Carbonic anhydrase in the human fetal kidney. *Pediatr Res*. 1983;17:390.
44. Fryckstedt J, Svensson LB, Linden M, Aperia A. The effect of dopamine on adenylate cyclase and Na$^+$,K$^+$-ATPase activity in the developing rat renal cortical and medullary tubule cells. *Pediatr Res*. 1993;34:308.
45. Schwartz GJ, Evan AP. Development of solute transport in rabbit proximal tubule. I. HCO-3 and glucose absorption. *Am J Physiol*. 1983;245:F382.
46. Baum M. Neonatal rabbit juxtamedullary proximal convoluted tubule acidification. *J Clin Invest*. 1990;85:499.
47. Felder CC, Campbell T, Albrecht F, Jose PA. Dopamine inhibits Na$^+$/H$^+$ exchanger activity in renal BBMV by stimulation of adenylate cyclase. *Am J Physiol*. 1990;259:F297.
48. Seri I. Cardiovascular, renal, and endocrine actions of dopamine in neonates and children. *J Pediatr*. 1995;126:333.
49. Bobulescu IA, Quiñones H, Gisler SM, et al. Acute regulation of renal Na+/H+ exchanger NHE3 by dopamine: role of protein phosphatase 2A. *Am J Physiol Renal Physiol*. 2010;298:F1205.
50. Ellison DH. Physiology and pathophysiology of diuretic action. In: Alpern RJ, Moe OW, Caplan M, eds. *Seldin and Giebisch's The Kidney*. 5th ed. Academic Press; 2013:1353–1404.
51. Hropot M, Fowler N, Karlmark B, Giebisch G. Tubular action of diuretics: distal effects on electrolyte transport and acidification. *Kidney Int*. 1985;28:477.
52. Seri I, Rudas G, Bors ZS, et al. Effects of low-dose dopamine on cardiovascular and renal functions, cerebral blood flow, and plasma catecholamine levels in sick preterm neonates. *Pediatr Res*. 1993;34:742.
53. Kerpel-Fronius E, Heim T, Sulyok E. The development of the renal acidifying processes and their relation to acidosis in low-birth-weight infants. *Biol Neonate*. 1970;15:156.
54. Sulyok E, Heim T. Assessment of maximal urinary acidification in premature infants. *Biol Neonate*. 1971;19:200.
55. Motoyama EK, Rivard G, Acheson F, Cook CD. Adverse effect of maternal hyperventilation on the foetus. *Lancet*. 1966;1:286.
56. Moya F, Morishima HO, Shnider SM, James L. Influence of maternal hypoventilation on the newborn infant. *Am J Obstet Gynecol*. 1965;91:76.
57. Ramiro-Tolentino SB, Markarian K, Kleinman LI. Renal bicarbonate excretion in extremely low birth weight infants. *Pediatrics*. 1996;98:256–261.
58. Appendix 2. Taeusch HW, Ballard RA, Gleason CA, eds. *Avery's Diseases of the Newborn*. 8th ed. 2005:1574.
59. Davies PSW. Energy requirements for growth and development in infancy. *Am J Clin Nutr*. 1998;68:939S.
60. Davies PSW, Clough H, Bishop N, et al. Total energy expenditure in small-for-gestational-age infants. *Arch Dis Child*. 1996;74:F208.
61. Hay WW, Catz CS, Grave GD, Yaffe SJ. Workshop summary: fetal growth: its regulation and disorders. *Pediatrics*. 1997;99:585.
62. Stearns MR, Jackson CGR, Landauer JA, et al. Small for gestational age: a new insight? *Med Hypotheses*. 1999;53:186.
63. Nicolaides KH, Economides DL, Soothill PW. Blood gasses, pH and lactate in appropriate- and small-for-gestational-age fetuses. *Am J Obstet Gynecol*. 1989;161:996.
64. Kaiser FE, Dirighi M, Muchnick J, et al. Regulation of gonadotropins and parathyroid hormone by nitric oxide. *Life Sci*. 1996;59:987.

65. Evans CH, Stefanovic-Racic M, Lancaster J. Nitric oxide and it role in orthopedic disease. *Clin Orthop Relat Res*. 1995;312:275.
66. Fleming I, Hecker M, Busse R. Intracellular alkalinization induced by bradykinin sustains activation of the constitutive nitric oxide synthase in endothelial cells. *Circ Res*. 1994;74:1220.
67. Kuhn NJ, Ward S, Piponski M, Young TW. Purification of human hepatic arginase and its manganese (II)-dependent and pH-dependent interconversion between active and inactive forms: a possible pH-sensing function of the enzyme on the ornithine cycle. *Arch Biochem Biophys*. 1995;320:24.
68. Perlman JF, Moore V, Siegel MJ, Dawson J. Is chloride depletion an important contributing cause of death in infants with bronchopulmonary dysplasia? *Pediatrics*. 1986;77:212.
69. Heinly MM, Wassner SJ. The effect of isolated chloride depletion on growth and protein turnover in young rats. *Pediatr Nephrol*. 1994;8:555.
70. Sulyok E, Kovacs L, Lichardus B, et al. Late hyponatremia in premature infants: role of aldosterone and arginine vasopressin. *J Pediatr*. 1985;106:990.
71. Rotmensch S, Liberati M, Celentano C, et al. The effect of betamethasone on fetal biophysical activities and Doppler velocimetry of umbilical and middle cerebral arteries. *Acta Obstet Gynecol Scand*. 1999;78:768.
72. Senat MV, Minoui S, Multon O, et al. Effect of dexamethasone and betamethasone on fetal heart rate variability in preterm labour: a randomized study. *Br J Obstet Gynaecol*. 1998;105:749.
73. Bennett L, Kozuma S, McGarrigle HH, Hanson MA. Temporal changes in fetal cardiovascular, behavioral, metabolic and endocrine responses to maternally administered dexamethasone in the late gestation fetal sheep. *Br J Obstet Gynaecol*. 1999;106:331.
74. Shenhav S, Volodarsky M, Anteby EY, Gemer O. Fetal acid-base balance after betamethasone administration: relation to fetal heart rate variability. *Arch Gynecol Obstet*. 2008;278:333.
75. Derks JB, Mulder EJ, Visser GH. The effects of maternal betamethasone administration on the fetus. *Br J Obstet Gynaecol*. 1995;102:40.
76. Simchen MJ, Alkazaleh F, Adamson SL, et al. The fetal cardiovascular response to antenatal steroids in severe early-onset intrauterine growth restriction. *Am J Obstet Gynecol*. 2004;190:296.
77. Miller SL, Supramaniam VG, Jenkin G, et al. Cardiovascular responses to maternal betamethasone administration in the intrauterine growth-restricted ovine fetus. *Am J Obstet Gynecol*. 2009;201:613.e1.
78. Wiberg N, Källén K, Olofsson P. Delayed umbilical cord clamping at birth has effects on arterial and venous blood gases and lactate concentrations. *BJOG*. 2008;115:697.
79. Hutchon DJ. Immediate cord clamping may increase neonatal acidaemia. *BJOG*. 2008;115:1190.
80. Ruangkit C, Moroney V, Viswanathan S, Bhola M. Safety and efficacy of delayed umbilical cord clamping in multiple and singleton premature infants—a quality improvement study. *J Neonatal Perinatal Med*. 2015;8:393.
81. Reynolds F, Seed PT. Anaesthesia for Caesarean section and neonatal acid-base status: a meta-analysis. *Anaesthesia*. 2005;60:636.
82. Tonni G, Ferrari B, De Felice C, Ventura A. Fetal acid-base and neonatal status after general and neuraxial anesthesia for elective cesarean section. *Int J Gynaecol Obstet*. 2007;97:143.

6

Glomerular Filtration Rate in Neonates

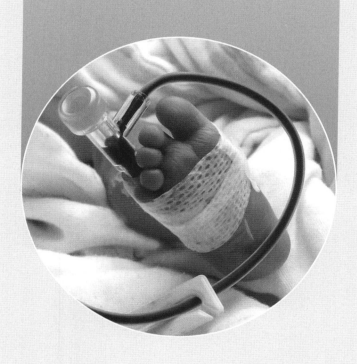

CHAPTER 7

Glomerular Filtration Rate in Neonates

Jean-Pierre Guignard, MD, Jean-Bernard Gouyon, MD

Ultrafiltration of plasma across permselective capillaries is the first step in urine formation. This process starts with the development of the metanephros around the 10th week of gestation. The glomerular filtration rate (GFR) increases progressively throughout fetal and postnatal life, reaching the "adult" mature levels by 1 year of life. During the period of maturation, the function of the kidney is characterized by elevated renal vascular resistance (RVR), low arterial renal perfusion pressure, and low renal blood flow (RBF). The ultrafiltration process is maintained by a delicate balance between vasoconstrictor and counteracting vasodilator forces. This balance can be easily disturbed by various factors, resulting in a transient or permanent impairment in GFR. This chapter briefly reviews the maturation of glomerular filtration, discusses the techniques available to assess GFR in neonates, and describes factors and agents that can impair or protect maturing glomerular filtration.

Development of Glomerular Filtration

Glomerular ultrafiltration depends on the net ultrafiltration pressure, which is the difference between the hydrostatic and oncotic pressures across glomerular capillaries. The low perfusion pressure and low glomerular plasma flow account, at least in part, for the low levels of GFR present during gestation. For any given ultrafiltration pressure, GFR will depend on the rate at which plasma flows through the glomerular capillaries, as well as on the ultrafiltration coefficient (K_f). K_f is a function of the total capillary surface area and of the permeability per unit of surface area.

During gestation, GFR increases in parallel with gestational age (GA), up to the end of nephrogenesis around the 35th week of gestation.[1] This pattern of development reflects both an increase in the number of nephrons and the growth of existing nephrons. From the 35th week of gestation, the development of GFR slows down up to the time of birth (Fig. 7.1). Postnatal maturation of renal function is characterized by a striking increase in GFR, the value of which doubles within the first 2 weeks of life (Fig. 7.2).[1] The velocity of this increase is somewhat slower in the most premature infants. An increase in both the net filtration pressure and the K_f accounts for the large postnatal increase in GFR. The increase in the glomerular capillary surface area represents the main factor responsible for the increase in the K_f.[2] Additional maturational changes that may contribute to the postnatal maturation of GFR include an increase in pore size and glomerular hydraulic permeability and a decrease in both the afferent and efferent arteriolar resistance.

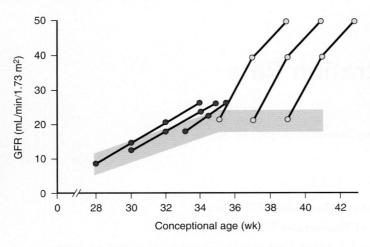

Fig. 7.1 Development of glomerular filtration rate (GFR) as a function of conceptional age during the last 3 months of gestation and the first month of postnatal life. The *shaded area* represents the range of normal values. The postnatal increase in GFR observed in preterm (●-●) and term neonates (o-o) is schematically represented. (Modified from Guignard JP, John EG. Renal function in the tiny, premature infant. *Clin Perinatol.* 1986;13:377.)

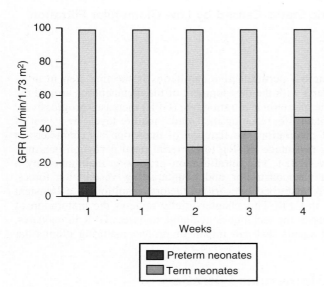

Fig. 7.2 Postnatal increase in glomerular filtration rate (GFR) in term and preterm infants. The upper part of each column represents the deficit between the neonate's GFR and mature levels (100 mL/min per 1.73 m²). Note that at the end of the first month of life, human neonates are in a state of relative renal insufficiency compared with adults. (Modified from Guignard JP, John EG. Renal function in the tiny, premature infant. *Clin Perinatol.* 1986;13:377.)

Vasoactive Factors

Several vasoactive agents and hormones modulate GFR and RBF.[2] By acting on the arcuate arteries, interlobular arteries, and afferent and efferent arterioles, they regulate the glomerular hydrostatic pressure and the glomerular transcapillary hydraulic pressure gradient. These agents can also modify the K_f by two mechanisms: a change in the capillary filtration area by contracting the mesangial cells and a change in hydraulic conductivity by decreasing the number or size (or both) of the filtration slit pores. The main vasoactive forces modulating single-nephron GFR (SNGFR) are listed in Table 7.1. Two vasoactive systems, the renin-angiotensin system and the prostaglandins (PGs) (Fig. 7.3), play key roles in maintaining GFR in the maturing kidney.

Angiotensin II

Angiotensin II (ATII) is a very potent vasoconstrictor of the afferent and efferent arterioles, acting on two types of receptors, the AT_1 and the AT_2 receptor subtypes. The AT_1 receptors are widely distributed and appear to mediate most of the biologic effects of ATII. Although AT_2 receptors appear essential for the ureteric branching and cell proliferation,[3] their exact role remains uncertain. ATII acts on both preglomerular and postglomerular resistance but appears to predominantly vasoconstrict

Table 7.1 VASOACTIVE FACTORS REGULATING THE GLOMERULAR MICROCIRCULATION

Vasoconstrictors	Vasodilators
Circulating hormones • Catecholamines • Angiotensin II • Vasopressin • Glucocorticoids	Circulating hormones • Dopamine
Paracrine + autocoïds • Endothelin • Thromboxane A_2 • Leukotrienes • Adenosine	Paracrine + autocoïds • Nitric oxide • Acetylcholine • PGI_2 + PGE_2 • Bradykinin • Adenosine

PG, Prostaglandin.

Fig. 7.3 The physiologic regulation of glomerular filtration rate (GFR) depends on two main factors: the afferent vasodilator prostaglandins and the efferent vasoconstrictor angiotensin II. *RBF,* Renal blood flow.

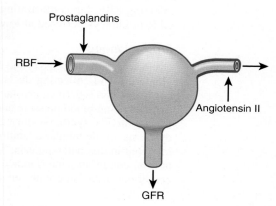

the efferent arteriole, thereby increasing the glomerular capillary hydrostatic pressure while decreasing the glomerular plasma flow rate.[4] This mechanism serves to maintain GFR when the renal perfusion pressure decreases to low levels. The action of ATII on the efferent arteriole is counterbalanced by intrarenal adenosine, an agent modulating the tubuloglomerular feedback mechanism. When both ATII and adenosine are overstimulated, their combined action results in afferent vasoconstriction.[5]

Prostaglandins

The renal PGs are potent vasoactive metabolites of arachidonic acid.[6,7] Under normal conditions, the renal PGs are present in low concentrations and exert only minor effects on the renal circulation and GFR. However, the vasodilator PGs are of major importance in protecting renal perfusion and GFR when vasoconstrictor forces are activated as, for instance, during hypotensive, hypovolemic, and sodium depletion states or during congestive heart failure. The PGs protect GFR by vasodilating the afferent arterioles and by dampening the renal vasoconstrictor effects of ATII, endothelin, and sympathetic nerve stimulation on the afferent arteriole.

Maturational Aspects of the Renin-Angiotensin and Prostaglandins Systems

Renin-Angiotensin System

Renin is found as early as the fifth week in the mesonephros and by the eighth week in the metanephros. The plasma renin concentration and activity generated by the fetal kidney are elevated.[8] The presence of an intact functional renin-angiotensin system is a key factor for the maintenance of blood pressure and RBF during fetal life. Acting through its AT_1 receptors, ATII is indeed the promoter of the postnatal expression of postglomerular capillaries and organization of vasa recta bundles, which are necessary for development of normal RBF.[9] Mutations in the genes encoding any of the components of the renin-angiotensin system result in severe tubular dysgenesis.[10] The plasma renin activity further increases after birth before slowly decreasing through infancy. The factors controlling renin release (macula densa, baroreceptor, sympathetic nervous system, and hormonal mechanisms) are active in the fetus.[8]

Elevated levels of ATII are present in the fetus and remain high in the neonatal period. Although AT_2 receptors predominate during embryonic and fetal life, they rapidly decline after birth.[11] AT_1 receptors predominate after birth and are found in glomeruli, macula densa and mesangial cells, resistance arteries, and vasa recta.[12] In addition to its AT_1-mediated vasoconstrictor effects, ATII promotes growth of the renal vasculature.[11] Blockade of the AT_1 receptors with losartan during fetal life interferes with normal renal development and results in vascular malformations, cystic dilatation of the tubules, and a decrease in the number of glomeruli.[12] Blockade of AT_1 receptor by losartan in newborn rabbits induces a decrease in GFR without affecting RBF,[13] thus illustrating the major role of ATII in regulating and protecting GFR in kidneys perfused at low systemic arterial pressures.

Prostaglandins

Cyclooxygenase 1 (COX-1) and 2 (COX-2) are expressed in the fetal renal vasculature, glomeruli, and collecting ducts. The COX-2 activity is highest after birth.[14] Renal cortical COX-2–derived prostanoids, particularly PGI_2 and PGE_2, play critical roles in maintaining blood pressure and renal function in volume-contracted states. Interference with PG synthesis during fetal life leads to renal dysgenesis with cortical dysplasia, cystic tubular dilatation, and impaired nephrogenesis.[15] COX-2 is probably involved in this pathogenesis.[16] Although the PGs probably do not regulate GFR in normal conditions, interference with PG synthesis may have deleterious effects in conditions associated with renal hypoperfusion.

Assessment of Glomerular Filtration Rate

Different methods using various markers have been used to assess GFR in neonates. The most common measurement of GFR is based on the concept of "clearance," which relates the quantitative urinary excretion of a substance per unit of time to the volume of plasma that, if "cleared" completely of the same contained substance, would yield a quantity equivalent to that excreted in the urine. The clearance C of a substance x is expressed by the formula:

$$C = U_X \bullet V/P_X$$

where U_X represents the urinary concentration of the substance, V the urine flow rate, and P_X the plasma concentration. For its clearance to be equal to the rate of glomerular filtration, a substance must have the following properties: (1) it must be freely filterable through the glomerular capillary membranes (i.e., not be bound to plasma proteins or sieved in the process of ultrafiltration); (2) it must not be excreted by an extrarenal route; and (3) it must be biologically inert and neither reabsorbed nor secreted by the renal tubules. Several substances, endogenous or exogenous, have been claimed to have these properties: inulin, creatinine, iohexol, ethylenediaminetetraacetic acid (EDTA), diethylenetriamine pentaacetic acid (DTPA), and sodium iothalamate. The experimental evidence that this is true has been produced only for inulin. To avoid the need for urine collection, various techniques have been developed to estimate GFR: the height/plasma creatinine (P_{creat}) formula; the plasma disappearance curve of an exogenous marker after a single injection; and the constant infusion of an exogenous glomerular marker without urine collection. Finally, cystatin C, a nonglycosylated basic protein, the concentration of which correlates with GFR, has been proposed as a surrogate marker of glomerular function. Different techniques

Table 7.2 CHARACTERISTICS OF THE GLOMERULAR MARKERS

	Inulin	Creatinine	Iohexol	DTPA	EDTA	Iothalamate
Molecular weight (Da)	5200	113	811	393	292	637
Elimination half-life (min)	70	200	90	110	120	120
Plasma protein binding (%)	0	0	<2	5	0	<5
Space of distribution	EC	TBW	EC	EC	EC	EC

DTPA, Diethylenetriamine pentaacetic acid; EC, extracellular space; EDTA, ethylenediaminetetraacetic acid; TBW, total body water.

have been used to assess GFR with the endogenous or exogenous markers listed in Table 7.2. These techniques and markers are discussed next.

Endogenous Markers

Creatinine

Creatinine, the normal metabolite of creatine phosphate present in skeletal muscle, has a molecular weight (MW) of 113 Da. The renal excretion of endogenous creatinine is fairly similar to that of inulin in humans and several animal species. However, in addition to being filtered through the glomerulus, creatinine is secreted in part by the renal tubular cells.

Overestimation of GFR by creatinine clearance (C_{creat}) is usually more evident at low GFRs. As GFR decreases progressively during the course of renal disease, the renal tubular secretion of creatinine contributes an increasing fraction to urinary excretion, so that C_{creat} may substantially exceed the actual GFR. Secretion of creatinine into the gut plays a role in this phenomenon.

Although creatinine has been used for decades, the methods available for its chemical determination are still biased by various interfering substances.[17] The coloric method described by Jaffe is still widely used in clinical laboratories. Its major drawback is the interference by noncreatinine chromogens such as bilirubin, pyruvate, uric acid, cotrimoxazole, and cyclosporins. The use of enzymatic methods has increased the specificity of creatinine determination.[17] Further improvement in measuring creatinine has been achieved by the use of newer techniques, such as high-performance liquid chromatography (HPLC), gas chromatography isotope dilution mass spectrometry (Gc-IDMS), and the HPLC-IDMS coupled technique.[17] Gc-IDMS is now considered the method of choice for measuring true creatinine. It has an excellent specificity and low relative standard deviation (SD) (<0.3%).[17] A method coupling HPLC with IDMS for the direct determination of creatinine has also been developed.[18] The procedure is simple and speedy. It appears to offer the same advantage as the Gc-IDMS technique. Although accurate and reproducible assessment of creatinine is mandatory, the calibration of its measurement is not yet standardized to a gold standard in most places, leading to substantial variations among laboratories.[17]

Creatinine as a Marker of Glomerular Filtration Rate in the Neonate

The handling of creatinine by immature kidneys is unique, with creatinine apparently undergoing glomerular filtration and partial tubular reabsorption. In newborn rabbits the urinary clearance of creatinine underestimates the concomitantly measured clearance of inulin with creatinine-to-inulin ratios less than 1 in the first days of life (Fig. 7.4).[19] Such ratios indicate that creatinine is actually reabsorbed at this stage of renal development. As the animals mature, the ratios increase to greater than 1, reflecting filtration and secretion of creatinine. Reabsorption of creatinine is present only in the first postnatal days and is probably explained by the passive reabsorption of the filtered creatinine across immature leaky tubules.[19,20] When water is reabsorbed along the nephron, the concentration of filtered creatinine rises so that creatinine back-diffuses into the blood according to its concentration gradient, thus raising its plasma concentration. The clearance of creatinine has also been shown to underestimate true GFR in very low birth weight (VLBW) human neonates, thus suggesting the occurrence of the same phenomenon in human immature kidneys.[20]

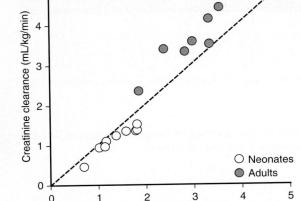

Fig. 7.4 The relationship between the clearances of creatinine and inulin in newborn and adult rabbits with comparable plasma levels of creatinine. (Modified from Matos P, Duarte-Silva M, Drukker A, Guignard JP. Creatinine reabsorption by the newborn rabbit kidney. *Pediatr Res.* 1998;44:639.)

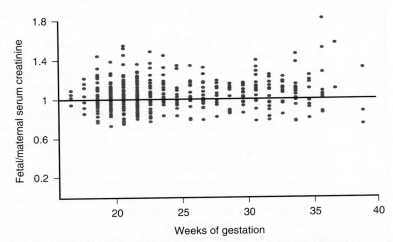

Fig. 7.5 Relationship between fetal cord and maternal serum creatinine during gestation. The ratio of the fetal to maternal serum creatinine remains close to 1 throughout gestation, indicating free diffusion of creatinine across the placental barrier. (Modified from Guignard JP, Drukker A. Why do newborn infants have a high plasma creatinine? *Pediatrics.* 1999;103(4):e49.)

The use of creatinine as a marker of GFR in neonates is not hampered only by its specific handling by the immature kidney but also, as previously mentioned, by the interference of noncreatinine chromogens, sometimes leading to spurious overestimation of the true P_{creat}.

Plasma Creatinine Concentration

The P_{creat} concentration of the neonate is elevated at birth, reflecting the maternal P_{creat} concentration. A near perfect equilibrium between the maternal and fetal P_{creat} concentrations has indeed been shown to occur throughout gestation (Fig. 7.5).[20] In preterm infants the elevated P_{creat} further increases transiently to reach a peak value between the second and fourth days of postnatal life (Fig. 7.6).[21,22] Peak P_{creat} concentrations as high as 195 to 247 μmol/L in 23 to 26 weeks' GA neonates and 99 to 140 μmol/L in 33 to 40 weeks' GA neonates have been recorded (Table 7.3).[22] This transient increase in the VLBW neonates' postnatal P_{creat} concentration is probably the result of creatinine reabsorption across leaky tubules. This phenomenon accounts for the observation that when measured during the first week of life, the P_{creat} is highest in the most premature infants.[23] Reference ranges for P_{creat} have been reported

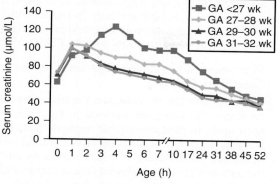

Fig. 7.6 Changes in serum creatinine in preterm neonates during the first 52 hours of postnatal life. Peak increases are observed on day 4 in the most premature infants. *GA*, Gestational age. (Modified from Gallini F, Maggio L, Romagnoli C, Marrocco G, Tortorolo G. Progression of renal function in preterm neonates with gestational age ≤32 weeks. *Pediatr Nephrol.* 2000;15:119.)

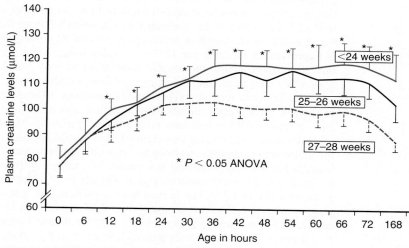

Fig. 7.7 Mean plasma creatinine level (95% confidence interval) and gestational age during the first week of life. (From Thayyil S, Sheik S, Kempley ST, Sinha A. A gestation- and postnatal age-based reference chart for assessing renal function in extremely premature infants. *J Perinatol.* 2008;28:226.)

Table 7.3 CHANGES IN PLASMA CREATININE OVER TIME FOR DIFFERENT GESTATION GROUPS

Group Gestation Age (Weeks)	Birth Creatinine (μmol/L)[a]	Peak Plasma Creatinine (μmol/L)[a]	Time to Peak Plasma Creatinine (h)[a]
23–26	67–92	195–247	40–78
27–29	65–89	158–200	28–51
30–32	60–69	120–158	25–40
33–45	67–79	99–140	8–23

[a]Range intervals.
From Miall LA, Henderson MJ, Turner, AJ, et al. Plasma creatinine rises dramatically in the first 48 hours of life in preterm infants. *Pediatrics.* 1999;6:104.

retrospectively in 218 appropriate-for-GA VLBW infants without risk factors for renal impairment[24] or established from a cohort of 161 extremely premature infants followed during the first 8 weeks of life (Fig. 7.7).[25] Normal values for P_{creat} (as measured by an enzymatic assay during the first year of life) are also available.[26] Factors affecting P_{creat} at birth and during the first postnatal weeks have been defined recently.[27,28] Hypertensive disease of pregnancy, ibuprofen-treated patent ductus arteriosus (PDA), low Apgar scores, ventilation, and low GA were prominent factors influencing P_{creat} at birth and later. In infants with hemodynamically significant PDA, P_{creat} levels before ibuprofen were significantly higher than those recorded in GA-matched control participants without PDA.

Estimation of Creatinine Clearance by the Length/Plasma Creatinine Ratio

The concentration of endogenous markers, such as creatinine, increases when GFR decreases. However, the increase in P_{creat} is not linear. Several attempts have thus been made to develop reliable methods that will allow a correct estimate of C_{creat} from its plasma concentration alone without urine collection. A formula has been developed for children,[29,30] which allows an estimate of C_{creat} (eC_{creat}) derived from the patient's creatinine plasma concentration and body length:

$$eC_{creat} = k \bullet Length/P_{creat}$$

where k is a constant, L represents the body length in centimeters, and P_{creat} the plasma creatinine concentration in mg/dL. This formula is based on the assumption that creatinine excretion is proportional to body length and inversely proportional to P_{creat}.[30] The value of the constant k can be obtained from the formula $k = eC_{creat} \bullet P_{creat}/Length$. When length is expressed in cm and P_{creat} in mg/dL, the resulting eC_{creat} is expressed in mL/min per 1.73 m^2. Under steady state conditions, k should be directly proportional to the muscle component of body weight, which corresponds reasonably well to the daily urinary creatinine excretion rate.

The Schwartz formula has been used in neonates.[30] The mean value of k, calculated in 118 low birth weight infants with corrected ages of 25 to 105 weeks, was 0.33 ± 0.01. It rose to 0.45 in full-term infants up to 18 months.[30] Despite a large scatter of normal values, the formula was claimed to be useful because it correlated well with the inulin single-injection technique.[30] It is only unfortunate that the k • Length/P_{creat} formula has not been validated in neonates by comparing its results with those given by the standard U • V/P inulin clearance. The accuracy of the k • Length/P_{creat} formula, as an estimate of GFR, has indeed been questioned. In a study in infants younger than 1 year of age, the k value ranged from 0.17 to 0.82 (15–72 when P_{creat} in μmol/L), and factor k was found to vary markedly with the state of hydration.[31] The k • Length/P_{creat} formula may be more informative clinically than P_{creat} alone because the creatinine value, in addition to renal function, is critically dependent on the percentage of muscle mass. However, caution should be exercised when using the formula as an estimate of GFR in studies aimed at defining renal pathophysiologic mechanisms in neonates.

U • V/P Urinary Clearance of Creatinine

The urinary clearance of creatinine has been claimed to approximate the urinary clearance of inulin in both preterm and term neonates. In premature infants a creatinine-to-inulin clearance ratio less than 1 has often been observed, suggesting that tubular reabsorption of creatinine also occurs in premature humans, as it does in immature animals.[19] Developmental studies based on the urinary clearance of creatinine have produced valuable information on the maturation of GFR.[23,32–34] Reference values for the urinary clearance of creatinine during the first month of life of premature infants with GA ranging from 27 to 31 weeks has been published.[35] The postnatal increase in C_{creat} observed in these preterm infants is illustrated in Fig. 7.8. At 28 days of postnatal age, C_{creat} remains significantly lower in preterm infants as compared with term neonates.[34] Regression lines for calculating the normal values of C_{creat} as a function of GA and postnatal day are given in Table 7.4.

Special Case of Cystatin C: A Nonclassical Glomerular Marker!

Cystatin C, a nonglycosylated 13-kDa basic protein, is a proteinase inhibitor involved in the intracellular catabolism of proteins.[36] It is produced by all nucleated cells,

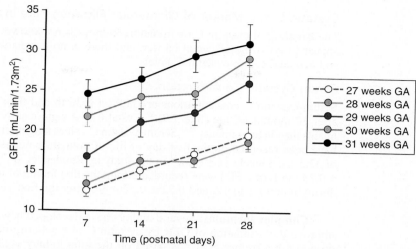

Fig. 7.8 Glomerular filtration rate (GFR) according to gestational age (GA) in the first month of life (n = 275). Data are means +/– SEM. (From Vieux R, Hascoet JM, Merdariu D, Fresson J, Guillemin F. Glomerular filtration rate reference values in very preterm infants. *Pediatrics.* 2010;125:e1186.)

Table 7.4 REGRESSION LINES TO CALCULATE THE REFERENCE MEDIAN NORMAL VALUE OF GLOMERULAR FILTRATION RATE AS A FUNCTION OF GESTATIONAL AGE (IN WEEKS) AND POSTNATAL DAY

Postnatal Day	Median GFR
7	$63.57 + 2.85 \times GA$
14	$60.73 + 2.85 \times GA$
21	$58.97 + 2.85 \times GA$
28	$55.93 + 2.85 \times GA$

GA, Gestational age; *GFR*, glomerular filtration rate.
Modified from Vieux R, Hascoet JM, Merdariu D, Fresson J, Guillemin F. Glomerular filtration rate reference values in very preterm infants. *Pediatrics.* 2010;125:e1186.

freely filtered across the glomerular capillaries, almost completely reabsorbed, and catabolized in the renal proximal tubular cells.[37] Being reabsorbed, cystatin C is not a classical marker of glomerular filtration, as strictly defined (see "Assessment of Glomerular Filtration Rate" section). When using the particle-enhanced immunonephelometry assay for its determination in blood, no interference from bilirubin, hemoglobin, triglycerides, and rheumatoid factor could be observed.[38] Cystatin C has been claimed to be a reliable marker of GFR independent of inflammatory conditions, muscle mass, and gender.[39,40] In children ages 1.8 to 18.8 years with various levels of GFR, serum cystatin C has been claimed to be broadly equivalent[41] or even superior[42] to P_{creat} as an estimate of GFR. However, a very large study of 8058 inhabitants of Groeningen questions the advantages of cystatin C.[43] In this study, male gender, older age, greater weight, higher serum C-reactive protein levels, and cigarette smoking were all independently associated with higher cystatin C levels after adjusting for eC_{creat}. Cystatin C has also been shown to be a poor marker of GFR in pregnancy,[44] in renal transplant patients, and in patients receiving corticosteroids,[45–47] as well as in intensive care unit patients.[48] In a recent study in children, cystatin C has also been shown to be less reliable than the Schwartz formula in distinguishing impaired from normal GFR.[49]

Cystatin C as a Marker of Glomerular Filtration Rate in the Neonate

The handling of cystatin C by immature kidneys is not known. Cystatin C does not appear to cross the placental barrier, and there is no correlation between maternal and neonatal serum cystatin C levels.[50]

Serum Cystatin Concentration

Serum cystatin C concentrations are highest at birth and then decrease to stabilize after 12 months of age (Fig. 7.9).[39] Cystatin C is significantly higher in premature infants than in term infants.[39,51] Serum cystatin C values ranging from 1.24 to 2.84 mg/L have been recorded on the first day of life of premature neonates, with a mean GA of 32.5 ± 2.6 weeks (x ± SD).[52] In the study by Randers et al.,[40] mean values of 1.63 ± 0.26 mg/L (x ± SD) were recorded during the first month of life, 0.95 ± 0.22 mg/L during months 1 to 12, and 0.72 ± 0.12 mg/L after the first year of life.

Complex formulas: Several authors have developed new complex formulas to improve the estimation of GFR by cystatin C in newborn infants.[53,54] The formula proposed by Treiber et al.[54] is based on the total kidney volume (as measured by three-dimensional ultrasound), birth weight, birth length, body surface area, and the serum cystatin C concentration. The eGFR calculated using this formula is said to be a reliable marker of GFR compared with neonatal reference clearance values. The so-called reference values are unfortunately all indirect formulas not validated by the urinary clearance of inulin, which remains the gold standard. The same criticism applies to the data provided by Abitbol et al.[53]

In an interesting recent review, Filler et al.[55] again asked the question whether creatinine is the best tool to assess GFR in neonates or whether cystatin C is superior. They conclude that "cystatin C may be the most suitable marker of neonatal renal function," but warn that "its ability is still limited, it is more costly, and the best method of reporting acute kidney injury and neonatal GFR remains to be established."

The claim that the concentration of cystatin C offers a greater sensitivity and reliability than creatinine in detecting an abnormal GFR in newborn infants and "that

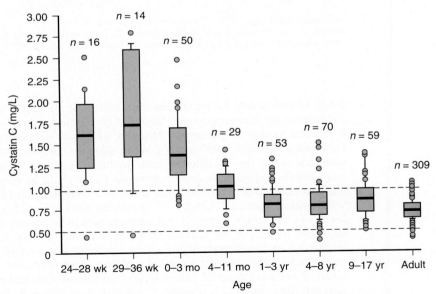

Fig. 7.9 Box plot distributions showing plasma cystatin C values across the age groups. *Dotted lines* indicate 95% confidence interval of the adult range. Preterm babies born between 24 and 36 weeks of gestation were 1 day old. (Modified from Finney H, Newman DJ, Thakkar H, Fell JM, Price CP. Reference ranges for plasma cystatin C and creatinine measurements in premature infants, neonates, and older children. *Arch Dis Child.* 2000;82:71.)

unlike creatinine, cystatin C can be used to assess GFR of the newborn and even the fetus"[56] may be somewhat illusive. There are indeed several reasons to question this conclusion: (1) the handling of cystatin C by the immature kidney is not known; (2) the scatter of the serum cystatin C concentrations in neonates is very large, so it is unlikely that a formula can be established to reliably estimate GFR at this early age; (3) because cystatin C is filtered and then reabsorbed and catabolized by the proximal tubular cells, its plasma concentration is obviously influenced by changes in the rate of degradation of cystatin C by injured renal proximal tubular cells; (4) the production and concentration of cystatin C may be influenced by factors other than GFR, such as the serum C-reactive protein levels, thyroid dysfunction, or corticosteroid administration; (5) the claim that cystatin C is a valuable marker of GFR has not been validated by comparison to the gold standard, either in neonates or in children; and (6) measurement of cystatin C is considerably more expensive than that of creatinine.[55]

Exogenous Markers of Glomerular Filtration Rate

Inulin

Inulin, an exogenous starchlike fructose polymer extracted from Jerusalem artichokes, has an Einstein-Stokes radius of 1.5 nm and an MW of approximately 5.2 kDa. It diffuses, as would a spherical body of such radius. Inulin is inert and is not metabolized, not reabsorbed, and not secreted by the renal tubular cells. Its clearance, consequently, reflects the rate of filtration only. Estimates of inulin clearance provide the basis for a standard reference against which the route or mechanisms of excretion of other substances can be ascertained.

Inulin as a Marker of Glomerular Filtration Rate in Neonates

The hypothesis that inulin may not be freely filtered by the immature glomerular barrier has never been confirmed, neither in animal nor in human studies.[57] Inulin has been used as a marker of GFR in human neonates using three different techniques to measure or estimate its clearance: (1) the urinary UV/P clearance (where U is the urine concentration, V is the urine flow rate, and P is the plasma concentration), (2) the single-injection (plasma disappearance curve) technique, and (3) the constant infusion technique without urine collection.

Urinary U • V/P Clearance of Inulin

The method based on the urinary clearance of inulin is the gold reference method for GFR. However, measurement of the urinary clearance of this exogenous marker is cumbersome because it requires constant intravenous infusion to maintain a steady state and the precise timed collection of urine. The method has been used successfully in early developmental studies[1] to define the maturation of GFR in relation to gestational and postnatal age (see Figs. 7.1 and 7.2).

Constant Infusion Technique Without Urine Collection

The constant infusion technique[58] assumes that the rate of infusion (IR) of a marker (x) needed to maintain constant its plasma concentration is equal to the rate of its excretion. After equilibration of the marker in its distribution space, the excretion rate must thus be equal to the IR, hence the derived clearance formula:

$$C_x = U_x \bullet V/P_x = IR_x \bullet P_x$$

The flow rate of the test solution containing the marker is expressed in mL/min per 1.73 m^2; so is the clearance C of the marker x.

The constant infusion technique without urine collection is attractive and has been used in newborn infants. The results obtained in short-term (a few hours) infusion studies have produced conflicting results. When inulin was constantly infused for 24 hours, the results obtained by this technique were in reasonable agreement with those obtained by the traditional urinary clearance.[59,60] As a whole, the infusion technique has the advantage of avoiding the need for urine collection but presents with the main disadvantage of requiring careful time-consuming supervision of the long-duration infusion of inulin.

Single-Injection (Plasma Disappearance Curve) Technique

The mathematical model for this technique is an open two-compartment system. The glomerular marker is injected in the first compartment, equilibrates with the second compartment, and is excreted from the first compartment by glomerular filtration. The plasma disappearance curve of the marker follows two consecutive patterns. In the first phase the agent diffuses in its distribution space and its plasma concentration falls rapidly. In the second phase, when the equilibration has been reached, the slope of the decline of the plasma concentration of the marker basically reflects its urinary excretion rate.

The plasma disappearance curve method has occasionally been used in neonates. A large overestimation of GFR by the single-injection technique during the first days of life has been repeatedly observed; it was ascribed to incomplete equilibration of inulin in its distribution space during the study period.[60,61]

Iohexol

Iohexol is a nonionic agent with a MW of 821 Da that appears to be eliminated exclusively by glomerular filtration. A significant correlation has been observed between the urinary clearance of inulin and both the urinary clearance of iohexol or its plasma disappearance clearance in a limited number of children.[62,63] Large studies to validate iohexol as a true glomerular marker are not yet available. Iohexol has not been validated in neonates.

Iothalamate Sodium

Iothalamate sodium has a MW of 637 Da. It can be used as ^{125}I-radiolabeled or without radioactive label, its plasma concentration then being assessed by x-ray fluorescence or by HPLC or, more recently, by capillary electrophoresis. It is only minimally bound to proteins, and its renal handling has some similarities with that of inulin. However, critical studies have unequivocally demonstrated that iothalamate is actively secreted by the renal tubules and perhaps also undergoes tubular reabsorption in humans and animal species.[64] The agreement between iothalamate and inulin clearances appears to be a fortuitous cancellation of errors between tubular excretion and protein binding of the agent. The substance does not consequently appear suitable for accurate estimation of GFR. The use of iothalamate has not been properly validated in neonates.[65] Radiolabeled iothalamate should not be used in the first month of life.

[99m]Tc-Diethylenetriamine Pentaacetic Acid and ^{51}Cr-Ethylenediaminetetraacetic Acid

The use of radiolabeled markers is not recommended during the neonatal period. This group of markers is thus not discussed here.

Assessment of Renal Function in Neonates: Which Method for Which Purpose?

Developmental Investigative Studies

When the purpose of performing clearance studies is to obtain basic information on the physiologic maturation of GFR, the use of reliable methods is mandatory. The urinary clearance of inulin remains the method of choice. This method requires constant inulin infusion to maintain steady state and timed urine collection by bladder catheterization or bag. The urinary clearance of creatinine also requires timed collection of urine and blood sampling in the middle of the urinary collection period. Valuable information has been obtained by this technique. The need for urine collection can be avoided by using the constant inulin infusion technique. In this case, inulin needs to be constantly infused for at least 24 hours, requiring careful supervision. When respecting the protocol strictly,[59,60] useful information can be obtained by this technique. The plasma inulin disappearance curve after a single injection significantly overestimates by 30% the urinary clearance of inulin in the first days of neonates.[66]

Other nonvalidated methods for measuring GFR should be avoided because they are unnecessarily complex without providing indisputable data.

Clinical Purposes

Simpler techniques can be used to estimate GFR for clinical purposes. When interpreted with caution, the serum creatinine concentrations can provide crude but valid information on the neonate's renal function. The transient "physiologic" increase in plasma concentrations occurring during the first days of very premature infants should be taken into account when interpreting such concentrations. The data published by Gallini et al.[21] and Miall et al.[22] should be used as reference values for creatinine levels in VLBW infants. In doing so, sequential measurements of the plasma concentration of creatinine can provide useful information on the putative presence of renal insufficiency.

When an approximate estimate of C_{creat} is needed, the Schwartz formula adapted for neonates[30] can be used. The formula is simple and requires only measurement of the neonate's P_{creat} and body length. The formula has indeed been shown to provide useful data on the level of GFR. The value of 0.33 ± 0.01 for constant k (when creatinine is expressed in mg/dL, and 29 when it is expressed in μmol/L) will, of course, only be valid if the reference values for creatinine are the same in the laboratory where creatinine is tested and in the laboratory where the value of factor k has been calculated.[31] Ideally, each laboratory should define its own value for constant k in a selected group of patients.

Measuring the serum concentration of cystatin C can also provide information on glomerular filtration in the neonatal period. Using complex nonvalidated formulas to ameliorate the accuracy of cystatin C as an index of GFR in an infant whose renal function is basically unstable does not seem worth the effort.

The use of more sophisticated techniques for clinical purpose is also not justified. Such is the case for the single-injection technique of inulin or sodium iothalamate. The information they give is not accurate enough to justify their complexity. They do not provide information that cannot be obtained by the simple Schwartz formula.

Conditions and Factors That Impair Glomerular Filtration Rate

In human neonates the major risk factors for developing acute renal insufficiency are severe respiratory disorders and perinatal exposure to PGs synthase inhibitors.[67–70]

Perinatal Asphyxia

Perinatal asphyxia is defined as a condition leading to progressive hypoxemia, hypercapnia, and metabolic acidosis with multiorgan failure, including the kidney. The pathogenesis of the hypoxia-induced vasomotor nephropathy has been studied in newborn rabbits and lambs. In the rabbit model, isolated hypoxemia induces intense renal vasoconstriction with a consequent decrease in GFR and in the filtration fraction (FF) and to less extent in RBF. The observed decrease in FF suggests efferent arteriolar vasodilation, presumably as a consequence of intrarenal activation of adenosine,[71] an endogenous vasoactive agent known to preferentially vasodilate the efferent arteriole and to decrease the intraglomerular pressure. The hypothesis that adenosine plays a key role in mediating the hypoxemic renal vasoconstriction was supported by the fact that theophylline, a nonspecific antagonist of adenosine cell surface receptors, prevented the decrease in GFR induced by hypoxemia in newborn rabbits.[71] Such an effect was not observed when enprofylline, a xanthine devoid of adenosine antagonistic properties, was administered instead of theophylline.[72] Clinical studies using prophylactic theophylline in high-risk asphyxiated neonates seem to confirm the putative beneficial effect of theophylline in protecting GFR (see Theophylline in Oliguric Neonates, later; Fig. 7.11).

Nonsteroidal Antiinflammatory Agents

Exposure to PG synthesis inhibitors during fetal development can lead to severe renal dysgenesis. Increased activity of the vasodilator PGs present during development is necessary to protect the function of immature kidneys. By blunting the effect of vasodilator PGs on the afferent arteriole, PG synthesis inhibitors can impair GFR in both fetuses and neonates. Indomethacin is sometimes used in pregnant women with polyhydramnios to reduce fetal urine output and consequently the production of amniotic fluid.[73] It should be realized that this "obstetric" benefit is achieved by producing a state of renal insufficiency in the fetus. Decreased GFR has been demonstrated in neonates whose mothers had been administered indomethacin shortly before birth,[74] as well as in neonates administered indomethacin for the closure of PDA.[75] This deleterious effect is usually transient, with renal function normalizing within 30 days,[76] but may have deleterious consequences for the elimination of drugs such as vancomycin, aminoglycosides, and digoxin, which are excreted mainly by glomerular filtration.

Ibuprofen, a COX nonselective inhibitor, has been claimed to be safer than indomethacin for newborn kidneys.[77] The efficacy and renal side effects of ibuprofen and indomethacin have been compared in two recent meta-analyses.[78,79] Although the efficacy of the two drugs in closing the PDA was similar, ibuprofen appeared to have fewer renal side effects than indomethacin. Ibuprofen-treated neonates presented with higher urine output (+0.74 mL/kg per min) and a lower increase of serum creatinine concentration (+0.44 ± 0.10 µmol/L). In contrast, in a well-controlled clinical study, the prophylactic administration of either acetylsalicylic acid (4 × 11 mg/kg per day for 2 days) or ibuprofen (10 mg/kg and 5 mg/kg at 24 hours and 48 hours, respectively) was associated with similar decreases in the clearance of amikacin administered concomitantly (Fig. 7.10).[80,81] Amikacin is eliminated almost exclusively by glomerular filtration, so that a decrease in its clearance indicates a decrease in GFR. This observation casts doubt on the renal innocuousness of ibuprofen. This doubt is supported by experimental studies failing to demonstrate a difference between various nonsteroidal antiinflammatory drugs, including the nonspecific COX inhibitors aspirin, indomethacin, and ibuprofen. All agents acutely decreased GFR and RBF when administered to newborn rabbits.[82,83]

In an excellent review describing the renal side effects of nonsteroidal antiinflammatory drugs (NSAIDs) in human neonates, Allegaert et al.[84] discuss the possible differences in the renal harmful effects of indomethacin and ibuprofen. They conclude, as did Ohlsson et al. from their Cochrane analysis,[79] that both agents had similar beneficial effects on the ductus arteriosus but a negative impact on GFR, this deleterious effect being more pronounced for indomethacin than for ibuprofen.

Differences in the renal side effects of indomethacin and ibuprofen may depend on the ratio of their respective activities on the two COX isoenzymes COX-1 and COX-2, with indomethacin inhibiting COX-1 more than COX-2. However, this hypothesis does not fit well with the observation made in newborn rabbits that the preferential COX-2 inhibitor nimesulide induced the same renal vasoconstriction as did the nonselective inhibitors.[85] If real, the potential advantage of using ibuprofen may have to be counterbalanced by a slight increase in the occurrence of chronic

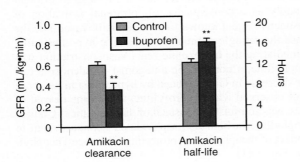

Fig. 7.10 Effect of prophylactic ibuprofen on the pharmacokinetics of amikacin. The decrease in amikacin clearance and the increase in amikacin half-life reflect the decrease in glomerular filtration rate (GFR) induced by ibuprofen. **, $P < 0.01$. (Modified from Allegaert K, Cossey V, Langhendries JP, et al. Effects of co-administration of ibuprofen-lysine on the pharmacokinetics of amikacin in preterm infants during the first days of life. *Biol Neonate.* 2004;86:207.)

lung disease at 28 days of age.[79] The warning that COX-2 selective inhibitors are also unsafe for human immature kidneys is supported by the occurrence of severe renal failure in several neonates born from mothers treated by nimesulide during pregnancy.[86,87]

Angiotensin-Converting Enzyme Inhibitors and Angiotensin II Receptor Antagonists

Angiotensin-converting enzyme (ACE) inhibitors and ATII receptor antagonists (ARAs) are potent hypotensive agents that act by interfering with the formation or the action of ATII. When administered to mothers with hypertension early in pregnancy, they can induce renal dysgenesis.[88] When administered later in pregnancy or to a neonate after birth, these agents can induce neonatal renal failure.[89–91] Renal abnormalities after brief intrauterine exposure to enalapril during late gestation have been detected in an adolescent girl.[92] In high-risk hypertensive neonates with bronchopulmonary dysplasia, whose renin-angiotensin system is overstimulated beyond the neonatal period, the administration of captopril has resulted in dramatic decreases in blood pressure and episodes of prolonged oliguria and seizures.[93] ACE inhibitors and ARAs must not be administered to pregnant mothers and should be administered with great caution to sick neonates.

Prevention of Oliguric States Caused by Low Glomerular Filtration Rate

Furosemide in Oliguric Neonates

Loop diuretics (furosemide, bumetanide) are commonly used to increase urine output in oliguric neonates, with the hope of improving GFR. This hope is based on the fact that furosemide stimulates the production of vasodilator PGs. When a diuretic response actually occurs following the administration of loop diuretics, it may give the illusory impression that GFR has been improved by the diuretic agent.[94] This is evidently rarely the case, because increased urine output usually induces hypovolemia with consequent vasoconstriction of the kidney and depression of GFR.

Loop diuretics are discussed in Chapter 15.

Dopaminergic Agents (Dopamine, Dopexamine) in Oliguric Neonates

Low doses of dopamine, the so-called renal doses (0.5–2.5 µg/kg per min), have been widely used in the hope that its selective actions on DA_1 dopaminergic receptors in the vascular bed would induce renal vasodilation and improve GFR in newborn infants. In initial uncontrolled clinical observations, increases in urine output, sodium excretion, and C_{creat} have been described after the administration of renal doses of dopamine to normotensive oliguric neonates[95] or to oliguric indomethacin-treated neonates.[96] However, these beneficial effects of low-dose dopamine on GFR have not been confirmed by a critical review of neonatal clinical studies[97,98] or by the meta-analysis of randomized trials, either in infants[99] or in adults.[100,101] The renal benefit of low-dose dopamine thus appears illusive.

Theophylline in Oliguric Neonates

Intrarenal adenosine is a physiologic regulator of GFR acting on the glomerular arteriolar tone.[102] When overstimulated, as for instance in hypoxemic states, adenosine dilates predominantly the efferent arteriole, thus decreasing the effective filtration pressure and GFR. Low-dose theophylline (0.5–1 mg/kg), a xanthine derivative with strong adenosine antagonistic properties, has been shown to prevent the hypoxemia-induced vasoconstriction in both newborn and adult rabbits.[71] It probably does so by blunting the efferent arteriolar adenosine-mediated vasodilation induced by hypoxia. A marked improvement in both urinary water excretion and GFR after theophylline administration was first observed in high-risk neonates with oliguric renal insufficiency (Fig. 7.11).[103] Well-controlled studies in severely asphyxiated term neonates have

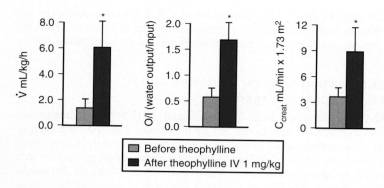

Fig. 7.11 Before theophylline and after theophylline IV 1 mg/kg. *, $p < 0.05$.

shown that a single dose of theophylline (5 or 8 mg/kg) given in the first hours of life significantly improved renal function and C_{creat}[104–107] without affecting the central nervous system. An improvement in urine output and C_{creat} has also been observed in a controlled study in preterm neonates with respiratory distress syndrome (RDS) given low-dose theophylline (1 mg/kg) for 3 days.[108] Low-dose aminophylline (1 mg/kg IV or orally, q 12 h), a compound of theophylline with ethylenediamine in a 2 : 1 ratio, has also been shown to improve renal function in neonates with nonoliguric renal failure[109] and in children with congenital or acquired heart disease.[110]

Interestingly enough, in the neonatal rabbit model the specific adenosine A_1 receptor antagonist DPCPX did not offer the same protection as theophylline during hypoxemic stress.[111]

Although the nonspecific adenosine antagonist theophylline appears to offer protection for the stressed hypoxemic kidney, additional studies are required before recommending the routine use of theophylline for preventive or curative purposes in neonates with perinatal asphyxia, RDS, or acute renal failure.

REFERENCES

1. Guignard JP, John EG. Renal function in the tiny, premature infant. *Clin Perinatol.* 1986;13:377.
2. Turner AJ, Brown RD, Carlström A, et al. Mechanisms of neonatal increase in glomerular filtration rate. *Am J Physiol Regul Integr Comp Physiol.* 2008;295:916.
3. Song R, Spera M, Garrett C, et al. Angiotensin II AT2 receptor regulates ureteric bud morphogenesis. *Am J Phsiol Renal Physiol.* 2010;298:F807.
4. Arendshorst WJ, Brännström K, Ruan X. Actions of angiotensin II on the renal microvasculature. *J Am Soc Nephrol.* 1999;10:S149.
5. Guignard JP, Gouyon JB, John E. Vasoactive factors in the immature kidney. *Pediatr Nephrol.* 1991;5:443.
6. Morris JL, Rosen DA, Rosen KR. Nonsteroidal anti-inflammatory agents in neonates. *Paediatr Drug.* 2003;5:385.
7. Hao CM, Breyer MD. Physiological regulation of prostaglandins in the kidney. *Ann Rev Physiol.* 2008;70:357.
8. Gomez RA, Pupilli C, Everett AD. Molecular and cellular aspects of renin during kidney ontogeny. *Pediatr Nephrol.* 1991;5:80.
9. Madsen K, Marcussen N, Pedersen M, et al. Angiotensin II promotes development of the renal microcirculation through its AT1 receptors. *J Am Soc Nephrol.* 2010;21:448.
10. Gubler MC, Antignac C. Renin-angiotensin system in kidney development: renal tubular dysgenesis. *Kidney Int.* 2010;77:400.
11. Norwood VF, Craig MR, Harris JM, et al. Differential expression of angiotensin II receptors during early renal morphogenesis. *Am J Physiol.* 1997;272:R662.
12. Tufro-McReddie A, Romano LM, Harris JM, et al. Angiotensin II regulates nephrogenesis and renal vascular development. *Am J Physiol.* 1995;269:F110.
13. Prévot A, Mosig D, Guignard JP. The effects of losartan on renal function in the newborn rabbit. *Pediatr Res.* 2002;51:728.
14. Khan KN, Paulson SK, Verburg KM, et al. Pharmacology of cyclooxygenase-2 inhibition in the kidney. *Kidney Int.* 2002;61:1210.
15. Kömoff M, Wang JL, Cheng HF, et al. Cyclooxygenase-2-selective inhibitors impair glomerulogenesis and renal cortical development. *Kidney Int.* 2000;57:14.
16. Norwood VF, Morham SG, Smithies O. Postnatal development and progression of renal dysplasia in cyclooxygenase-2 null-mice. *Kidney Int.* 2000;58:2291.

17. Myers GL, Miller WG, Coresh J, et al. Recommendations for improving serum creatinine measurement: a report from the Laboratory Working Group of the National Kidney Disease Education Program. *Clin Chem.* 2006;52:169.
18. Stokes P, O'Connor G. Development of a liquid chromatography-mass spectrometry method for high-accuracy determination of creatinine in serum. *J Chromatogr B Analyt Technol Biomed Life Sci.* 2003;794:125.
19. Matos P, Duarte-Silva M, Drukker A, Guignard JP. Creatinine reabsorption by the newborn rabbit kidney. *Pediatr Res.* 1998;44:639.
20. Guignard JP, Drukker A. Why do newborn infants have a high plasma creatinine? *Pediatrics.* 1999;103:e49.
21. Gallini F, Maggio L, Romagnoli C, et al. Progression of renal function in preterm neonates with gestational age ≤32 weeks. *Pediatr Nephrol.* 2000;15:119.
22. Miall LS, Henderson MJ, Turner AJ, et al. Plasma creatinine rises dramatically in the first 48 hours of life in preterm infants. *Pediatrics.* 1999;6:104.
23. Bueva A, Guignard JP. Renal function in preterm neonates. *Pediatr Res.* 1994;36:572.
24. Bateman DA, Thomas W, Parravicini E, et al. Serum creatinine concentration in ery low-birth-weight infants from birth to 34–36 wk postmentrual age. *Pediatr Res.* 2015;77:696.
25. Thayyil S, Sheik S, Kempley ST, et al. A gestation- and postnatal age-based reference chart for assessing renal function in extremely premature infants. *J Perinatol.* 2008;28:226.
26. Boer DP, de Rijke YB, Hop WC, et al. Reference values for serum creatinine in children younger than 1 year of age. *Pediatr Nephrol.* 2010;25:2010.
27. Iacobelli S, Bonsante F, Ferdinus C, et al. Factors affecting postnatal changes in serum creatinine in preterm infants with gestational <32 weeks. *J Perinatol.* 2009;29:232.
28. George I, Mekahli D, Rayyan M, et al. Postnatal trends in creatininemia and its covariates in extremely low birth weigh (ELBW) neonates. *Pediatr Nephrol.* 2011;26:1843.
29. Counahan R, Chantler C, Ghazali S, et al. Estimation of glomerular filtration rate from plasma creatinine concentration in children. *Arch Dis Child.* 1976;51:875.
30. Schwartz GJ, Brion LP, Spitzer A. The use of plasma creatinine concentration for estimating glomerular filtration rate in infants, children, and adolescents. *Pediatr Clin North Am.* 1987;34:571.
31. Haenggi MH, Pelet J, Guignard JP. Estimation of glomerular filtration rate by the formula GFR=K x T/Pc. *Arch Pediatr.* 1999;6:165.
32. Stonestreet BS, Bell EF, Oh W. Validity of endogenous creatinine clearance in low birthweight infants. *Pediatr Res.* 1979;13:1002.
33. Coulthard MG, Hey EN, Ruddock V. Creatinine and urea clearances compared to inulin clearance in preterm and mature babies. *Early Hum Dev.* 1985;11:11.
34. Gubhaju L, Sutherland MR, Horne RSC, et al. Assessment of renal functional maturation and injury in preterm neonates during the first month of life. *Am J Physiol Renal Physiol.* 2014;307:F149.
35. Vieux R, Hascoet JM, Merdariu D, et al. Glomerular filtration rate reference values in very premature infants. *Pediatrics.* 2010;125:e1186.
36. Olafsson I. The human cystatin C gene promotor: functional analysis and identification of heterogeneous mRNA. *Scand J Clin Lab Invest.* 1995;55:597.
37. Tenstad O, Roald AB, Grubb A. Renal handling of radiolabelled human cystatin C in the rat. *Scand J Clin Lab Invest.* 1996;56:409.
38. Erlandsen EJ, Randers E, Kristensen JH. Evaluation of the N Latex Cystatin C assay on the Dade Behring Nephelometer II system. *Scand J Clin Lab Invest.* 1999;59:1.
39. Finney H, Newman DJ, Thakkar H, et al. Reference ranges for plasma cystatin C and creatinine measurements in premature infants, neonates, and older children. *Arch Dis Child.* 2000;82:71.
40. Randers E, Krue S, Erlandsen EJ, et al. Reference interval for serum cystatin C in children. *Clin Chem.* 1999;45:1856.
41. Stickle D, Cole B, Hock K, et al. Correlation of plasma concentrations of cystatin C and creatinine to inulin clearance in a pediatric population. *Clin Chem.* 1998;44:1334.
42. Bökenkamp A, Domanetzki M, Zinck R, et al. Reference values for cystatin C serum concentrations in children. *Pediatr Nephrol.* 1998;12:125.
43. Knight EL, Verhave JC, Spiegelman D, et al. Factors influencing serum cystatin C levels other than renal function and the impact on renal function measurement. *Kidney Int.* 2004;65:777.
44. Akbari A, Lepage N, Keely E, et al. Cystatin-C and beta trace protein as markers of renal function in pregnancy. *BJOG.* 2005;112:575.
45. Podraacka L, Feber J, Lepage N, et al. Intra-individual variation of cystatin C and creatinine in pediatric solid organ transplant recipients. *Pediatr Transplant.* 2005;9:28.
46. Mendiluce A, Bustamante J, Martin D, et al. Cystatin C as a marker of renal function in kidney transplant patients. *Transplant Proc.* 2005;37:3844.
47. Bökenkamp A, van Wijk JAE, Lentze MJ, et al. Effects of corticosteroid therapy on serum cystatin C and beta 2-microglobulin concentrations. *Clin Chem.* 2002;48:1123.
48. Wulkan R, den Hollander J, Berghout A. Cystatin C unsuited to use as a marker of kidney function in the intensive care unit. *Crit Care.* 2005;9:531.
49. Martini S, Prévot A, Mosig D, Guignard JP. Glomerular filtration rate: measure creatinine and height rather than cystatin C! *Acta Paediatr.* 2003;92:1052.
50. Cataldi L, Mussap M, Bertelli N, et al. Cystatin C in healthy women at term pregnancy and in their infant newborns: relationship between maternal and neonatal serum levels and reference values. *Am J Perinatol.* 1999;16:287.

51. Harmoinen A, Ylinen E, Ala-Houhala M, et al. Reference intervals for cystatin C in pre-and full-term infants and children. *Pediatr Nephrol*. 2000;15:105.
52. Armangil D, Yurka M, Canpolat FE, et al. Determination of reference values for plasma cystatin C and comparison with creatinine in premature infants. *Pediatr Nephrol*. 2008;23:2081.
53. Abitbol C, Seeherunvong W, Galarza MG, et al. Neonatal kidney size and function in preterm infants: what is a true estimate of glomerular filtration rate? *J Pediatr*. 2014;164:1026.
54. Treiber M, Pecovnic Balon B, Gorenjak M. A new serum cystatin C formula for estimating glomerular filtration rate in newborns. *Pediatr Nephrol*. 2015;30:1297.
55. Filler G, Guerrero-Kanan R, Alvarez-Elias AC. Assessment of glomerular filtration rate: is creatinine the best tool? *Curr Opin Pediatr*. 2016;28:173.
56. Filler G, Bökenkamp A, Hofmann W, et al. Cystatin C as a marker of GFR: history, indications, and future research. *Clin Biochem*. 2005;38:1.
57. Coulthard MG, Ruddock V. Validation of inulin as a marker for glomerular filtration in preterm babies. *Kidney Int*. 1983;23:407.
58. Cole BR, Giangiacomo J, Ingelfinger JR, et al. Measurement of renal function without urine collection. A critical evaluation of the constant-infusion technique for determination of inulin and para-aminohippurate. *N Engl J Med*. 1972;287:1109.
59. vd Heijden AJ, Grose WF, Ambagtsheer JJ, et al. Glomerular filtration rate in the preterm infant: the relation to gestational and postnatal age. *Eur J Pediatr*. 1988;148:24.
60. Coulthard MG. Comparison of methods of measuring renal function in preterm babies using inulin. *J Pediatr*. 1983;102:923.
61. Fawer CL, Torrado A, Guignard JP. Single injection clearance in the neonate. *Biol Neonate*. 1979;35:321.
62. Lindblad HG, Berg HB. Comparative evaluation of iohexol and inulin clearance for glomerular filtration rate determinations. *Acta Paediatr*. 1994;83:418.
63. Berg UB, Bäck R, Celsi G, et al. Comparison of plasma clearance of iohexol and urinary clearance of inuline for measurement of GFR in children. *Am J Kidney Dis*. 2011;57:55.
64. Odlind B, Hallgren R, Sohtell M, et al. Is 125I iothalamate an ideal marker for glomerular filtration? *Kidney Int*. 1985;27:9.
65. Holliday MA, Heilbron D, al-Uzri A, et al. Serial measurements of GFR in infantsb using the continuous iothalamate infusion technique. *Kidney Int*. 1993;43:893.
66. Fawer CL, Torrado A, Guignard JP. Maturation of renal function in full-term and premature neonates. *Helv Paediatr Acta*. 1979;34:11.
67. Toth-Heynh P, Drukker A, Guignard JP. The stressed neonatal kidney: from pathophysiology to clinical management of neonatal vasomotor nephropathy. *Pediatr Nephrol*. 2000;14:227.
68. Gouyon JB, Guignard JP. Management of acute renal failure in newborns. *Pediatr Nephrol*. 2000;14:1037.
69. Choker G, Gouyon JB. Diagnosis of acute renal failure in very preterm infants. *Biol Neonate*. 2004;86:212.
70. Cataldi L, Leone R, Moretti U, et al. Potential risk factors for the development of acute renal failure in preterm newborn infants: a case-control study. *Arch Dis Child Fetal Neonatal Ed*. 2005;90:F514.
71. Gouyon JB, Guignard JP. Theophylline prevents the hypoxemia-induced hemodynamic changes in rabbits. *Kidney Int*. 1988;33:1078.
72. Gouyon JB, Arnaud M, Guignard JP. Renal effects of low-dose aminophylline and enprofylline in newborn rabbits. *Life Sci*. 1988;42:1271.
73. Abhyankar S, Salvi VS. Indomethacin therapy in hydrammios. *J Postgrad Med*. 2000;46:176.
74. vd Heijden AJ, Provoost AP, Nauta J, et al. Renal function impairment in preterm neonates related to intrauterine indomethacin exposure. *Pediatr Res*. 1988;24:644.
75. Catterton Z, Sellers B, Gray B. Inulin clearance in the premature infant receiving indomethacin. *J Pedriatr*. 1980;96:737.
76. Akima S, Kent A, Reynolds GJ, et al. Indomethacin and renal impairment in neonates. *Pediatr Nephrol*. 2004;19:490.
77. Van Overmeire B, Smets K, Lecoutere D, et al. A comparison of ibuprofen and indomethacin for closure of patent ductus arteriosus. *N Engl J Med*. 2000;343:674.
78. Thomas RL, Parker GC, Van Overmeire B, et al. A meta-analysis of ibuprofen versus indomethacin for closure of patent ductus arteriosus. *Eur J Pediatr*. 2005;164:135.
79. Ohlsson A, Walia R, Shah S. Ibuprofen for the treatment of patent ductus arteriosus in preterm or low birth weight (or both) infants. *Cochrane Database Syst Rev*. 2015;(3):CD003481.
80. Allegaert K, Cossey V, Langhendries JP, et al. Effects of co-administration of ibuprofen-lysine on the pharmacokinetics of amikacin in preterm infants during the first days of life. *Biol Neonate*. 2004;86:20.
81. Vieux R, Desandes R, Boubred F, et al. Ibuprofen in very preterm infants impairs renal function for the first month of life. *Pediatr Nephrol*. 2009;25:267.
82. Guignard JP. The adverse renal effects of prostaglandin-synthesis inhibitors in the newborn rabbit. *Semin Perinatol*. 2002;26:398.
83. Chamaa NS, Mosig D, Drukker A, et al. The renal hemodynamic effects of ibuprofen in the newborn rabbit. *Pediatr Res*. 2000;48:600.
84. Allegaert K, de Hoon J, Debeer A, et al. Renal side effects of non-steroidal anti-inflammatory drugs in neonates. *Pharmaceuticals (Basel)*. 2010;3:393.

85. Prevot A, Mosig D, Martini S, et al. Nimesulide, a cyclooxygenase-2 preferential inhibitor, impairs renal function in the newborn rabbit. *Pediatr Res*. 2004;55:254.

86. Peruzzi L, Gianoglio B, Porcellini M, et al. Neonatal end-stage renal failure associated with maternal ingestion of cyclo-oxygenase type I selective inhibitor nimesulide as tocolytic. *Lancet*. 1999; 354:9190.

87. Ali US, Khubchandani S, Andankar P, et al. Renal tubular dysgenesis associated with in utero exposure to nimesulide. *Pediatr Nephrol*. 2006;21:274.

88. Cunniff C, Jones KL, Phillipson J, et al. Oligohydramnios sequence and renal tubular malformation associated with maternal enalapril use. *Am J Obstet Gynecol*. 1990;162:187.

89. Guignard JP, Burgener F, Calame A. Persistent anuria in a neonate: a side effect of captopril? *Int J Pediatr Nephrol*. 1981;2:133.

90. Vendemmia M, Garcia-Méric P, Rizzoti A, et al. Fetal and neonatal consequences of antenatal exposure to type 1 angiotensin II receptor-antagonists. *J Matern Fetal Neonatal Med*. 2005;18:137.

91. Gersak K, Cvijic M, Cerar LK. Angiotensin II receptor blockers in pregnancy: a report of five cases. *Reprod Toxicol*. 2009;28:109.

92. Guron G, Mölne J, Swerkersson S, et al. A 14-year-old girl with renal abnormalities after brief intrauterine exposure to enalapril during late gestation. *Nephrol Dial Transplant*. 2006;21:522.

93. Tack ED, Perlman JM. Renal failure in sick hypertensive premature infants receiving captopril therapy. *J Pediatr*. 1988;112:805.

94. Dubourg L, Drukker A, Guignard JP. Failure of the loop diuretic torasemide to improve renal function of hypoxemic vasomotor nephropathy in the newborn rabbit. *Pediatr Res*. 2000;47:504.

95. Lynch SK, Lemley KV, Polak MJ. The effect of dopamine on glomerular filtration rate in normotensive, oliguric premature neonates. *Pediatr Nephrol*. 2003;18:649.

96. Seri I, Abbasi S, Wood DC, et al. Regional hemodynamic effects of dopamine in the indomethacin-treated preterm infant. *J Perinatol*. 2002;22:300.

97. Prins I, Plötz FB, Cuno SPM, et al. Low-dose dopamine in neonatal and pediatric intensive care: a systematic review. *Intensive Care Med*. 2001;27:206.

98. Cuevas L, Yeh TF, John E, et al. The effect of low-dose dopamine infusion on cardiopulmonary and renal status in premature newborns with respiratory distress syndrome. *Am J Dis Child*. 1991; 145:799.

99. Barrington K, Brion LP. Dopamine versus no treatment to prevent renal dysfunction in indomethacin-treated preterm newborn infants. *Cochrane Database Syst Rev*. 2002;(3):CD003213.

100. Lauschke A, Teichgraber UK, Frei U, Eckhardt KU. "Low-dose" dopamine worsens renal perfusion in patients with acute renal failure. *Kidney Int*. 2004;65:1416.

101. Kellum JA, Decker J. Use of dopamine in acute failure: a meta-analysis. *Crit Care Med*. 2001;29(8):1526–1531.

102. Gouyon JB, Guignard JP. Adenosine in the immature kidney. *Dev Pharmacol Ther*. 1989;13:113.

103. Huet F, Semama D, Grimaldi M, et al. Effects of theophylline on renal insufficiency in neonates with respiratory distress syndrome. *Intensive Care Med*. 1995;21:511.

104. Jenik AG, Ceriani Cernadas JM, Gorenstein A, et al. A randomized, double blind, placebo-controlled trial of the effects of prophylactic theophylline on renal function in term neonates with perinatal asphyxia. *Pediatrics*. 2000;105(4):e45.

105. Bakr AF. Prophylactic theophylline to prevent renal dysfunction in newborns exposed to perinatal asphyxia—a study in a developing country. *Pediatr Nephrol*. 2005;20:1249.

106. Bhat MA, Shah ZA, Makhdoomi MS, Mufti MH. Theophylline for renal function in term neonates with perinatal asphyxia: a randomized, placebo-controlled trial. *J Pediatr*. 2006;149:e180–e184.

107. Eslami Z, Shajari A, Kheirandish M, et al. Theophylline for prevention of kidney dysfunction in neonates with severe asphyxia. *Iran J Kidney Dis*. 2009;3:222.

108. Cattarelli D, Spandrio M, Gasparoni A, et al. A randomized, double blind, placebo controlled trial of the effect of theophylline in prevention of vasomotor nephropathy in very preterm neonates with respiratory distress syndrome. *Arch Dis Child Fetal Neonatal Ed*. 2006;91:F80.

109. Lynch BA, Gal P, Ransom JL, et al. Low-dose aminophylline for the treatment of neonatal non-oliguric renal failure—case series and review of the litteature. *J Pediatr Pharmacol Ther*. 2008;13:80.

110. Axelrod DM, Sutherland SM, Anglemyer A, et al. A double-blinded, randomized, placebo-controlled clinical trial of aminophylline to prevent acute kidney injury in children following congenital heart surgery with cardiopulmonary bypss. *Pediatr Crit Care Med*. 2016;17:135.

111. Prévot A, Mosig D, Rijtema M, et al. Renal effects of adenosine A1-receptor blockade with 7-cyclopentyl-1, 3-dipropylxanthine in hypoxemic newborn rabbits. *Pediatr Res*. 2003;54:400.

Normal and Abnormal Renal Development and Abnormalities of Fluid and Electrolyte Homeostasis

CHAPTER 8

Renal Development and Molecular Pathogenesis of Renal Dysplasia

Carlton Bates, MD, Jacqueline Ho, MD, Debora Malta Cerqueira, PhD, Pawan Puri, PhD, DVM

- Human Renal Dysplasia
- Ureteric Bud
- Stromal Mesenchyme
- Vasculature
- Nephrogenic Mesenchyme

Introduction

Renal dysplasia is one of the leading causes of chronic kidney disease and end-stage kidney disease in children.[1] Elucidating the molecular pathogenesis of renal maldevelopment began in the 1950s with classical studies by Clifford Grobstein, who isolated and characterized primordial tissues that interact to form the metanephric (adult) kidney.[2,3] Since then, studies have shown that four embryonic tissues develop and send reciprocal signaling to form the kidney: the nephrogenic mesenchyme, ureteric bud, stromal mesenchyme, and renal vasculature (see reference 4). Evolving molecular biology and gene targeting techniques have also identified many genes and signaling pathways required for proper kidney formation in animal models.[4] Epigenetic mechanisms have also been described as necessary for renal development in animal models (see reference 5). Studies in patients with syndromic and nonsyndromic renal dysplasia and other congenital renal malformations have identified many causative genetic defects that were previously identified in animal models (see reference 6). This chapter will first review the molecular control of the embryonic tissues that form the kidney and then discuss the genes known to contribute to renal dysplasia in patients.

Nephrogenic Mesenchyme

The development of the human kidney begins in the fifth week of gestation, and the process of new nephron formation continues until approximately 32 to 36 weeks gestational age.[7-9] The process begins with reciprocal inductive signals that cause outgrowth of the ureteric bud from the mesonephric duct and, in turn, the metanephric mesenchyme (from Osr1+ cells in the intermediate mesoderm) to condense around the ureteric bud to form nephrogenic mesenchyme (nephron progenitors). These progenitor cells self-renew throughout kidney development to generate an appropriate number of nephrons and have the capacity to form the multiple epithelial cell types of the nephron from the glomerular podocytes to the distal tubule. How these progenitor cells are specified and regulated in their self-renewal or differentiation is the subject of intense study because these processes are critical for determining nephron endowment, nephron pattern, and therefore long-term kidney health.

Following formation of the nephrogenic mesenchyme around ureteric bud tips, a subset of these cells receive spatiotemporal cues to begin differentiating into epithelialized renal vesicles (Fig. 8.1).[10] The renal vesicle then goes on to sequentially

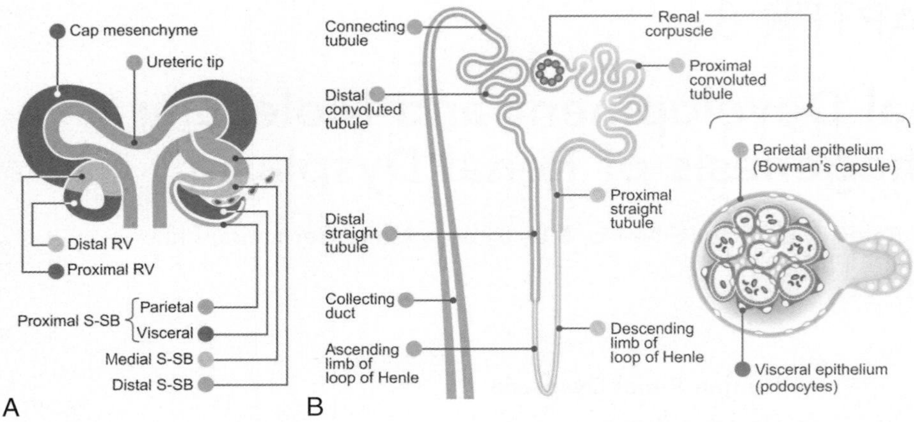

Fig. 8.1 The developing mouse kidney. The adult mouse kidney is patterned into a renal cortex, medulla, and a single papilla. (A) The mammalian kidney arises from the ureteric bud *(brown)* and the metanephric mesenchyme. Nephron progenitors condense around the tips of the ureteric bud to form the cap (nephrogenic) mesenchyme *(purple)*. They undergo a mesenchymal to epithelial transition to form the renal vesicle *(green and purple)*, then elongate to and segment to form the S-shaped body *(blue-green-purple)*. (B) The S-shaped body ultimately differentiates into a nephron with a mature glomerulus. (From McMahon AP. Development of the mammalian kidney. *Curr Top Dev Biol.* 2016;117:31 [Figure 3]).

form the comma-shaped body and then the S-shaped body. The lower limb of the S-shaped body differentiates into glomerular podocytes, and both endothelial and mesangial cells migrate into the cleft of the lower limb of the S-shaped body to form the immature glomerulus.[11,12] Concurrently, the middle and upper limbs of the S-shaped body elongate and differentiate into nephron tubules, including proximal tubules, loops of Henle, and distal convoluted tubules. The terminal ends of the distal convoluted tubules eventually connect to the ureteric epithelia. Nephrogenesis occurs in a radial fashion, such that the most mature nephrons exist in juxtamedullary regions and the most immature nephrons in the cortex (where nephron induction occurs), until the full complement of nephrons is reached.

Nephrons continue to mature structurally (nephron elongation and growth) and functionally (transport functions) prenatally and postnatally. For example, the loops of Henle begin in the renal cortex, elongate in utero through the corticomedullary boundary in term infants, and eventually reach the inner renal medulla.[13–15] As a result, the urinary concentrating capacity of newborn infants is limited by a reduced medullary tonicity gradient, due to the relatively shorter loops of Henle. In the next subsections, we will review the molecular control of the process of nephron development.

Specification of Nephrogenic Mesenchyme

The differentiation of the metanephric mesenchyme to become nephrogenic mesenchyme is marked by the expression of several growth factors, cell adhesion molecules, and transcription factors. Thus the nephrogenic mesenchyme expresses a secreted peptide growth factor, glial-derived neurotrophic factor (Gdnf), which induces ureteric bud outgrowth and branching.[16] The differentiation of the nephrogenic mesenchyme to the renal vesicle involves changes in cell motility, which is at least partly marked by changes in the expression of transmembrane molecules, such as cadherin-11 in the nephron progenitors to cadherin-6 in the renal vesicle.[17] High-resolution expression studies have demonstrated that the nephrogenic mesenchyme is a spatially and temporally heterogeneous population.[18,19] Thus the nephrogenic mesenchyme that exists nearer to the renal capsule around the ureteric tip represent a self-renewing population of nephron progenitors, whereas those located underneath the ureteric tip appear to be committed to differentiate into renal vesicles. Moreover, nephron progenitors that are present at midgestation versus late gestation in the mouse appear to have different capacities with respect to self-renewal or differentiation.[19] The molecular mechanisms that regulate the cessation of nephrogenesis remain ill defined.

The use of tissue-specific gene knockouts in the mouse has revealed the functional importance of several transcription factors in nephron progenitors. Conditional deletion of *Eyes absent homolog 1 (Eya1)*,[20] *Sine oculis homeobox homolog 1 (Six1)*,[21] *Paired box gene 2 (Pax2)*,[22,23] *Wilms tumor 1 (Wt1)*,[24] *Sal-like 1 (Sall1)*,[25] *Sine oculis homeobox homolog 2 (Six2)*,[26] or *Lim homeobox 1 (Lhx1)*[27,28] leads to severe bilateral kidney disease (absent or small and nonfunctional) from defects in nephron progenitor specification and/or differentiation. *Pax2*-mutant mice generate a metanephric mesenchyme that is incompetent to differentiate into nephrons and fail to form the mesonephric duct, which is required for ureteric bud induction.[23] In *Lhx1*[27,29] and *Sall1*[25] mutants, the metanephric mesenchyme does induce the ureteric bud, but it fails to elongate and branch, and the mesenchyme is also unable to differentiate. In *Wt1* mutants a defective metanephric mesenchyme forms and rapidly undergoes apoptosis.[24] Deletion of *Six2* in mice results in the formation of ectopic nephron tubules and depletion of nephron progenitors.[26]

The balance between self-renewal and differentiation of nephron progenitors is at least partly driven by differential wingless-related integration site (Wnt) signaling (low levels promote self-renewal and high levels stimulate differentiation of nephron progenitors). Secreted Wnt9b from the ureteric bud appears to be required for the differentiation of nephron progenitors; deletion of *Wnt9b* results in a failure of progenitors to undergo the mesenchymal to epithelial transition that is required to form the renal vesicle.[30] In contrast, the fibroblast growth factor (Fgf) signaling pathway promotes the survival and proliferation of nephron progenitors. Nephrogenic zone cell culture studies revealed that addition of Fgf1, 2, 9, and 20 ligands promote nephron progenitor proliferation.[31] This is corroborated by in vivo mouse studies that show that *Fgf9* and *Fgf20* are critical for maintaining nephron progenitor survival, proliferation, and competence to respond to inductive signals[32] and that deletion of the Fgf receptors, *Fgfr1* and *Fgfr2,* in the metanephric mesenchyme leads to small and poorly functioning kidneys.[33–35] Other growth factors that have been implicated in progenitor survival include transforming growth factor-β2 (Tgf-β2), leukemia inhibitory factor (Lif), epidermal growth factor (Egf), Fgf2, and bone morphogenetic protein 7 (Bmp7).[36–39]

Emerging evidence has implicated epigenetic mechanisms in the regulation of nephron progenitor specification, survival, and differentiation. For example, histone deacetylases (HDACs) function by removing acetyl groups from histones, which usually results in the stimulation of gene transcription. A study has revealed that class I HDACs are highly expressed in nephron progenitors and are required for normal expression of several key genes, including *Osr1, Eya1, Pax2, Wt1,* and *Wnt9b.*[40] MicroRNAs (miRNAs) are small noncoding RNAs that bind to specific mRNA targets to block translation and promote mRNA degradation. Conditional deletion of a specific miRNA cluster, the miR-17–92 complex, in nephron progenitors leads to a decrease in progenitor proliferation, fewer nephrons, proteinuria, and chronic kidney disease.[41]

Nephron Induction

Nephron progenitors undergo a mesenchymal to epithelial transition to form the renal vesicle, the most immature nephron. In vitro experiments have implicated several growth factors that stimulate nephron progenitors to undergo tubuloepithelial differentiation, including Fgf2,[42] Lif,[39,43,44] Tgf-β2,[39,45] growth/differentiation factor-11 (Gdf-11),[39,46] and Wnt1/4.[47,48] Moreover, transgenic mouse models have identified critical endogenous pathways necessary for this mesenchymal to epithelial transition. For example, global deletion of *Wnt4* (normally expressed in renal vesicles) results in an inability of the mutant nephron progenitors to epithelialize.[30] Conditional deletion of *Fgf8* in the metanephric mesenchyme (nephrogenic and stromal) leads to a block of nephrogenesis beyond the renal vesicle stage.[49,50] Interestingly, global deletion of *Fgfr-like 1,* a membrane-bound Fgf receptor that lacks intracellular signaling, leads to a block in nephrogenesis similar to *Fgf8* conditional mutants.[51]

Nephron Segmentation

Shortly after renal vesicle formation, the developing nephron undergoes a series of morphologic changes to form the comma-shaped and then S-shaped body. These changes reflect the initial establishment of the proximal-distal axis required for nephron segmentation and patterning. Reciprocal repressive interactions between Wt1 and Pax2 appear vital to proximal-distal axis patterning.[52–54] In the S-shaped body, Wt1 is localized to the lower limb and inhibits Pax2 expression, which together promotes a podocyte cell fate.[55] In contrast, Pax2 is present in the upper limb and represses Wt1, stimulating these cells to become proximal and distal tubules.[49,56]

Two other transcription factors important for proximal/distal axis patterning of the nephron are Lhx1 and brain-specific homeobox 1 (Brn1), both of which are expressed in the renal vesicle. Conditional deletion of *Lhx1* leads to a loss of *Brn1* expression.[27] Conditional targeting of *Brn1* results in failure of the loop of Henle to form and the distal convoluted tubules to terminally differentiate.[14] These results suggest that Lhx1 acts upstream of Brn1, which is critical for distal nephron patterning. In contrast, Notch receptor signaling, mediated largely by the recombining binding protein suppressor of hairless (Rbpsuh), appears critical for proximal nephron patterning.[57–59] Use of a Notch inhibitor in mouse metanephric kidney explants led to a loss of proximal cell fates, including glomeruli and proximal tubules.[57] In vivo, conditional deletion of *Notch2* or *Rbpsuh* leads to an absence of proximal tubules and glomerular podocytes.[58] Finally, ectopic Notch expression in nephron progenitors results in premature differentiation into proximal nephron epithelia.[60]

Podocyte Differentiation

Formation of the glomerulus begins at the S-shaped body stage, with the lower limb of the S-shape body committed to becoming podocytes. Initially, the immature podocytes are highly proliferative and have a columnar shape and a single-layer basement membrane.[61] As the S-shaped body matures, the lower cleft transforms into a cup shape. This is accompanied by podocyte differentiation, forming foot processes and slit diaphragms (specialized intracellular junctions critical for proper glomerular filtration).[62,63] This differentiation is associated with a transition in the glomerular basement membrane from laminin-1 to laminin-11, and from α-1 and α-2 type IV collagen chains to α-3, α-4, and α-5 type IV collagen chains.[64] Several mouse models have shown that failure in these transitions leads to glomerular basement membrane defects.[65–67]

Several transcription factors are known to be critical for podocyte differentiation, including Wt1, Lim homeobox transcription factor 1b (Lmx1b), and Mafb. Several studies using transgenic mouse models altering *Wt1* expression have demonstrated its critical roles in mediating podocyte differentiation, in addition to its role in nephron progenitors.[68–71] In addition, genetic deletion of *Lmx1b* or *Mafb* leads to podocyte differentiation defects after the capillary loop stage.[72,73] Finally, three studies have demonstrated the importance of miRNAs in the maintenance of differentiated podocytes in the mouse by targeted ablation of *Dicer* (required for the production of mature miRNAs) in podocytes.[74–76]

Ureteric Bud

As noted previously, the development of the mammalian kidney begins when signals from the metanephric mesenchyme elicit outgrowth of the ureteric bud from the caudal region of the nephric duct. The nephric duct itself is induced from the rostral region of the intermediate mesoderm and begins to elongate caudally. As the embryo develops, cells in the rostral portion of the nephric duct undergo apoptosis, whereas the caudal region of the nephric duct grows towards the cloaca. It is from this region of the nephric duct that the ureteric bud is induced to invade the adjacent metanephric mesenchyme. The ureteric bud elongates and branches, initially forming a T-shaped bifurcation and subsequently undergoing repetitive cycles of branching and elongation to form the collecting system of the kidney.[77,78]

Development of the Nephric Duct

Genetically engineered mouse models have provided important insights into the mechanisms underlying nephric duct formation. For example, *Pax2* knockout *(Pax2−/−)* mice lack kidneys and other structures derived from the intermediate mesoderm, including the ureters. Although the nephric duct starts to form in *Pax2−/−* mice, it fails to extend and reach the cloaca, which results in its eventual degeneration. Because the ureteric bud cannot be induced from the nephric duct, no further kidney development occurs.[79] *Pax8,* like *Pax2,* is expressed in precursors of the nephric duct, and these two transcription factors together specify the nephric duct lineage.[80] Simultaneous deletion of *Pax2* and *Pax8* results in the failure of the intermediate mesoderm to commit to the nephric duct's fate, and it undergoes massive apoptosis. Thus *Pax2−/−Pax8−/−* mice are incapable of forming a kidney.[80]

Interestingly, Pax2 and Pax8 regulate the expression of a third gene that is indispensable for nephric duct development, the transcription factor *Gata3.*[81,82] *Gata3−/−* mice form multiple disorganized nephric ducts that extend toward the surface ectoderm (rather than a single nephric duct that elongates towards the cloaca). The absence of *Gata3* results in increased proliferation of nephric duct cells that also lack expression of *Ret,* a receptor tyrosine kinase for Gdnf.[82] Studies in Axolotl *(Ambystoma mexicanum)* demonstrated that Gdnf is chemoattractant for nephric duct cells that fail to migrate properly when Gdnf expression is disrupted.[83] As expected, genetic deletion of *Gdnf, Ret,* and *retinaldehyde dehydrogenase 2−/−* *(Raldh2,* an upstream regulator of *Gata3)* in mice results in nephric ducts that fail to fuse with the cloaca and ultimately urinary tract obstruction and hydronephrosis.[84,85] The downstream molecular mechanisms activated by Ret/Gdnf signaling and its effects on kidney morphogenesis will be discussed later in this section.

The transcription factor genes *hepatocyte nuclear factor-1β (HNF1β;* also known as *vHNF1)* and *Lhx1* are other important regulators of nephric duct development. In *HNF1β* mutants, the nephric duct forms initially but subsequently degenerates. Because *HNF1β* is necessary for maintenance of *Pax2* and *Lhx1* expression, the phenotype is likely due to reduced levels of these genes in the nephric duct.[86] Lhx1 is necessary for the differentiation of the intermediate mesoderm, as well as the formation and extension of the nephric duct towards the urogenital sinus.[87,88] Therefore *Lhx1*-deficient mice exhibit renal agenesis and lack reproductive tract structures.[88,89]

In summary, the concerted action between *Pax2, Pax8, HNF1β,* and *Lhx1* is necessary to specify the nephric duct lineage. Subsequently, downstream effectors such as *Gata3, Gdnf, Ret,* and *Raldh2* act in parallel to regulate the elongation of the nephric duct and its correct insertion in the cloaca. Dysregulation of any step in this molecular network can lead to urinary tract defects, such as absent kidneys, urinary tract obstruction, and hydronephrosis.[79,80,84,86,88,89]

Ureteric Bud Outgrowth

After specification and elongation, the nephric duct reaches the cloaca as a simple cuboidal epithelium. Shortly afterwards, the epithelium becomes pseudostratified and will soon give rise to the ureteric bud. At this point, the expression of Ret and its coreceptor Gfrα-1 becomes restricted to the caudal portion of the nephric duct, and Gdnf expression is restricted to the nephrogenic mesenchyme.[85,90–93] The binding of Gdnf to Gfrα-1 (facilitated by heparan sulphate glycosaminoglycans)[78,94] activates Ret, which in turn elicits a number of intracellular pathways that promote cell adhesion, proliferation, and migration. Among these are phosphatidylinositol 3-kinase (PI3K)/ AKT, p38 mitogen-activated protein kinase (MAPK), RAS/extracellular signal-related kinase (ERK), and phospholipase Cγ (PLCγ)/Ca$^+$ (see reference 95). A critical step in the Ret/Gdnf signaling pathway is the activation (via PI3K) of the ETS transcription factor genes, *Etv4* and *Etv5,* which drive the expression of a number of transcripts required for ureteric bud outgrowth.[96]

An elegant study by Chi et al. elucidated the cellular basis of Ret/Gdnf-mediated ureteric bud outgrowth. Using time-lapse imaging and chimeric embryos containing both $Ret^{+/+}$ and $Ret^{-/-}$ cells, they demonstrated that $Ret^{+/+}$ cells contribute preferentially to form the ureteric bud tip, whereas the $Ret^{-/-}$ cells form the ureteric trunk. This preferential positioning of $Ret^{+/+}$ cells in the nascent ureteric bud tip facilitates their response to Gdnf signals to proliferate and branch and prevents an indiscriminate ureteric bud induction site.[97] A similar scenario occurs in chimeric embryos containing Etv4- or Etv5-deficient cells, confirming a critical role for these ETS transcription factors in ureteric bud outgrowth and branching.[98]

A complex signaling network is necessary for controlling the correct spatiotemporal execution of ureteric bud outgrowth and its precise positioning on the nephric duct (Fig. 8.2). In this regard, Six1, Pax2, Sall1, Hox11, and Eya1 act in concert to positively modulate the expression of Gdnf in the nephrogenic mesenchyme (see reference 99). Mutations in these genes result in failure of ureteric bud outgrowth, as would be expected.[79,100–103] Conversely, Gdnf/Ret feedback inhibitors, such as

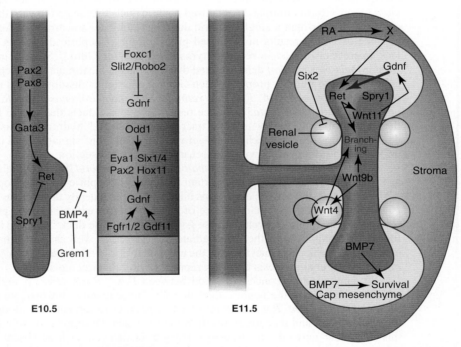

Fig. 8.2 Molecular mechanisms underlying early kidney organogenesis. At embryonic day 10.5 in the mouse, the expression of glial-derived neurotrophic factor (Gdnf) is restricted to the metanephric mesenchyme (MM; *dark brown*), a subset of the caudal portion of the nephrogenic cord *(light brown)*. Gdnf induces the ureteric bud (UB) by binding to Ret receptors expressed by cells in the caudal region of the nephric duct (ND). The expression of Ret in the ND is positively modulated by the transcription factor *Gata3*. Conversely, Gdnf/Ret signaling is negatively modulated by Spry1. Bmp4 also antagonizes Gdnf signaling, and its expression is regulated by the Grem1 binding protein. At embryonic day 11.5, the UB has branched, generating a T-shaped structure in which each ureteric tip is surrounded by a subpopulation of condensed MM cells, called cap (nephrogenic) mesenchyme or nephron progenitors *(light brown)*. The expression of Ret (in the UB) and Gdnf (in nephron progenitors) is sustained by reciprocal inductive interactions between these two compartments and by signals from stromal cell mesenchymal cells *(dark brown)*. The nephron progenitors give rise to renal vesicles (RVs) on either side of each UB tip. Wnt9b and Wnt4 instruct nephron formation from the RVs and are required to maintain ureteric branching. Bmp7 promotes survival of the cap mesenchyme cells, and ectopic nephron formation is prevented by the Six2 transcription factor. See the text for a more comprehensive list of genes involved in metanephric development. *Red arrows* represent interactions between Gdnf and Ret. Epistasis between genes is indicated *by black arrows*, but, in most cases, it is not clear if these interactions are direct. T-shaped symbols represent inhibitory crosstalk. *BMP,* Bone morphogenetic protein; *Eya,* eyes absent homolog; *Fgfr,* fibroblast growth factor receptors; *Gdf,* growth/differentiation factor. (From Davidson AJ. Mouse kidney development (January 15, 2009), StemBook, ed. The Stem Cell Research Community, StemBook, doi/10.3824/stembook.1.34.1, http://www.stembook.org. The specific figure is Fig. 5.)

Sprouty1 (Spry1), Foxc1, Bmp4, and Slit2 (and its receptor Robo2), restrict Gdnf/Ret-mediated ureteric bud outgrowth. If mutated, these aforementioned genes lead to the development of multiple ureters and multiplex kidneys due to the formation of ectopic ureteric buds.[104–108]

Mutations that disrupt Gdnf/Ret signaling also cause renal developmental abnormalities. $Ret^{-/-}$, $GFR\alpha$-$1^{-/-}$ and $Gdnf^{-/-}$ mice have absent kidneys due to failure of ureteric bud formation.[84,85,93,109–112] The same kidney phenotypes occur in $Etv4/5^{-/-}$ mice[96] and mice lacking *heparan sulfate 2-sulfotransferase (HS2ST),* a key enzyme in heparan sulfate biosynthesis.[113] Moreover, *Ret* mutations in the critical tyrosine residues Y^{1062} (activates MAPK and PI3K pathways) or Y^{1015} (activates PLCγ/Ca$^+$) result in absent kidneys or nonfunctional kidneys with megaureters, respectively.[114,115]

Although Gdnf/Ret signaling is critical to the induction of ureteric bud outgrowth, other signaling pathways also have roles. This is supported by the observation that occasionally $Ret^{-/-}$, $Gfr\alpha$-$1^{-/-}$, and $Gdnf^{-/-}$ mice form some kidney tissue, albeit nonfunctional. Subsequent studies have demonstrated that Fgf signaling (likely Fgf10) can compensate for the combined loss of *Ret, Gdnf,* and *Spry.* This occurs because Fgfs can activate the same downstream signaling pathways stimulated by Gdnf/Ret (e.g., PI3K-AKT and RAS/MAPK), which are normally negatively regulated by Spry.[99,116,117]

Ureteric Bud Branching Morphogenesis and Collecting Duct Elongation

Many of the regulators of bud outgrowth are also critical for ureteric bud branching morphogenesis, including Gdnf, Ret, and Etv4/5.[91,93,96,97,99,114] Wnt signaling also plays a critical role in ureteric bud branching and collecting duct elongation. During embryonic kidney development, *Wnt11* is present in the tips of the branching ureteric epithelium. Wnt11 functions as a positive feedback regulator of Gdnf/Ret signaling; *Wnt11* deletion leads to a reduction in *Gdnf* expression and in the number of ureteric tips, resulting in development of small and poorly functioning kidneys.[118] $Wnt9b^{-/-}$ mice exhibit a defective pattern of branching, in addition to nephron induction defects (outlined earlier).[119] In addition, deletion of β-catenin in the ureteric lineage results in either absent or very small kidneys, due to dysregulation of hierarchical circuitry, involving Emx2, Lim1, Pax2, Ret, and Wnt11, all of which are required for appropriate ureteric branching.[120]

Members of the Bmp family regulate ureteric bud branching and collecting duct morphogenesis, via activation of type I Bmp receptors (also known as Alk).[121] *Bmp4* is expressed in the mesenchymal cells surrounding the nephric duct and ureteric bud trunks. Genetic studies have demonstrated that Bmp4 antagonizes Gdnf/Ret signaling and ureteric outgrowth, preventing ectopic budding, and later regulates collecting duct elongation. $Bmp4^{-/-}$ mice have a wide array of kidney and urinary tract defects, including dilated ureters, duplicated collecting system, and small or abnormally patterned kidneys.[107] Mice with deletion of *Alk3* have similar kidney and urinary tract defects.[121]

The Fgf signaling pathway also regulates ureteric branching morphogenesis. Fgf7 and Fgf10, expressed in renal stroma, bind to and activate their cognate receptor, Fgfr2, expressed in the ureteric lineage. Global deletion of *Fgf7, Fgf10,* and the IIIb isoform (epithelial isoform) of *Fgfr2* developing nephrons leads to small kidneys due to presumed ureteric branching defects.[122–124] Conditional deletion of *Fgfr2* in the ureteric lineage confirms that the small kidneys result from ureteric branching defects, due to changes in expression of other downstream genes critical for ureteric branching morphogenesis, such as *Gdnf, Ret, Wnt11,* and *Etv4/5.*[125,126]

Stromal Mesenchyme

Origin and Development

Renal stromal progenitors likely originate from the Osr1+ cells of intermediate mesoderm that are also precursors of nephrogenic mesenchyme.[77] Stromal progenitors are

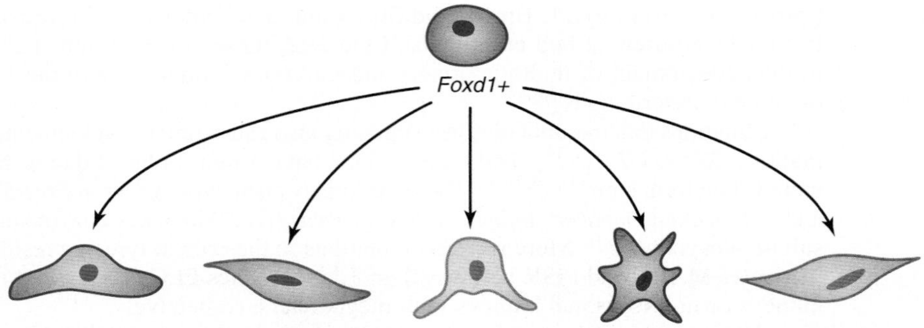

Fig. 8.3 Cell types derived from Foxd1+ renal stromal progenitors. Diagram showing the various cell types derived from the renal cortical stromal progenitors. (From Li W, Hartwig S, Rosenblum ND. Developmental origins and functions of stromal cells in the normal and diseased mammalian kidney. *Dev Dyn.* 2014;243(7):853-863. The specific figure is Fig. 4, used with permission from Wiley Periodicals, Inc.)

identified by their spindle-shaped appearance and the expression of the transcription factor Foxd1.[127,128] At E10.5 in the mouse, stromal progenitors surround the nephrogenic mesenchyme, but as metanephric kidney development progresses, the stromal population expands and is distributed in the capsular, cortical, and medullary regions.[127,128] Lineage tracing studies have shown that the renal stromal population gives rise to interstitial fibroblasts, pericytes, erythropoietin-producing cells, vascular smooth muscle cells, mesangial cells, and subsets of peritubular capillary endothelia of the kidney (Fig. 8.3).[128–130] Many of the signaling pathways that regulate the commitment of stromal progenitors towards these different lineages are yet to be defined.

Stromal Genetics (and Epigenetics) Implicated in Renal Development

Studies have shown that stromal progenitors are critical in patterning interstitial and vascular tissues and have nonautonomous effects on developing nephron progenitors and ureteric bud lineages. Mouse models that ablate expression of genes such as *Foxd1, Hox10,* and *Ctnb1* in the stromal compartment reveal their critical roles in kidney development.[129,131–134] Mice with global deletion of *Foxd1* develop an abnormal renal capsule due to mispatterning of capsular stromal cells, resulting in fused kidneys that are unable to detach from the peritoneum and are trapped in the pelvic region.[129,131] Mutant mice that lack the expression of *Hox10* paralogs (*Hoxa10, Hoxc10,* and *Hoxd10*) in renal stroma also develop severally malformed kidneys with impaired differentiation of capsular stromal cells that fail to integrate into the developing metanephric anlagen.[132] Deletion of *Ctnb1,* encoding for β-catenin, an effector of canonical Wnt signaling, in Foxd1+ stroma progenitors impairs the development of renal medulla; conversely, expression of constitutively active β-catenin in the renal stromal compartment results in expansion of the stroma with disrupted nephrogenesis and ureteric branching morphogenesis.[134]

Many studies have established that stroma directly signals to and regulates the size of the nephrogenic mesenchyme. Diphtheria toxin-mediated ablation of Foxd1+ stromal cells results in the increase in size of the nephron progenitor pool.[135] Other studies have shown that the stromally expressed transcription factors *Foxd1, Pbx1, Pod1,* and *Sall1* and atypical cadherin *Fat4* regulate size of the cap (nephrogenic) mesenchyme.[129,133,136–139] Mice with germline deletion of *Foxd1, Pbx1,* and *Pod1* or with conditional deletion of *Sall1* or *Fat4* in the cortical stroma have an increase in the size of nephron progenitor pool.[131,133,136,138,139] Interestingly, Fat4-mediated crosstalk with nephron progenitors is restricted to cortical stroma because deletion of *Fat4* specifically in the medullary stroma does not affect the size of the nephron progenitor pool.[138] The downstream mechanisms and targets of *Fat4* in stromal cells remain controversial.[138,140] In contrast, Decorin, a proteoglycan that is expressed in cortical stroma, appears to regulate the size of nephron progenitor pool. Decorin levels are increased in *Foxd1*- and *Sall1*-deficient stromal progenitors, which may lead to sequestration of Bmp4, which is required for the differentiation of nephron progenitors (thereby increasing the pool of self-renewing progenitors). Notably, concomitant deletion of Decorin partially rescues the nephron progenitor expansion defects in *Foxd1* mutants.[133,141] Studies have determined that miRNAs in stromal cells also regulate the size of nephron progenitor pool.[142] Deletion of *Dicer* (required for the production of mature miRNAs) in Foxd1+ stromal cells leads to expansion of nephron progenitors and disrupts nephrogenesis (presumably due to upregulation of yet to be identified miRNA target genes).[142]

As mentioned, studies have also identified signaling molecules emanating from the renal stroma that affect ureteric morphogenesis. Ablation of Foxd1+ stromal progenitors with diphtheria toxin not only results in nephron progenitor expansion but also in ureteric bud branching defects suggesting the role of stromal-ureteric bud crosstalk during kidney development.[135] In vitro studies have shown that stromal cell production of retinoic acid, renin, and angiotensinogen triggers pathways that modulate the Gdnf/Ret/Wnt11 axis, which is critical for ureteric bud branching.[143–145] Elegant in vivo studies by the Mendelsohn group showed how simultaneous knockout of two retinoic acid receptors, *Rara* and *Rarb2,* led to impaired Ret expression and subsequent ureteric branching defects, providing strong evidence that stromal signals crosstalk with the ureteric lineage.[146]

Vasculature

A highly intricate network of blood vessels traverses through the kidney to ensure efficient filtration and tubular transport, as well as sufficient nutrient supply for metabolic demands of renal cells. Both angiogenesis (new vessels sprouting from existing vessels) and vasculogenesis (de novo vessel formation) contribute to the development of renal vasculature.[77] Endothelial cells and mural cells (vascular smooth muscle cells and pericytes) constitute the main components of renal blood vessels. Renal blood vessels exhibit some features that are common to or in other cases distinct from the vascular beds of other organs; for example, fenestrated endothelia of glomerular capillaries are supported by mesangial cells that are specialized pericytes, whereas renal peritubular capillaries are surrounded by typical pericytes that enfold capillaries and venules throughout the body.[147] Renal arteriolar endothelia are lined by layers of vascular smooth muscle cells and pericytes but also contact renin cells, specialized smooth muscle cells, at juxtaglomerular locations.[147]

Origin and Development of Renal Endothelial Cells

Most of the renal endothelial cells are thought to be derived from hemangioblasts, common precursors for blood cells and endothelial cells, that express the transcription factor stem cell leukemia (Scl).[148] Lineage tracing studies have shown that Scl+ cells are precursors to endothelial cells that line arteries, veins, arterioles, glomerular, and many peritubular capillaries of the kidney.[148] A conditional knockout mouse model shows that G protein–coupled sphingosine-1-phosphate receptor signaling in Scl+ cells is essential for the proper development of the renal vasculature.[148] Another group discovered that Foxd1+ stromal progenitors give rise to endothelial cells that line subsets of peritubular capillaries.[149] One marker of Foxd1+ stromal-derived endothelial precursors is CD146, a coreceptor for vascular endothelial growth factor receptor 2.[150]

Renal Vascular Mural Cell Development, Genetics, and Epigenetics

Mural cells include vascular smooth muscle cells, pericytes, and renin-producing cells that surround the renal endothelia. Lineage tracing studies have established that mural cells originate from the Foxd1+ stromal progenitor population and that much of the endothelial cell network develops within the stroma; moreover, diphtheria toxin–mediated deletion of Foxd1+ stromal progenitors during embryonic stages leads to severe vascular mispatterning.[135] Other studies have shown that expression of transcription factor genes *Foxd1* and *Pbx1* in stromal progenitors is critical for the normal development of renal vasculature.[129,151] Mutant mouse models lacking *Foxd1* or *Pbx1* expression show severe vascular patterning defects in which renal artery branching occurs in a random pattern in contrast to the stereotypical fashion observed in controls; this marked disruption in spatiotemporal vascular morphogenesis in *Foxd1* and *Pbx1* mutants leads to kidney failure resulting in perinatal lethality.[129,151] Interestingly, Pbx1 mutants exhibit ectopic expression of platelet-derived growth factor receptor beta (Pdgfrβ), leading to premature differentiation of stromal progenitors and vascular defects, all of which can be at least partially rescued by a simultaneous one allele loss of *Pdgfβ*. The downstream targets of Foxd1 in stromal progenitors and mural cells are yet to be identified.

Foxd1+ stromal cells are also precursors of mesangial cells, a specialized pericyte population that attaches to glomerular endothelial cells that (together with podocytes) form an assembly critical for glomerular filtration. The Notch signaling pathway is essential for mesangial cell formation by regulating their specification, proliferation, and survival. Foxd1-cre mediated deletion of RBPJ, a well-established downstream target of Notch 1 and Notch 2 signaling, results in the failure of differentiation of stromal progenitors into mesangial cells.[152] Another pathway essential for mesangial cell formation is Pdgfβ signaling.[153] Glomerular endothelial cells secrete Pdgfβ that binds to its receptor, Pdgfrβ, expressed by mesangial cells; disruption of Pdgfβ/Pdgfrβ signaling leads to the failure of mesangial precursors to migrate to their proper position within glomeruli.[153] As expected, the failure of mesangial cell formation in mutant mice with disrupted Notch and Pdgf signaling results in perinatal lethality due to kidney failure.[152,153] Finally, conditional deletion of *Dicer* in the Foxd1+ stromal population leads to an absence of mesangial cells, showing that miRNAs are also critical for mesangial cell development from the stroma.[142]

Renin-secreting cells are specialized vascular smooth muscle cells localized in the juxtaglomerular apparatus; these cells regulate blood pressure by secreting renin and also originate from Foxd1+ stromal progenitors.[144] Although renin is also expressed in collecting ducts, conditional knockout studies have shown that deletion of the renin gene in collecting duct epithelium is dispensable for renal development; however, deletion of renin in Foxd1+ progenitors disrupts renal vasculature development resulting in hypertrophic arteries and arterioles with marked increased expression of smooth muscle actin.[154]

Studies have also shown that tubular epithelial cells communicate with renal vascular cells and regulate their development. Wnt7b, a growth factor that is secreted by the developing ureteric bud, regulates proliferation of medullary peritubular capillary mural cells and ultimately vessel lumen diameter.[155] Deletion of *vascular endothelial growth factor a (Vegfa)* in renal epithelial cells leads to reduction in the density of peritubular capillaries resulting in small kidneys.[156]

Signaling pathways, such as angiopoietin, ephrin, and Tgf-β1, that are known to regulate vasculature development in other organ systems likely play crucial roles in the development of renal vasculature, and future studies will define their functions specifically in the endothelial and mural cells of the kidney.[147] Identification of specific miRNAs involved in the regulation of renal vasculature is of significant interest based upon the aforementioned studies showing that stromal-specific *Dicer* deletion leads to progressive loss of mesangial cells.[142] The identification and detailed understanding of the molecular networks that regulate the development of renal vasculature are crucial in defining the role of renal maldevelopment in pediatric and adult kidney disease and for the success of regenerative efforts to build a kidney.

Human Renal Dysplasia

Congenital anomalies of the kidney and urinary tract (CAKUTs) are the leading causes of chronic and end-stage kidney disease in children.[1] Intrinsic defects in kidney formation are included among the top causes of CAKUTs. These intrinsic kidney formation defects can be classified by the type of structural defect. Renal aplasia

Fig. 8.4 Magnetic resonance image (MRI) of a multicystic dysplastic kidney. T2-weighted coronal image showing multicystic dysplastic kidney on the left and a normal kidney on the right. (From Wood CG 3rd, Stromberg LJ 3rd, Harmath CB, et al. CT and MR imaging for evaluation of cystic renal lesions and diseases. *Radiographics.* 2015;35(1):125-141. The specific figure is Fig. 13 panel b, used with permission from the Radiological Society of North America.)

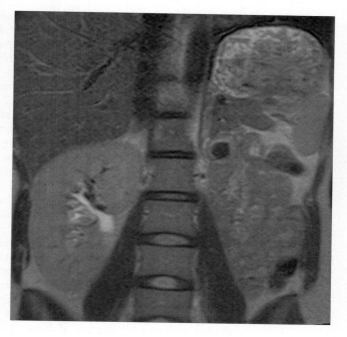

8

means that there is no identifiable kidney present in the patient. This contrasts with the term agenesis, in which there were never any embryonic elements present (and likely occurs very rarely because in animal models of aplasia, there are almost always embryonic kidney elements present that fail to form an identifiable kidney). Dysplasia means that the tissue elements within a kidney formed incorrectly and do not function. Renal dysplasia can be global or regional (focal abnormal areas disbursed among normal functioning elements). Dysplastic kidneys can also be cystic or noncystic; the extreme form of renal cystic dysplasia is a multicystic dysplastic kidney, which is completely nonfunctional and features noncommunicating epithelial cysts surrounded by stromal elements (Fig. 8.4). Finally, kidneys may be hypoplastic, or smaller than normal, meaning that fewer functioning nephrons are present. Frequently the same genetic defect within a family can result in aplasia, dysplasia, or hypoplasia. An example extrapolated from animal studies would be genetic mutations that led to variable ureteric induction defects, which could include no ureteric bud (resulting in aplasia), abnormal interaction with the metanephric mesenchyme (dysplasia), or displacement from the usual induction site (hypoplasia). Often one may even see combinations of defects within the same kidney (regional dysplasia in a hypoplastic kidney). Genetic defects resulting in human kidney dysplasia (taken to include aplasia or hypoplasia as well) can occur as part of syndromes or as isolated kidney abnormalities.

Syndromic Renal Dysplasia

There are now many human syndromes with kidney developmental defects that have had causative gene mutations identified. The most common monogenic syndrome that results in human renal developmental abnormalities is called renal cysts and diabetes syndrome (RCAD), resulting from mutations in the gene encoding for the transcription factor HNF1B (see reference 157). Patients with a single allele mutation in *HNF1B* (inherited in autosomal dominant fashion or arising as a spontaneous mutation) have a wide spectrum of variably penetrant phenotypes, most commonly renal cysts and early onset diabetes mellitus.[157] The kidney defects in these patients include renal dysplasia, hypoplasia, aplasia, cysts, duplex collecting systems, hydronephrosis, and hyperuricemic nephropathy.[157] HNF1B appears to act in both nephrogenic mesenchyme and the ureteric bud to regulate early nephrogenesis, tubular development, and ureteric branching.[157] It also appears to directly or indirectly regulate transcription of many genes, including *WNT9b, UMOD, PKHD1,* and *PKD2* (which explains the wide range of renal and nonrenal phenotypes).[157] Among several studies examining patients with congenital renal anomalies, *HNF1B* mutations have been identified in 5% to 12% of these patients.[157]

Another common monogenic syndrome that results in congenital kidney defects arises from single allele mutations in *PAX2* (see reference 158). In the early 1990s, families with renal coloboma syndrome, an autosomal dominant disease featuring renal and optic nerve developmental defects, were found to have inactivating mutations in PAX2.[158] *PAX2* encodes for a DNA-binding protein with transcription factor activities, as well as links to epigenetic regulation of gene activation.[158] PAX2 acts in the nephric duct/ureteric lineage early (required for nephric duct formation and ureteric induction) and then later in nephrogenic mesenchymal lineages (required for nephron differentiation).[158] Patients with defects in one *PAX2* allele can have a wide spectrum of renal anomalies, including renal dysplasia, hypoplasia, aplasia, and/or multicystic dysplastic kidneys (sometimes with variable renal phenotypes within the same family).[158] Extrarenal manifestations such as colobomas (common) or hearing defects (less common) can be completely absent.[158] Mutations in *PAX2* are likely the second most common monogenic cause of isolated renal developmental anomalies.[159]

There are numerous examples of other syndromes with renal developmental defects in which causative mutations in genes have been identified. One example is branchio-oto-renal (and branchio-oto-ureteral) syndrome, an autosomal dominant disease with variable degrees of renal maldevelopment (including family members with and without kidney disease); the known disease-causing mutations are in *EYA1, SIX1,* or *SIX5,* whose gene products are known to form complexes that interact with promoter regions of target genes in the early developing nephrogenic mesenchyme and other affected tissues.[160] Mutations in *SALL1,* which encodes for a transcription factor critical for early kidney mesenchyme patterning, are associated with Townes-Brocks syndrome; this is an autosomal dominant disease, leading to a spectrum of congenital renal anomalies, as well as imperforate anus, malformed ears, and thumb defects.[161] Pallister-Hall syndrome, an autosomal dominant disease that includes renal aplasia, dysplasia, and/or hypoplasia, occurs secondary to mutations in *GLI3,* which encodes for an effector of the Hedgehog pathway that regulates other earlier mentioned genes, such as *PAX2* and *SALL1.*[162] Finally, Apert syndrome, in which there are activating mutations in *FGFR2,* and Feingold syndrome, in which there are mutations in either *MYCN* (encoding for a transcription factor) or *MIR17HG* (encoding for the miR-17-92 miRNA cluster), often feature renal malformations.[163,164] The latter is an example of an epigenetic defect (in miRNA cluster) that is linked to renal dysplasia.[164] The list of syndromes with known genetic (or epigenetic) defects associated with renal dysplasia is ever growing and often identifies genes that were first characterized in animal models as having critical roles in kidney development (as noted in earlier sections of this chapter).

In addition to syndromes with renal dysplasia, there have been many genetic mutations identified in patients with nonsyndromic/isolated renal anomalies. One of the first studies examining candidate gene sequences within a cohort of 99 unrelated patients with renal hypoplasia (with only five suspected to have a syndrome such as RCAD) found mutations in *HNF1β, PAX2, EYA1, SIX1,* and *SALL1* in 17% of unrelated families, with most being mutations being in *HNF1β* or *PAX2.*[165] A later study from the same group examined 250 patients with apparently nonsyndromic renal dysplasia and using a candidate approach again identified what appear to be causative mutations in *SIX2* or *BMP4* (10 total mutations).[166] A separate smaller study examining stillborn fetuses with congenital renal aplasia or severe renal dysplasia used a candidate approach to identify a relatively high number of *RET* mutations, including 37% of those with bilateral aplasia/severe dysplasia (7 of 19 fetuses) and in 20% of those with unilateral aplasia (2 of 10 fetuses); the group also identified one mutation in *GDNF,* the gene encoding the RET ligand.[167] More recently, consanguineous patients with two mutations in *FGF20,* encoding for a ligand for Fgf receptors, were found to have isolated renal dysplasia.[168] Thus many gene mutations that are associated with syndromes featuring renal dysplasia appear to also cause isolated kidney malformations.

As sequencing techniques have become more high throughput, investigators are beginning to examine larger numbers of patients and families with renal anomalies for monogenic causes. A study from the Hildebrandt lab examined 749 patients (among 650 families) with renal congenital anomalies and, using a candidate approach, identified 37 single allele mutations in 47 total patients (from 41 families); these mutations include (number of families in parentheses): *BMP7* (1), *CDC5L* (1), *CHD1L* (5), *EYA1* (3), *GATA3* (2), *HNF1β* (6), *PAX2* (5), *RET* (3), *ROBO2* (4), *SALL1* (9), *SIX2* (1), and *SIX5* (1).[159] Another study from the same group used high-throughput sequencing in 574 patients with isolated congenital kidney malformations for candidate gene mutations and in 15, identified likely causative recessive mutations in *FRAS1, FREM2, GRIP1, FREM1, ITGA8,* and *GREM1;* based on animal studies, these genes are known to regulate interactions between the ureteric bud and metanephric mesenchyme.[169] Finally, the same group used whole exome sequencing to identify likely disease causing recessive mutations in patients with isolated renal hypodysplasia in 33 consanguineous families; notably, the group identified recessive mutations in nine families including: *ZBTB24, WFS1, HPSE2, ATRX, ASPH, AGXT, AQP2, CTNS,* and *PKHD1.*[170] Moreover, mutations in these genes were previously known to cause either syndromes that featured renal anomalies or isolated renal congenital defects (but were not suspected in any of these patients).[170]

In conclusion, many genes and signaling pathways have been identified as having critical roles in renal development in many different animal models. As more studies are performed in patients with either syndromic and/or nonsyndromic forms of renal dysplasia, we are finding that many of these genes have similar roles in human kidney development. Moreover, a surprisingly large number of human renal dysplasia appears to be caused by monogenic mutations. As high-throughput sequencing continues to identify novel mutations in patients with renal dysplasia, using animal models to prove causality for those mutations will continue to be invaluable.

REFERENCES

1. Becherucci F, Roperto RM, Materassi M, Romagnani P. Chronic kidney disease in children. *Clin Kidney J.* 2016;9(4):583–591.
2. Grobstein C. Inductive epithelio-mesenchymal interaction in cultured organ rudiments of the mouse. *Science.* 1953;118:52–55.
3. Grobstein C. Trans-filter induction of tubules in mouse metanephrogenic mesenchyme. *Exp Cell Res.* 1956;10:424–440.
4. McMahon AP. Development of the Mammalian Kidney. *Curr Top Dev Biol.* 2016;117:31–64.
5. Hilliard SA, El-Dahr SS. Epigenetics mechanisms in renal development. *Pediatr Nephrol.* 2016;31(7):1055–1060.
6. Phua YL, Ho J. Renal dysplasia in the neonate. *Curr Opin Pediatr.* 2016;28(2):209–215.
7. Osathanondh V, Potter EL. Development of human kidney as shown by microdissection. *Arch Pathol.* 1966;82:391–402.
8. Potter EL. *Normal and Abnormal Development of the Kidney.* Chicago: Year Book Medical Publishers Inc; 1972.
9. Hinchliffe SA, Sargent PH, Howard CV, et al. Human intrauterine renal growth expressed in absolute number of glomeruli assessed by the disector method and Cavalieri principle. *Lab Invest.* 1991;64(6):777–784.
10. Clark AT, Bertram JF. Molecular regulation of nephron endowment. *Am J Physiol.* 1999;276(4 Pt 2):F485–F497.
11. Schrijvers BF, Flyvbjerg A, De Vriese AS. The role of vascular endothelial growth factor (VEGF) in renal pathophysiology. *Kidney Int.* 2004;65(6):2003–2017.
12. Simon M, Rockl W, Hornig C, et al. Receptors of vascular endothelial growth factor/vascular permeability factor (VEGF/VPF) in fetal and adult human kidney: localization and [125I]VEGF binding sites. *J Am Soc Nephrol.* 1998;9(6):1032–1044.
13. Neiss WF. Histogenesis of the loop of Henle in the rat kidney. *Anat Embryol (Berl).* 1982;164(3):315–330.
14. Nakai S, Sugitani Y, Sato H, et al. Crucial roles of Brn1 in distal tubule formation and function in mouse kidney. *Development.* 2003;130(19):4751–4759.
15. Neiss WF, Klehn KL. The postnatal development of the rat kidney, with special reference to the chemodifferentiation of the proximal tubule. *Histochemistry.* 1981;73(2):251–268.
16. Hellmich HL, Kos L, Cho ES, et al. Embryonic expression of glial cell-line derived neurotrophic factor (GDNF) suggests multiple developmental roles in neural differentiation and epithelial-mesenchymal interactions. *Mech Dev.* 1996;54:95–105.

D

17. Cho EA, Patterson LT, Brookhiser WT, et al. Differential expression and function of cadherin-6 during renal epithelium development. *Development*. 1998;125(5):803–812.

18. Mugford JW, Sipila P, Kobayashi A, et al. Hoxd11 specifies a program of metanephric kidney development within the intermediate mesoderm of the mouse embryo. *Dev Biol*. 2008;319(2):396–405.

19. Chen S, Brunskill EW, Potter SS, et al. Intrinsic Age-Dependent Changes and Cell-Cell Contacts Regulate Nephron Progenitor Lifespan. *Dev Cell*. 2015;35(1):49–62.

20. Xu P-X, Adams J, Peters H, et al. Eya1-deficient mice lack ears and kidneys and show abnormal apoptosis of organ primordia. *Nat Genet*. 1999;23:113–117.

21. Xu PX, Zheng W, Huang L, et al. Six1 is required for the early organogenesis of mammalian kidney. *Development*. 2003;130(14):3085–3094.

22. Rothenpieler UW, Dressler GR. Pax-2 is required for mesenchyme-to-epithelium conversion during kidney development. *Development*. 1993;119:711–720.

23. Torres M, Gomez-Pardo E, Dressler GR, Gruss P. *Pax-2* controls multiple steps of urogenital development. *Development*. 1995;121:4057–4065.

24. Kreidberg JA, Sariola H, Loring JM, et al. WT-1 is required for early kidney development. *Cell*. 1993;74:679–691.

25. Nishinakamura R, Matsumoto Y, Nakao K, et al. Murine homolog of SALL1 is essential for ureteric bud invasion in kidney development. *Development*. 2001;128:3105–3115.

26. Self M, Lagutin OV, Bowling B, et al. Six2 is required for suppression of nephrogenesis and progenitor renewal in the developing kidney. *EMBO J*. 2006;25(21):5214–5228.

27. Kobayashi A, Kwan KM, Carroll TJ, et al. Distinct and sequential tissue-specific activities of the LIM-class homeobox gene Lim1 for tubular morphogenesis during kidney development. *Development*. 2005;132(12):2809–2823.

28. Tsang TE, Shawlot W, Kinder SJ, et al. Lim1 activity is required for intermediate mesoderm differentiation in the mouse embryo. *Dev Biol*. 2000;223(1):77–90.

29. Shawlot W, Behringer RR. Requirement for *Lim1* in head-organizer function. *Nature*. 1995;374:425–430.

30. Carroll TJ, Park JS, Hayashi S, et al. Wnt9b plays a central role in the regulation of mesenchymal to epithelial transitions underlying organogenesis of the mammalian urogenital system. *Dev Cell*. 2005;9(2):283–292.

31. Brown AC, Adams D, de Caestecker M, et al. FGF/EGF signaling regulates the renewal of early nephron progenitors during embryonic development. *Development*. 2011;138(23):5099–5112.

32. Barak H, Huh SH, Chen S, et al. FGF9 and FGF20 maintain the stemness of nephron progenitors in mice and man. *Dev Cell*. 2012;22(6):1191–1207.

33. Hains D, Sims-Lucas S, Kish K, et al. Role of fibroblast growth factor receptor 2 in kidney mesenchyme. *Pediatr Res*. 2008;64(6):592–598.

34. Poladia DP, Kish K, Kutay B, et al. Role of fibroblast growth factor receptors 1 and 2 in the metanephric mesenchyme. *Dev Biol*. 2006;291(2):325–339.

35. Sims-Lucas S, Cusack B, Baust J, et al. Fgfr1 and the IIIc isoform of Fgfr2 play critical roles in the metanephric mesenchyme mediating early inductive events in kidney development. *Dev Dyn*. 2011;240(1):240–249.

36. Barasch J, Qiao J, McWilliams G, et al. Ureteric bud cells secrete multiple factors, including bFGF, which rescue renal progenitors from apoptosis. *Am J Physiol*. 1997;273:F757–F767.

37. Dudley AT, Godin RE, Robertson EJ. Interaction between FGF and BMP signaling pathways regulates development of metanephric mesenchyme. *Genes Dev*. 1999;13:1601–1613.

38. Koseki C, Herzlinger D, Al-Awqati Q. Apoptosis in metanephric development. *J Cell Biol*. 1992;119(5):1327–1333.

39. Plisov SY, Yoshino K, Dove LF, et al. TGF beta 2, LIF and FGF2 cooperate to induce nephrogenesis. *Development*. 2001;128(7):1045–1057.

40. Chen S, Bellew C, Yao X, et al. Histone deacetylase (HDAC) activity is critical for embryonic kidney gene expression, growth, and differentiation. *J Biol Chem*. 2011;286(37):32775–32789.

41. Marrone AK, Stolz DB, Bastacky SI, et al. MicroRNA-17~92 is required for nephrogenesis and renal function. *J Am Soc Nephrol*. 2014;25(7):1440–1452.

42. Karavanov AA, Karavanova I, Perantoni A, Dawid IB. Expression pattern of the rat Lim-1 homeobox gene suggests a dual role during kidney development. *Int J Dev Biol*. 1998;42:61–66.

43. Stewart CL, Kaspar P, Brunet LJ, et al. Blastocyst implantation depends on maternal expression of leukaemia inhibitory factor. *Nature*. 1992;359(6390):76–79.

44. Barasch J, Yang J, Ware CB, et al. Mesenchymal to epithelial conversion in rat metanephros is induced by LIF. *Cell*. 1999;99(4):377–386.

45. Sanford LP, Ormsby I, Gittenberger-de Groot AC, et al. TGFb2 knockout mice have multiple developmental defects that are non-overlapping with other TGFb knockout phenotypes. *Development*. 1997;124:2659–2670.

46. McPherron AC, Lawler AM, Lee SJ. Regulation of anterior/posterior patterning of the axial skeleton by growth/differentiation factor 11. *Nat Genet*. 1999;22(3):260–264.

47. Herzlinger D, Qiao J, Cohen D, et al. Induction of kidney epithelial morphogenesis by cells expressing Wnt-1. *Dev Biol*. 1994;166:815–818.

48. Kispert A, Vainio S, McMahon AP. Wnt-4 is a mesenchymal signal for epithelial transformation of metanephric mesenchyme in the developing kidney. *Development*. 1998;125:4225–4234.

49. Grieshammer U, Cebrian C, Ilagan R, et al. FGF8 is required for cell survival at distinct stages of nephrogenesis and for regulation of gene expression in nascent nephrons. *Development*. 2005;132(17):3847–3857.

50. Perantoni AO, Timofeeva O, Naillat F, et al. Inactivation of FGF8 in early mesoderm reveals an essential role in kidney development. *Development*. 2005;132(17):3859–3871.
51. Gerber SD, Steinberg F, Beyeler M, et al. The murine Fgfrl1 receptor is essential for the development of the metanephric kidney. *Dev Biol*. 2009;335(1):106–119.
52. Majumdar A, Lun K, Brand M, Drummond IA. Zebrafish no isthmus reveals a role for pax2.1 in tubule differentiation and patterning events in the pronephric primordia. *Development*. 2000;127(10): 2089–2098.
53. Wallingford JB, Carroll TJ, Vize PD. Precocious expression of the Wilms' tumor gene xWT1 inhibits embryonic kidney development in Xenopus laevis. *Dev Biol*. 1998;202(1):103–112.
54. Ryan G, Steele-Perkins V, Morris JF, et al. Repression of Pax-2 by WT1 during normal kidney development. *Development*. 1995;121(3):867–875.
55. Pelletier J, Schalling M, Buckler AJ, et al. Expression of the Wilms' tumor gene WT1 in the murine urogenital system. *Genes Dev*. 1991;5:1345–1356.
56. Dressler GR, Douglass EC. Pax-2 is a DNA-binding protein expressed in embryonic kidney and Wilms tumor. *Proc Natl Acad Sci USA*. 1992;89:1179–1183.
57. Cheng HT, Miner JH, Lin M, et al. Gamma-secretase activity is dispensable for mesenchyme-to-epithelium transition but required for podocyte and proximal tubule formation in developing mouse kidney. *Development*. 2003;130(20):5031–5042.
58. Cheng HT, Kim M, Valerius MT, et al. Notch2, but not Notch1, is required for proximal fate acquisition in the mammalian nephron. *Development*. 2007;134(4):801–811.
59. Wang P, Pereira FA, Beasley D, Zheng H. Presenilins are required for the formation of comma- and S-shaped bodies during nephrogenesis. *Development*. 2003;130(20):5019–5029.
60. Boyle SC, Kim M, Valerius MT, et al. Notch pathway activation can replace the requirement for Wnt4 and Wnt9b in mesenchymal-to-epithelial transition of nephron stem cells. *Development*. 2011;138(19):4245–4254.
61. Kreidberg JA. Podocyte differentiation and glomerulogenesis. *J Am Soc Nephrol*. 2003;14(3):806–814.
62. Garrod DR, Fleming S. Early expression of desmosomal components during kidney tubule morphogenesis in human and murine embryos. *Development*. 1990;108(2):313–321.
63. Pavenstadt H, Kriz W, Kretzler M. Cell biology of the glomerular podocyte. *Physiol Rev*. 2003;83(1):253–307.
64. Miner JH, Sanes JR. Collagen IV alpha 3, alpha 4, and alpha 5 chains in rodent basal laminae: sequence, distribution, association with laminins, and developmental switches. *J Cell Biol*. 1994;127(3):879–891.
65. Miner JH, Li C. Defective glomerulogenesis in the absence of laminin alpha5 demonstrates a developmental role for the kidney glomerular basement membrane. *Dev Biol*. 2000;217(2):278–289.
66. Miner JH, Sanes JR. Molecular and functional defects in kidneys of mice lacking collagen alpha 3(IV): implications for Alport syndrome. *J Cell Biol*. 1996;135(5):1403–1413.
67. Noakes PG, Miner JH, Gautam M, et al. The renal glomerulus of mice lacking s-laminin/laminin ß2: nephrosis despite molecular compensation by laminin ß1. *Nat Genet*. 1995;10:400–406.
68. Gao F, Maiti S, Sun G, et al. The Wt1+/R394W mouse displays glomerulosclerosis and early-onset renal failure characteristic of human Denys-Drash syndrome. *Mol Cell Biol*. 2004;24(22):9899–9910.
69. Patek CE, Little MH, Fleming S, et al. A zinc finger truncation of murine WT1 results in the characteristic urogenital abnormalities of Denys-Drash syndrome. *Proc Natl Acad Sci USA*. 1999;96(6):2931–2936.
70. Hammes A, Guo JK, Lutsch G, et al. Two splice variants of the Wilms' tumor 1 gene have distinct functions during sex determination and nephron formation. *Cell*. 2001;106(3):319–329.
71. Guo JK, Menke AL, Gubler MC, et al. WT1 is a key regulator of podocyte function: reduced expression levels cause crescentic glomerulonephritis and mesangial sclerosis. *Hum Mol Genet*. 2002;11(6):651–659.
72. Sadl V, Jin F, Yu J, et al. The mouse Kreisler (Krml1/MafB) segmentation gene is required for differentiation of glomerular visceral epithelial cells. *Dev Biol*. 2002;249(1):16–29.
73. Miner JH, Morello R, Andrews KL, et al. Transcriptional induction of slit diaphragm genes by Lmx1b is required in podocyte differentiation. *J Clin Invest*. 2002;109(8):1065–1072.
74. Ho J, Ng KH, Rosen S, et al. Podocyte-specific loss of functional microRNAs leads to rapid glomerular and tubular injury. *J Am Soc Nephrol*. 2008;19(11):2069–2075.
75. Harvey SJ, Jarad G, Cunningham J, et al. Podocyte-specific deletion of dicer alters cytoskeletal dynamics and causes glomerular disease. *J Am Soc Nephrol*. 2008;19(11):2150–2158.
76. Shi S, Yu L, Chiu C, et al. Podocyte-selective deletion of dicer induces proteinuria and glomerulosclerosis. *J Am Soc Nephrol*. 2008;19(11):2159–2169.
77. Little MH, McMahon AP. Mammalian kidney development: principles, progress, and projections. *Cold Spring Harb Perspect Biol*. 2012;4(5):pii: a008300.
78. Davidson AJ. Mouse kidney development. *StemBook*. Cambridge, MA; 2008.
79. Torres M, GomezPardo E, Dressler GR, Gruss P. Pax-2 controls multiple steps of urogenital development. *Development*. 1995;121(12):4057–4065.
80. Bouchard M, Souabni A, Mandler M, et al. Nephric lineage specification by Pax2 and Pax8. *Genes Dev*. 2002;16(22):2958–2970.
81. Grote D, Boualia SK, Souabni A, et al. Gata3 acts downstream of beta-catenin signaling to prevent ectopic metanephric kidney induction. *PLoS Genet*. 2008;4(12):e1000316.
82. Grote D, Souabni A, Busslinger M, Bouchard M. Pax2/8-regulated Gata3 expression is necessary for morphogenesis and guidance of the nephric duct in the developing kidney. *Development*. 2006; 133(1):53–61.

8

83. Drawbridge J, Meighan CM, Mitchell EA. GDNF and GFR alpha-1 are components of the axolotl pronephric duct guidance system. *Dev Biol*. 2000;228(1):116–124.
84. Chia I, Grote D, Marcotte M, et al. Nephric duct insertion is a crucial step in urinary tract maturation that is regulated by a Gata3-Raldh2-Ret molecular network in mice. *Development*. 2011; 138(10):2089–2097.
85. Pichel JG, Shen LY, Sheng HZ, et al. Defects in enteric innervation and kidney development in mice lacking GDNF. *Nature*. 1996;382(6586):73–76.
86. Lokmane L, Heliot C, Garcia-Villalba P, et al. vHNF1 functions in distinct regulatory circuits to control ureteric bud branching and early nephrogenesis. *Development*. 2010;137(2):347–357.
87. Tsang TE, Shawlot W, Kinder SJ, et al. Lim1 activity is required for intermediate mesoderm differentiation in the mouse embryo. *Dev Biol*. 2000;223(1):77–90.
88. Pedersen A, Skjong C, Shawlot W. Lim1 is required for nephric duct extension and ureteric bud morphogenesis. *Dev Biol*. 2005;288(2):571–581.
89. Kobayashi A, Shawlot W, Kania A, Behringer RR. Requirement of Lim1 for female reproductive tract development. *Development*. 2004;131(3):539–549.
90. Durbec P, Marcos-Gutierrez CV, Kilkenny C, et al. GDNF signalling through the Ret receptor tyrosine kinase. *Nature*. 1996;381(6585):789–793.
91. Pachnis V, Mankoo B, Costantini F. Expression of the c-ret proto-oncogene during mouse embryogenesis. *Development*. 1993;119(4):1005–1017.
92. Hellmich HL, Kos L, Cho ES, et al. Embryonic expression of glial cell-line derived neurotrophic factor (GDNF) suggests multiple developmental roles in neural differentiation and epithelial-mesenchymal interactions. *Mech Dev*. 1996;54(1):95–105.
93. Sainio K, Suvanto P, Davies J, et al. Glial-cell-line-derived neurotrophic factor is required for bud initiation from ureteric epithelium. *Development*. 1997;124(20):4077–4087.
94. Tanaka M, Xiao HY, Kiuchi K. Heparin facilitates glial cell line-derived neurotrophic factor signal transduction. *Neuroreport*. 2002;13(15):1913–1916.
95. Takahashi M. The GDNF/RET signaling pathway and human diseases. *Cytokine Growth Factor Rev*. 2001;12(4):361–373.
96. Lu BC, Cebrian C, Chi X, et al. Etv4 and Etv5 are required downstream of GDNF and Ret for kidney branching morphogenesis. *Nat Genet*. 2009;41(12):1295–1302.
97. Chi X, Michos O, Shakya R, et al. Ret-dependent cell rearrangements in the Wolffian duct epithelium initiate ureteric bud morphogenesis. *Dev Cell*. 2009;17(2):199–209.
98. Kuure S, Chi X, Lu B, Costantini F. The transcription factors Etv4 and Etv5 mediate formation of the ureteric bud tip domain during kidney development. *Development*. 2010;137(12):1975–1979.
99. Costantini F. Genetic controls and cellular behaviors in branching morphogenesis of the renal collecting system. *Wiley Interdiscip Rev Dev Biol*. 2012;1(5):693–713.
100. Xu PX, Zheng WM, Huang L, et al. Six1 is required for the early organogenesis of mammalian kidney. *Development*. 2003;130(14):3085–3094.
101. Sajithlal G, Zou D, Silvius D, Xu PX. Eya1 acts as a critical regulator for specifying the metanephric mesenchyme. *Dev Biol*. 2005;284(2):323–336.
102. Nishinakamura R, Matsumoto Y, Nakao K, et al. Murine homolog of SALL1 is essential for ureteric bud invasion in kidney development. *Development*. 2001;128(16):3105–3115.
103. Wellik DM, Hawkes PJ, Capecchi MR. Hox11 paralogous genes are essential for metanephric kidney induction. *Genes Dev*. 2002;16(11):1423–1432.
104. Basson MA, Akbulut S, Watson-Johnson J, et al. Sprouty1 is a critical regulator of GDNF/RET-mediated kidney induction. *Dev Cell*. 2005;8(2):229–239.
105. Grieshammer U, Ma L, Plump AS, et al. SLIT2-mediated ROBO2 signaling restricts kidney induction to a single site. *Dev Cell*. 2004;6(5):709–717.
106. Kume T, Deng KY, Hogan BLM. Murine forkhead/winged helix genes Foxc1 (Mf1) and Foxc2 (Mfh1) are required for the early organogenesis of the kidney and urinary tract. *Development*. 2000;127(7):1387–1395.
107. Miyazaki Y, Oshima K, Fogo A, et al. Bone morphogenetic protein 4 regulates the budding site and elongation of the mouse ureter. *J Clin Invest*. 2000;105(7):863–873.
108. Miyazaki Y, Oshima K, Fogo A, Ichikawa I. Evidence that bone morphogenetic protein 4 has multiple biological functions during kidney and urinary tract development. *Kidney Int*. 2003;63(3):835–844.
109. Schuchardt A, DAgati V, Pachnis V, Costantini F. Renal agenesis and hypodysplasia in ret-k(-) mutant mice result from defects in ureteric bud development. *Development*. 1996;122(6):1919–1929.
110. Moore MW, Klein RD, Farinas I, et al. Renal and neuronal abnormalities in mice lacking GDNF. *Nature*. 1996;382(6586):76–79.
111. Sanchez MP, Silos-Santiago I, Frisen J, et al. Renal agenesis and the absence of enteric neurons in mice lacking GDNF. *Nature*. 1996;382(6586):70–73.
112. Enomoto H, Araki T, Jackman A, et al. GFR alpha 1-deficient mice have deficits in the enteric nervous system and kidneys. *Neuron*. 1998;21(2):317–324.
113. Bullock SL, Fletcher JM, Beddington RSP, Wilson VA. Renal agenesis in mice homozygous for a gene trap mutation in the gene encoding heparan sulfate 2-sulfotransferase. *Genes Dev*. 1998;12(12):1894–1906.
114. Jain S, Encinas M, Johnson EM, Milbrandt J. Critical and distinct roles for key RET tyrosine docking sites in renal development. *Genes Dev*. 2006;20(3):321–333.
115. Wong A, Bogni S, Kotka P, et al. Phosphotyrosine 1062 is critical for the in vivo activity of the Ret9 receptor tyrosine kinase isoform. *Mol Cell Biol*. 2005;25(21):9661–9673.

116. Maeshima A, Sakurai H, Choi Y, et al. Glial cell-derived neurotrophic factor-independent ureteric bud outgrowth from the Wolffian duct. *J Am Soc Nephrol.* 2007;18(12):3147–3155.

117. Michos O, Cebrian C, Hyink D, et al. Kidney development in the absence of Gdnf and Spry1 requires Fgf10. *PLoS Genet.* 2010;6(1):e1000809.

118. Majumdar A, Vainio S, Kispert A, et al. Wnt11 and Ret/Gdnf pathways cooperate in regulating ureteric branching during metanephric kidney development. *Development.* 2003;130(14): 3175–3185.

119. Carroll TJ, Park JS, Hayashi S, et al. Wnt9b plays a central role in the regulation of mesenchymal to epithelial transitions underlying organogenesis of the mammalian urogenital system. *Dev Cell.* 2005;9(2):283–292.

120. Bridgewater D, Cox B, Cain J, et al. Canonical WNT/beta-catenin signaling is required for ureteric branching. *Dev Biol.* 2008;317(1):83–94.

121. Hartwig S, Bridgewater D, Di Giovanni V, et al. BMP receptor ALK3 controls collecting system development. *J Am Soc Nephrol.* 2008;19(1):117–124.

122. Qiao J, Uzzo R, Obara-Ishihara T, et al. FGF-7 modulates ureteric bud growth and nephron number in the developing kidney. *Development.* 1999;126(3):547–554.

123. Ohuchi H, Hori Y, Yamasaki M, et al. FGF10 acts as a major ligand for FGF receptor 2 IIIb in mouse multi-organ development. *Biochem Biophys Res Commun.* 2000;277(3):643–649.

124. Revest JM, Spencer-Dene B, Kerr K, et al. Fibroblast growth factor receptor 2-IIIb acts upstream of Shh and Fgf4 and is required for limb bud maintenance but not for the induction of Fgf8, Fgf10, Msx1, or Bmp4. *Dev Biol.* 2001;231(1):47–62.

125. Zhao HT, Kegg H, Grady S, et al. Role of fibroblast growth factor receptors 1 and 2 in the ureteric bud. *Dev Biol.* 2004;276(2):403–415.

126. Bates CM. Role of fibroblast growth factor receptor signaling in kidney development. *Pediatr Nephrol.* 2011;26(9):1373–1379.

127. Kobayashi A, Mugford JW, Krautzberger AM, et al. Identification of a multipotent self-renewing stromal progenitor population during mammalian kidney organogenesis. *Stem Cell Reports.* 2014;3(4):650–662.

128. Li W, Hartwig S, Rosenblum ND. Developmental origins and functions of stromal cells in the normal and diseased mammalian kidney. *Dev Dyn.* 2014;243(7):853–863.

129. Sequeira-Lopez ML, Lin EE, Li M, et al. The earliest metanephric arteriolar progenitors and their role in kidney vascular development. *Am J Physiol Regul Integr Comp Physiol.* 2015;308(2):R138–R149.

130. Kobayashi H, Liu Q, Binns TC, et al. Distinct subpopulations of FOXD1 stroma-derived cells regulate renal erythropoietin. *J Clin Invest.* 2016;126(5):1926–1938.

131. Levinson RS, Batourina E, Choi C, et al. Foxd1-dependent signals control cellularity in the renal capsule, a structure required for normal renal development. *Development.* 2005;132(3):529–539.

132. Yallowitz AR, Hrycaj SM, Short KM, et al. Hox10 genes function in kidney development in the differentiation and integration of the cortical stroma. *PLoS ONE.* 2011;6(8):e23410.

133. Ohmori T, Tanigawa S, Kaku Y, et al. Sall1 in renal stromal progenitors non-cell autonomously restricts the excessive expansion of nephron progenitors. *Sci Rep.* 2015;5:15676.

134. Boivin FJ, Sarin S, Evans JC, Bridgewater D. The Good and Bad of beta-Catenin in Kidney Development and Renal Dysplasia. *Front Cell Dev Biol.* 2015;3:81.

135. Hum S, Rymer C, Schaefer C, et al. Ablation of the renal stroma defines its critical role in nephron progenitor and vasculature patterning. *PLoS ONE.* 2014;9(2):e88400.

136. Schnabel CA, Godin RE, Cleary ML. Pbx1 regulates nephrogenesis and ureteric branching in the developing kidney. *Dev Biol.* 2003;254(2):262–276.

137. Cui S, Schwartz L, Quaggin SE. Pod1 is required in stromal cells for glomerulogenesis. *Dev Dyn.* 2003;226(3):512–522.

138. Bagherie-Lachidan M, Reginensi A, Pan Q, et al. Stromal Fat4 acts non-autonomously with Dchs1/2 to restrict the nephron progenitor pool. *Development.* 2015;142(15):2564–2573.

139. Quaggin SE, Schwartz L, Cui S, et al. The basic-helix-loop-helix protein pod1 is critically important for kidney and lung organogenesis. *Development.* 1999;126(24):5771–5783.

140. Das A, Tanigawa S, Karner CM, et al. Stromal-epithelial crosstalk regulates kidney progenitor cell differentiation. *Nat Cell Biol.* 2013;15(9):1035–1044.

141. Fetting JL, Guay JA, Karolak MJ, et al. FOXD1 promotes nephron progenitor differentiation by repressing decorin in the embryonic kidney. *Development.* 2014;141(1):17–27.

142. Phua YL, Chu JY, Marrone AK, et al. Renal stromal miRNAs are required for normal nephrogenesis and glomerular mesangial survival. *Physiol Rep.* 2015;3(10).

143. Rosselot C, Spraggon L, Chia I, et al. Non-cell-autonomous retinoid signaling is crucial for renal development. *Development.* 2010;137(2):283–292.

144. Sequeira Lopez ML, Pentz ES, Robert B, et al. Embryonic origin and lineage of juxtaglomerular cells. *Am J Physiol Renal Physiol.* 2001;281(2):F345–F356.

145. Iosipiv IV, Schroeder M. A role for angiotensin II AT1 receptors in ureteric bud cell branching. *Am J Physiol Renal Physiol.* 2003;285(2):F199–F207.

146. Batourina E, Gim S, Bello N, et al. Vitamin A controls epithelial/mesenchymal interactions through Ret expression. *Nat Genet.* 2001;27(1):74–78.

147. Sequeira Lopez ML, Gomez RA. Development of the renal arterioles. *J Am Soc Nephrol.* 2011;22(12):2156–2165.

148. Hu Y, Li M, Gothert JR, et al. Hemovascular Progenitors in the Kidney Require Sphingosine-1-Phosphate Receptor 1 for Vascular Development. *J Am Soc Nephrol.* 2016;27(7):1984–1995.

149. Sims-Lucas S, Schaefer C, Bushnell D, et al. Endothelial Progenitors Exist within the Kidney and Lung Mesenchyme. *PLoS ONE*. 2013;8(6):e65993.
150. Halt KJ, Parssinen HE, Junttila SM, et al. CD146(+) cells are essential for kidney vasculature development. *Kidney Int*. 2016;90(2):311–324.
151. Hurtado R, Zewdu R, Mtui J, et al. Pbx1-dependent control of VMC differentiation kinetics underlies gross renal vascular patterning. *Development*. 2015;142(15):2653–2664.
152. Boyle SC, Liu Z, Kopan R. Notch signaling is required for the formation of mesangial cells from a stromal mesenchyme precursor during kidney development. *Development*. 2014;141(2):346–354.
153. Lindahl P, Hellstrom M, Kalen M, et al. Paracrine PDGF-B/PDGF-Rbeta signaling controls mesangial cell development in kidney glomeruli. *Development*. 1998;125(17):3313–3322.
154. Sequeira-Lopez ML, Nagalakshmi VK, Li M, et al. Vascular versus tubular renin: role in kidney development. *Am J Physiol Regul Integr Comp Physiol*. 2015;309(6):R650–R657.
155. Roker LA, Nemri K, Yu J. Wnt7b Signaling from the Ureteric Bud Epithelium Regulates Medullary Capillary Development. *J Am Soc Nephrol*. 2017;28(1):250–259.
156. Dimke H, Sparks MA, Thomson BR, et al. Tubulovascular cross-talk by vascular endothelial growth factor a maintains peritubular microvasculature in kidney. *J Am Soc Nephrol*. 2015;26(5):1027–1038.
157. Clissold RL, Hamilton AJ, Hattersley AT, et al. HNF1B-associated renal and extra-renal disease-an expanding clinical spectrum. *Nat Rev Nephrol*. 2015;11(2):102–112.
158. Sharma R, Sanchez-Ferras O, Bouchard M. Pax genes in renal development, disease and regeneration. *Semin Cell Dev Biol*. 2015;44:97–106.
159. Hwang DY, Dworschak GC, Kohl S, et al. Mutations in 12 known dominant disease-causing genes clarify many congenital anomalies of the kidney and urinary tract. *Kidney Int*. 2014;85(6):1429–1433.
160. Castiglione A, Melchionda S, Carella M, et al. EYA1-related disorders: two clinical cases and a literature review. *Int J Pediatr Otorhinolaryngol*. 2014;78(8):1201–1210.
161. Miller EM, Hopkin R, Bao L, Ware SM. Implications for genotype-phenotype predictions in Townes-Brocks syndrome: case report of a novel SALL1 deletion and review of the literature. *Am J Med Genet A*. 2012;158A(3):533–540.
162. Hall JG. The early history of Pallister-Hall syndrome-Buried treasure of a sort. *Gene*. 2016;589(2):100–103.
163. Cohen MM Jr, Kreiborg S. Visceral anomalies in the Apert syndrome. *Am J Med Genet*. 1993;45(6):758–760.
164. de Pontual L, Yao E, Callier P, et al. Germline deletion of the miR-17 approximately 92 cluster causes skeletal and growth defects in humans. *Nat Genet*. 2011;43(10):1026–1030.
165. Weber S, Moriniere V, Knuppel T, et al. Prevalence of mutations in renal developmental genes in children with renal hypodysplasia: results of the ESCAPE study. *J Am Soc Nephrol*. 2006;17(10):2864–2870.
166. Weber S, Taylor JC, Winyard P, et al. SIX2 and BMP4 mutations associate with anomalous kidney development. *J Am Soc Nephrol*. 2008;19(5):891–903.
167. Skinner MA, Safford SD, Reeves JG, et al. Renal aplasia in humans is associated with RET mutations. *Am J Hum Genet*. 2008;82(2):344–351.
168. Barak H, Huh SH, Chen S, et al. FGF9 and FGF20 maintain the stemness of nephron progenitors in mice and man. *Dev Cell*. 2012;22(6):1191–1207.
169. Kohl S, Hwang DY, Dworschak GC, et al. Mild recessive mutations in six Fraser syndrome-related genes cause isolated congenital anomalies of the kidney and urinary tract. *J Am Soc Nephrol*. 2014;25(9):1917–1922.
170. Vivante A, Hwang DY, Kohl S, et al. Exome Sequencing Discerns Syndromes in Patients from Consanguineous Families with Congenital Anomalies of the Kidneys and Urinary Tract. *J Am Soc Nephrol*. 2017;28(1):69–75.

CHAPTER 9

Prenatal Programming of Hypertension and Kidney and Cardiovascular Disease

Michel Baum, MD

Epidemiologic studies have solidified the association of a number of factors, such as smoking, obesity, diabetes mellitus, elevated serum cholesterol, hypertension, and a sedentary lifestyle, with the development of cardiovascular disease. David Barker made a number of seminal observations demonstrating an association of low birth weight as another factor that can predispose to cardiovascular disease in later life. The first clue that led Barker and his colleagues to this association was rather tenuous. He divided England and Wales into 212 areas and examined if there was an association between infant mortality between 1921 and 1925 and death from cardiovascular disease between 1968 and 1978.[1] They found that areas with high infant mortality were by and large the poorer areas of England and Wales where limited resources led to poor living conditions and poor infant nutrition. Infant mortality usually occurred within the first week of life and was associated with low birth weight.[2] Survivors of these adverse conditions were predisposed or programmed to develop cardiovascular disease in later life. Thus there was a potential link between infant mortality due predominantly to low birth weight and cardiovascular disease. Animal models have confirmed this association and provided insights into the pathogenesis of prenatal programming. This chapter focuses on the current evidence that poor maternal nutrition leading to fetal and infant low birth weight leads to premature death due to cardiovascular and renal disease.

Prenatal Programming of Hypertension and Cardiovascular Disease

Barker and colleagues focused on the association of small-for-gestational-age infants and cardiovascular outcomes in several studies. These investigators focused on cities in England where there were excellent birth and death records. In Hertfordshire there were 5654 male births between 1911 and 1930. The death rates from cardiovascular disease in the ensuing 70 years was greatest in men who were less than 5.5 pounds at birth.[3] There appeared to be a protective effect of being a large baby. At 1 year of age, those children who were less than 18 pounds had a threefold greater risk of death from ischemic heart disease than those greater than 27 pounds.[3] A similar relationship between low birth weight and death from cardiovascular disease, but not other diseases, was also found for women born in Hertfordshire during this time.[4] In studies performed in Preston, England, examining the relationship between birth weight and blood pressure measured in men and women aged 46 to 54 found that infants born less than 5.5 pounds had on average an 11 mm Hg greater blood pressure than those born at 7.5 pounds or more.[5] The effect of being small for gestational age on blood pressure is even apparent in children. For every 1-kg decrease in birth weight, there is a 1.3-mm Hg increase in systolic blood pressure and 0.7-mm Hg increase in diastolic blood pressure at 7 years of age.[6]

It does not appear that one can compensate for fetal undernutrition with postnatal caloric supplementation. Nutrient supplementation in small-for-gestational-age neonates by increasing the protein content of their formula resulted in higher blood pressures when measured at 6 to 8 years of age compared with nonsupplemented infants.[7] Another study also found that accelerated early postnatal weight gain resulted in an increase in blood pressure in small-for-gestational-age infants when blood pressure was measured as adults.[8] The greatest risk for hypertension is in those who are small at birth and who have rapid catch-up growth in childhood.[9]

Perhaps the best studied population is adult offspring whose mothers were exposed to the Dutch famine that occurred between late November 1944 to early May 1945. During World War II the Germans cut the daily rations on the Dutch population from 1600 Kcal to 400 to 800 Kcal, in retaliation for a railroad strike that was imposed by the Dutch government in exile to prevent the Germans from reenforcing their troops after the invasion at Normandy. The offspring of the mothers who endured the famine have been compared with those whose mothers were pregnant before or after the famine.[10] Approximately 50 years after the famine the offspring were found to have an increased likelihood of glucose intolerance,[11] microalbuminuria (a harbinger of renal disease),[12] an atherogenic lipid profile,[13] and obesity.[14] Although not all neonates exposed prenatally to the famine were small for gestational age, those who were of low birth weight had a 2.7-mm Hg increase in blood pressure for every 1-kg decrease in birth weight.[15] Thus, in total, exposure to the Dutch famine increased the likelihood of having the metabolic syndrome, although the severity of the organs involved was dependent on the time during gestation when maternal exposure to the famine occurred.[10] Importantly, those with prenatal exposure to the Dutch famine had a threefold increase in death from coronary artery disease.[16] Similarly, those exposed to the Holocaust during early life have an increased incidence of congestive heart failure, angina, dyslipidemia, diabetes mellitus, and malignancy compared with those who were not Holocaust survivors.[17] The observation that small-for-gestational-age infants are at risk for hyperlipidemia, hypertension, noninsulin-dependent diabetes mellitus, and cardiovascular disease has been extended to insults from multiple different causes and in diverse ethnic populations.[11,16,18–36]

Prenatal Programming of Nephron Endowment: Chronic Kidney Disease and Hypertension

The dogma that there are 1 million nephrons in each kidney is likely not correct.[37] Determining nephron endowment with any precision is technically challenging and complicated by the fact that there is a loss of glomeruli as we age. It is apparent that the number of glomeruli is affected by sex, race, age, and importantly by birth weight. Rather than the 1 million nephrons in each kidney in every human, as reviewed by Hoy et al., there is a tremendous variability in the number of nephrons per kidney, ranging from just over 225,000 to more than 2 million.[37] For each kilogram increase in birth weight, there is approximately a 250,000 increase in glomerular number.[38] A study examined the effect of birth weight on kidney development in neonates born after 36 weeks of gestation, a point when nephrogenesis is complete, in infants who died within the first 2 weeks after birth from nonrenal causes.[39] As shown in Fig. 9.1, there was a direct relationship between glomerular number and birth weight and an inverse relationship between birth weight and glomerular volume. The increase in glomerular capillary surface area and glomerular volume in the remaining nephrons compensates for the reduction in nephron mass.

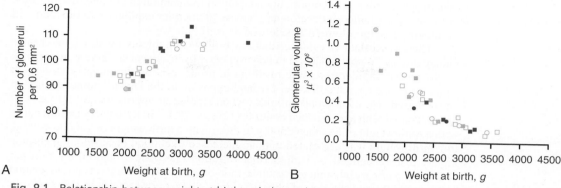

Fig. 9.1 Relationship between weight at birth and glomerular number (A) and glomerular volume (B) in infants of various weights born after 36 weeks' gestation when nephrogenesis is complete. (From Manalich R, Reyes L, Herrera M, Melendi C, Fundora I. Relationship between weight at birth and number and size of renal glomeruli in humans: a histomorphometric study. *Kidney Int.* 2000;58:770-773.)

Fig. 9.2 Pathogenesis of chronic kidney disease and hypertension as a result of reduced glomerular number. (Adapted from Brenner BM, Garcia DL, Anderson S. Glomeruli and blood pressure. Less of one, more the other? *Am J Hypertens.* 1988;1: 335-347.)

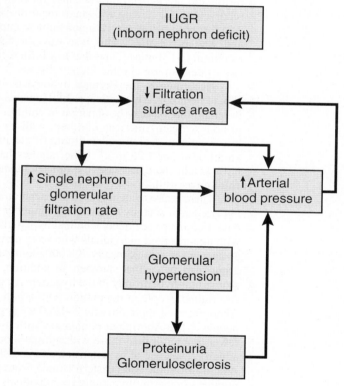

A decreased nephron number has been postulated to be a harbinger for hypertension and a progressive fall in glomerular filtration rate.[40,41] The Brenner hypothesis is depicted in Fig. 9.2, which shows that a reduction in nephron number from any means, including a reduction of nephron endowment from low birth weight, sets up a progressive process leading to further nephron loss. The mechanism for the effect of renal mass on glomerular hemodynamics has been studied in rats because some strains have surface glomeruli that are amenable to micropuncture. A reduction in nephron number has been shown to increase glomerular capillary pressure, resulting in proteinuria and eventually glomerular sclerosis.[40–43] Glomerular sclerosis leads to a further fall in glomerular capillary surface area, leading to a vicious cycle resulting in progressive decline in glomerular filtration rate. The remaining unaffected glomeruli hypertrophy, which is a temporizing adaptation to maintain the glomerular filtration rate, but these glomeruli develop an increase glomerular capillary pressure and will eventually undergo glomerular sclerosis as well.[44]

There is substantive evidence that low birth weight infants are at risk for chronic kidney disease. With a reduction in nephron mass from any cause, there is an increase in glomerular capillary pressure resulting in proteinuria or albuminuria as the first sign of progressive renal disease. Prenatal exposure to the Dutch famine resulted in an increased risk of microalbuminuria when studied at approximately 50 years of age compared with age-matched controls (12% vs. 7%).[12] In a study comparing males with a birth weight of less than 2500 g to those with a birth weight of 2500 to 4499 g, low birth weight was associated with an increased likelihood of developing chronic kidney disease defined as a glomerular filtration rate of less than 60 mL/min per 1.73 m^2 or a urinary albumin to creatinine ratio of $\geq$30 mg/g.[45] There was no association of birth weight and the risk of chronic kidney disease for females in this study. In the southeastern United States a study examined the birth weight of adult dialysis patients and compared the weight with age-, sex-, and race-matched controls. A birth weight less than 2.5 kg was associated with a 1.4-fold greater risk of developing end-stage renal disease compared with those weighing 3 to 3.5 kg at birth.[46] The results did not depend on the cause for the end-stage renal disease. In Norway the relative risk for having end-stage renal disease was 1.7 (confidence interval 1.4 to 2.2) for those below the 10th percentile compared with those born between the 10th and 90th percentile.[47] This was true for both men and women. A meta-analysis examining 31 studies found that low birth weight was associated with a 70% greater risk of developing chronic kidney disease.[48]

According to the Brenner hypothesis the decline in glomerular filtration rate should be progressive with age.[40,41] However, there is some evidence that a decrease in renal function may be apparent in children. In African-American children but not in non–African-American children, with an average age of 1.5 years, there was a lower estimated glomerular filtration rate in children of low birth weight (82 vs. 95 mL/min per 1.73 m^2).[49] Other studies have found an association between low birth weight and a decrease in estimated glomerular filtration rate in white school-age children as well.[50]

There is also evidence that a low nephron endowment is a risk factor for developing hypertension. A study examined the number of glomeruli in 10 people age 35 to 59 who died in car accidents who had hypertension and/or left ventricular hypertrophy with age-matched individuals who were normotensive. The hypertensive group had an average of approximately 700,000 glomeruli per kidney, whereas the normotensive group had twice that number. In addition, there was evidence of compensatory glomerular hypertrophy in the hypertensive group.[51] Similar findings were shown in Aboriginal people, a population with a high prevalence of chronic kidney disease. Aborigines had approximately 200,000 fewer glomeruli per kidney than non-Aboriginal people.[52] The Aboriginal population with hypertension had approximately 250,000 fewer glomeruli than those with normal blood pressures.[52] Another population with a high prevalence of hypertension and end-stage renal disease is African Americans. A study from the southeastern United States did not find a difference in glomerular number comparing hypertensive individuals to controls. This same study examined whites and found a reduction in glomerular number in the hypertensive group, but it was only approximately 20% less than controls.[52] These data are consistent with an association between glomerular number and hypertension in some populations but not others. The significance of the reduction in glomerular number in mediating the increase in blood pressure is not clear because the hypertension could be a factor in medicating the reduction in nephron number.

Thrifty Phenotype Hypothesis

Why would a prenatal insult leading to small-for-gestational-age infants result in changes that would predispose to early death from cardiovascular or renal disease? One possible teleologic explanation lies in the thrifty phenotype hypothesis, which

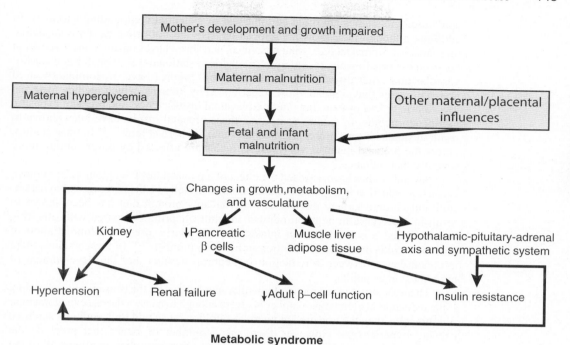

Fig. 9.3 Pathogenesis of the metabolic syndrome according to the thrifty phenotype hypothesis. (From Hales CN, Barker DJP. The thrifty phenotype hypothesis. *Br Med Bull.* 2001;60:5-20.)

states that adaptation at one point in time may lead to changes that are maladaptive at a later time point. This phenomenon occurs because of plasticity, which allows us to adapt to our environment during specific periods of time, usually during prenatal or early neonatal development. These early adaptive changes result in permanent phenotypic changes despite the fact that our genotype does not change.[2] The changes are advantageous for the time surrounding when they are programmed but may become disadvantageous in later life. Thus, if a neonate is born small for gestational age and then becomes an obese adult, the settings established as a neonate or fetus are maladaptive to the adult.[53,54] The thrifty phenotype hypothesis is depicted in Fig. 9.3. As an example, if there is a prenatal insult such as fetal malnutrition, one may shift resources from nephron development to brain and cardiovascular development, which are vital at the time. During this point in life there is an adequate number of nephrons for fluid and electrolyte homeostasis, but as we age the paucity of nephrons at birth may lead to progressive chronic kidney disease in later life. The same argument can be made for the pancreas, where the number of islets may be compromised during development if nutrition is inadequate. Indeed, low birth weight infants who become obese as adults are also at substantial risk for the development of type 2 diabetes as adults.[20,34,53,55,56] The mechanism whereby one can alter the phenotype without a change in the DNA sequence is due to epigenetic changes that affect transcription and translation. During discrete times during development, changes in the environment can cause changes in methylation of CpG islands in the promoter of some genes affecting transcription and there can also be environmental changes in histones and micro-RNAs. These changes can have permanent effects on the phenotype of the organism and in some cases can be passed on to the next generation.

Animal Models of Prenatal Programming

The previous human epidemiologic studies show an association between small-for-gestational-age infants and the development of hypertension and cardiovascular and chronic kidney disease. However, although the previous data are very compelling, epidemiologic studies are often complicated by potential confounding variables. In addition, although they show an association, they do not prove causality or define mechanisms. Animal studies using rats, mice, and sheep have cemented the association between maternal insults resulting in small-for-gestational-age neonates and cardio-vascular and renal disease in mature offspring. Studies have predominantly used prenatal insults that simulate those experienced by humans, which include maternal low calorie or low protein diet, uterine-placental insufficiency, and prenatal exposure to glucocorticoids. In studies using rats, these prenatal insults have been shown to result in small-for-gestational-age neonates that are born at term.[57–60] In most studies, unless the prenatal insult is very severe, males are affected by programming more severely than females.[61]

Several studies have assessed the effect of a prenatal insult on glomerular number, because a reduction in nephron number could potentially be the harbinger of hypertension and chronic kidney disease. A maternal low protein diet has been shown to result in a decrease in nephron number in adult offspring compared with offspring that were fed a normal protein intake.[60,62–65] Similarly, prenatal administration of glucocorticoids produces a reduction in nephron number.[66–68] In these studies, there is concordance between a reduction in nephron number and the development of hypertension as adults.

Theoretically, a reduction in glomerular number can be the cause for hypertension. If the reduction in glomerular number is severe enough to cause a decrease in glomerular filtration rate, then the impaired glomerular filtration rate could limit sodium excretion, causing hypertension. However, there are a number of issues that preclude the hypertension being mediated by a reduction in nephron number. In almost all of the studies examining the effect of a low protein diet or prenatal administration of dexamethasone on glomerular number, there is only a 20% to 30% reduction in glomeruli, which is far too low to cause impaired sodium excretion. Furthermore, in some studies examining programming, there are rats that are hypertensive but do not have a decrease in glomerular number.[68,69] Some studies have found a significant reduction in nephron number by perinatal programming, but that the rats and mice did not develop hypertension.[70,71] Direct measurement of glomerular filtration rate has been found to be normal in several studies at a time when programmed rats are hypertensive.[61,67,68] Other studies using different models have also demonstrated that there is a poor correlation between glomerular number and the development of hypertension.[72]

However, the reduction in nephron endowment with programming could be a predisposing factor for chronic kidney disease. Studies looking at the effect of prenatal programming by administration of dexamethasone to rats did not show a decrease in glomerular filtration rate when compared with vehicle-treated controls at 2 months and at 6 to 9 months of age.[67,68] In rats whose mothers had surgically induced uteroplacental insufficiency, there was an increase in blood pressure at 3 months but no decrease in glomerular filtration rate.[58] Several studies have examined the effect of a maternal low protein diet on glomerular filtration rate. Compared with offspring whose mothers were fed a normal protein diet, offspring whose mothers were fed a low protein diet did not have a reduction in glomerular filtration rate when corrected for body weight at 4 to 5 months of age.[62,73] There are compensatory mechanisms that maintain a normal glomerular filtration rate with a loss in nephron number comparable with that seen with programming. The reduction in glomerular filtration rate may only manifest when the rats age. Two studies have examined the effect of maternal low protein diet on glomerular filtration rate in rats at 1.5 years of age, and both found an approximately 50% reduction in glomerular filtration rate.[74,75] There was no reduction in glomerular filtration rate in rats whose mothers were fed a low protein diet compared with controls at 3 months of age.[75] Thus these studies solidify the epidemiologic studies and show a direct effect of programming on the kidney that results in a progressive decrease in glomerular filtration rate.

Because a reduction in glomerular number does not seem to be the predominant factor mediating the hypertension, investigators have looked at other potential factors that could mediate the increase in blood pressure in programmed animals. Several studies have examined the role of the renin-angiotensin system in the prenatal programming of hypertension. The renin-angiotensin system can act to cause vasoconstriction and an increase in tubular transport, which can both affect blood pressure. Many studies have examined the effect of programming on the systemic renin-angiotensin system, and the results have been reviewed elsewhere.[18,76] To summarize, although an increase in renin-angiotensin-aldosterone activity could explain the hypertension with programming, the results are quite variable, depending on the cause of the prenatal insult resulting in small for gestational age, the age and sex of the offspring studied, and which components of the system were assayed. Dysregulation of the systemic renin-angiotensin system, although clearly present in some studies, does not provide a unifying cause for hypertension with programming.

An increase in salt transport could explain the hypertension with prenatal programming. In a study comparing renal transporter protein abundance in several nephron segments, rats whose mothers were fed a low protein diet had an increase in NKCC2 and NCC protein abundance.[77] These are the apical membrane sodium transporters in the thick ascending limb and distal convoluted tubule, respectively. More direct assessment of transport was performed using isolated perfused tubules, where sodium transport was measured in programmed and control rat nephron segments. Rats whose mothers were administered dexamethasone had an increase in proximal tubule and thick ascending limb sodium transport compared with vehicle-treated controls.[78,79] A maternal low protein diet also programmed an increase sodium transport in the thick ascending limb and cortical collecting duct compared with offspring of rats whose mothers were fed a normal protein diet.[79,80]

The kidney is richly innervated, and sodium transport in several nephron segments is regulated by renal sympathetic nerve activity. Renal denervation normalized the blood pressure in programmed rats to control levels resulting from both maternal uteroplacental insufficiency and prenatal administration of dexamethasone, whereas denervation did not affect the blood pressure of control rats.[81,82] Prenatal administration of dexamethasone increased proximal tubule NHE3 (the apical membrane Na^+/H^+ exchanger responsible for the majority of proximal tubule sodium transport), the thick limb NKCC2, and the distal convoluted tubule NCC protein abundance.[82] The abundance of these transporters was normalized to control levels with denervation, whereas denervation had no effect on the expression of the transporters in offspring of mothers who received that vehicle.[82] Subsequent studies measured renal sympathetic nerve activity directly, which demonstrated an increase in renal sympathetic nerve activity with leg muscle contraction.[83,84] These results were consistent with prenatal programming increasing transport via an increase in sodium transport mediated by an increase in sympathetic nerve activity. Other factors, such as reactive oxygen species, the systemic and intrarenal renin-angiotensin system, and vascular changes, may contribute to programming of hypertension. These have been reviewed elsewhere.[76,85–89]

Postnatal Modulation of Prenatal Insults

Barker et al. examined the growth trajectories of people born in Helsinki from 1934 to 1944 where growth records were kept.[90] People who were small at birth and remained thin at 2 years, but subsequently gained weight rapidly to an average weight at 11 years, were compared with controls. The small-for-gestational-age children with rapid weight gain were at increased risk for insulin resistance and coronary artery disease as adults. This study suggests that not just the prenatal or early neonatal weight but also the weight trajectory in childhood may be risk factors for cardiac disease and diabetes. As discussed previously, accelerated weight gain in small-for-gestational-age neonates results in higher blood pressure than the effect of small-for-gestational-age infants alone.[9]

Rats have been used to determine the impact of rapid postnatal weight gain on blood pressure and renal function. In studies in which rats were overfed by reducing the litter size to 3 pups on day 3 of life compared with controls from a litter of 10 pups, the overfed pups weighed substantively more than control rats even into adulthood. The overfed pups had a 20% greater nephron number than controls but nonetheless developed hypertension and proteinuria. At 22 months of age the kidneys from the postnatal overfed group had higher urinary protein excretion and greater glomerulosclerosis than the controls.[91] This group also looked at overfeeding in rats by reducing the litter to three pups whose mothers were fed a low protein diet compared with offspring that were overfed after mothers were fed a control diet. As with the overfed group, the programmed male overfed group was hypertensive, had glomerulosclerosis, and had proteinuria. However, only the programmed overfed group and not the overfed only group had a decrease in creatinine clearance compared with controls that were not programmed or overfed at 12 months. Neither overfeeding nor programming affected any of these parameters in females.[92]

There is accumulating evidence that the result of prenatal programming is not written in stone and that manipulating the postnatal environment can prevent the adverse outcome of a maternal insult leading for small-for-gestational-age offspring. Rats programmed by administration of prenatal dexamethasone developed hypertension and hyperleptinemia.[93] In those rats cross-fostered to a mother fed a diet enriched in ω-3 fatty acids and continued on this diet after weaning did not develop hypertension or hyperleptinemia.[93] Administration of a low salt diet or enalapril for 3 weeks near the time of weaning can result in normalization of blood pressure weeks after the drug has been discontinued.[94–96] The mechanism for the reprogramming of hypertension has recently been studied. Transient administration of enalapril to programmed rats by maternal dietary protein deprivation normalized the blood pressure 3 months after the drug had been administered to programmed rats. There was no effect of enalapril on control rats. Transient enalapril did not affect the systemic renin-angiotensin system which was not found to be affected at 6 months in programmed rats. Programming caused an increase in the intrarenal renin-angiotensin system which was normalized by transient administration of enalapril.[96]

Very Premature Infants and Programming

Small-for-gestational-age neonates are often the result of maternal malnutrition that impacts the nutrition of the fetus. This is a problem that has occurred for centuries but came to the forefront by and large from the work of David Barker and colleagues examining adults who were of low birth weight due to caloric deprivation. Currently, a new population of infants may also be at risk, the very premature infant. Similar to the small-for-gestational-age neonate who had intrauterine caloric deprivation, the very premature infant in the neonatal intensive care unit does not receive the same nutrition that would be present if in the womb. In addition, the very premature infant is exposed to a number of drugs and an intrusive environment which may have an impact in later life. The very premature infant is now surviving the neonatal intensive care unit, and many very premature infants are now adults; studies are now emerging showing that the risk factors for chronic disease in later life for the very premature infant are comparable with the small-for-gestational-age infant. However, it should be appreciated that only in the past 30 years are very premature infants surviving into adulthood and thus we do not know the full impact of being born very premature.

Meta-analyses examining the effect of prematurity on blood pressure demonstrate that as with small for gestational age, prematurity is a risk factor for high blood pressure. In one study in which the average birth weight was 1280 g and gestation 30.2 weeks, the systolic blood pressure was 2.5 mm Hg higher at approximately 18 years of age.[97] Another study compared adults who were born at less than 37 weeks' gestation with those at term and found a 4.2-mm Hg systolic and 2.6-mm Hg diastolic blood pressure increase in adults born preterm. Blood pressure assessed in young adults born less than 1.5 kg, compared with term infants that were age, sex, and birth hospital matched using 24-hour blood pressure monitoring found that those adults who were very premature had an average 2.4 mm Hg higher blood pressure and a higher prevalence of hypertension than term controls.[98] As with small-for-gestational-age offspring, premature infants are at increased risk for developing type 2 diabetes and may be at risk for metabolic syndrome.[99]

In utero nephrogenesis in the human starts at approximately 10 weeks' gestation and continues until 36 weeks. Although nephron endowment is usually dependent on several factors discussed previously, it is impacted significantly by prematurity. Nephrogenesis occurs predominantly in the third trimester and can continue to occur in neonates born before 36 weeks' gestation.[100] However, postnatal accrual of nephrons occurs only for 40 days postnatally.[100] Thus, if a premature neonate is born at 24 weeks' gestation and has 40 days to accrue nephrons, the number of nephrons formed will likely be only half of the number if the neonate had remained in the womb.

Renal biopsies performed in patients who were born very low birth weight between 22 and 30 weeks' gestation were evaluated for proteinuria (1.3 to 6 g/day) at an average age of 32 years. Although the patients had normal or mildly impaired renal function, all patients had evidence of focal and segmental glomerulosclerosis, a harbinger of progressive renal disease.[101] Although this was a series of a handful of patients, it is unclear what the prognosis for progressive renal disease will be for very low birth weight infants as they age.

REFERENCES

1. Barker DJ, Osmond C. Infant mortality, childhood nutrition, and ischaemic heart disease in England and Wales. *Lancet.* 1986;1:1077–1081.
2. Barker DJ. The origins of the developmental origins theory. *J Intern Med.* 2007;261:412–417.
3. Barker DJ, Winter PD, Osmond C, et al. Weight in infancy and death from ischaemic heart disease. *Lancet.* 1989;2:577–580.
4. Osmond C, Barker DJ, Winter PD, et al. Early growth and death from cardiovascular disease in women. *BMJ.* 1993;307:1519–1524.
5. Barker DJ, Bull AR, Osmond C, Simmonds SJ. Fetal and placental size and risk of hypertension in adult life. *BMJ.* 1990;301:259–262.
6. Yiu V, Buka S, Zurakowski D, et al. Relationship between birthweight and blood pressure in childhood. *Am J Kidney Dis.* 1999;33:253–260.
7. Singhal A, Cole TJ, Fewtrell M, et al. Promotion of faster weight gain in infants born small for gestational age: is there an adverse effect on later blood pressure? *Circulation.* 2007;115:213–220.
8. Ben-Shlomo Y, McCarthy A, Hughes R, et al. Immediate postnatal growth is associated with blood pressure in young adulthood: the Barry Caerphilly Growth Study. *Hypertension.* 2008;52:638–644.
9. Law CM, Shiell AW, Newsome CA, et al. Fetal, infant, and childhood growth and adult blood pressure: a longitudinal study from birth to 22 years of age. *Circulation.* 2002;105:1088–1092.
10. Painter RC, Roseboom TJ, Bleker OP. Prenatal exposure to the Dutch famine and disease in later life: an overview. *Reprod Toxicol.* 2005;20:345–352.
11. Ravelli AC, van der Meulen JH, Michels RP, et al. Glucose tolerance in adults after prenatal exposure to famine. *Lancet.* 1998;351:173–177.
12. Painter RC, Roseboom TJ, van Montfrans GA, et al. Microalbuminuria in adults after prenatal exposure to the Dutch famine. *J Am Soc Nephrol.* 2005;16:189–194.
13. Roseboom TJ, van der Meulen JH, Osmond C, et al. Plasma lipid profiles in adults after prenatal exposure to the Dutch famine. *Am J Clin Nutr.* 2000;72:1101–1106.
14. Ravelli AC, van der Meulen JH, Osmond C, et al. Obesity at the age of 50 y in men and women exposed to famine prenatally. *Am J Clin Nutr.* 1999;70:811–816.
15. Roseboom TJ, van der Meulen JH, Ravelli AC, et al. Blood pressure in adults after prenatal exposure to famine. *J Hypertens.* 1999;17:325–330.
16. Roseboom TJ, van der Meulen JH, Osmond C, et al. Coronary heart disease after prenatal exposure to the Dutch famine, 1944–45. *Heart.* 2000;84:595–598.
17. Bercovich E, Keinan-Boker L, Shasha SM. Long-term health effects in adults born during the Holocaust. *Isr Med Assoc J.* 2014;16:203–207.
18. Alexander BT, Dasinger JH, Intapad S. Fetal programming and cardiovascular pathology. *Compr Physiol.* 2015;5:997–1025.
19. Liew G, Wang JJ, Mitchell P. Which is the better marker for susceptibility to disease later in life—low birthweight or prematurity? *Arch Dis Child.* 2008;93:450.
20. Barker DJ, Hales CN, Fall CH, et al. Type 2 (non-insulin-dependent) diabetes mellitus, hypertension and hyperlipidaemia (syndrome X): relation to reduced fetal growth. *Diabetologia.* 1993;36:62–67.
21. Barker DJ, Godfrey KM, Osmond C, Bull A. The relation of fetal length, ponderal index and head circumference to blood pressure and the risk of hypertension in adult life. *Paediatr Perinat Epidemiol.* 1992;6:35–44.
22. Campbell DM, Hall MH, Barker DJ, et al. Diet in pregnancy and the offspring's blood pressure 40 years later. *Br J Obstet Gynaecol.* 1996;103:273–280.
23. Curhan GC, Willett WC, Rimm EB, et al. Birth weight and adult hypertension, diabetes mellitus, and obesity in US men. *Circulation.* 1996;94:3246–3250.

24. Curhan GC, Chertow GM, Willett WC, et al. Birth weight and adult hypertension and obesity in women. *Circulation.* 1996;94:1310–1315.
25. Fall CH, Osmond C, Barker DJ, et al. Fetal and infant growth and cardiovascular risk factors in women. *BMJ.* 1995;310:428–432.
26. Forrester TE, Wilks RJ, Bennett FI, et al. Fetal growth and cardiovascular risk factors in Jamaican schoolchildren. *BMJ.* 1996;312:156–160.
27. Hinchliffe SA, Lynch MR, Sargent PH, et al. The effect of intrauterine growth retardation on the development of renal nephrons. *Br J Obstet Gynaecol.* 1992;99:296–301.
28. Hinchliffe SA, Sargent PH, Howard CV, et al. Human intrauterine renal growth expressed in absolute number of glomeruli assessed by the disector method and Cavalieri principle. *Lab Invest.* 1991;64:777–784.
29. Law CM, Barker DJ, Bull AR, Osmond C. Maternal and fetal influences on blood pressure. *Arch Dis Child.* 1991;66:1291–1295.
30. Lithell HO, McKeigue PM, Berglund L, et al. Relation of size at birth to non-insulin dependent diabetes and insulin concentrations in men aged 50-60 years. *BMJ.* 1996;312:406–410.
31. Moore VM, Miller AG, Boulton TJ, et al. Placental weight, birth measurements, and blood pressure at age 8 years. *Arch Dis Child.* 1996;74:538–541.
32. Rich-Edwards JW, Colditz GA, Stampfer MJ, et al. Birthweight and the risk for type 2 diabetes mellitus in adult women. *Ann Intern Med.* 1999;130:278–284.
33. Stein CE, Fall CH, Kumaran K, et al. Fetal growth and coronary heart disease in south India. *Lancet.* 1996;348:1269–1273.
34. Fall CH, Stein CE, Kumaran K, et al. Size at birth, maternal weight, and type 2 diabetes in South India. *Diabet Med.* 1998;15:220–227.
35. Yajnik CS, Fall CH, Vaidya U, et al. Fetal growth and glucose and insulin metabolism in four-year-old Indian children. *Diabet Med.* 1995;12:330–336.
36. Whincup PH, Kaye SJ, Owen CG, et al. Birth weight and risk of type 2 diabetes: a systematic review. *JAMA.* 2008;300:2886–2897.
37. Hoy WE, Hughson MD, Bertram JF, et al. Nephron number, hypertension, renal disease, and renal failure. *J Am Soc Nephrol.* 2005;16:2557–2564.
38. Hughson M, Farris AB III, Douglas-Denton R, et al. Glomerular number and size in autopsy kidneys: the relationship to birth weight. *Kidney Int.* 2003;63:2113–2122.
39. Manalich R, Reyes L, Herrera M, et al. Relationship between weight at birth and the number and size of renal glomeruli in humans: a histomorphometric study. *Kidney Int.* 2000;58:770–773.
40. Brenner BM, Chertow GM. Congenital oligonephropathy and the etiology of adult hypertension and progressive renal injury. *Am J Kidney Dis.* 1994;23:171–175.
41. Brenner BM, Chertow GM. Congenital oligonephropathy: an inborn cause of adult hypertension and progressive renal injury? *Curr Opin Nephrol Hypertens.* 1993;2:691–695.
42. Anderson S, Rennke HG, Brenner BM. Therapeutic advantage of converting enzyme inhibitors in arresting progressive renal disease associated with systemic hypertension in the rat. *J Clin Invest.* 1986;77:1993–2000.
43. Brenner BM, Garcia DL, Anderson S. Glomeruli and blood pressure. Less of one, more the other? *Am J Hypertens.* 1988;1:335–347.
44. Zandi-Nejad K, Luyckx VA, Brenner BM. Adult hypertension and kidney disease: the role of fetal programming. *Hypertension.* 2006;47:502–508.
45. Li S, Chen SC, Shlipak M, et al. Low birth weight is associated with chronic kidney disease only in men. *Kidney Int.* 2008;73:637–642.
46. Lackland DT, Bendall HE, Osmond C, et al. Low birth weights contribute to high rates of early-onset chronic renal failure in the Southeastern United States. *Arch Intern Med.* 2000;160:1472–1476.
47. Vikse BE, Irgens LM, Leivestad T, et al. Low birth weight increases risk for end-stage renal disease. *J Am Soc Nephrol.* 2008;19:151–157.
48. White SL, Perkovic V, Cass A, et al. Is low birth weight an antecedent of CKD in later life? A systematic review of observational studies. *Am J Kidney Dis.* 2009;54:248–261.
49. Cassidy-Bushrow AE, Wegienka G, Barone CJ, et al. Race-specific relationship of birth weight and renal function among healthy young children. *Pediatr Nephrol.* 2012;27:1317–1323.
50. Lopez-Bermejo A, Sitjar C, Cabacas A, et al. Prenatal programming of renal function: the estimated glomerular filtration rate is influenced by size at birth in apparently healthy children. *Pediatr Res.* 2008;64:97–99.
51. Keller G, Zimmer G, Mall G, et al. Nephron number in patients with primary hypertension. *N Engl J Med.* 2003;348:101–108.
52. Hughson MD, Douglas-Denton R, Bertram JF, Hoy WE. Hypertension, glomerular number, and birth weight in African Americans and white subjects in the southeastern United States. *Kidney Int.* 2006;69:671–678.
53. Hales CN, Barker DJ. The thrifty phenotype hypothesis. *Br Med Bull.* 2001;60:5–20.
54. Simeoni U, Ligi I, Buffat C, Boubred F. Adverse consequences of accelerated neonatal growth: cardiovascular and renal issues. *Pediatr Nephrol.* 2011;26:493–508.
55. Forsen T, Eriksson J, Tuomilehto J, et al. The fetal and childhood growth of persons who develop type 2 diabetes. *Ann Intern Med.* 2000;133:176–182.
56. Hales CN, Barker DJ. Type 2 (non-insulin-dependent) diabetes mellitus: the thrifty phenotype hypothesis. *Diabetologia.* 1992;35:595–601.
57. Habib S, Zhang Q, Baum M. Prenatal programming of hypertension in the rat: effect of postnatal rearing. *Nephron Extra.* 2011;1:157–165.

58. Alexander BT. Placental insufficiency leads to development of hypertension in growth-restricted offspring. *Hypertension*. 2003;41:457–462.
59. Somm E, Vauthay DM, Guerardel A, et al. Early metabolic defects in dexamethasone-exposed and undernourished intrauterine growth restricted rats. *PLoS ONE*. 2012;7:e50131.
60. Vehaskari VM, Aviles DH, Manning J. Prenatal programming of adult hypertension in the rat. *Kidney Int*. 2001;59:238–245.
61. Woods LL, Weeks DA. Prenatal programming of adult blood pressure: role of maternal corticosteroids. *Am J Physiol Regul Integr Comp Physiol*. 2005;289:R955–R962.
62. Woods LL, Weeks DA, Rasch R. Programming of adult blood pressure by maternal protein restriction: role of nephrogenesis. *Kidney Int*. 2004;65:1339–1348.
63. Langley-Evans SC, Welham SJ, Jackson AA. Fetal exposure to a maternal low protein diet impairs nephrogenesis and promotes hypertension in the rat. *Life Sci*. 1999;64:965–974.
64. Habib S, Gattineni J, Twombley K, Baum M. Evidence that prenatal programming of hypertension by dietary protein deprivation is mediated by fetal glucocorticoid exposure. *Am J Hypertens*. 2011;24:96–101.
65. Wlodek ME, Westcott K, Siebel AL, et al. Growth restriction before or after birth reduces nephron number and increases blood pressure in male rats. *Kidney Int*. 2008;74:187–195.
66. Celsi G, Kistner A, Aizman R, et al. Prenatal dexamethasone causes oligonephronia, sodium retention, and higher blood pressure in the offspring. *Pediatr Res*. 1998;44:317–322.
67. Ortiz LA, Quan A, Weinberg A, Baum M. Effect of prenatal dexamethasone on rat renal development. *Kidney Int*. 2001;59:1663–1669.
68. Ortiz LA, Quan A, Zarzar F, et al. Prenatal dexamethasone programs hypertension and renal injury in the rat. *Hypertension*. 2003;41:328–334.
69. Wlodek ME, Mibus A, Tan A, et al. Normal lactational environment restores nephron endowment and prevents hypertension after placental restriction in the rat. *J Am Soc Nephrol*. 2007;18:1688–1696.
70. Moritz KM, Mazzuca MQ, Siebel AL, et al. Uteroplacental insufficiency causes a nephron deficit, modest renal insufficiency but no hypertension with ageing in female rats. *J Physiol*. 2009;587:2635–2646.
71. Hoppe CC, Evans RG, Bertram JF, Moritz KM. Effects of dietary protein restriction on nephron number in the mouse. *Am J Physiol Regul Integr Comp Physiol*. 2007;292:R1768–R1774.
72. Black MJ, Briscoe TA, Constantinou M, et al. Is there an association between level of adult blood pressure and nephron number or renal filtration surface area? *Kidney Int*. 2004;65:582–588.
73. Woods LL, Ingelfinger JR, Nyengaard JR, Rasch R. Maternal protein restriction suppresses the newborn renin-angiotensin system and programs adult hypertension in rats. *Pediatr Res*. 2001;49:460–467.
74. Regina S, Lucas R, Miraglia SM, et al. Intrauterine food restriction as a determinant of nephrosclerosis. *Am J Kidney Dis*. 2001;37:467–476.
75. Lozano G, Elmaghrabi A, Salley J, et al. Effect of prenatal programming and postnatal rearing on glomerular filtration rate in adult rats. *Am J Physiol Renal Physiol*. 2015;308:F411–F419.
76. Moritz KM, Cuffe JS, Wilson LB, et al. Review: sex specific programming: a critical role for the renal renin-angiotensin system. *Placenta*. 2010;31(suppl):S40–S46.
77. Manning J, Beutler K, Knepper MA, Vehaskari VM. Upregulation of renal BSC1 and TSC in prenatally programmed hypertension. *Am J Physiol Renal Physiol*. 2002;283:F202–F206.
78. Dagan A, Gattineni J, Cook V, Baum M. Prenatal programming of rat proximal tubule Na+/H+ exchanger by dexamethasone. *Am J Physiol Regul Integr Comp Physiol*. 2007;292:R1230–R1235.
79. Dagan A, Habbib S, Gattineni J, et al. Prenatal programming of rat thick ascending limb chloride transport by low protein diet and dexamethasone. *Am J Physiol Regul Integr Comp Physiol*. 2009;297:R93–R99.
80. Cheng CJ, Lozano G, Baum M. Prenatal programming of rat cortical collecting tubule sodium transport. *Am J Physiol Renal Physiol*. 2012;302:F674–F678.
81. Alexander BT, Hendon AE, Ferril G, Dwyer TM. Renal denervation abolishes hypertension in low-birth-weight offspring from pregnant rats with reduced uterine perfusion. *Hypertension*. 2005;45:754–758.
82. Dagan A, Kwon HM, Dwarakanath V, Baum M. Effect of renal denervation on prenatal programming of hypertension and renal tubular transporter abundance. *Am J Physiol Renal Physiol*. 2008;295:F29–F34.
83. Mizuno M, Siddique K, Baum M, Smith SA. Prenatal programming of hypertension induces sympathetic overactivity in response to physical stress. *Hypertension*. 2013;61:180–186.
84. Mizuno M, Lozano G, Siddique K, et al. Enalapril attenuates the exaggerated sympathetic response to physical stress in prenatally programmed hypertensive rats. *Hypertension*. 2014;63:324–329.
85. Vehaskari VM, Woods LL. Prenatal programming of hypertension: lessons from experimental models. *J Am Soc Nephrol*. 2005;16:2545–2556.
86. Baum M. Role of the kidney in the prenatal and early postnatal programming of hypertension. *Am J Physiol Renal Physiol*. 2010;298:F235–F247.
87. Alexander BT. Fetal programming of hypertension. *Am J Physiol Regul Integr Comp Physiol*. 2006;290:R1–R10.
88. Ingelfinger JR, Woods LL. Perinatal programming, renal development, and adult renal function. *Am J Hypertens*. 2002;15:46S–49S.
89. Rasch R, Skriver E, Woods LL. The role of the RAS in programming of adult hypertension. *Acta Physiol Scand*. 2004;181:537–542.
90. Barker DJP, Osmond C, Forsen TJ, et al. Trajectories of growth among children who have coronary events as adults. *N Engl J Med*. 2005;353:1802–1809.

91. Boubred F, Buffat C, Feuerstein JM, et al. Effects of early postnatal hypernutrition on nephron number and long-term renal function and structure in rats. *Am J Physiol Renal Physiol.* 2007;293:F1944–F1949.

92. Boubred F, Daniel L, Buffat C, et al. Early postnatal overfeeding induces early chronic renal dysfunction in adult male rats. *Am J Physiol Renal Physiol.* 2009;297:F943–F951.

93. Wyrwoll CS, Mark PJ, Mori TA, et al. Prevention of programmed hyperleptinemia and hypertension by postnatal dietary omega-3 fatty acids. *Endocrinology.* 2006;147:599–606.

94. Sherman RC, Langley-Evans SC. Early administration of angiotensin-converting enzyme inhibitor captopril, prevents the development of hypertension programmed by intrauterine exposure to a maternal low-protein diet in the rat. *Clin Sci.* 1998;94:373–381.

95. Manning J, Vehaskari VM. Postnatal modulation of prenatally programmed hypertension by dietary Na and ACE inhibition. *Am J Physiol Regul Integr Comp Physiol.* 2005;288:R80–R84.

96. Mansuri A, Elmaghrabi A, Legan SK, et al. Transient Exposure of Enalapril Normalizes Prenatal Programming of Hypertension and Urinary Angiotensinogen Excretion. *PLoS ONE.* 2015;10:e0146183.

97. de Jong F, Monuteaux MC, van Elburg RM, et al. Systematic review and meta-analysis of preterm birth and later systolic blood pressure. *Hypertension.* 2012;59:226–234.

98. Hovi P, Andersson S, Raikkonen K, et al. Ambulatory blood pressure in young adults with very low birth weight. *J Pediatr.* 2010;156:54–59.

99. Kajantie E, Hovi P. Is very preterm birth a risk factor for adult cardiometabolic disease? *Semin Fetal Neonatal Med.* 2014;19:112–117.

100. Rodriguez MM, Gomez AH, Abitbol CL, et al. Histomorphometric analysis of postnatal glomerulogenesis in extremely preterm infants. *Pediatr Dev Pathol.* 2004;7:17–25.

101. Hodgin JB, Rasoulpour M, Markowitz GS, D'Agati VD. Very low birth weight is a risk factor for secondary focal segmental glomerulosclerosis. *Clin J Am Soc Nephrol.* 2009;4:71–76.

CHAPTER 10

Fluid and Electrolyte Management of High-Risk Infants

Jeffrey Segar, MD

- **Changes in Body Water in the Fetus and Newborn**
- **Fetal Water Balance**
- **Newborn Water Balance**
- **Insensible Water Loss**
- **Fetal Sodium Balance**
- **Neonatal Sodium Balance**
- **Aldosterone**
- **Atrial Natriuretic Peptide**
- **Renin-Angiotensin System**
- **Principles of Fluid and Electrolyte Therapy**
- **Calculations of Fluid Requirement**
- **Calculations of Electrolyte Requirements**

Changes in Body Water in the Fetus and Newborn

Fetal Water Balance

Water is the major component of cells and tissues and "is the basis for the physical and chemical conditions of life."[1] Within the body, water is distributed into two major compartments, intracellular water (ICW) and extracellular water (ECW). ECW is further divided into the plasma water (intravascular water) and interstitial water.[2,3] The total amount of body water, as well as the distribution within the two major compartments, is developmentally regulated. During the first few months of fetal development, total body water (TBW) comprises over 90% of total body weight. By 6 months of gestation, TBW has decreased to approximately 86% and by term is approximately 76% of the body weight.[2] During the last trimester, distribution of body water also changes; ECW decreases from 54% to 44% of body weight while ICW increases from 27% to 34% (Fig. 10.1).

Fluid balance in the fetus is dependent upon the movement of water from the maternal circulation across the placenta, primarily at the level of the syncytiotrophoblast.[4,5] This water flow increases with advancing gestation to meet increasing fetal water needs for sustaining fetal cell growth and plasma volume, as well as amniotic fluid volume. Osmotic and hydrostatic forces promote placental water flow, although the contribution of each of these mechanisms during normal pregnancy is not known.[6] Transcellular flow of solute-free water involves a family of cell membrane water channel proteins named aquaporins (AQPs), many of which appear to be developmentally regulated.[7] Water exchange between the placenta, fetus, and amniotic fluid is poorly understood, although intramembranous flow across the amnion to the fetal circulation is important.[8]

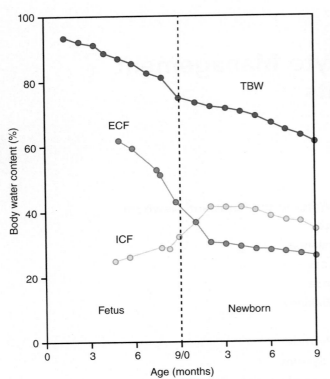

Fig. 10.1 Total body water *(TBW)* content and fluid distribution between extracellular fluid *(ECF)* and intracellular fluid *(ICF)* compartments during fetal and postnatal life. (Data modified from Friis-Hansen B. Body water compartments in children: changes during growth and selected changes in body composition. *Pediatrics.* 1961; 28:169-181.)

In humans the fetal metanephric kidney develops and begins to produce urine by 8 to 10 weeks of gestation.[9] Fetal urine is the primary contributor to amniotic fluid volume during the last half of gestation. It has been estimated that in the healthy fetus, urine flow rate increases 10-fold, from 0.1 mL/min at 20 weeks to 1 mL/min at 40 weeks' gestation.[10,11] Fetal urine is typically hypotonic with respect to fetal plasma, the range of osmolality being 100 to 250 mOsm/kg H_2O. Although capable of producing diluted urine, the concentrating capacity of the fetal kidney is limited. Decreased sensitivity to arginine vasopressin (AVP), structural immaturity of the kidney, as well as the distribution of blood flow within the kidney likely contribute to this inability to concentrate urine.[12]

Newborn Water Balance

Maintaining water and sodium balance following birth poses a unique challenge because the kidney is relatively immature, lacking fully functional regulatory systems. The ability to concentrate urine develops progressively during postnatal life.[13,14] The term neonate can maximally concentrate urine to approximately half that of the older child or adult. Maturation of concentrating abilities occurs over the first 2 years of life, with urine osmolality exceeding 600 mOsm/L within a week of life, greater than 1000 mOsm/L by 1 month of age, and reaching adult values of 1300 to 1400 mOsm/L by 2 years of age.[15] This limited concentrating ability of the infant kidney is of little importance unless the infant is provided formula with a high solute load, as occurred with some milk-based formulas in the 1950s to 1960s,[16] in the presence of excessive water loss from diarrhea and/or fever or if intake is insufficient to cover obligatory water loss (e.g., insensible water loss, IWL). The preterm infant has a greater impairment of urine concentrating ability than the term infant likely related to a variety of functional and anatomic factors, although functional maturation progresses at a greater rate ex utero than in utero.

Infants born prematurely have higher TBW and ECW per kilogram than do term infants, whereas small-for-gestational-age infants have higher TBW and ECW than appropriate-for-gestational-age infants.[17] After birth, TBW content continues to fall, primarily due to contraction of the extracellular space.[18] The degree of contraction of the ECW compartment is inversely proportional to gestational age and greater in small-for-gestational-age than appropriate-for-gestational-age infants. Preterm infants may exhibit a 10% to 15% weight loss during the first week of life related to loss of ECW, whereas term infants generally exhibit a 5% to 7% weight loss.[19–22] Failure to allow the normal postnatal contraction in ECW and weight loss in preterm infants may increase the risk of patent ductus arteriosus, necrotizing enterocolitis, and bronchopulmonary dysplasia.[23–27] However, the optimal amount of weight loss is not known. ICW increases, decreases, or remains unchanged immediately after birth, although ICW increases approximately in proportion to body weight in the first few weeks of postnatal life. ICW continues to increase as a percent of body weight until exceeding that of ECW by 3 months of life.

Newborn water loss may occur by sensible (urine and stool) and insensible (evaporation from skin and with respiration) mechanisms. Urine production is necessitated by the need to excrete soluble waste products. The amount of urine produced is therefore governed by the renal solute load, comprised primarily of nitrogenous compounds and electrolytes, as well as the ability of the kidney to concentrate urine.[12,28] Urine water loss is primarily regulated by water channels, or AQPs, which allow transcellular water reabsorption along the nephron segment.[29,30] The majority of water from glomerular ultrafiltrate is reabsorbed in the proximal nephron via AQP1.[31] Further refinement of water absorption and urinary concentrating ability is regulated by AQP2, located on collecting duct principal cells. AQP2 is the primary target for AVP, an antidiuretic hormone produced by the posterior pituitary gland in response to activation of osmoreceptors in the hypothalamus or baroreceptors in selected vasculature. The ontogenic pattern of AQP2 in the kidney parallels the development of AVP responsiveness and urinary-concentrating ability.[32] The limited ability of the newborn kidney to concentrate urine in the presence of elevated AVP levels likely reflects the decreased number of AVP receptors or decreased responsiveness of downstream mechanisms following vasopressin receptor activation. The lack of concentration ability of the immature kidney results in higher obligate water losses and may predispose to hypertonic dehydration.

Insensible Water Loss

In addition to the production of urine, obligate water losses result from evaporation from the respiratory tract and the skin. Approximately 30% of IWL occurs through the respiratory tract, although respiratory losses are decreased by approximately ⅓ in intubated infants receiving humidified gas compared with breathing room air.[33–35] Insensible water loss from the skin is inversely proportional to birth weight and gestational age, a function of the increased ratio of surface area to body weight, as well as thinner skin and greater skin blood flow.[36,37] Transepidermal water loss of a 24-week appropriate-for-gestational-age infant is 10 to 15 times greater than that of a term neonate on the first day of life.[38] As gestational age and postnatal age increase, transepidermal water loss decreases, although it remains elevated on a per kilogram basis in premature compared with term infants, even beyond a month of age.

Numerous factors affect insensible skin water loss in the neonate.[39] Elevated environmental and body temperatures increase water loss in proportion to the increase in temperature. Exposure to nonionizing radiant energy, such as that originating from radiant warmers or phototherapy, may increase IWL by approximately 50%. Increased motor activity and crying may also significantly increase IWL. Alternatively, use of plastic heat shields or blankets, semipermeable membranes, and high ambient or inspired humidity reduce IWL by at least 30%.

Fetal Sodium Balance

The fetus experiences an intake (net transplacental transfer) of sodium that greatly exceeds that of the newborn. Using a sodium tracer method, sodium transfer across the human placenta has been estimated to be approximately 130 mEq/day at term.[40] Although a certain amount of water and sodium is retained by the fetus for growth, the healthy fetus excretes a large amount of sodium because renal mechanisms to retain sodium are relatively immature.[41–43] Urinary excretion of sodium ($U_{Na}V$), and $U_{Na}V$ normalized to glomerular filtration rate (GFR) and expressed as fractional excretion of sodium (FE_{Na}), is greater in the fetus than the newborn. In fact, FE_{Na} is greater in the fetal sheep at 0.75 gestation (14%–15%) than 0.9 gestation (11%) or near term (5%, 145 days), suggesting developmental changes in renal tubular sodium transport occurs in utero.[44]

Limited data regarding human fetal renal function are available, although they provide important insight into maturational changes in renal sodium metabolism. Analysis of fetal urine obtained from infants diagnosed prenatally with obstructive uropathy demonstrated that urine sodium concentration decreases whereas creatinine increases as gestational age advances between 20 and 38 weeks.[45] Urine sodium concentrations ranged from 60 to 65 mmol/L before 25 weeks' gestation to 40 to 50 mmol/L near term. In contrast, protein and phosphorus concentrations are low and remain unchanged over this period of time. Similar developmental changes in urine sodium concentration were reported from fetuses whose urine was obtained prior to elective termination or red blood cell transfusion for Rh isoimmunization.[46] Along with a decreasing urine sodium concentration, the fractional excretion of sodium similarly decreases during the second half of gestation.[47]

Neonatal Sodium Balance

Following birth, significant changes in renal sodium handling occur, the extent of which is dependent upon gestational age as well as postnatal age. Studies in term fetal sheep delivered by cesarean section demonstrate $U_{Na}V$ and FE_{Na} are initially maintained at fetal levels, although they rapidly decrease during the first few hours of postnatal life.[48] This rapid increase in renal tubular absorption was associated with increased GFR but not aldosterone levels.

In term infants, FE_{Na} decreases from 3.4% to 1.5% in the first few hours of life and continues to decrease to adult values (<1%) over subsequent days.[49] Several studies have shown in preterm infants that FE_{Na} and $U_{Na}V$ are inversely associated with gestational age at birth and postnatal age (Fig. 10.2).[50–52] Siegel and Oh found

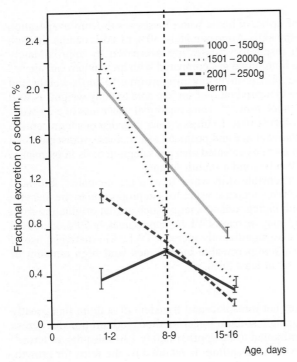

Fig. 10.2 Fractional excretion of sodium during the first weeks of life. (Reprinted by permission from Macmillan Publishers Ltd: *Pediatr Res.* 1994;36:572-577 copyright [1994].)

the magnitude of urinary sodium excretion decreased from approximately 200 μEq/ kg per hour in infants at 27 weeks' gestation to less than 25 μEq/kg per hour at term.[51] In addition, Gubhaju and coworkers reported FE_{Na} exceeded 6% in infants less than 28 weeks' gestation on day of life 3, decreasing to approximately 4% by the end of the first week of life and 2% at a month of age.[52] Less premature infants (29–36 weeks' gestation at birth) had lower FE_{Na} at 3 days of age and showed a similar maturational decrease in FE_{Na} over the first month of life. By 28 days of life, there was no statistically significant difference in FE_{Na} among the gestation age groups, although infants born at less than 28 weeks' gestation appeared to have an FE_{Na} twice that of older infants.

Term infants have a diminished ability to excrete a sodium load compared with adults, as a result of the inability of the newborn to increase GFR to the similar extent as an adult.[53] In term infants provided an oral sodium load, the urinary sodium excretion rate is only approximately 10% of that found in older children.[54] Preterm infants demonstrate a greater ability to excrete a sodium load compared with term infants because a lower percentage of the sodium load presented to the distal tubule is reabsorbed in preterm infants than in term infants.[55]

Multiple factors likely contribute to the changes in renal sodium excretion with development, including but not limited to a redistribution of renal blood flow, increased oxygen availability, increased proximal tubular length, increased expression and activity of the basolateral sodium-potassium ATPase and luminal membrane sodium-hydrogen exchanger, and response to hormones.[56,57] Relative to the newborn, the fetus displays a state of high renal vascular resistance.[48] In the first day after birth, there is little change in total renal blood flow or renal vascular resistance, although GFR increases significantly as a result of the redistribution of intrarenal blood flow in favor of outer cortical nephrons.[48] The rise in arterial oxygen content and renal oxygen delivery, with an associated increase in available renal energy, likely enhances the ability of the newborn kidney to reabsorb sodium. Oxygen delivered to the newborn sheep kidney is five to seven times that to the fetal kidney, and there is a positive relationship between the quantities of sodium reabsorbed and renal oxygen delivery and consumption. In fetal sheep, in utero ventilation, which increased fetal arterial pO_2 values from 18 to 86 mm Hg, decreased urine flow rate and FE_{Na} without changes in atrial natriuretic peptide (ANP), vasopressin, angiotensin II, or GFR.[58]

Aldosterone

Aldosterone, a potent mineralocorticoid produced by the adrenal cortex, increases sodium reabsorption in the distal collecting duct system by activating a number of sodium cotransporters, including ENaC and Na^+,K^+-ATPase.[59,60] Following birth, there is increasing renal responsiveness to aldosterone, likely related to developmental changes in mineralocorticoid receptor expression, downstream effector mechanisms, and activity of the Na^+,K^+-ATPase.[61] Preterm infants, and to a lesser degree term newborn infants, have a variable degree of aldosterone resistance, as evidenced by their large urinary sodium losses despite high levels of aldosterone.[62] Plasma aldosterone levels at birth increase significantly with gestational age, although levels in preterm infants (<33 weeks' gestation) are still significantly higher than those in adults.[62]

Atrial Natriuretic Peptide

ANP, synthesized primarily within the cardiac atria and released in response to stretch, is detectable in the fetus and newborn, with circulating levels increasing throughout gestation to levels significantly higher than found in the mother.[63,64] Plasma ANP levels are higher in premature infants than in term neonates, with peak levels 48 to 72 hours after birth, coinciding with the timing of peak postnatal diuresis, postnatal weight loss, and contraction of the extracellular space.[65] It is likely that the increase in pulmonary blood flow and resultant left atrial stretch as blood fills the left side of the heart contributes to the elevation in ANP immediately after birth.

Renal effects of ANP are blunted in the fetus and newborn compared with the adult.[66,67] In a number of systems, ANP has been shown to induce natriuresis by increasing GFR, glomerular permeability, and thus filtration fraction, inhibiting the proximal tubule Na/H exchanger, Na^+,K^+-ATPase, the type II Na-Pi cotransporter, and distal tubule NKCC2 activity.[68] Whether the blunted renal response to ANP early in life is related to developmental differences in any of these mechanisms is not known.

Renin-Angiotensin System

In the adult, angiotensin II mediates control of sodium tubular transport directly by activating luminal and basolateral Na transport mechanisms in the proximal tubule and indirectly through stimulation of aldosterone release.[69] However, there is little evidence of angiotensin II being functional in fetal or newborn renal tubules. Rather, the effects of angiotensin II on sodium excretion in the fetus are primarily related to the stimulation of aldosterone production and effects on renal blood flow and GFR.[70,71]

Principles of Fluid and Electrolyte Therapy

Calculations of Fluid Requirement

Water is life's matter and matrix, mother and medium. There is no life without water.

—Albert Szent-Gyorgi (Nobel Laureate 1937)

The provision of water is the most basic concept in sustaining life. Although hundreds of thousands of infants receive parenteral fluids each year, studies to guide the clinicians approach are limited. Recent Cochrane reviews highlight that, although more than 4000 infants were involved in more than 20 trials of antenatal steroids to decrease the incidence of respiratory distress syndrome, fewer than 600 preterm infants have been involved in a total of five randomized controlled trials of restricted versus liberal water intake for preventing morbidity and mortality.[23,72]

To determine daily maintenance water requirements, one must consider IWL, urine volume, fecal water loss, metabolically derived water, and water retained for growth. For practical purposes, stool water need not be included in calculations of initial fluid needs because stool water losses are minimal in the first few days of life. Water produced by oxidation is approximately 5 to 10 mL/kg per day and is ignored in fluid calculations because it essentially offsets fecal losses.[73] Water necessary for growth is approximately 10 to 15 mL/kg per day, assuming a weight gain of 10 to 20 mL/kg per day and 60% to 70% of cellular growth is water. However, in the first week of life, during which time there is a physiologic weight loss and minimal somatic growth, the calculation of maintenance fluid is based primarily on IWL and urine water loss.

The volume of water needed in the first few days of life is that which is necessary to avoid hypernatremia but also allows for the contraction of the extracellular space and physiologic weight loss. For the term infant under basal conditions, respiratory water loss is approximately 7 to 10 mL/kg per day and evaporative water loss is 10 to 30 mL/kg depending upon environmental conditions. Thus total IWL is approximately 20 to 40 mL/kg per day, and urine output also averages approximately 5 to 10 mL/kg per day for the first few days of life.[74,75] The breastfed term infant loses on average 1% to 2% of his or her birth weight daily for the first few days of life, with a target weight loss of 7% to 10% of birth weight. Because 60% to 80% of this weight loss is likely extracellular fluid, a mild increase in extracellular sodium concentration develops. Although increased, serum sodium values remain in the "normal" range because newborns are often mildly hyponatremic at birth.[61] However, excessive weight loss resulting from limited enteral intake, IWL and ongoing urine output increases the risk for development of dehydration and clinical hypernatremia. With hypernatremic dehydration, the extracellular fluid compartment becomes relatively less contracted than the intracellular compartment, making diagnosis on clinical evaluation more difficulty.

Moritz and coworkers reported up to 2% of neonatal hospital admissions of infants ≥35 weeks' gestation are for breastfeeding-associated hypernatremic dehydration (serum sodium concentration ≥150 mEq/L), the vast majority of cases associated with primiparous mothers.[76] Despite education and support from a lactation consultant, 16% of exclusively breastfed infants born to primiparous woman had greater than 10% weight loss by day 3 of life. Providers need to be aware of breastfeeding-associated hypernatremia and increased risk for hyperbilirubinemia and provide follow-up monitoring of those infants most at risk. Although there is a reluctance to provide supplemental formula to breastfed infants with insufficient lactation, judicious use of supplementation has been demonstrated to decrease the incidence of excessive weight loss (>10%).[77,78] Although additional studies are needed to best identify infants at risk for breastfeeding-associated hypernatremia, consideration of supplemental feeds to breastfed infants may be given for greater than 7% to 8% weight loss.

Term infants receiving intravenous fluids soon after birth are typically provided sufficient water to replace IWL plus urine output. Initially, 50 to 60 mL/kg per day of fluid, often provided as 10% dextrose in water, is sufficient to meet these needs. With the provision of enteral or parenteral nutritional, which increases the renal solute load, fluid requirements increase. After the first few days of life, a need for water for growth (deposition in to new tissues) also exists. For example, a 3.5-kg infant receiving parenteral nutrition that provides 3.5 g protein/kg, 3 mEq NaCl/kg, 2 mEq KCl/kg, and 1 mEq NaPO$_4$/kg needs to excrete a potential renal solute load of 112 mOsm (70 mOsm urea [1 g protein = 5.7 mOsm urea], 14 mOsm Na$^+$, 7 Osm K$^+$, 17.5 mOsm Cl$^-$, 3.5 mOsm PO$_4^{-3}$). Assuming a urine concentration of 300 mOsm/L, approximately 375 mL of urinary water is necessary. When 15 mL/kg are provided for growth and 30 mL/kg per day for IWL, approximately 375 + 52 + 105 = 532 mL, or 150 mL/kg per day, of water intake is necessary. Stool water loss and metabolically derived water are excluded from this calculation because they essentially offset each other.

The development of parenteral fluid therapy for preterm infants in the 1960s was a major turning point for the care of this population and generated several randomized and nonrandomized trials of early parenteral therapy versus no fluids for 24 to 72 hours. Meta-analysis of these trials showed a lower death rate in fluid-treated infants, with a relative risk of death of approximately 0.8, although the difference did not reach statistical significance.[79] Premature infants have larger maintenance water requirements than term infants because of increased IWL, as discussed previously. Most often these fluids are provided by the parenteral route. The IWL replacement component of maintenance water should be increased with decreasing birth weight or gestation age and decreased with advancing postnatal age (Table 10.1). However, careful attention to the prevention of excessive IWL is as important as the replacement of increased IWL. These efforts include maintenance environmental temperature in the thermoneutral zone and use of plastic shields/chambers/barriers and semipermeable membranes.

A number of small clinical trials provide some guidance regarding the amount of water to provide this population. Bell and coworkers randomized infants with birth weights 750 to 2000 g to "high" or "low" maintenance fluid therapy beginning on

Table 10.1 ESTIMATED DAILY INSENSIBLE WATER LOSS OVER FIRST 48 HOURS OF LIFE IN PRETERM INFANTS OF DIFFERING BIRTH WEIGHTS CARED FOR UNDER RADIANT WARMERS OR IN INCUBATORS[39]

Birth Weight (g)	Insensible Water Loss (mL/kg per day)	
	Radiant Warmer	Incubator
<750	125–200	100–150
750–1000	100–150	75–100
1000–1500	75–100	50
1500–2000	50	25–50
>2000	40	25–40

day of life 3 and continuing until day of life 30.[25] The upper limits of intake for each group were constructed by considering (1) urine volume necessary to excrete a solute load allowing urine concentration to be 200 to 250 mOsm/L; (2) insensible water loss; and (3) water for growth. Infants in the "high" group were provided at least 20 mL/kg per day of fluid greater than the upper limit of the "low" volume group. During the study period, average fluid intake in the high group averaged 169 mL/kg per day and in the low group 122 mL/kg. Rates of patent ductus arteriosus were significantly lower in the "low" volume group. Lorenz and coworkers randomized infants with birth weights 750 to 1500 g to two different fluid management regimes distinguished by rate and extent of weight loss in the first 5 days of life.[20] No difference in clinical outcomes was seen between the groups, although the sample size was small and both groups demonstrated a significant decrease in weight from birth over the first 5 days of life. Of interest, the difference in weight loss was less than ⅕ the difference in fluid intake, indicating infant water balance was maintained by regulating water excretion. Thus variation in fluid intake that does not overwhelm the infant's capacity to remain within a range of negative water balance has little to no effect on clinical outcomes. In a Cochrane review, Bell and Acarregui found restricted water intake significantly reduced the risks of patent ductus arteriosus and necrotizing enterocolitis with nonsignificant trends toward reduced risks of bronchopulmonary dysplasia, intracranial hemorrhage, and death.[23] These authors concluded that the most prudent prescription for water intake to premature infants would seem to be careful restriction of water intake so that physiologic needs are met without allowing significant dehydration.

In a case-control study, Vuohelainen and coworkers found decreased free water clearance was associated with worse pulmonary outcomes.[80] Although cause and effect were not established, the findings emphasize the importance of individualized management of fluid intake. Finally, a post hoc multivariate logistic regression analysis of a parenteral glutamine supplementation trial of 1382 infants with birth weights 400 to 1000 g demonstrated higher fluid intake and lack of weight loss were significantly associated with death or bronchopulmonary dysplasia.[21]

It is difficult, if not inappropriate, to provide a "recipe" for the amount of fluid that should be provided to premature infants over the first few days of life, given large variations in gestational age, physiologic maturity of skin, and local practices with use or avoidance of radiant warmers, ambient humidity, etc. A short-term goal of therapy is the achievement of a daily weight loss of 2% to 3% of birth weight for the first 3 to 5 days of life, after which time weight loss should plateau. Early protein intake (≤2 g/kg per day) beginning on the first day of life may limit the degree of postnatal weight loss and shorten the time to regain birth weight.[81] Weight gain should begin to occur at the start of the second week of life. Any approach should consider estimated IWL and an allowance for urinary water of 1 to 2 mL/kg per hour or 25 to 50 mL/kg per day. Table 10.1 provides a range of IWL across a range of birth weights and environmental conditions. Based upon these values, the approach for initial provision of fluids at our institution, which uses radiant warmers, is provided in Table 10.2. The delivery of glucose is adjusted based upon serum glucose values. Careful attention is directed a serial determinations of serum sodium and chloride values, which provide assessment of TBW status. Hypernatremia is most frequently caused by intake of water insufficient to meet ongoing losses rather than excessive administration of sodium. Conversely, hyponatremia in the first few days of life frequently results from an excessive supply of water rather than deficient sodium intake. Urine output also needs to be monitored. Extremely premature infants (≤26 weeks' gestation) may demonstrate an inability to concentrate urine that results in obligate urine losses and ongoing urine production despite dehydration and decreasing intravascular volume.

Calculations of Electrolyte Requirements

After parturition, there is a significant contraction of the extracellular fluid compartment manifested by natriuresis and diuresis. In term infants, achievement of negative sodium balance during this time is enabled by obligate renal sodium losses and the

Table 10.2 RECOMMENDED INITIAL FLUID INTAKE ACCORDING TO GESTATIONAL AGE

GA (weeks)	Total Fluids (mL/kg per day)	Additional Fluid
≥34	60–70	$D_{10}W$
30–33	60–80	
29	80–90	$D_{10}W$
28	90–100	
27	100–120	
26	130–140	D_5W
25	140–150	
24	150	
22–23	175–200	$D_{2.5}W$

D_xW represents percent dextrose concentration in sterile water.
Total fluid intake consists of neonatal venous nutrition (NVN) fluid plus additional fluid outlined in Table 10.1. Initial NVN: (D10, 5% amino acids, AA) for infants <30 weeks' gestational age, GA.
22–26 6/7 weeks' gestation receive 30 to 60 mL/kg per day (1.5 g/kg per day protein, glucose rate of 2.1 mg/kg per minute) NVN plus additional fluid.
27–29 weeks' gestation receive 60 mL/kg per day (3 g/kg per day AA, glucose rate of 4.2 mg/kg per minute) NVN plus additional fluid.

limited intake of breast milk coupled with the low sodium content of breast milk.[82,83] For term infants requiring parenteral fluid therapy, initial therapy should, with few exceptions, consist of dextrose containing fluids devoid of electrolytes.

In contrast to term infants, electrolyte intake of preterm infants is most often determined by medical providers. Although the fluid requirements of these infants are higher than those of term infants, related primarily to increased IWL, there remains little reason to provide sodium in the first 24 to 48 hours of life and the use of electrolyte-free nutritional solutions is recommended. Delaying sodium supplementation allows for the physiologic loss of body water that is part of normal postnatal adaptation. In a trial involving preterm infants of 25 to 30 weeks' gestation age, delaying sodium supplementation until a weight loss of 6% of birth weight compared with initiating sodium administration of 4 mmol/k per day on the second day of life resulted in a significantly greater percentage of infants on room air at 7 days of life without changes in time to regain birth weight and weight at 36 weeks and 6 months of postmenstrual age.[84] Avoidance of sodium may be difficult because many centers administer sodium acetate solutions through umbilical arterial catheters to (1) avoid extreme hypotonic fluids and (2) to provide a base to compensate mild respiratory acidosis resulting from hypercapnia secondary to gentler ventilation.

Beyond the immediate postnatal period, preterm infants have higher sodium requirements (mEq/kg) than term infants and older children, primarily related to the inability of the preterm kidney to retain salt.[52,85] The decision regarding the timing and the quantity of sodium supplementation for preterm infants differs among practitioners. Many sources recommend a sodium intake of 3 to 5 mEq/kg per day for preterm infants beyond the first week of life, although agreement is not universal.[86] The decision to provide supplemental sodium to preterm infants beyond that found in milk or formula is often based on the serum sodium concentration, although there is little uniformity in this approach. Furthermore, there is limited physiologic basis for this practice, given the poor relationship between serum sodium concentration and body sodium content.[87–89] The issue of sodium supplementation becomes more relevant when one recognizes the significant impact of total body sodium status on somatic growth. In young, growing rats, feeding a sodium-deficient diet impairs weight and length growth, diminishes nitrogen retention, and decreases muscle protein synthesis and RNA concentrations.[90] Salt supplementation to sodium-depleted animals restored normal rates of weight and length growth and protein synthesis.[91] Sodium deficiency reduces the compensatory growth on the contralateral lung following pneumonectomy in young rats.[92] Taken together, these findings raise the question of

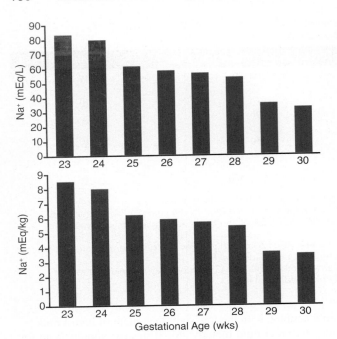

Fig. 10.3 Estimated urine sodium concentrations *(top)* and daily urine sodium losses *(bottom)* in sodium-replete preterm infants of various gestational ages at 2 weeks of postnatal age. Values based upon calculations by author using data provided in the literature.[52,93]

whether salt restriction and use of diuretics in preterm infants with chronic lung disease may in fact impede tissue reparative processes.

The preterm infant displays an obligate urine sodium loss that may result in a negative sodium balance even when recommended levels of sodium are provided. Using published data of renal hemodynamics and function in preterm infants, we have calculated expected urinary sodium losses in preterm infants with advancing postnatal age.[52,93] Assumptions were necessary regarding weight, length, urine volume, and serum sodium values at each time point. These data demonstrate that the preterm infant has urine sodium losses ranging from approximately 8 mEq/kg per day (23 weeks' gestation infant at 2 weeks postnatal age) to slightly less than 4 mEq/kg per day (Fig. 10.3). These calculations are in accord with data Siegel and Oh reported on a limited number of preterm infants ≥27 weeks' gestation.[51] Recognition of this degree of obligate sodium loss is important because currently recommended intakes of Na in preterm infants (3–5 mEq/kg per day) likely do not meet the needs for many preterm infants to ensure optimal growth and development.[86]

In human infants, improved weight gain has been demonstrated in infants given 3 to 5 mEq/kg per day sodium supplements administered from as early as the fourth day of life for as long as 5 weeks.[94,95] Isemann and coworkers reported that sodium supplementation to infants less than 32 weeks' gestation at a dose of 4 mEq/kg per day from days 7 to 35 of life enhanced weight gain (26.9 ± 3.1 vs. 22.9 ± 4.7 g/kg per day).[96] Importantly, 79% of patients in the supplemented group maintained their Fenton growth curve birth centile at 6 weeks of age compared with 13% in the nonsupplemented group. Salt supplementation to increase sodium intake in preterm infants (<33 weeks' gestation) to 4 to 5 mEq/kg per day compared with 1 to 1.5 mEq/kg per day for the 4th to 14th postnatal day resulted in improved neurodevelopmental outcome at 10 to 13 years of age.[97]

Hyperkalemia with or without oliguria is a common problem in extremely premature infants during the first week of life. This potentially dangerous condition likely results from immaturity of the Na⁺,K⁺-ATPase, allowing for a potassium shift from the intracellular to extracellular fluid space and potassium release from catabolized cells in the presence of immature distal renal tubular function.[98–100] Early caloric and amino acid intake appears to modify potassium metabolism and may reduce nonoliguric hyperkalemia.[101] Exposure to antenatal steroids appears protective against nonoliguric hyperkalemia during the first few days of life, despite decreasing potassium excretion.[102] Hyperkalemia is exacerbated if dehydration and oliguria occur as a result of inadequate water intake. Potassium administration should likely be avoided in premature infants until the serum potassium concentration falls to less than 4.5 to 5 mEq/L and urine output is established. If the serum potassium concentration exceeds 7 mEq/L, therapeutic measures to redistribute potassium within body water compartments (insulin plus glucose, albuterol administration) should be considered. Attempts at removal of potassium from the body, through the use of diuretics or ion exchange resins, present risk without well-proven benefit in the premature infant.

REFERENCES

1. Friis-Hansen B. Body water metabolism in early infancy. *Acta Paediatr Scand Suppl*. 1982;296:44–48.
2. Friis-Hansen B. Changes in body water compartments during growth. *Acta Paediatr Suppl*. 1957; 46(suppl 110):1–68.
3. Friis-Hansen B. Water distribution in the foetus and newborn infant. *Acta Paediatr Scand Suppl*. 1983;305:7–11.
4. Jansson T, Illsley NP. Osmotic water permeabilities of human placental microvillous and basal membranes. *J Membr Biol*. 1993;132(2):147–155.
5. Stulc J. Placental transfer of inorganic ions and water. *Physiol Rev*. 1997;77(3):805–836.
6. Beall MH, van den Wijngaard JP, van Gemert MJ, Ross MG. Regulation of amniotic fluid volume. *Placenta*. 2007;28(8–9):824–832.
7. Liu H, Zheng Z, Wintour EM. Aquaporins and fetal fluid balance. *Placenta*. 2008;29(10):840–847.
8. Brace RA, Cheung CY. Regulation of amniotic fluid volume: evolving concepts. *Adv Exp Med Biol*. 2014;814:49–68.
9. Matsell DG, Hiatt MJ. Functional development of the kidney in utero. In: Polin RA, Abman SH, Rowitch DH, et al, eds. *Fetal and Neonatal Physiology*. Vol. 2. 5th ed. Philadelphia, PA: Elsevier/ Saunders; 2017:965–976.
10. Hedriana HL. Ultrasound measurement of fetal urine flow. *Clin Obstet Gynecol*. 1997;40(2):337–351.
11. Lee SM, Park SK, Shim SS, et al. Measurement of fetal urine production by three-dimensional ultrasonography in normal pregnancy. *Ultrasound Obstet Gynecol*. 2007;30(3):281–286.
12. Iacobelli S, Guignard JP. Concentration and dilution of urine. In: Polin RA, Abman SH, Rowitch DH, et al, eds. *Fetal and Neonatal Physiology*. Vol. 2. 5th ed. Philadelphia, PA: Elsevier/Saunders; 2017:1046–1066.
13. Aperia A, Broberger O, Herin P, Zetterstrom R. Sodium excretion in relation to sodium intake and aldosterone excretion in newborn pre-term and full-term infants. *Acta Paediatr Scand*. 1979;68(6): 813–817.
14. Calcagno PL, Rubin MI, Weintraub DH. Studies on the renal concentrating and diluting mechanisms in the premature infant. *J Clin Invest*. 1954;33(1):91–96.
15. Polacek E, Vocel J, Neugebauerova L, et al. The osmotic concentrating ability in healthy infants and children. *Arch Dis Child*. 1965;40:291–295.
16. Fomon S. Infant feeding in the 20th century: formula and beikost. *J Nutr*. 2001;131(2):409S–420S.
17. Hartnoll G, Betremieux P, Modi N. Body water content of extremely preterm infants at birth. *Arch Dis Child Fetal Neonatal Ed*. 2000;83(1):F56–F59.
18. Shaffer SG, Bradt SK, Hall RT. Postnatal changes in total body water and extracellular volume in the preterm infant with respiratory distress syndrome. *J Pediatr*. 1986;109(3):509–514.
19. Hansen JD, Smith CA. Effects of withholding fluid in the immediate postnatal period. *Pediatrics*. 1953;12(2):99–113.
20. Lorenz JM, Kleinman LI, Kotagal UR, Reller MD. Water balance in very low-birth-weight infants: relationship to water and sodium intake and effect on outcome. *J Pediatr*. 1982;101(3):423–432.
21. Oh W, Poindexter BB, Perritt R, et al. Association between fluid intake and weight loss during the first ten days of life and risk of bronchopulmonary dysplasia in extremely low birth weight infants. *J Pediatr*. 2005;147(6):786–790.
22. Shaffer SG, Quimiro CL, Anderson JV, Hall RT. Postnatal weight changes in low birth weight infants. *Pediatrics*. 1987;79(5):702–705.
23. Bell EF, Acarregui MJ. Restricted versus liberal water intake for preventing morbidity and mortality in preterm infants. *Cochrane Database Syst Rev*. 2014;(12):CD000503.
24. Bell EF, Warburton D, Stonestreet BS, Oh W. High-volume fluid intake predisposes premature infants to necrotising enterocolitis. *Lancet*. 1979;2(8133):90.
25. Bell EF, Warburton D, Stonestreet BS, Oh W. Effect of fluid administration on the development of symptomatic patent ductus arteriosus and congestive heart failure in premature infants. *N Engl J Med*. 1980;302(11):598–604.
26. Van Marter LJ, Leviton A, Allred EN, et al. Hydration during the first days of life and the risk of bronchopulmonary dysplasia in low birth weight infants. *J Pediatr*. 1990;116(6):942–949.
27. Wadhawan R, Oh W, Perritt R, et al. Association between early postnatal weight loss and death or BPD in small and appropriate for gestational age extremely low-birth-weight infants. *J Perinatol*. 2007;27(6):359–364.
28. Fomon SJ, Ziegler EE. Renal solute load and potential renal solute load in infancy. *J Pediatr*. 1999;134(1):11–14.

10

29. King LS, Kozono D, Agre P. From structure to disease: the evolving tale of aquaporin biology. *Nat Rev Mol Cell Biol.* 2004;5(9):687–698.

30. Zelenina M, Zelenin S, Aperia A. Water channels (aquaporins) and their role for postnatal adaptation. *Pediatr Res.* 2005;57(5 Pt 2):47R–53R.

31. Holtback U, Aperia AC. Molecular determinants of sodium and water balance during early human development. *Semin Neonatol.* 2003;8(4):291–299.

32. Yasui M, Marples D, Belusa R, et al. Development of urinary concentrating capacity: role of aquaporin-2. *Am J Physiol.* 1996;271(2 Pt 2):F461–F468.

33. Hey EN, Katz G. Evaporative water loss in the new-born baby. *J Physiol.* 1969;200(3):605–619.

34. Riesenfeld T, Hammarlund K, Sedin G. Respiratory water loss in relation to gestational age in infants on their first day after birth. *Acta Paediatr.* 1995;84(9):1056–1059.

35. Sosulski R, Polin RA, Baumgart S. Respiratory water loss and heat balance in intubated infants receiving humidified air. *J Pediatr.* 1983;103(2):307–310.

36. Okken A, Jonxis JH, Rispens P, Zijlstra WG. Insensible water loss and metabolic rate in low birthweight newborn infants. *Pediatr Res.* 1979;13(9):1072–1075.

37. Wu PY, Hodgman JE. Insensible water loss in preterm infants: changes with postnatal development and non-ionizing radiant energy. *Pediatrics.* 1974;54(6):704–712.

38. Hammarlund K, Sedin G, Stromberg B. Transepidermal water loss in newborn infants. VIII. Relation to gestational age and post-natal age in appropriate and small for gestational age infants. *Acta Paediatr Scand.* 1983;72(5):721–728.

39. Bell EF, Segar JL, Oh W. Fluid and electrolyte management. In: MacDonald MG, Seshia MMK, eds. *Avery's Neonatology: Pathophysiology & Management of the Newborn.* 7th ed. Philadelphia, PA: Wolters Kluwer; 2016:265–279.

40. Cox LW, Chalmers TA. The transfer of sodium to the placental blood during the third stage of labour determined by Na24 tracer methods. *J Obstet Gynaecol Br Emp.* 1953;60(2):226–229.

41. Guyton AC, Cowley AW Jr, Young DB, et al. Integration and control of circulatory function. *Int Rev Physiol.* 1976;9:341–385.

42. Robillard JE, Nakamura KT, Matherne GP, Jose PA. Renal hemodynamics and functional adjustments to postnatal life. *Semin Perinatol.* 1988;12(2):143–150.

43. Rudolph AM, Heymann MA. Circulatory changes during growth in the fetal lamb. *Circ Res.* 1970;26(3):289–299.

44. Segar JL, Smith FG, Guillery EN, et al. Ontogeny of renal response to specific dopamine DA1-receptor stimulation in sheep. *Am J Physiol.* 1992;263(4 Pt 2):R868–R873.

45. Muller F, Dommergues M, Bussieres L, et al. Development of human renal function: reference intervals for 10 biochemical markers in fetal urine. *Clin Chem.* 1996;42(11):1855–1860.

46. Nicolini U, Fisk NM, Rodeck CH, Beacham J. Fetal urine biochemistry: an index of renal maturation and dysfunction. *Br J Obstet Gynaecol.* 1992;99(1):46–50.

47. Haycock GB. Development of glomerular filtration and tubular sodium reabsorption in the human fetus and newborn. *Br J Urol.* 1998;81(suppl 2):33–38.

48. Nakamura KT, Matherne GP, McWeeny OJ, et al. Renal hemodynamics and functional changes during the transition from fetal to newborn life in sheep. *Pediatr Res.* 1987;21(3):229–234.

49. Wilkinson AW, Stevens LH, Hughes EA. Metabolic changes in the newborn. *Lancet.* 1962;1(7237):983–987.

50. Bueva A, Guignard JP. Renal function in preterm neonates. *Pediatr Res.* 1994;36(5):572–577.

51. Siegel SR, Oh W. Renal function as a marker of human fetal maturation. *Acta Paediatr Scand.* 1976;65(4):481–485.

52. Gubhaju L, Sutherland MR, Horne RS, et al. Assessment of renal functional maturation and injury in preterm neonates during the first month of life. *Am J Physiol Renal Physiol.* 2014;307(2):F149–F158.

53. Dean RF, Mc CR. The renal responses of infants and adults to the administration of hypertonic solutions of sodium chloride and urea. *J Physiol.* 1949;109(1–2):81–97.

54. Aperia A, Broberger O, Thodenius K, Zetterstrom R. Renal response to an oral sodium load in newborn full term infants. *Acta Paediatr Scand.* 1972;61(6):670–676.

55. Aperia A, Broberger O, Thodenius K, Zetterstrom R. Developmental study of the renal response to an oral salt load in preterm infants. *Acta Paediatr Scand.* 1974;63(4):517–524.

56. Gattineni J, Baum M. Developmental changes in renal tubular transport-an overview. *Pediatr Nephrol.* 2015;30(12):2085–2098.

57. Petershack JA, Nagaraja SC, Guillery EN. Role of glucocorticoids in the maturation of renal cortical Na+-K+-ATPase during fetal life in sheep. *Am J Physiol.* 1999;276(6 Pt 2):R1825–R1832.

58. Ogundipe OA, Kullama LK, Stein H, et al. Fetal endocrine and renal responses to in utero ventilation and umbilical cord occlusion. *Am J Obstet Gynecol.* 1993;169(6):1479–1486.

59. Derfoul A, Robertson NM, Lingrel JB, et al. Regulation of the human Na/K-ATPase beta1 gene promoter by mineralocorticoid and glucocorticoid receptors. *J Biol Chem.* 1998;273(33):20702–20711.

60. Mick VE, Itani OA, Loftus RW, et al. The alpha-subunit of the epithelial sodium channel is an aldosterone-induced transcript in mammalian collecting ducts, and this transcriptional response is mediated via distinct cis-elements in the 5′-flanking region of the gene. *Mol Endocrinol.* 2001;15(4):575–588.

61. Martinerie L, Viengchareun S, Delezoide AL, et al. Low renal mineralocorticoid receptor expression at birth contributes to partial aldosterone resistance in neonates. *Endocrinology.* 2009;150(9):4414–4424.

62. Martinerie L, Pussard E, Yousef N, et al. Aldosterone-Signaling Defect Exacerbates Sodium Wasting in Very Preterm Neonates: The Premaldo Study. *J Clin Endocrinol Metab.* 2015;100(11):4074–4081.

63. Cheung CY, Gibbs DM, Brace RA. Atrial natriuretic factor in maternal and fetal sheep. *Am J Physiol.* 1987;252(2 Pt 1):E279–E282.
64. Weil J, Bidlingmaier F, Dohlemann C, et al. Comparison of plasma atrial natriuretic peptide levels in healthy children from birth to adolescence and in children with cardiac diseases. *Pediatr Res.* 1986;20(12):1328–1331.
65. Modi N, Betremieux P, Midgley J, Hartnoll G. Postnatal weight loss and contraction of the extracellular compartment is triggered by atrial natriuretic peptide. *Early Hum Dev.* 2000;59(3):201–208.
66. Robillard JE, Nakamura KT, Varille VA, et al. Ontogeny of the renal response to natriuretic peptide in sheep. *Am J Physiol.* 1988;254(5 Pt 2):F634–F641.
67. Robillard JE, Smith FG, Segar JL, et al. Mechanisms regulating renal sodium excretion during development. *Pediatr Nephrol.* 1992;6(2):205–213.
68. Theilig F, Wu Q. ANP-induced signaling cascade and its implications in renal pathophysiology. *Am J Physiol Renal Physiol.* 2015;308(10):F1047–F1055.
69. Lopez MLSS, Gomez RA. Development of the renin-angiotensin sytstem. In: Polin RA, Fox WW, Abman SH, eds. *Fetal and Neonatal Physiology.* Vol. 2. 4th ed. Philadelphia: Elsevier/Saunders; 2011:1330–1339.
70. Lumbers ER. Functions of the renin-angiotensin system during development. *Clin Exp Pharmacol Physiol.* 1995;22(8):499–505.
71. Vinturache AE, Smith FG. Renal effects of angiotensin II in the newborn period: role of type 1 and type 2 receptors. *BMC Physiol.* 2016;16:3.
72. Roberts D, Dalziel S. Antenatal corticosteroids for accelerating fetal lung maturation for women at risk of preterm birth. *Cochrane Database Syst Rev.* 2006;(3):CD004454.
73. Lemoh JN, Brooke OG. Frequency and weight of normal stools in infancy. *Arch Dis Child.* 1979;54(9):719–720.
74. Cort RL, Pribylova H. Placental Transfusion and Fluid Metabolism on the First Day of Life. *Arch Dis Child.* 1964;39:363–370.
75. Karoum F, Ruthven CR, Sandler M. Urinary phenolic acid and alcohol excretion in the newborn. *Arch Dis Child.* 1975;50(8):586–594.
76. Moritz ML, Manole MD, Bogen DL, Ayus JC. Breastfeeding-associated hypernatremia: are we missing the diagnosis? *Pediatrics.* 2005;116(3):e343–e347.
77. Konetzny G, Bucher HU, Arlettaz R. Prevention of hypernatraemic dehydration in breastfed newborn infants by daily weighing. *Eur J Pediatr.* 2009;168(7):815–818.
78. Moritz ML. Preventing breastfeeding-associated hypernatraemia: an argument for supplemental feeding. *Arch Dis Child Fetal Neonatal Ed.* 2013;98(5):F378–F379.
79. Bell EF. Fluid therapy. In: Sinclair JC, Bracken MB, eds. *Effective Care of the Newborn Infant.* Oxford; New York: Oxford University Press; 1992:59–72.
80. Vuohelainen T, Ojala R, Virtanen A, et al. Decreased free water clearance is associated with worse respiratory outcomes in premature infants. *PLoS ONE.* 2011;6(2):e16995.
81. Maggio L, Cota F, Gallini F, et al. Effects of high versus standard early protein intake on growth of extremely low birth weight infants. *J Pediatr Gastroenterol Nutr.* 2007;44(1):124–129.
82. Casey CE, Neifert MR, Seacat JM, Neville MC. Nutrient intake by breast-fed infants during the first five days after birth. *Am J Dis Child.* 1986;140(9):933–936.
83. Santoro W Jr, Martinez FE, Ricco RG, Jorge SM. Colostrum ingested during the first day of life by exclusively breastfed healthy newborn infants. *J Pediatr.* 2010;156(1):29–32.
84. Hartnoll G, Betremieux P, Modi N. Randomised controlled trial of postnatal sodium supplementation on oxygen dependency and body weight in 25-30 week gestational age infants. *Arch Dis Child Fetal Neonatal Ed.* 2000;82(1):F19–F23.
85. Al-Dahhan J, Haycock GB, Chantler C, Stimmler L. Sodium homeostasis in term and preterm neonates. I. Renal aspects. *Arch Dis Child.* 1983;58(5):335–342.
86. American Academy of Pediatrics Committee on Nutrition. Nutritional needs of low-birth-weight infants. *Pediatrics.* 1985;75(5):976–986.
87. Edelman IS, Leibman J, O'Meara MP, Birkenfeld LW. Interrelations between serum sodium concentration, serum osmolarity and total exchangeable sodium, total exchangeable potassium and total body water. *J Clin Invest.* 1958;37(9):1236–1256.
88. Kurtz I, Nguyen MK. Evolving concepts in the quantitative analysis of the determinants of the plasma water sodium concentration and the pathophysiology and treatment of the dysnatremias. *Kidney Int.* 2005;68(5):1982–1993.
89. Warner GF, Sweet NJ, Dobson EL. Sodium space and body sodium content, exchangeable with sodium24, in normal individuals and patients with ascites. *Circ Res.* 1953;1(6):486–490.
90. Wassner SJ. Altered growth and protein turnover in rats fed sodium-deficient diets. *Pediatr Res.* 1989;26(6):608–613.
91. Wassner SJ. The effect of sodium repletion on growth and protein turnover in sodium-depleted rats. *Pediatr Nephrol.* 1991;5(4):501–504.
92. Gallaher KJ, Wolpert E, Wassner S, Rannels DE. Effect of diet-induced sodium deficiency on normal and compensatory growth of the lung in young rats. *Pediatr Res.* 1990;28(5):455–459.
93. Vieux R, Hascoet JM, Merdariu D, et al. Glomerular filtration rate reference values in very preterm infants. *Pediatrics.* 2010;125(5):e1186–e1192.
94. Al-Dahhan J, Haycock GB, Nichol B, et al. Sodium homeostasis in term and preterm neonates. III. Effect of salt supplementation. *Arch Dis Child.* 1984;59(10):945–950.
95. Vanpee M, Herin P, Broberger U, Aperia A. Sodium supplementation optimizes weight gain in preterm infants. *Acta Paediatr.* 1995;84(11):1312–1314.

10

96. Isemann B, Mueller EW, Narendran V, Akinbi H. Impact of Early Sodium Supplementation on Hyponatremia and Growth in Premature Infants: A Randomized Controlled Trial. *JPEN J Parenter Enteral Nutr.* 2016;40(3):342–349.

97. Al-Dahhan J, Jannoun L, Haycock GB. Effect of salt supplementation of newborn premature infants on neurodevelopmental outcome at 10-13 years of age. *Arch Dis Child Fetal Neonatal Ed.* 2002;86(2):F120–F123.

98. Gruskay J, Costarino AT, Polin RA, Baumgart S. Nonoliguric hyperkalemia in the premature infant weighing less than 1000 grams. *J Pediatr.* 1988;113(2):381–386.

99. Shaffer SG, Kilbride HW, Hayen LK, et al. Hyperkalemia in very low birth weight infants. *J Pediatr.* 1992;121(2):275–279.

100. Stefano JL, Norman ME. Nitrogen balance in extremely low birth weight infants with nonoliguric hyperkalemia. *J Pediatr.* 1993;123(4):632–635.

101. Bonsante F, Iacobelli S, Chantegret C, et al. The effect of parenteral nitrogen and energy intake on electrolyte balance in the preterm infant. *Eur J Clin Nutr.* 2011;65(10):1088–1093.

102. Omar SA, DeCristofaro JD, Agarwal BI, LaGamma EF. Effect of prenatal steroids on potassium balance in extremely low birth weight neonates. *Pediatrics.* 2000;106(3):561–567.

CHAPTER 11

Renal Modulation: The Renin-Angiotensin System

Aruna Natarajan, MD, DCH, PhD, Van Anthony M. Villar, MD, PhD, Pedro A. Jose, MD, PhD

- **Components of the Renin-Angiotensin-Aldosterone System**
- **Ontogeny**

The renin-angiotensin-aldosterone system (RAAS) plays a critical role in the maintenance of salt and water homeostasis by the kidneys, particularly in hypovolemic and salt-depleted states. However, the inappropriate activation of this system results in abnormal sodium retention, potassium loss, and an increase in blood pressure. In addition, excess angiotensin II (Ang II) and aldosterone can cause inflammation and oxidative stress, both of which can cause chronic kidney disease and aggravate the increase in blood pressure.[1–4]

Components of the Renin-Angiotensin-Aldosterone System

Angiotensin Generation

The renin-angiotensin system (RAS) is currently divided into the classical RAS and the nonclassical RAS pathways.[1–6] The classical pathway comprises angiotensin converting enzyme (ACE), Ang II, and Ang II type 1 receptor (AT_1R) (Fig. 11.1). The nonclassical pathway is composed of two components: one pathway comprises the Ang II/Ang III/Ang IV/AT_2R, and the other pathway comprises ACE2, Ang 1-7, and alamandine/Mas1/MrgD (Fig. 11.2).[2,3,5,6]

Both the classical and nonclassical RAS pathways are initiated by renin (see Figs. 11.1 and 11.2), which is primarily synthesized in renal juxtaglomerular cells (smooth muscle cells in the walls of the afferent arteriole as it enters the glomerulus) and stored as prorenin.[1–3] The principal cells and intercalated cells of the renal collecting duct also synthesize renin and prorenin, respectively.[7,8] Renin is also synthesized in the connecting segment.[1] Renin enzymatically causes the formation of Ang I (Ang 1-10) from angiotensinogen, its only substrate, with the liver as the major source. The binding of renin and prorenin to the (pro)renin receptor (PRR) activates prorenin and markedly enhances renin activity. In the classical pathway, Ang I is acted upon by ACE to form Ang II. The rate-limiting step in the activation of the RAS is the release of renin, which is the most well-regulated component of the RAS. Renal renin secretion is stimulated by three primary pathways: (1) stimulation of renal baroreceptors by a decrease in afferent arterial stretch (pressure)[9–11]; (2) stimulation of renal β_1-adrenergic receptors, partly through increased renal sympathetic nerve activity[12–16]; and (3) a decrease in sodium and chloride delivery to, and transport by, the macula densa.[15,16] Renin secretion can also be regulated by several endocrine and paracrine hormones,[1,3,17] hypoxia,[18] and gases (e.g., H_2S).[19] It should be mentioned that angiotensinogen may have Ang II-independent effects, including the regulation of body weight and the induction of atherosclerosis.[20]

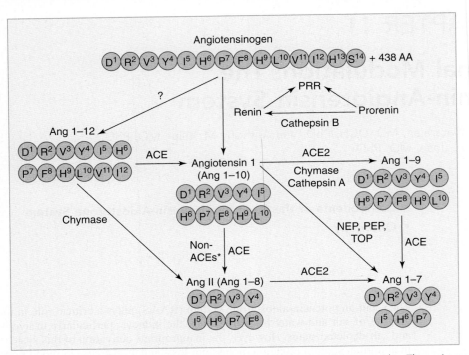

Fig. 11.1 Pathways of angiotensin (Ang) generation showing the generation of Ang peptides. The renin-angiotensin system is currently divided into the classical renin-angiotensin system (RAS) and the nonclassical RAS pathways. Both the classical and nonclassical pathways are initiated by renin cleaving angiotensinogen to Ang I. The classical pathway is initiated mainly by angiotensin converting enzyme (ACE) with contributions from non-ACEs. The nonclassical pathway is composed of two components: one pathway is initiated by ACE2 and the other component has three pathways (see Fig. 11.2). Angiotensinogen may also be cleaved to Ang 1-12 by an unknown enzyme. The letters are the symbols of the specific amino acid. *PRR*, (Pro)renin receptor. *Non-ACE enzymes include: carboxypeptidase, cathepsin G, chymase, elastase-2, metallo-proteinase 8, and tonin.

Renin-Angiotensin System Outside Juxtaglomerular Cells

The RAS has been demonstrated in tissues other than the kidney. Synthesis of certain components of the RAAS occurs to a greater extent in some organs relative to others, such as ACE in the lung, aldosterone in the adrenal glands, angiotensinogen in the liver, and renin in the kidney, which function together as an endocrine system. Some or all of the RAAS components are expressed in the adipose tissue, blood vessel, brain, heart, kidney, pancreas, and placenta, among others, exerting autocrine, intracrine, and paracrine effects. This adds complexity to the understanding of the regulatory effects of the RAAS in maintaining body homeostasis.[1-4] Extraglomerular sites of prorenin synthesis include the adrenal cortex and medulla,[21] adipocyte,[3,22] brain,[21] eye (retina and vitreous humor),[23] heart,[3,21] mast cells,[19,24] ovarian follicle,[25] chorionic villus of the placenta,[26] renal collecting duct cell,[1,7,8] submandibular gland,[21] testis and male reproductive system,[26,27] uterus (endometrium, decidua basalis, and decidua vera),[28,29] and vascular wall,[3] among others. The sites of synthesis of components of the RAS are species specific.[30,31] The components of the RAAS can also be trapped from the circulation, renin is trapped in the brain of mice, for example.[30] Angiotensinogen is produced in extrahepatic sites, such as the adrenal gland, brain, cardiac atrium, kidney, large intestine, lung, mesentery, ovary, spinal cord, stomach, and spleen and is also expressed in the ventricle and conducting tissue of the heart.[1,3,32,33] ACE is ubiquitously expressed. However, the conversion of circulating Ang I to Ang II by ACE occurs mainly in the lung. ACE2 has been consistently identified in the human heart, kidney, and testis, and may be present in other tissues as well.[34]

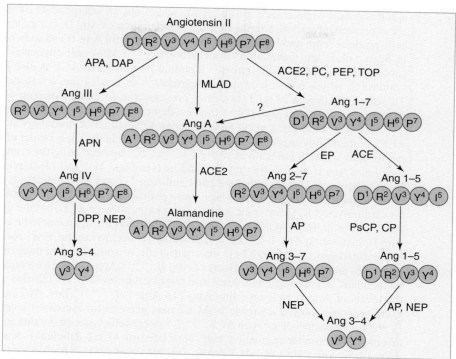

Fig. 11.2 Angiotensin II (Ang II) has at least three metabolites, Ang III (Ang 2-8), Ang A (Ala1-Ang 1-8), and Ang 1-7. Ang III (Ang 2-8) differs from Ang II by absence of aspartate (D^1). Ang A differs from Ang II because of a change in the first amino acid from Asp to Ala (Ala^1-Ang 1-8). Ang 1-7 differs from Ang II by the absence of phenylalanine (F^8). *ACE*, Angiotensin converting enzyme; *ACE2*, angiotensin converting enzyme 2; *AP*, aminopeptidase; *APA*, aminopeptidase A; *APN*, aminopeptidase N; *CP*, carboxypeptidase; *DAP*, aspartyl aminopeptidase; *DPP*, dipeptidyl peptidase; *EP*, endopeptidase; *MLAD*, mononuclear leucocyte aspartate decarboxylase; *NEP*, neprilysin; *PC*, prolyl carboxypeptidase; *PEP*, prolyl endopeptidase; *PsCP*, Plummer's sensitive carboxypetidase; *TOP*, thimet oligopeptidase. (Figure is adapted from Dias J, Axelband F, Lara LS, et al. Is angiotensin-(3-4) (Val-Tyr), the shortest angiotensin II-derived peptide, opening new vistas on the renin-angiotensin system? *J Renin Angiotensin Aldosterone Syst.* 2017;18(1):1470320316689338, Figure 4.)

Effects of Angiotensin Converting Enzyme and Nonangiotensin-Converting Enzymes Other Than the Production of Angiotensin II

As mentioned earlier, the RAS is currently divided into the classical and the nonclassical RAS.[1–6] The activation of the classical pathway results in an increase in blood pressure, directly, by vasoconstriction and extracellular volume expansion, and by an increase in renal and intestinal electrolyte transport and water flux, and indirectly by stimulation of the synthesis of mineralocorticoids, especially aldosterone. Ang II acting in brain centers (e.g., lateral paraventricular, median preoptic, lateral parabrachial, and supraoptic nuclei) can also increase salt and water intake.[36] Inappropriate, excessive, or prolonged stimulation of the classical RAS can lead to abnormal cell growth, fibrosis, inflammation, myocardial ischemia, obesity, and oxidative stress, among others.[1–6,34,37,38] By contrast, the nonclassical pathway is perceived to oppose the nonbeneficial effects of the classical pathway, with exceptions, to be discussed subsequently.[1–6]

ACE acts on Ang I (Ang 1-10) to cleave off the active octapeptide, Ang II (Ang 1-8), which is a more potent vasoconstrictor than Ang I (see Fig. 11.1).[1–6] Ang II can also be formed from Ang I by non-ACE enzymes and nonrenin enzymes, such as carboxypeptidase, cathepsin G, chymase, elastase-2, metallo-proteinase 8, and tonin.[5,39–41] The roles of these enzymes in humans need elucidation, as tonin has not been reported in humans.[40] Nevertheless, these non-ACE, nonrenin enzymes assume greater significance in the organs where not all components of the RAAS are expressed, providing alternate means of generation of Ang II. For example, mast cells produce renin and have chymases, which help form Ang II and may play a role in heart failure and generation of arrhythmias.[19,24,42] Mast cell chymases limit the cardiac efficacy of ACE inhibitors.[43] It should be noted that ACE is also known as kininase 2, which is involved in the degradation of bradykinin, a vasodepressor.[44] Therefore, inhibition of ACE not only prevents the formation of Ang II with its vasopressor effect, but also allows the vasodepressor effect of bradykinin to persist.

ACE2 is a homolog of ACE, with about 42% sequence homology in humans. ACE2 is abundantly expressed in the kidney, specifically in the brush border of proximal tubule cells where it colocalizes with ACE.[45] ACE2, by catalyzing the conversion of Ang I and Ang II to Ang 1-7 and alamandine (see Figs. 11.1 and 11.2), provides the balance between Ang II on the one hand and Ang 1-7 and alamandine, on the other, in the kidney and other tissues where these pathways may occur.[1-5,46,47] In neonatal rat cardiomyocytes, aldosterone increases the expression of ACE, but the opposite is observed for ACE2.[48] ACE2 is a carboxypeptidase and the main catabolic enzyme of Ang II, generating Ang 1-7. Ang 1-7, probably by occupying the Mas1 receptor and Mas-related gene receptor, MrgD, has natriuretic, vasodilator, and antiproliferative properties and counteracts the effects of Ang II.[2-6,46-48] Ang 1-7 can also regulate lipid metabolism, decreasing cholesterol and triglyceride levels.[49] ACE2 also decreases the levels of Ang II by converting Ang I to Ang 1-9.[2-6,45,50] Thus, ACE and ACE2 exert opposing roles; a decrease in ACE2 may account for increased levels of Ang II, and the opposite occurs with ACE.[1-6,48,50] Sympathetic vasoconstriction in systemic disorders of vascular regulation may be related to ACE2 deficiency, leading to a decrease in Ang 1-7.[51] The ACE2-Ang 1-7–Mas axis plays a protective role in the pathogenesis of hypertension, regulation of renal function, and progression of renal disease, including diabetic nephropathy.[52] A decrease in the expression or function of this system may play a critical role in the progression of cardiovascular diseases, as elucidated below.[6,47,53] Ang 1-7 can also act as a biased AT_1R agonist, resulting in the recruitment of β-arrestin 2, antagonizing the detrimental effects of Ang II.[53] A homologue of ACE2, collectrin, which does not have a catalytic domain, may also be protective against hypertension.[54]

The processing and effects of angiotensins are also species-, tissue-, and sex-specific.[2-6,55]

Cardiovascular System

Ang I can be converted to Ang 1-9 by ACE2, chymase, and cathepsin A (aka carboxypeptidase A).[2-6,45,48] The main products of Ang 1 due to ACE and chymase are Ang 1-9 and Ang II in the heart,[56] as well as arteries,[57] and Ang 1-9, via cathepsin A,[56] but not Ang II in platelets.[58] Circulating Ang 1-9 levels are increased after myocardial infarction[59] and inhibit cardiac hypertrophy.[60] Whereas Ang 1-9 is prothrombotic,[61] Ang 1-7 is antithrombotic.[62]

Adipocyte

In adipocytes, Ang 1-7 derived from Ang 1-9 is the main degradation product, and Ang III inhibits insulin-regulated amino peptidase (IRAP), which also possesses a binding site for Ang IV.[2,22] White adipose tissue is the major site of angiotensinogen synthesis outside the liver, contributing to about 20% of circulating angiotensinogen.[63] Ang II increases adipose tissue angiotensinogen expression, a case of positive feedback.[64] ACE2, which converts Ang 1 to Ang (1-9) and Ang II to Ang (1-7),[2-6,48] is upregulated by high-fat diet and decreases adipocyte inflammation.[65] Mice lacking angiotensinogen or AT_2R are protected from high-fat-diet–induced obesity and featured adipose tissue hypotrophy.[38] Therefore, it seems that Ang II via AT_2R and Ang (1-7) via Mas1 or MrgD counteract each other.[2-6,38,45,48,65]

Kidney

In rat glomeruli, Ang I is mainly converted to Ang 1-7 via neprilysin and Ang 2-10 via aminopeptidase A (APA), in one study,[66] and to Ang II, Ang 1-9, Ang 1-7, and

Ang 3-8, enzyme(s) not determined, in another study.[67] In mouse podocytes, the main product of Ang I is Ang 1-7, via neprilysin.[68] Podocytes can also convert Ang II to Ang III; angiotensinogen, renin, AT_1R, AT_2R, and PRR are also expressed in podocytes.[68,69] By contrast, human mesangial cells mainly convert Ang I to Ang II.[68] In several animal models, renal intratubular Ang II has been found to be higher than that found in the circulation.[70] In the mouse, components of the RAS, except ACE, are expressed in the proximal tubule; renin is also expressed in the distal convoluted tubule and cortical collecting duct, and angiotensinogen is also expressed in the thin descending and thick ascending limbs of Henle.[71,72] Prorenin is expressed in the intercalated cells of the collecting duct.[73,74] Thus, angiotensinogen can be converted to Ang I in the proximal and distal convoluted tubules and cortical collecting duct and, in turn, converted into Ang II by ACE from the renal vasculature or systemic circulation.[72] However, liver-derived rather than proximal tubule–derived angiotensinogen may be the primary source of intrarenal angiotensinogen, under physiologic conditions.[75–80] On normal sodium intake, angiotensinogen within the S1 and S2 segments of the proximal tubule comes from the systemic circulation, while angiotensinogen in the S3 comes from endogenous synthesis.

Blood Vessel

Vascular smooth muscles can also synthesize Ang II,[4] in which the primary source of renin and angiotensinogen is from the plasma.[79,81] However, all the other components of the RAS are expressed in the vascular wall.[4,79–84] Ang 1 is produced from angiotensinogen via cathepsin D, rather than renin, and chymase rather than ACE converts Ang I to Ang II in injured vessels.[4,81,84] Ang 1-7 formed in the vascular smooth muscle interacts with Mas1 in the endothelial cells.[79,84] In rat mesenteric arteries, Ang I is converted by cathepsin A1 to Ang 1-7, with Ang 1-9 and Ang II as intermediates. By contrast, Ang 1 is converted by cathepsin A2 to Ang 1-9.[82]

Renin-Angiotensin System and Brain

The existence of local brain RAS was suggested by the demonstration of renin within the brain of nephrectomized dogs.[85] Although there are studies suggesting that brain renin represents trapped plasma renin,[86] there are more studies that attest to the presence of a local brain RAS.[87] In the brain, angiotensinogen is expressed more than renin, and ACE is expressed in brain areas that are important in cardiovascular regulation. The subfornical organ is important in angiotensin-mediated drinking and blood pressure regulation. Drinking and whole body metabolism may be regulated by a brain-specific isoform of renin, which negatively regulates the brain RAS.[88] In the subfornical organ, the AT_1R increases fluid intake while the AT_1R increases blood pressure. In the arcuate nucleus, the AT_1R and leptin receptor interact to regulate resting metabolic rate.[89] In the brain, Ang II may be the primary AT_1R agonist.[90]

Angiotensin II and Its Metabolites

Ang II has at least three metabolites: Ang III (Ang 2-8), Ang A (Ala^1-Ang 1-8), and Ang 1-7 (see Fig. 11.2).[2,46,91] Ang III (Ang 2-8) differs from Ang II by absence of Asp^1 and by the action of APA on Ang II. Ang III, as with Ang II, participates in the classical effects on body fluid and electrolyte homeostasis, such as drinking behavior, vasopressin release, and sodium appetite in brain centers.[3,46,83,88] However, Ang III has been shown to exert a natriuretic effect via its interaction with the AT_2R.[3,92,93] Aminopeptidase N (APN) acts on Ang III to form Ang IV (Ang 3-8).[3,48,94–96] Ang IV stimulates AT_4R[95] and AT_2R[97] and inhibits AT_1R in one study.[97] Ang IV negatively regulates APA and thus influences the generation of Ang III.[98] Ang IV can be cleaved to Ang 3-4 by dipeptidyl peptidase or neprilysin.[99] Ang 3-4 can also be formed from Ang 1-7 by the action of a series of enzymes (see Fig. 11.2); Ang 3-4 is natriuretic by occupying AT_2R.[99]

Ang A differs from Ang II because of a change in the first amino acid from Asp to Ala (Ala^1-Ang 1-8), presumably by decarboxylation of Ang II that may involve the mononuclear leucocyte aspartate decarboxylase.[5,46,100] Although Ang A may have affinity for both AT_1R and AT_2R, Ang A, via AT_1R, is mainly a vasoconstrictor and increases blood pressure, although at much higher concentrations than Ang II.[101] Unlike Ang II, Ang A does not increase the amplitude of the calcium transient in isolated rat ventricular myocytes, acting as a biased agonist.[46]

Ang 1-7 differs from Ang II by the absence of Phe[8]; it is derived from Ang II by the action of ACE2, as well as prolyl carboxypeptidase, prolyl endopeptidase, and thimet oligopeptidase.[6,96,99,102–105] In the central nervous system, Ang 1-7 may also inhibit norepinephrine synthesis and release.[102] The physiologic effects of Ang 1-7, such as vasodilation, natriuresis, and antiangiogenesis, counteract the effects of Ang II by occupying the AT_2R and MrdG.[106–108] Ang 1-7 also inhibits Ang II-stimulated phosphorylation of mitogen-activated protein (MAP) kinase in rat renal proximal tubule cells.[109] The ability of Ang 1-7 to counteract the effects of Ang II (e.g., cell proliferation and extracellular matrix synthesis) in rat renal mesangial cells is exerted via Mas1.[110] However, Ang 1-7, by itself, can mimic the ability of Ang II to stimulate cell proliferation and extracellular matrix synthesis in these cells.[110] The significance of this apparently detrimental effect of Ang 1-7 remains to be determined.

Alamandine is a heptapeptide, which is derived from Ang A by the cleavage of phenylalanine (Ala^1-Ang 1-7) by the action of ACE2. Alamandine also can be derived from Ang 1-7 by the decarboxylation of its aspartate residue; the specific enzyme has not been definitely determined but may involve ACE.[5,46,111] There are similarities and differences between Ang 1-7 and alamandine.[46,106] As with Ang 1-7, alamandine is a vasodilator, in part by activating nitric oxide.[48,106] Both alamandine and Ang 1-7 can inhibit the vasoconstriction of the rabbit aorta induced by Ang A but not that caused by Ang II. In the diseased aorta, neither Ang 1-7 nor alamandine had any effect on Ang A-induced vasoconstriction; however Ang 1-7, but not alamandine, increased Ang II-mediated vasoconstriction.[107] However, in the human internal mammary artery, Ang 1-7 has been reported to antagonize the vasoconstrictor effect of Ang II.[112] While alamandine reduces leptin expression in peri-renal adipocytes, Ang 1-7 increases it.[113] Unlike Ang 1-7, which can activate both Mas1 and MrgD receptors, alamandine activates only the MrgD receptor.[46,111] Alamandine can also exert is vaosodepressor effect by acting at the rostral ventrolateral medulla.[111]

In summary, the RAS is now accepted to be present in many tissues. There are two pathways: the classical RAS comprises ACE, Ang II, and AT_1R, whereas the non-RAS is composed of two components: Ang II/Ang III/Ang IV and AT_2R component; and the ACE2, Ang 1-7, and alamandine component.[2,3,5,6,46,91] The classical pathway is responsible for increasing water and sodium intake, sodium retention, and vasoconstriction; overactivation of the classical pathway leads to oxidative stress, inflammation, fibrosis, and cell growth, while the nonclassical pathway, in general, opposes the actions of the classical pathway. However, not all members of the nonclassical pathway oppose the classical pathway because while Ang IV, via AT_4R, has been reported to inhibit inflammation in the heart with ischemia/reperfusion injury,[95] it may also promote vasoconstriction, cell proliferation, and inflammation.[48,114] In a model of Ang II-induced abdominal aneurysm, a medium dose but not a high dose of Ang IV exerted a beneficial effect, in part by decreasing inflammation.[115] The RAS also could be viewed as an ACE pathway and is composed of two distinct and opposing arms: the ACE pathway, which generates Ang II, acting via the AT_1R to subserve the biologic effects of vasoconstriction and the increase in renal sodium transport, and the ACE2 pathway, which generates an endogenous antagonist to Ang II, namely Ang 1-7 activating the oncogene Mas1 receptor protein to subserve vasodilatory and antiproliferative effects on the vasculature and decreased epithelial ion transport. In the brain, ACE2 activation also opposes the effects of Ang II exerted via the AT_1R. The RAS has also been suggested to be divisible into five axes: (1) classic angiotensinogen/renin/ACE/Ang II/AT_1R; (2) Ang II/APA/Ang III/AT_2R/NO/cyclic guanosine monophosphate (cGMP); (3) Ang I/Ang II/ACE2/Ang 1-7/Mas1 receptor; (4) prorenin/renin/(pro)renin receptor (PRR or Atp6ap2)/MAP kinases ERK1/2/V-ATPase; and (5) Ang III/APN/Ang IV/IRAP/AT_4R.[2]

Aldosterone

Aldosterone secretion by the zona glomerulosa cells of the adrenal gland is normally regulated by Ang II and potassium, which is mediated by an increase in intracellular calcium.[116-118] ACTH becomes a very important stimulus of aldosterone secretion under conditions of volume depletion.[118] Mast cells located in the subcapsular region of the human adrenal cortex also stimulate aldosterone secretion by releasing serotonin.[119] Extraadrenal sites of aldosterone synthesis include the adipose tissue that secretes aldosterone-releasing factors.[117] An increase in circulating aldosterone increases local aldosterone production in hypothalamic nuclei (e.g., supraoptic nucleus and parventricular nucleus), which participates in aldosterone-induced increase in salt and water intake.[120-122] The brain AT_1R may preferentially respond to Ang III that is critical for the hypertensinogenic effect of Ang II.[123] The RAS in cardiac myocytes plays a role in the ventricular remodeling associated with salt retention.[124] In neurons and cardiomyocytes, the effects of aldosterone are opposed by glucocorticoids.[125] However, under conditions of cardiac damage, corticosterone, rather than aldosterone, may be the activator of mineralocorticoid receptors.[126] Both corticosterone and aldosterone increase cardiac contractility; however, corticosterone increases, whereas aldosterone decreases, coronary flow.[127] Depending on the species and experimental conditions, aldosterone may have positive (rat heart) or negative (human heart) inotropic effect.[127] Aldosterone promotes salt and water retention by stimulating sodium transport mediated by the epithelial sodium channel (ENaC) in the distal nephron.[128] Aldosterone can also increase sodium transport in the renal proximal tubule by the stimulation of the Na^+/H^+ exchanger types 1 and 3 (NHE1 and NHE3, respectively), as well as $Na^+,K^+/ATPase$.[129,130]

Gene Targeting of Angiotensin Synthesis: Lessons From Genetically Manipulated Rodents

Genetic ablation of angiotensinogen and ACE in separate lines of mice uniformly results in low blood pressure, abnormal renal development, renal malfunction, and low hematocrit.[131] Tissue-specific targeted ablation helps to elucidate the paracrine and autocrine effects of tissue RAS. As indicated earlier, the main source of renal angiotensinogen is the liver; liver-specific but not renal-specific deletion of angiotensinogen decreases renal angiotensinogen and Ang II proteins.[132,133] Blood pressure is decreased in both instances. However, the reduction in urinary angiotensinogen in renal- but not liver-specific deletion of angiotensinogen needs to be explained.[1] Glial-specific ablation of angiotensinogen in mice decreases blood pressure and causes diabetes insipidus.[134,135] As aforementioned, there is a report indicating that brain renin represents trapped plasma.[86] However, ablation of the brain-specific promoter (renin-b) but not preprorenin caused hypertension, via the renin, ACE, and AT_1R pathway in the brain.[136] These genetic manipulations support the notion that the central nervous system contributes to the regulation of blood pressure via the RAS. Ablation of the renin gene in mice reduces aldosterone secretion in the zona glomerulosa and impairs aldosterone production.[137] Systemic genetic ablation of many genes of the RAS (e.g., angiotensinogen, ACE) results in normal mice at birth; however, death generally ensues before 3 weeks of age.[138,139] In addition to gene-targeted deletion, tissue-specific targeting of RAS overexpression has been accomplished.[138,139] Transgenic mice overexpressing the human angiotensinogen and renin, specifically in renal proximal tubules, develop hypertension.[140] The introduction of the mouse *Ren-2* gene into normotensive rats creates a transgenic strain that expresses *Ren-2* mRNA in the adrenal gland, heart, and kidney.[140] This transgenic rat is a monogenic model for a form of sodium-dependent malignant hypertension.[140] These transgenic rats are characterized by high plasma prorenin but unchanged or even suppressed concentrations of active renin, Ang 1, Ang II, and angiotensinogen, compared with transgene-negative littermates. Renal renin is suppressed while adrenal renin and corticosteroid production is increased. Transgenic mice, with selective overexpression of angiotensinogen in the renal proximal tubule, are also hypertensive despite having normal plasma angiotensinogen levels and renin activity. However,

11

urinary angiotensinogen and Ang II concentrations are increased.[141] Blockade of the ET_A receptor in young *Ren-2* transgenic rats decreases blood pressure and ameliorates end-organ damage, suggesting a potential application in the management of hypertension in newborn babies.[142]

ACE-deficient mice have low blood pressure and severe renal disease characterized by vascular hyperplasia of the intrarenal arteries, perivascular infiltrates, paucity of renal papillae,[143] and impaired concentrating ability, which highlight the critical role of ACE in the development of the kidneys.[139,143,144] Inhibitors of ACE have been identified in hypoallergenic infant milk formulas containing hydrolyzed milk proteins, which could potentially affect renal function later in life.[145] ACE inhibition in young rats has been reported to cause retardation of glomerular growth (see below). Mice with renal-specific ablation of ACE have normal serum Ang II, blood pressure, and renal architecture under basal conditions.[146] However, there is a marked attenuation of the hypertensinogenic effect of intravenously administered Ang II and inhibition of nitric oxide synthesis with L-NAME, as well as a decrease in the expression of renal sodium transporters.

ACE2-deficient mice develop dilated cardiomyopathy,[147,148] as well as severe hypertensive nephropathy in response to chronic Ang II infusion, with impairment of renal function that is related to progressive renal fibrosis and inflammation.[149] ACE2-deficient mice develop impaired endothelium-dependent and -independent relaxation in vitro and in vivo, which is associated with a decrease in eNOS expression and nitric oxide (NO) concentration in the aorta.[150] Lack of ACE2 also predisposes to high-fat-diet–induced nephropathy, atherosclerosis, and arterial neointima formation.[151] A decrease in ACE2 expression has been implicated in the delayed hypertension observed in sheep treated antenatally with betamethasone,[152] which needs further elucidation in humans, given the widespread use of antenatal steroids to enhance lung maturity in infants born prematurely. ACE2 effects extend beyond the renal and cardiovascular systems; ACE2 has been reported to be a key regulator of dietary amino acid homeostasis, innate immunity, and gut microbial ecology, which may increase a susceptibility to develop colitis.[153] ACE2 deficiency also impairs glucose tolerance and may predispose to the development of diabetes.[154] However, the β-cell defect of the pancreas with ACE2 deficiency is not dependent on Ang II but rather on the collectrin-like action of ACE2.[155] There are no reports of organ/tissue-selective deletion of ACE2. However, gonadectomy prevents the increase in blood pressure and glomerular injury in diabetic male mice lacking ACE2.[156]

Renin is no longer expressed after removal of the kidneys but prorenin is still present in the blood; renin in anephric subjects has been suggested to be "open" prorenin. Therefore, the kidney may be the only renin-secreting organ while prorenin is secreted from nonrenal tissues (see later).[157] The consequences on blood pressure on the deletion of non-ACE genes related to the RAS have not been reported.

Gene Targeting of Angiotensin Receptors: Lessons From Genetically Manipulated Rodents

Angiotensin Receptors

The effects of the angiotensinogen metabolites, such as Ang II (Ang 1-8), Ang III (Ang 2-8), and Ang IV (Ang 3-8), Ang 1-7, Ang A (Ala1-8), alamandine (Ala1-7), and Ang 3-4 and prorenin, are mediated by their occupation of specific angiotensin receptors.[1–6,46,91] There are six receptors of the RAS: AT_1R, AT_2R, Mas1, and MrgD, all of which are G protein–coupled receptors with seven transmembrane domains[1–6,46]; AT_4R and PRR have one transmembrane domain.[158] An AT_3R was cloned from the rat adrenal cortex.[159]

Ang II interacts mainly with two receptors, AT_1R and AT_2R. Adult human renal vasculature, glomeruli, and tubules (proximal and distal convoluted tubule, ascending limb of Henle, and collecting duct) express AT_1R; AT_2R is expressed in the vasculature and glomeruli, but not in the tubules.[160] In rodents, AT_2R is expressed in most segments of the nephron. Whereas human Ang II, Ang III, and Ang A are full agonists at the human AT_1R, Ang IV binds to this receptor with low affinity.[161,162] The conversion

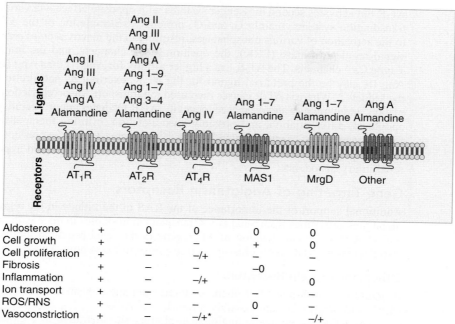

Effect	AT$_1$R	AT$_2$R	AT$_4$R	MAS1	MrgD/Other
Aldosterone	+	0	0	0	0
Cell growth	+	−	−	+	0
Cell proliferation	+	−	−/+	−	
Fibrosis	+	−	−	−0	−
Inflammation	+	−	−/+		0
Ion transport	+	−	−	−	−
ROS/RNS	+	−	−	0	−
Vasoconstriction	+	−	−/+*	−	−/+

Fig. 11.3 Effects of angiotensin (Ang) peptides via their receptors. Positive action is depicted as +, and the opposite effect is depicted as −. The absence of an effect is depicted as 0. *RNS,* Reactive nitrogen species; *ROS,* reactive oxygen species.

of Ang II to Ang III is necessary for its interaction with the AT$_2$R to cause natriuresis.[163] However, Ang III is also a full agonist of AT$_2$R; Ang IV, Ang A, Ang 1-9, Ang 1-7, and Ang 3-4 are AT$_2$R agonists (see Fig. 11.3).[99,106,107,162] The human AT$_1$R gene *(AGTR1)* is located in chromosome 3q24. The human AT$_2$R gene *(AGTR2)* is located in chromosome Xq23.[161,164]

The current understanding that AT$_2$R expression is higher in fetal life than in newborns or adults has been challenged by recent observations in rats, wherein AT$_2$R protein expression is lower and AT$_1$R expression is higher in the fetal and neonatal brain and kidneys than in adults, but the expression of AT$_2$R is higher in the fetal and neonatal liver compared with adults.[165]

Occupation of the AT$_1$R by Ang II triggers the generation of various second messengers via heterotrimeric G proteins, mainly G$_{q/11}$. Phospholipase C (PLC) β1 is activated, leading to the formation of 1,4,5-inositol trisphosphate (IP$_3$) and diacyl glycerol (DAG) from the hydrolysis of phosphatidylinositol-4,5-bisphosphonate. IP$_3$ activates IP$_3$ receptors in the endoplasmic reticulum, releasing Ca^{2+}. Ca^{2+} released from the endoplasmic reticulum causes the Ca^{2+}-sensing stromal interaction molecule protein to interact with Orai1 in the plasma membrane. This interaction, together with the activation of IP$_3$ receptors at the plasma membrane, allows the influx of extracellular calcium.[166,167] The increase in intracellular calcium and the stimulation of protein kinase C (PKC) by DAG lead to vasoconstriction.[168] Activation of the AT$_1$R stimulates growth factor pathways, such as tyrosine phosphorylation and PLCγ activation, leading to the activation of downstream proteins, including MAP kinases, and signal transducers and activators of transcription (STAT protein). These cellular proliferative pathways, mediated by the AT$_1$R, have been implicated in the proliferative changes seen in cardiovascular and renal diseases.[169] AT$_1$R signaling may also be positively affected by reactive oxygen species (ROS) and reactive nitrogen species, but NO may decrease AT$_1$R signaling by cysteine modification of the nuclear transcription factor, NFκB.[170]

The AT$_1$R and AT$_2$R are differentiated based on their affinity for various non-peptide antagonists.[162] The human AT$_2$R has 34% sequence homology with the human

AT_1R but activates second messenger systems with opposite effects via various signal transduction systems, mainly G_i and G_o proteins.[171] Stimulation of the AT_2R leads to the activation of various phosphatases, resulting in the inactivation of extracellular signal-regulated kinase (ERK), the opening of K^+ channels, and the inhibition of T-type Ca^{2+} channels. The AT_2R has a higher affinity for Ang III than Ang II; indeed, Ang III may be the preferred ligand for the AT_2R, exerting its natriuretic effect in the kidney.[163] Whereas AT_1R causes increased ion transport, vasoconstriction, inflammation, and immunity and decreased longevity, AT_2R mediates antiproliferative effects, apoptosis, differentiation, and possibly vasodilatation, offering therapeutic targets for the treatment of cardiovascular diseases.[172] An increase in the expression of AT_1R and a decrease in the expression of AT_2R are associated with increased hypertensive renal injury in rodents.[173]

Gene Targeting of Angiotensin Receptors

Additional support of the importance of the RAS in the kidney in the regulation of blood pressure comes from renal cross-transplantation studies in mice with or without the AT_1R gene.[174] The deletion of AT_1R gene in the renal proximal tubule of mice also decreases basal blood pressure and response to exogenous Ang II.[175]

Other Angiotensin Receptors

In addition to AT_1R and AT_2R, there are three other angiotensin receptors (i.e., AT_4R, Mas1, and MrgD)[1-6,46] and possibly a fourth one, AT_3R.

The AT_3R represents an angiotensin-binding site identified in a mouse neuroblastoma cell line.[176] The AT_3R has a high affinity for Ang II but a low affinity for Ang III. An AT_3R was cloned from the rat adrenal cortex.[159] However, its existence in humans has not been shown.[177]

The AT_4R is an angiotensin-binding site with a high affinity for Ang IV.[177,178] Unlike the AT_1R and AT_2R, the AT_4R is a class II receptor and has one transmembrane domain[162] and is not coupled to heterotrimeric G proteins. AT_4R has been identified as IRAP.[177-179] Human IRAP is in chromosome 5q21.[180] However, IRAP may not be the only receptor for Ang IV.[177,181]

Mas1 receptor, encoded by *MAS1,* has been identified as the receptor for Ang 1-7.[6,37,182] The human *MAS1* is located at chromosome 6q25.3-q26.[162] As aforementioned, Ang 1-7 can also activate the MrgD receptor (see below).[46,111] Ang 1-7 has kinin-like effects that are transduced by the Mas1 receptor, apparently because of heterodimerizaton of Mas1 with the bradykinin 2 receptor (B_2R).[6,183] The ability of Ang 1-7 to inhibit noradrenergic neurotransmission[184] and stimulate nitric oxide production may be due to stimulation of B_2R.[6,185] Ang 1-7 may also stimulate the production of prostaglandins, via Mas1.[41]

Human *MRGD* is a single copy gene located in chromosome 11q13.3.[162,186] As aforementioned, it belongs to the G protein-coupled receptor family with seven transmembrane domains. MrgD is a receptor for both alamandine[2,4,111] and Ang 1-7.[6,47,187] Alamandine increases NO production[111] whereas Ang 1-7 increases arachidonic acid synthesis.[47] MrgD couples to Gq/11 and pertussis toxin (PTX)-sensitive Gi/o proteins.[186,188] MrgD-deficient mice have been generated,[187] but their blood pressure phenotype has not been reported. However, in the two-kidney, one-clipped kidney model, the intravenous infusion of alamandine initially increases blood pressure, via the AT_1R, and subsequently decreases blood pressure, via MrgD.[189] By contrast, alamandine increases the blood pressure in normotensive rats.[189] The hypotensive effect of alamandine injected into the caudal ventrolateral medulla may be via the Mas1 and AT_2R.[190]

(Pro)Renin Receptor

The discovery of the PRR adds another layer of complexity to the understanding of the scope and extent of the RAAS. PRR is a receptor for both renin and prorenin.[1,191] Circulating levels of prorenin are 10 times higher than levels of renin. The PRR, so called because it binds to renin and prorenin, regulates intracellular profibrotic and cyclooxygenase genes independent of Ang II. The binding affinity of prorenin for the PRR is two to three times the affinity of renin for the PRR.[192] The PRR has catalytic (generation of Ang II) and non-catalytic signal transduction effects (which lead to hypertension and glomerulosclerosis). Furthermore, the myriad of intracellular signaling pathways mediated by this receptor may hold the key to the mechanisms underlying important developmental processes and the progression of diseases, such as hypertension and diabetes.[191] For example, ablation of the prorenin *ATP6ap2* gene results in embryonic lethality.[192,193] By associating with vacuolar H^+-ATPase, the PRR is essential for the Wnt/β catenin signaling molecular pathways, now known to be responsible for neural and renal embryonic development (see Fig. 11.1).[194–198]

Whole body overexpression of human PRR in mice causes slowly progressive glomerulosclerosis that is independent of tissue Ang II.[198] Inducible renal-tubular specific knockout of PRR in mice does not change basal blood pressure. However, the absence of renal tubular PRR promotes sodium wasting and attenuates the hypertensive response to Ang II. PRR, via direct prorenin/renin stimulation of PKA/Akt-dependent pathways, stimulates ENaC activity in the collecting duct.[199] A similar renal tubular-specific deletion of PRR in another strain of mice has no effect on the RAS but the mice have renal concentration defect and distal renal tubular acidosis, caused by impaired V-ATPase activity.[200] Low concentrations (nM) of prorenin increase ENaC activity that is not affected by AT_1R blockade in cultured mouse medullary collecting ducts cells and microdissected renal collecting ducts.[201] The specificity of these studies has been questioned because the concentrations of prorenin used is much higher than the EC50 for renin.[202] Nevertheless, renal collecting duct-selective silencing of PRR or renin similarly blunts the Ang II-mediated increase in urinary renin activity and the increase in ENaC, relative to control floxed mice.[203,204] The silencing of PRR in the subfornical organ of the brain attenuates Ang II-induced hypertension in human renin-angiotensinogen double-transgenic mice and prevents deoxycorticosterone acetate/salt-induced hypertension by inhibiting brain Ang II formation.[205] The intracerebroventricular infusion of a PRR antagonist also prevents prorenin-induced hypertension in C57Bl6/J mice.[206] The hypertension mediated by brain PRR also may be related to an increased sodium appetite.[207]

Physiologic Effects of Angiotensin II

Via the Ang II Type 1 Receptor

Ang II exerts most of its effects via the AT_1R.[1–6,46] Ang II has pleiotropic actions,[208] including direct and indirect vasopressor effects. In response to sodium depletion, hypotension, or hypovolemia, Ang II synthesis is increased, which causes immediate vasoconstriction of arteries and veins, and activates the sympathetic nervous system, increasing peripheral vascular resistance and venous return, respectively, and raising blood pressure. The effect of Ang II on blood pressure secondary to increased ion transport by the renal tubule and intestines is more gradual. Ang II increases sodium and chloride reabsorption directly in several segments of the nephron. In the proximal tubule, low concentrations of Ang II play a central role in ion transport by increasing the activity of renal tubular luminal NHE3, Na-glucose cotransporter,[209] sodium phosphate cotransporter (NaPi-II),[210] and basolateral Na^+,K^+-ATPase[211,212] and Na^+-HCO_3^- cotransporter.[213] AT_1R stimulates NHE3[214–217] but not NHE2[217] activity in brush-border membranes of renal proximal tubules. High concentrations of Ang II can inhibit proximal tubule sodium transport via the stimulation of PLA2- and cytochrome P450–dependent metabolites of arachidonic acid.[213,217–222] Ang II also affects ion transport in the medullary thick ascending limb of the loop of Henle in a biphasic manner.[223] In this nephron segment, low concentrations of Ang II increase sodium, potassium, and chloride transport by stimulating NHE3 and Na^+,K^+, $2Cl^-$ cotransporter activities.[223] The inositol 1,4,5-trisphosphate receptor-binding protein released with inositol 1,4,5-trisphosphate is important in the stimulatory effect of Ang II on ion transport in renal proximal tubules.[224] Ang II stimulates NHE1 activity in the macula densa.[225] Ang II also stimulates ENaC activity in the collecting duct[226–228] and NHE2 in the distal convoluted tubule, but not in the proximal tubule.[217] Ang II also stimulates water transport in the collecting duct by regulating aquaporin II.[229] All of these effects are mediated by the AT_1R.

Via the Ang II Type 2 Receptor

The role of the AT_2R in influencing sodium transport is not well established. AT_2R inhibits sodium transport. As mentioned previously, the natriuresis mediated by the AT_2R occurs because of its interaction with Ang III.[163] AT_2R is coupled to the sodium/hydrogen exchanger type 6 (NHE6),[230] but NHE6 is not involved in renal tubular sodium reabsorption.[231] Ang 1-7 has been reported to inhibit Na^+,K^+-ATPase in pig outer cortical nephrons[232] and Na^+-HCO_3^- exchanger in mouse renal proximal tubules.[233] However, an increase in sodium transport via the AT_2R in rat proximal tubules has also been reported.[234] These discrepancies may be related to the condition of the animal. For example, AT_2R inhibits Na^+/K^+-ATPase activity in renal proximal tubules of obese, but not lean, rats[235] and during AT_1R blockade.[236] In human renal proximal tubule cells, the relatively low expression of AT_2R is increased with its heterodimerization with the dopamine D_1 receptor (D_1R). This results in a cooperative increase in cyclic adenosine monophosphate (cAMP) and cGMP production, protein phosphatase 2A activation, Na^+/K^+-ATPase internalization, and sodium transport inhibition.[237] The ability of Ang II to increase NO production via the AT_2R has been shown to be the mechanism by which Ang II can decrease sodium transport in rat thick ascending limb[238] and renal proximal tubule cells.[239]

Indirect Effects

Ang II indirectly increases sodium transport, partly by stimulating the synthesis of aldosterone in the zona glomerulosa of the adrenal cortex. Aldosterone increases ENaC activity by inducing the transcription of α-ENaC and redistribution of α-ENaC in the connecting tubule and collecting duct from a cytoplasmic to an apical location. However, Ang II can stimulate the expression of α, β, and γ ENaC independent of aldosterone.[240] Aldosterone also activates Na^+/K^+-ATPase in the basolateral membrane of the principal cells of the collecting duct. Aldosterone, similar to Ang II, can act in an autocrine and paracrine manner. Aldosterone has been reported to be produced by aldosterone-producing cells other than the adrenal glomerulosa, such as neuronal glial cells and cardiac myocytes.[241] Aldosterone can also stimulate NHE1 activity in the renal proximal tubule of spontaneously hypertensive (SHR), but not normotensive Wistar-Kyoto rats.[130] Aldosterone and Ang II may act in ligand-independent ways to affect cell signaling, cell–cell communication, and growth. Some components of the RAS may have effects opposite to those of aldosterone and among the products of the RAS and their receptors.[242] Although the AT_1R can be stimulated by stretch, independent of Ang II,[243,244] Ang II can have intracellular effects independent of the AT_1R.[245] The effects of the Ang II metabolites on sodium transport are described in the Ang II metabolites section.

Regulators of the Intrarenal Renin-Angiotensin System

The renal RAS is under tight control by a complex network of both positive and negative regulators. The positive regulators include Wnt/β-catenin and prostaglandin E2 receptor 4 pathways. The negative regulators included fibroblast growth factor 23/Klotho, vitamin D receptor, and liver X receptor.[1]

Ontogeny

Development of the Renin-Angiotensin System: Structure of the Kidney and Urinary Tract

Postnatal Changes in Renin-Angiotensin-Aldosterone System Structure and Function in Humans

Studies in Humans

In humans, Ang-related genes are activated at stage 11 of the developing embryo,[246] which corresponds to 23 to 24 days of gestation. AT_1R and AT_2R are expressed very early (24 days of gestation), indicating that Ang II may play a role in organogenesis. Whereas the AT_1R is expressed in the glomeruli, the AT_2R is found in the undifferentiated mesonephros that surrounds the primitive tubules and glomeruli. The AT_2R is maximally expressed at about 8 weeks of gestation followed by decreasing but persistent expression until about 20 weeks of gestation.[247] At stages 12 to 13, which corresponds to 25 to 30 days of gestation, angiotensinogen is expressed in the proximal part of the primitive tubule, and renin is expressed in glomeruli and juxtaglomerular arterioles. ACE is detected in the mesonephric tubules at stage 14. By 30 to 35 days, all components of the RAAS are expressed in the human embryonic mesonephros. Expression of these proteins in the future collecting system occurs later, at about 8 weeks of gestation.

ACE has a role in fetal growth and development. ACE inhibitor-induced fetopathy, consisting of oligohydramnios, intrauterine growth restriction (IUGR), hypocalvaria, renal dysplasia, anuria, and death, has been described in mothers exposed to ACE inhibitors during the second and third trimesters of pregnancy.[248] These effects were initially believed to arise from a decrease in organ perfusion.[249] More recent evidence indicates that ACE inhibition has teratogenic effects during development. Fetuses exposed to ACE inhibitors during the first trimester have an increased risk of congenital malformations, with an incidence of 7.1%, compared with those with no maternal exposure to antihypertensive medications during the same time period. The congenital anomalies are major and include cardiovascular defects, such as atrial septal defect, patent ductus arteriosus, ventricular septal defect, and pulmonary stenosis; skeletal malformations, including polydactyly, upper limb defects, and craniofacial anomalies; gastrointestinal malformations, such as pyloric stenosis and intestinal atresia; central nervous system malformations, such as hydrocephalus, spina bifida, and microcephaly; and genitourinary malformations, including renal malformations.[250] Angiotensin receptor blockers (ARBs) have also been reported to be fetotoxic.[251] Inhibition of the activity of the RAAS in pregnancy may have effects on the fetus that manifest later on in life, such as hypertension, which are addressed later.

The expression patterns of the RAS components in the embryonic kidney are similar in rodents and humans.[246,252] In rodents, mutations of genes encoding renin, angiotensinogen, ACE, or the AT_1R are associated with skull ossification defects,[253] as well as autosomal recessive renal tubular dysgenesis.[254–256] AT_1R-deficient mice do not develop renal pelves.[254] AT_2R-deficient mice have congenital abnormalities of the kidney and urinary tract, such as multicystic dysplastic and aplastic kidneys.[256] The more dramatic phenotypes seen in mice with deficient AT_2R compared with humans with similar defects are attributed to the fact that human nephrogenesis is completed in utero, but morphogenesis of rodent nephrons continues for up to 10 days after birth. However, the phenotypes of AT_1R gene *(Agtr1/AGTR1)* deficiency are similar in rodents and humans. As indicated earlier, mutations in Ang-related genes in humans are associated with renal tubular dysgenesis[255] characterized by early onset and persistent fetal anuria leading to oligohydramnios and the Potter sequence. Whereas increased renin production is noted in the kidneys of patients with mutations in the genes encoding angiotensinogen, ACE, or AT_1R, the effect of defects in the human renin gene *(REN)* on renin production is variable with loss-of-function mutation associated with absence of renin production, and *REN* missense mutations are associated with increased renin production.[257] These studies demonstrate the importance of the RAAS in the development and maturation of the kidneys and collecting systems.[258] The importance of the PRR in embryonic development has been discussed previously.

Postnatal Changes in Renin-Angiotensin-Aldosterone System Structure and Function in Humans

The RAAS is more active in the neonatal period and infancy than later in childhood.[259] Plasma renin activity and plasma aldosterone levels are markedly increased in preterm human infants in the first 3 weeks of life.[260] Although fetal ACE levels remain stable during gestation in rats,[261] serum ACE activity has been reported by some to be higher in late fetal than in early neonatal life in humans,[261–263] lambs, and guinea pigs.[264,265] By contrast, renal ACE activity may increase with age, at least in pigs and horses.[266,267] A similar pattern may be found in humans, based on the measurement of urine ACE isoforms.[268] One study reported that plasma Ang II levels are similar among human infants with normal and low birth weights. However, at 7 days of life, plasma Ang II levels are markedly increased in very low birth weight infants.[269] Small for gestational age boys (8–13 years) may have increased circulating Ang II and ACE activity relative to those with birth weights appropriate for gestational age.[270] High serum aldosterone levels are seen at 2 hours of age and gradually decrease over the first year of life.[271]

Unconventional Behavior of Renin-Angiotensin System Components

Although the canonical scheme of activation of the RAS components from renin to Ang II and its effects on Ang receptors is well recognized, recent evidence of other effects merits discussion. Both Ang I and Ang II may lead to effects that are independent of, or even antagonistic to, the accepted effects of the RAS.[242] ACE may also function as a "receptor" that initiates intracellular signaling and influences gene expression.[272] AT_1R and AT_2R have been shown to form heterodimers with other 7-transmembrane receptors and to influence signal transduction pathways with physiologic and pathologic consequences.[237,273–277] For example, the high glucose-induced dimerization between adiponectin and AT_1R leads to tubulointerstitial injury.[278]

Intracellular Ang II affects cell communication, cell growth, and gene expression via the AT_1R, but also has RAS-related independent effects.[243,244,279]

Fetal Programming for Hypertension: Failure of Renoprotection?

The association of low birth weight with the development of hypertension later in life has been validated epidemiologically[280] and, more recently, has been demonstrated experimentally in animal models.[281] A suboptimal fetal environment may lead to maladaptive responses, including failure of renal autoregulation and the development of hypertension. A reduction in nephron number during development may contribute to a reduction in the glomerular filtration rate, but this is not always borne out in experimental studies. Multiple factors may contribute to the development of hypertension, but this chapter is restricted to the role of renal mechanisms. The RAAS may play a more important role than other factors because it is expressed early and is associated with nephrogenesis. Blockade of the AT_1R during the nephrogenic period after birth in rats led to a decrease in nephron number, a reduction in renal function, and hypertension.[282] The consequences of impairment of the RAS in utero and during development have been discussed earlier. Protein-restricted diets have also been shown to increase ACE levels in pregnant ewes.[283] A general stimulation of all components of the systemic RAS, in response to protein restriction, is blocked by treatment with an ACE inhibitor or an ARB. Thus, the adverse environment in utero, which programs the fetus to develop hypertension, could be critically linked to abnormalities in the RAS.[284] There are sex differences in fetal programming that may be related to hormonal milieu, which affect the RAS, with testosterone having a permissive effect and estrogen having a protective effect.[285] A high fructose diet in pregnant Sprague-Dawley rats also increases blood pressure and aggravates the increase in blood pressure caused by a high-salt diet in male offspring that may involve the RAS.[286,287] Other aspects of fetal programming and the effect on blood pressure have been recently reviewed.[288]

Clinical Aspects

As discussed earlier, the development of the kidney occurs during the first 35 days postconception in humans. The integrity of the RAAS is essential for normal development, and Ang II is essential for normal structural development of the kidney and collecting system. The excretory function of the kidney begins soon after clamping of the umbilical cord at birth. It follows that the neonate is exquisitely sensitive to stressors, which activate the RAAS and lead to profound oligoanuric states. Disruption of the production or action of Ang II by genetic manipulation or pharmacologic blockade results in renal tubular agenesis and anemia in fetuses. More recently, the recognition of ACE2 as an important player in vasodilation by generation of alternative metabolites of Ang II has led to the discovery that blunting of the ACE2 effect is responsible for the postural orthostatic tachycardia syndrome—a syndrome of widespread vasoconstriction.[51] This is probably the first human illness that is directly related to ACE2 and is applicable to the wider field of disordered vasoregulation, extending to fetal and neonatal life.[51] The recognition of the importance of the PRR in hypertension has paved the way for the use of new antihypertensive drugs based on their ability to block the PRR.[191,289] Ischemia and asphyxia generate renin by sympathetic stimulation. Drugs, such as furosemide, that increase distal delivery of sodium and water, decrease NKCC2 activity and should decrease renin secretion. However, decreased cotransporter activity impairs tubuloglomerular feedback and in the face of continued ion and water excretion may result in hypovolemia and activation of the RAS, which may result in oliguria. Indomethacin, and to a lesser extent ibuprofen, which is used to treat patent ductus arteriosus in neonates, could lead to decreased renal blood flow and renal insufficiency.[290,291] Congenital abnormalities in steroid synthesis that lead to deficiencies in aldosterone production cause profound salt wasting.[292] In type 1 pseudohypoaldosteronism, mutations in ENaC cause profound neonatal salt wasting.[293] To counter the heightened activity of the RAAS in neonates, adenosine receptor antagonists may offer new avenues of therapy. The association between maternal ACE inhibition and renal abnormalities in fetuses has been described earlier in this chapter. Recent observations of increased fetal renin levels in hydronephrosis lend credence to the developmental significance of an intact RAAS in developing embryos.[294] Preterm birth alters the development of the RAAS that can result in deleterious consequences.[295] However, ACE2 may have a protective role in the heart and kidney.[296]

In summary, the RAAS is an important developmental and physiologic system, which is involved in many aspects of renal function and blood pressure regulation. Moreover, drugs that interfere with the RAAS, given to developing fetuses, can program the development of renal abnormalities and hypertension. In addition to genetics, epigenetics, paternal and maternal nutrition, and health-related activities affect the development of the RAAS. A better understanding of these mechanisms would translate to better care for premature and full-term newborns with renal dysregulation, hyponatremia, and oligoanuric renal failure.

REFERENCES

1. Yang T, Xu C. Physiology and pathophysiology of the intrarenal renin-angiotensin system: an update. *J Am Soc Nephrol.* 2017;28(4):1040–1049.
2. Li XC, Zhang J, Zhuo JL. The vasoprotective axes of the renin-angiotensin system: physiological relevance and therapeutic implications in cardiovascular, hypertensive and kidney diseases. *Pharmacol Res.* 2017;125(Pt A):21–38.
3. Te Riet L, van Esch JH, Roks AJ, et al. Hypertension: renin-angiotensin-aldosterone system alterations. *Circ Res.* 2015;116(6):960–975.
4. Aroor AR, Demarco VG, Jia G, et al. The role of tissue Renin-Angiotensin-aldosterone system in the development of endothelial dysfunction and arterial stiffness. *Front Endocrinol (Lausanne).* 2013;4:161.
5. Etelvino GM, Peluso AA, Santos RA. New components of the renin-angiotensin system: alamandine and the MAS-related G protein-coupled receptor D. *Curr Hypertens Rep.* 2014;16(6):433.
6. McKinney CA, Fattah C, Loughrey CM, et al. Angiotensin-(1-7) and angiotensin-(1-9): function in cardiac and vascular remodelling. *Clin Sci.* 2014;126(12):815–827.
7. Gonzalez AA, Cifuentes-Araneda F, Ibaceta-Gonzalez C, et al. Vasopressin/V2 receptor stimulates renin synthesis in the collecting duct. *Am J Physiol Renal Physiol.* 2016;310(4):F284–F293.
8. Ramkumar N, Kohan DE. Role of the collecting duct renin angiotensin system in regulation of blood pressure and renal function. *Curr Hypertens Rep.* 2016;18(4):29.
9. Krieger MH, Moreira ED, Oliveira EM, et al. Dissociation of blood pressure and sympathetic activation of renin release in sinoaortic-denervated rats. *Clin Exp Pharmacol Physiol.* 2006;33(5–6):471–476.
10. Schweda F, Segerer F, Castrop H, et al. Blood pressure-dependent inhibition of renin secretion requires A1 adenosine receptors. *Hypertension.* 2005;46(4):780–786.
11. Seghers F, Yerna X, Zanou N, et al. TRPV4 participates in pressure-induced inhibition of renin secretion by juxtaglomerular cells. *J Physiol.* 2016;594(24):7327–7340.
12. Milavec-Krizman M, Evenou JP, Wagner H, et al. Characterization of beta-adrenoceptor subtypes in rat kidney with new highly selective beta 1 blockers and their role in renin release. *Biochem Pharmacol.* 1985;34(22):3951–3957.

11

13. DiBona GF. Neural regulation of renal tubular sodium reabsorption and renin secretion. *Fed Proc.* 1985;44(13):2816–2822.

14. Goldsmith SR. Interactions between the sympathetic nervous system and the RAAS in heart failure. *Curr Heart Fail Rep.* 2004;1(2):45–50.

15. Schweda F. Salt feedback on the renin-angiotensin-aldosterone system. *Pflugers Arch.* 2015;467(3):565–576.

16. Schnermann J, Briggs JP. Tubular control of renin synthesis and secretion. *Pflugers Arch.* 2013;465(1):39–51.

17. Bai J, Chow BK. Secretin is involved in sodium conservation through the renin-angiotensin-aldosterone system. *FASEB J.* 2017;31(4):1689–1697.

18. Krämer BK, Ritthaler T, Schweda F, et al. Effects of hypoxia on renin secretion and renal renin gene expression. *Kidney Int Suppl.* 1998;67:S155–S158.

19. Liu YH, Lu M, Xie ZZ, et al. Hydrogen sulfide prevents heart failure development via inhibition of renin release from mast cells in isoproterenol-treated rats. *Antioxid Redox Signal.* 2014;20(5):759–769.

20. Lu H, Cassis LA, Kooi CW, Daugherty A. Structure and functions of angiotensinogen. *Hypertens Res.* 2016;39(7):492–500.

21. Markus MA, Goy C, Adams DJ, et al. Renin enhancer is crucial for full response in renin expression to an in vivo stimulus. *Hypertension.* 2007;50(5):933–938.

22. Weiland F, Verspohl EJ. Local formation of angiotensin peptides with paracrine activity by adipocytes. *J Pept Sci.* 2009;15(11):767–776.

23. Danser AH, van den Dorpel MA, Deinum J, et al. Renin, prorenin, and immunoreactive renin in vitreous fluid from eyes with and without diabetic retinopathy. *J Clin Endocrinol Metab.* 1989;68(1):160–167.

24. Mackins CJ, Kano S, Seyedi N, et al. Cardiac mast cell-derived renin promotes local angiotensin formation, norepinephrine release, and arrhythmias in ischemia/reperfusion. *J Clin Invest.* 2006;116(4):1063–1070.

25. Itskovitz J, Sealey JE, Glorioso N, et al. Plasma prorenin response to human chorionic gonadotropin in ovarian-hyperstimulated women: correlation with the number of ovarian follicles and steroid hormone concentrations. *Proc Natl Acad Sci USA.* 1987;84(20):7285–7289.

26. Leung PS, Sernia C. The renin-angiotensin system and male reproduction: new functions for old hormones. *J Mol Endocrinol.* 2003;30(3):263–270.

27. Sealey JE, Goldstein M, Pitarresi T, et al. Prorenin secretion from human testis: no evidence for secretion of active renin or angiotensinogen. *J Clin Endocrinol Metab.* 1988;66(5):974–978.

28. Nielsen AH, Schauser KH, Poulsen K. Current topic: the uteroplacental renin-angiotensin system. *Placenta.* 2000;21(5–6):468–477.

29. Lumbers ER, Wang Y, Delforce SJ, et al. Decidualisation of human endometrial stromal cells is associated with increased expression and secretion of prorenin. *Reprod Biol Endocrinol.* 2015;13:129.

30. van Thiel BS, Góes Martini A, Te Riet L, et al. Brain Renin-angiotensin system: does it exist? *Hypertension.* 2017;69(6):1136–1144.

31. Niimura F, Okubo S, Fogo A, Ichikawa I. Temporal and spatial expression pattern of the angiotensinogen gene in mice and rats. *Am J Physiol.* 1997;272(1 Pt 2):R142–R147.

32. Agassandian K, Grobe JL, Liu X, et al. Evidence for intraventricular secretion of angiotensinogen and angiotensin by the subfornical organ using transgenic mice. *Am J Physiol Regul Integr Comp Physiol.* 2017;312(6):R973–R998.

33. Gavras I, Gavras H. Angiotensin II as a cardiovascular risk factor. *J Hum Hypertens.* 2002;16(suppl 2):S2–S6.

34. Danilczyk U, Penninger JM. Angiotensin-converting enzyme II in the heart and kidney. *Circ Res.* 2006;98(4):463–471.

35. Deleted in review.

36. Speth RC, Vento PJ, Carrera EJ, et al. Acute repeated intracerebroventricular injections of angiotensin II reduce agonist and antagonist radioligand binding in the paraventricular nucleus of the hypothalamus and median preoptic nucleus in the rat brain. *Brain Res.* 2014;1583:132–140.

37. Patel VB, Basu R, Oudit GY. ACE2/Ang 1-7 axis: A critical regulator of epicardial adipose tissue inflammation and cardiac dysfunction in obesity. *Adipocyte.* 2016;5(3):306–311.

38. Yvan-Charvet L, Quignard-Boulangé A. Role of adipose tissue renin-angiotensin system in metabolic and inflammatory diseases associated with obesity. *Kidney Int.* 2011;79(2):162–168.

39. Becari C, Teixeira FR, Oliveira EB, Salgado MC. Angiotensin-converting enzyme inhibition augments the expression of rat elastase-2, an angiotensin II-forming enzyme. *Am J Physiol Heart Circ Physiol.* 2011;301:H565–H570.

40. Ribeiro AA, Palomino Z, Lima MP, et al. Characterization of the renal renin-angiotensin system in transgenic mice that express rat tonin. *J Renin Angiotensin Aldosterone Syst.* 2015;16(4):947–955.

41. Laxton RC, Hu Y, Duchene J, et al. A role of matrix metalloproteinase-8 in atherosclerosis. *Circ Res.* 2009;105(9):921–929.

42. Mackins CJ, Kano S, Seyedi N, et al. Cardiac mast cell-derived renin promotes local angiotensin formation, norepinephrine release, and arrhythmias in ischemia/reperfusion. *J Clin Invest.* 2006;116(4):1063–1070.

43. Wei CC, Hase N, Inoue Y, et al. Mast cell chymase limits the cardiac efficacy of Ang I-converting enzyme inhibitor therapy in rodents. *J Clin Invest.* 2010;120(4):1229–1239.

44. Stone C Jr, Brown NJ. Angiotensin-converting enzyme inhibitor and other drug-associated angioedema. *Immunol Allergy Clin North Am.* 2017;37(3):483–495.

45. Mizuiri S, Ohashi Y. ACE and ACE2 in kidney disease. *World J Nephrol.* 2015;4(1):74–82.
46. Hrenak J, Paulis L, Simko F. Angiotensin A/alamandine/MrgD axis: another clue to understanding cardiovascular pathophysiology. *Int J Mol Sci.* 2016;17(7):pii: E1098.
47. Gembardt F, Grajewski S, Vahl M, et al. Angiotensin metabolites can stimulate receptors of the Mas-related genes family. *Mol Cell Biochem.* 2008;319(1–2):115–123.
48. Yamamuro M, Yoshimura M, Nakayama M, et al. Aldosterone, but not angiotensin II, reduces angiotensin converting enzyme 2 gene expression levels in cultured neonatal rat cardiomyocytes. *Circ J.* 2008;72(8):1346–1350.
49. Santos SH, Braga JF, Mario EG, et al. Improved lipid and glucose metabolism in transgenic rats with increased circulating angiotensin-(1–7). *Arterioscler Thromb Vasc Biol.* 2010;30:953–961.
50. Donoghue M, Hsieh F, Baronas E, et al. A novel angiotensin-converting enzyme-related carboxy-peptidase (ACE2) converts angiotensin I to angiotensin 1-9. *Circ Res.* 2000;87(5):E1–E9.
51. Stewart JM, Ocon AJ, Clarke D, et al. Defects in cutaneous angiotensin-converting enzyme 2 and angiotensin-(1-7) production in postural tachycardia syndrome. *Hypertension.* 2009;53(5):767–774.
52. Ferrario CM. ACE2: more of Ang-(1-7) or less Ang II? *Curr Opin Nephrol Hypertens.* 2011;20(1):1–6.
53. Galandrin S, Denis C, Boularan C, et al. Cardioprotective angiotensin-(1-7) peptide acts as a natural-biased ligand at the angiotensin II type 1 receptor. *Hypertension.* 2016;68(6):1365–1374.
54. Chu PL, Le TH. Role of collectrin, an ACE2 homologue, in blood pressure homeostasis. *Curr Hypertens Rep.* 2014;16(11):490.
55. Boschmann M, Jordan J, Adams F, et al. Tissue-specific response to interstitial angiotensin II in humans. *Hypertension.* 2003;41(1):37–41.
56. Jackman HL1, Massad MG, Sekosan M, et al. Angiotensin 1-9 and 1-7 release in human heart: role of cathepsin A. *Hypertension.* 2002;39(5):976–981.
57. Richard V, Hurel-Merle S, Scalbert E, et al. Functional evidence for a role of vascular chymase in the production of angiotensin II in isolated human arteries. *Circulation.* 2001;104(7):750–752.
58. Snyder RA, Watt KW, Wintroub BU. A human platelet angiotensin I-processing system. Identification of components and inhibition of angiotensin-converting enzyme by product. *J Biol Chem.* 1985;260(13):7857–7860.
59. Ocaranza MP, Godoy I, Jalil JE, et al. Enalapril attenuates downregulation of angiotensin-converting enzyme 2 in the late phase of ventricular dysfunction in myocardial infracted heart. *Hypertension.* 2006;48(4):572–578.
60. Ocaranza MP, Lavandero S, Jalil JE, et al. Angiotensin-(1-9) regulates cardiac hypertrophy in vivo and in vitro. *J Hypertens.* 2010;28(5):1054–1064.
61. Kramkowski K, Mogielnicki A, Leszczynska A, et al. Angiotensin-(1-9), the product of angiotensin I conversion in platelets, enhances arterial thrombosis in rats. *J Physiol Pharmacol.* 2010;61(3):317–324.
62. Kucharewicz I, Pawlak R, Matys T, et al. Antithrombotic effect of captopril and losartan is mediated by angiotensin-(1-7). *Hypertension.* 2002;40(5):774–779.
63. Massiéra F, Bloch-Faure M, Ceiler D, et al. Adipose angiotensinogen is involved in adipose tissue growth and blood pressure regulation. *FASEB J.* 2001;15(14):2727–2729.
64. Lu H, Boustany-Kari CM, Daugherty A, et al. Angiotensin II increases adipose angiotensinogen expression. *Am J Physiol Endocrinol Metab.* 2007;292(5):E1280–E1287.
65. Patel VB, Basu R, Oudit GY. ACE2/Ang 1-7 axis: A critical regulator of epicardial adipose tissue inflammation and cardiac dysfunction in obesity. *Adipocyte.* 2016;(3):306–311.
66. Velez JC, Ryan KJ, Harbeson CE, et al. Angiotensin I is largely converted to angiotensin (1-7) and angiotensin (2-10) by isolated rat glomeruli. *Hypertension.* 2009;53(5):790–797.
67. Singh R, Singh AK, Alavi N, et al. Mechanism of increased angiotensin II levels in glomerular mesangial cells cultured in high glucose. *J Am Soc Nephrol.* 2003;14(4):873–880.
68. Velez JC, Bland AM, Arthur JM, et al. Characterization of renin-angiotensin system enzyme activities in cultured mouse podocytes. *Am J Physiol Renal Physiol.* 2007;293(1):F398–F407.
69. Wennmann DO, Hsu HH, Pavenstädt H. The renin-angiotensin-aldosterone system in podocytes. *Semin Nephrol.* 2012;32(4):377–384.
70. Satou R, Shao W, Navar LG. Role of stimulated intrarenal angiotensinogen in hypertension. *Ther Adv Cardiovasc Dis.* 2015;9(4):181–190.
71. Rohrwasser A, Morgan T, Dillon HF, et al. Elements of a paracrine tubular renin-angiotensin system along the entire nephron. *Hypertension.* 1999;34(6):1265–1274.
72. Reinhold SW, Krüger B, Barner C, et al. Nephron-specific expression of components of the renin-angiotensin-aldosterone system in the mouse kidney. *J Renin Angiotensin Aldosterone Syst.* 2012;13(1):46–55.
73. Advani A, Kelly DJ, Cox AJ, et al. The (Pro)renin receptor: site-specific and functional linkage to the vacuolar H+-ATPase in the kidney. *Hypertension.* 2009;54(2):261–269.
74. Gonzalez AA, Prieto MC. Roles of collecting duct renin and (pro)renin receptor in hypertension: mini review. *Ther Adv Cardiovasc Dis.* 2015;9(4):191–200.
75. Kobori H, Nishiyama A, Harrison-Bernard LM, et al. Urinary angiotensinogen as an indicator of intrarenal angiotensin status in hypertension. *Hypertension.* 2003;41(1):42–49.
76. Matsusaka T, Niimura F, Shimizu A, et al. Liver angiotensinogen is the primary source of renal angiotensin II. *J Am Soc Nephrol.* 2012;23(7):1181–1189.
77. Li XC, Zhuo JL. Recent updates on the proximal tubule renin-angiotensin system in angiotensin II-dependent hypertension. *Curr Hypertens Rep.* 2016;18(8):63.
78. Schulz WW, Hagler HK, Buja LM, et al. Ultrastructural localization of angiotensin I-converting enzyme (EC 3.4.15.1) and neutral metalloendopeptidase (EC 3.4.24.11) in the proximal tubule of the human kidney. *Lab Invest.* 1988;59(6):789–797.

79. Bader M. Tissue renin-angiotensin-aldosterone systems: targets for pharmacological therapy. *Annu Rev Pharmacol Toxicol*. 2010;50:439–465.

80. De Mello WC. Local renin angiotensin aldosterone systems and cardiovascular diseases. *Med Clin North Am*. 2017;101(1):117–127.

81. Lavrentyev EN, Estes AM, Malik KU. Mechanism of high glucose induced angiotensin II production in rat vascular smooth muscle cells. *Circ Res*. 2007;101(5):455–464.

82. Pereira HJ, Souza LL, Costa-Neto CM, et al. Carboxypeptidases A1 and A2 from the perfusate of rat mesenteric arterial bed differentially process angiotensin peptides. *Peptides*. 2012;33(1):67–76.

83. Yugandhar VG, Clark MA. Angiotensin III: a physiological relevant peptide of the renin angiotensin system. *Peptides*. 2013;46:26–32.

84. Bihl JC, Zhang C, Zhao Y, et al. Angiotensin-(1-7) counteracts the effects of Ang II on vascular smooth muscle cells, vascular remodeling and hemorrhagic stroke: role of the NFκB inflammatory pathway. *Vascul Pharmacol*. 2015;73:115–123.

85. Ganten D, Marquez-Julio A, Granger P, et al. Renin in dog brain. *Am J Physiol*. 1971;221(6):1733–1737.

86. van Thiel BS, Góes Martini A, Te Riet L, et al. Brain renin-angiotensin system: does it exist? *Hypertension*. 2017;69(6):1136–1144.

87. Sigmund CD, Diz DI, Chappell MC. No brain renin-angiotensin system: déjà vu all over again? *Hypertension*. 2017;69(6):1007–1010.

88. Coble JP, Grobe JL, Johnson AK, et al. Mechanisms of brain renin angiotensin system-induced drinking and blood pressure: importance of the subfornical organ. *Am J Physiol Regul Integr Comp Physiol*. 2015;308(4):R238–R249.

89. Claflin KE, Sandgren JA, Lambertz AM, et al. Angiotensin AT1A receptors on leptin receptor-expressing cells control resting metabolism. *J Clin Invest*. 2017;127(4):1414–1424.

90. Leenen F, Blaustein MP, Hamlyn J. Update on angiotensin II: new endocrine connections between the brain, adrenal glands and the cardiovascular system. *Endocr Connect*. 2017;6:R131–R145.

91. Chappell MC. Biochemical evaluation of the renin-angiotensin system: the good, bad, and absolute? *Am J Physiol Heart Circ Physiol*. 2016;310(2):H137–H152.

92. Padia SH, Howell NL, Kemp BA, et al. Intrarenal aminopeptidase N inhibition restores defective angiotensin II type 2-mediated natriuresis in spontaneously hypertensive rats. *Hypertension*. 2010;55(2):474–480.

93. Carey RM. Blood pressure and the renal actions of AT2 receptors. *Curr Hypertens Rep*. 2017;19(3):21.

94. Wong AH, Zhou D, Rini JM. The X-ray crystal structure of human aminopeptidase N reveals a novel dimer and the basis for peptide processing. *J Biol Chem*. 2012;287(44):36804–36813.

95. Park BM, Cha SA, Lee SH, Kim SH. Angiotensin IV protects cardiac reperfusion injury by inhibiting apoptosis and inflammation via AT4R in rats. *Peptides*. 2016;79:66–74.

96. Velez JC. Prolyl carboxypeptidase: a forgotten kidney angiotensinase. Focus on "Identification of prolyl carboxypeptidase as an alternative enzyme for processing of renal angiotensin II using mass spectrometry." *Am J Physiol Cell Physiol*. 2013;304(10):C939–C940.

97. Kong J, Zhang K, Meng X, et al. Dose-dependent bidirectional effect of angiotensin IV on abdominal aortic aneurysm via variable angiotensin receptor stimulation. *Hypertension*. 2015;66(3):617–626.

98. Goto Y, Hattori A, Ishii Y, et al. Enzymatic properties of human aminopeptidase A. Regulation of its enzymatic activity by calcium and angiotensin IV. *J Biol Chem*. 2006;281(33):23503–23513.

99. Dias J, Axelband F, Lara LS, et al. Is angiotensin-(3-4) (Val-Tyr), the shortest angiotensin II-derived peptide, opening new vistas on the renin-angiotensin system? *J Renin Angiotensin Aldosterone Syst*. 2017;18(1):1470320316689338.

100. Jankowski V, Vanholder R, van der Giet M, et al. Mass-spectrometric identification of a novel angiotensin peptide in human plasma. *Arterioscler Thromb Vasc Biol*. 2007;27(2):297–302.

101. Yang R, Smolders I, Vanderheyden P, et al. Pressor and renal hemodynamic effects of the novel angiotensin A peptide are angiotensin II type 1A receptor dependent. *Hypertension*. 2011;57(5):956–964.

102. Gironacci MM, Carbajosa NA, Goldstein J, et al. Neuromodulatory role of angiotensin-(1-7) in the central nervous system. *Clin Sci*. 2013;125(2):57–65.

103. Souza ÁP, Sobrinho DB, Almeida JF, et al. Angiotensin II type 1 receptor blockade restores angiotensin-(1-7)-induced coronary vasodilation in hypertrophic rat hearts. *Clin Sci*. 2013;125(9):449–459.

104. Xue H, Zhou L, Yuan P, et al. Counteraction between angiotensin II and angiotensin-(1-7) via activating angiotensin type I and Mas receptor on rat renal mesangial cells. *Regul Pept*. 2012;177(1–3):12–20.

105. Grobe N, Weir NM, Leiva O, et al. Identification of prolyl carboxypeptidase as an alternative enzyme for processing of renal angiotensin II using mass spectrometry. *Am J Physiol Cell Physiol*. 2013;304(10):C945–C953.

106. Qaradakhi T, Apostolopoulos V, Zulli A. Angiotensin (1-7) and Alamandine: similarities and differences. *Pharmacol Res*. 2016;111:820–826.

107. Habiyakare B, Alsaadon H, Mathai ML, et al. Reduction of angiotensin A and alamandine vasoactivity in the rabbit model of atherogenesis: differential effects of alamandine and Ang(1-7). *Int J Exp Pathol*. 2014;95(4):290–295.

108. Mansoori A, Oryan S, Nematbakhsh M. Role of Mas receptor antagonist (A779) on pressure diuresis and natriuresis and renal blood flow in the absence of angiotensin II receptors type 1 and 2 in female and male rats. *J Physiol Pharmacol*. 2014;65(5):633–639.

109. Su Z, Zimpelmann J, Burns KD. Angiotensin-(1-7) inhibits angiotensin II-stimulated phosphorylation of MAP kinases in proximal tubular cells. *Kidney Int*. 2006;69(12):2212–2218.

110. Xue H, Zhou L, Yuan P, et al. Counteraction between angiotensin II and angiotensin-(1-7) via activating angiotensin type I and Mas receptor on rat renal mesangial cells. *Regul Pept*. 2012;177(1–3):12–20.

111. Lautner RQ, Villela DC, Fraga-Silva RA, et al. Discovery and characterization of alamandine: a novel component of the renin-angiotensin system. *Circ Res.* 2013;112(8):1104–1111.
112. Roks AJ, van Geel PP, Pinto YM, et al. Angiotensin-(1-7) is a modulator of the human renin-angiotensin system. *Hypertension.* 1999;34:296–301.
113. Uchiyama T, Okajima F, Mogi C, et al. Alamandine reduces leptin expression through the c-Src/p38 MAP kinase pathway in adipose tissue. *PLoS ONE.* 2017;12(6):e0178769.
114. Esteban V, Ruperez M, Sánchez-López E, et al. Angiotensin IV activates the nuclear transcription factor-kappaB and related proinflammatory genes in vascular smooth muscle cells. *Circ Res.* 2005;96(9):965–973.
115. Kong J, Zhang K, Meng X, et al. Dose-dependent bidirectional effect of angiotensin IV on abdominal aortic aneurysm via variable angiotensin receptor stimulation. *Hypertension.* 2015;66(3):617–626.
116. Lalli E, Barhanin J, Zennaro MC, Warth R. Local control of aldosterone production and primary aldosteronism. *Trends Endocrinol Metab.* 2016;27(3):123–131.
117. Kawarazaki W, Fujita T. The role of aldosterone in obesity-related hypertension. *Am J Hypertens.* 2016;29(4):415–423.
118. Bollag WB. Regulation of aldosterone synthesis and secretion. *Compr Physiol.* 2014;4(3):1017–1055.
119. Duparc C, Moreau L, Dzib JF. Mast cell hyperplasia is associated with aldosterone hypersecretion in a subset of aldosterone-producing adenomas. *J Clin Endocrinol Metab.* 2015;100(4):E550–E560.
120. Joëls M, de Kloet ER. 30 Years of the mineralocorticoid receptor: the brain mineralocorticoid receptor: a saga in three episodes. *J Endocrinol.* 2017;234(1):T49–T66.
121. Wang HW, Huang BS, Chen A, et al. Role of brain aldosterone and mineralocorticoid receptors in aldosterone-salt hypertension in rats. *Neuroscience.* 2016;314:90–105.
122. Xue B, Zhang Z, Roncari CF, et al. Aldosterone acting through the central nervous system sensitizes angiotensin II-induced hypertension. *Hypertension.* 2012;60(4):1023–1030.
123. Wright JW, Tamura-Myers E, Wilson WL, et al. Conversion of brain angiotensin II to angiotensin III is critical for pressor response in rats. *Am J Physiol Regul Integr Comp Physiol.* 2003;284(3):R725–R733.
124. Delcayre C, Swynghedauw B. Molecular mechanisms of myocardial remodeling. The role of aldosterone. *J Mol Cell Cardiol.* 2002;34(12):1577–1584.
125. Colombo L, Dalla Valle L, Fiore C, et al. Aldosterone and the conquest of land. *J Endocrinol Invest.* 2006;29(4):373–379.
126. Funder JW. Aldosterone and mineralocorticoid receptors-physiology and pathophysiology. *Int J Mol Sci.* 2017;18(5):pii: E1032.
127. Chai W, Hofland J, Jansen PM, et al. Steroidogenesis vs. steroid uptake in the heart: do corticosteroids mediate effects via cardiac mineralocorticoid receptors? *J Hypertens.* 2010;28(5):1044–1053.
128. Terker AS, Yarbrough B, Ferdaus MZ, et al. Direct and indirect mineralocorticoid effects determine distal salt transport. *J Am Soc Nephrol.* 2016;27(8):2436–2445.
129. Salyer SA, Parks J, Barati MT, et al. Aldosterone regulates Na(+), K(+) ATPase activity in human renal proximal tubule cells through mineralocorticoid receptor. *Biochim Biophys Acta.* 2013;1833(10):2143–2152.
130. Pinto V, Pinho MJ, Hopfer U, et al. Oxidative stress and the genomic regulation of aldosterone stimulated NHE1 activity in SHR renal proximal tubular cells. *Mol Cell Biochem.* 2008;310(1–2):191–201.
131. Doan TN, Gletsu N, Cole J, et al. Genetic manipulation of the renin-angiotensin system. *Curr Opin Nephrol Hypertens.* 2001;10(4):483–491.
132. Matsusaka T, Niimura F, Shimizu A, et al. Liver angiotensinogen is the primary source of renal angiotensin II. *J Am Soc Nephrol.* 2012;23(7):1181–1189.
133. Matsusaka T, Niimura F, Pastan I, et al. Podocyte injury enhances filtration of liver-derived angiotensinogen and renal angiotensin II generation. *Kidney Int.* 2014;85(5):1068–1077.
134. Sherrod M, David DR, Zhou X, et al. Glial-specific ablation of angiotensinogen lowers arterial pressure in renin and angiotensin transgenic mice. *Am J Physiol Regul Integr Comp Physiol.* 2005;289(6):R1763–R1769.
135. Schinke M, Baltatu O, Böhm M, et al. Blood pressure reduction and diabetes insipidus in transgenic rats deficient in brain angiotensinogen. *Proc Natl Acad Sci USA.* 1999;96(7):3975–3980.
136. Shinohara K, Liu X, Morgan DA, et al. Selective deletion of the brain-specific isoform of renin causes neurogenic hypertension. *Hypertension.* 2016;68:1385–1392.
137. Raff H, Gehrand A, Bruder ED, et al. Renin knockout rat: control of adrenal aldosterone and corticosterone synthesis in vitro and adrenal gene expression. *Am J Physiol Regul Integr Comp Physiol.* 2015;308(1):R73–R77.
138. Sigmund CD. Genetic manipulation of the renin-angiotensin system in the kidney. *Acta Physiol Scand.* 2001;173(1):67–73.
139. Gonzalez-Villalobos RA, Shen XZ, et al. Rediscovering ACE: novel insights into the many roles of the angiotensin-converting enzyme. *J Mol Med.* 2013;91(10):1143–1154.
140. Langheinrich M, Lee MA, Böhm M, et al. The hypertensive Ren-2 transgenic rat TGR (mREN2)27 in hypertension research. Characteristics and functional aspects. *Am J Hypertens.* 1996;9(5):506–512.
141. Ramkumar N, Kohan DE. Proximal tubule angiotensinogen modulation of arterial pressure. *Curr Opin Nephrol Hypertens.* 2013;22(1):32–36.
142. Vernerová Z, Kujal P, Kramer HJ, et al. End-organ damage in hypertensive transgenic Ren-2 rats: influence of early and late endothelin receptor blockade. *Physiol Res.* 2009;58(suppl 2):S69–S78.
143. Esther CR Jr, Howard TE, Marino EM, et al. Mice lacking angiotensin-converting enzyme have low blood pressure, renal pathology, and reduced male fertility. *Lab Invest.* 1996;74(5):953–965.

144. Bernstein KE. Views of the renin-angiotensin system: brilling, mimsy and slithy tove. *Hypertension.* 2006;47(3):509–514.

145. Martin M, Wellner A, Ossowski I, et al. Identification and quantification of inhibitors for angiotensin-converting enzyme in hypoallergenic infant milk formulas. *J Agric Food Chem.* 2008;56(15):6333–6338.

146. Cole J, Quach DL, Sundaram K, et al. Mice lacking endothelial angiotensin-converting enzyme have a normal blood pressure. *Circ Res.* 2002;90(1):87–92.

147. Yamamoto K, Ohishi M, Katsuya T, et al. Deletion of angiotensin-converting enzyme 2 accelerates pressure overload-induced cardiac dysfunction by increasing local angiotensin II. *Hypertension.* 2006;47(4):718–726.

148. Crackower MA, Sarao R, Oudit GY, et al. Angiotensin-converting enzyme 2 is an essential regulator of heart function. *Nature.* 2002;417(6891):822–828.

149. Liu Z, Huang XR, Chen HY, et al. Deletion of angiotensin-converting enzyme-2 promotes hypertensive nephropathy by targeting Smad7 for ubiquitin degradation. *Hypertension.* 2017;70:822–830.

150. Rabelo LA, Todiras M, Nunes-Souza V, et al. Genetic deletion of ACE2 induces vascular dysfunction in C57BL/6 mice: role of nitric oxide imbalance and oxidative stress. *PLoS ONE.* 2016;11(4):e0150255.

151. Sahara M, Ikutomi M, Morita T, et al. Deletion of angiotensin-converting enzyme 2 promotes the development of atherosclerosis and arterial neointima formation. *Cardiovasc Res.* 2014;101(2):236–246.

152. Shaltout HA, Figueroa JP, Rose JC, et al. Alterations in circulatory and renal angiotensin-converting enzyme and angiotensin-converting enzyme 2 in fetal programmed hypertension. *Hypertension.* 2009;53(2):404–408.

153. Hashimoto T, Perlot T, Rehman A, et al. ACE2 links amino acid malnutrition to microbial ecology and intestinal inflammation. *Nature.* 2012;487(7408):477–481.

154. Yuan L, Wang Y, Lu C, et al. Angiotensin-converting enzyme 2 deficiency aggravates glucose intolerance via impairment of islet microvascular density in mice with high-fat diet. *J Diabetes Res.* 2013;2013:405284.

155. Bernardi S, Tikellis C, Candido R, et al. ACE2 deficiency shifts energy metabolism towards glucose utilization. *Metabolism.* 2015;64(3):406–415.

156. Clotet S, Soler MJ, Rebull M, et al. Gonadectomy prevents the increase in blood pressure and glomerular injury in angiotensin-converting enzyme 2 knockout diabetic male mice. Effects on renin-angiotensin system. *J Hypertens.* 2016;34(9):1752–1765.

157. Krop M, de Bruyn JH, Derkx FH, et al. Renin and prorenin disappearance in humans post-nephrectomy: evidence for binding? *Front Biosci.* 2008;13:3931–3939.

158. Burcklé C, Bader M. Prorenin and its ancient receptor. *Hypertension.* 2006;48(4):549–551.

159. Sandberg K, Ji H, Clark AJ, et al. Cloning and expression of a novel angiotensin II receptor subtype. *J Biol Chem.* 1992;267(14):9455–9458.

160. Mifune M, Sasamura H, Nakazato Y, et al. Examination of Ang II type 1 and type 2 receptor expression in human kidneys by immunohistochemistry. *Clin Exp Hypertens.* 2001;23(3):257–266.

161. Gardiner SM, Kemp PA, March JE, Bennett T. Regional haemodynamic effects of angiotensin II (3-8) in conscious rats. *Br J Pharmacol.* 1993;110(1):159–162.

162. Karnik S, Bernstein KE, Kemp J, et al Angiotensin receptors. Accessed September 15, 2017. IUPHAR/BPS Guide to PHARMACOLOGY, http://www.guidetopharmacology.org/GRAC/FamilyDisplayForward?familyId=6.

163. Padia SH, Kemp BA, Howell NL, et al. Conversion of renal angiotensin II to angiotensin III is critical for AT2 receptor-mediated natriuresis in rats. *Hypertension.* 2008;51(2):460–465.

164. http://www.genecards.org/.

165. Yu L, Zheng M, Wang W, et al. Developmental changes in AT1 and AT2 receptor-protein expression in rats. *J Renin Angiotensin Aldosterone Syst.* 2010;11(4):214–221.

166. Gill DL, Spassova MA, Soboloff J. Signal transduction. Calcium entry signals–trickles and torrents. *Science.* 2006;313(5784):183–184.

167. Sandberg K, Ji H. Comparative analysis of amphibian and mammalian angiotensin receptors. *Comp Biochem Physiol A Mol Integr Physiol.* 2001;128(1):53–75.

168. Wynne BM, Chiao CW, Webb RC. Vascular smooth muscle cell signaling mechanisms for contraction to angiotensin II and endothelin-1. *J Am Soc Hypertens.* 2009;3(2):84–95.

169. Kalantarinia K, Okusa MD. The renin-angiotensin system and its blockade in diabetic renal and cardiovascular disease. *Curr Diab Rep.* 2006;6(1):8–16.

170. Nishida M, Kitajima N, Saiki S. Regulation of angiotensin II receptor signaling by cysteine modification of NF-κB. *Nitric Oxide.* 2011;25(2):112–117.

171. Zhang J, Pratt RE. The AT2 receptor selectively associates with Giα2 and Giα3 in the rat fetus. *J Biol Chem.* 1996;271(25):15026–15033.

172. Stegbauer J, Coffman TM. New insights into angiotensin receptor actions: from blood pressure to aging. *Curr Opin Nephrol Hypertens.* 2011;20(1):84–88.

173. Landgraf SS, Wengert M, Silva JS, et al. Changes in angiotensin receptors expression play a pivotal role in the renal damage observed in spontaneous hypertensive rats. *Am J Physiol Renal Physiol.* 2011;300(2):F499–F510.

174. Crowley SD, Gurley SB, Oliverio MI, et al. Distinct roles for the kidney and systemic tissues in blood pressure regulation by the renin-angiotensin system. *J Clin Invest.* 2005;115(4):1092–1099.

175. Gurley SB, Riquier-Brison ADM, Schnermann J, et al. AT1A angiotensin receptors in the renal proximal tubule regulate blood pressure. *Cell Metab.* 2011;13(4):469–475.

176. Chaki S, Inagami T. Identification and characterization of a new binding site for angiotensin II in mouse neuroblastoma neuro-2A cells. *Biochem Biophys Res Commun.* 1992;182(1):388–394.

177. Singh KD, Karnik SS. Angiotensin receptors: structure, function, signaling and clinical applications. *J Cell Signal.* 2016;1(2):pii: 111.

178. Albiston AL, McDowall SG, Matsacos D, et al. Evidence that the angiotensin IV (AT(4)) receptor is the enzyme insulin-regulated aminopeptidase. *J Biol Chem.* 2001;276:48623–48626.

179. Davis CJ, Kramár EA, De A, et al. AT4 receptor activation increases intracellular calcium influx and induces a non-N-methyl-D-aspartate dependent form of long-term potentiation. *Neuroscience.* 2006;137(4):1369–1379.

180. Rasmussen TE, Pedraza-Díaz S, Hardré R, et al. Struture of the human oxytocinase/insulin-regulated aminopeptidase gene and localization to chromosome 5q21. *Eur J Biochem.* 2000;267(8):2297–2306.

181. Wright JW, Yamamoto BJ, Harding JW. Angiotensin receptor subtype mediated physiologies and behaviors: new discoveries and clinical targets. *Prog Neurobiol.* 2008;84(2):157–181.

182. Santos RA, Simoes e Silva AC, Maric C, et al. Angiotensin-(1-7) is an endogenous ligand for the G protein-coupled receptor Mas. *Proc Natl Acad Sci USA.* 2003;100(14):8258–8263.

183. Cerrato BD, Carretero OA, Janic B, et al. Heteromerization between the bradykinin B2 receptor and the angiotensin-(1-7) Mas receptor: functional consequences. *Hypertension.* 2016;68(4):1039–1048.

184. Gironacci MM, Valera MS, Yujnovsky I, et al. Angiotensin-(1-7) inhibitory mechanism of norepinephrine release in hypertensive rats. *Hypertension.* 2004;44(5):783–787.

185. Costa MA, Lopez Verrilli MA, Gomez KA, et al. Angiotensin-(1-7) upregulates cardiac nitric oxide synthase in spontaneously hypertensive rats. *Am J Physiol Heart Circ Physiol.* 2010;299(4):H1205–H1211.

186. Ajit SK1, Pausch MH, Kennedy JD, et al. Development of a FLIPR assay for the simultaneous identification of MrgD agonists and antagonists from a single screen. *J Biomed Biotechnol.* 2010; 2010:pii: 326020.

187. Solinski HJ, Gudermann T, Breit A. Pharmacology and signaling of MAS-related G protein-coupled receptors. *Pharmacol Rev.* 2014;66(3):570–597.

188. Shinohara T, Harada M, Ogi K, et al. Identification of a G protein-coupled receptor specifically responsive to beta-alanine. *J Biol Chem.* 2004;279(22):23559–23564.

189. Soltani Hekmat A, Javanmardi K, Kouhpayeh A, et al. Differences in cardiovascular responses to alamandine in two-kidney, one clip hypertensive and normotensive rats. *Circ J.* 2017;81(3):405–412.

190. Soares ER, Barbosa CM, Campagnole-Santos MJ, et al. Hypotensive effect induced by microinjection of Alamandine, a derivative of angiotensin-(1-7), into caudal ventrolateral medulla of 2K1C hypertensive rats. *Peptides.* 2017;96:67–75.

191. Nguyen G. Renin, (pro)renin and receptor: an update. *Clin Sci.* 2011;120(5):169–178.

192. Batenburg WW, Krop M, Garrelds IM, et al. Prorenin is the endogenous agonist of the (pro)renin receptor. Binding kinetics of renin and prorenin in rat vascular smooth muscle cells overexpressing the human (pro)renin receptor. *J Hypertens.* 2007;25(12):2441–2453.

193. Amsterdam A, Nissen RM, Sun Z, et al. Identification of 315 genes essential for early zebrafish development. *Proc Natl Acad Sci USA.* 2004;101(35):12792–12797.

194. Burckle C, Bader M. Prorenin and its ancient receptor. *Hypertension.* 2006;48(4):549–551.

195. Ille F, Sommer L. Wnt signaling: multiple functions in neural development. *Cell Mol Life Sci.* 2005;62(10):1100–1108.

196. Falk S, Wurdak H, Ittner LM, et al. Brain area-specific effect of TGF-beta signaling on Wnt-dependent neural stem cell expansion. *Cell Stem Cell.* 2008;2(5):472–483.

197. Schmidt-Ott KM, Barasch J. WNT/beta-catenin signaling in nephron progenitors and their epithelial progeny. *Kidney Int.* 2008;74(8):1004–1008.

198. Kaneshiro Y, Ichihara A, Sakoda M, et al. Slowly progressive, angiotensin II-independent glomerulosclerosis in human (pro)renin receptor-transgenic rats. *J Am Soc Nephrol.* 2007;18(6):1789–1795.

199. Ramkumar N, Stuart D, Mironova E, et al. Renal tubular epithelial cell prorenin receptor regulates blood pressure and sodium transport. *Am J Physiol Renal Physiol.* 2016;311(1):F186–F194.

200. Trepiccione F, Gerber SD, Grahammer F, et al. Renal Atp6ap2/(Pro)renin receptor is required for normal vacuolar H+-ATPase function but not for the renin-angiotensin system. *J Am Soc Nephrol.* 2016;27(11):3320–3330.

201. Lu X, Wang F, Liu M, et al. Activation of ENaC in collecting duct cells by prorenin and its receptor PRR: involvement of Nox4-derived hydrogen peroxide. *Am J Physiol Renal Physiol.* 2016;310(11): F1243–F1250.

202. Danser AH. The role of the (pro)renin receptor in hypertensive disease. *Am J Hypertens.* 2015; 28(10):1187–1196.

203. Ramkumar N, Stuart D, Rees S, et al. Collecting duct-specific knockout of renin attenuates angiotensin II-induced hypertension. *Am J Physiol Renal Physiol.* 2014;307(8):F931–F938.

204. Peng K, Lu X, Wang F. Collecting duct (pro)renin receptor targets ENaC to mediate angiotensin II-induced hypertension. *Am J Physiol Renal Physiol.* 2017;312(2):F245–F253.

205. Li W, Peng H, Mehaffey EP, et al. Neuron-specific (pro)renin receptor knockout prevents the development of salt-sensitive hypertension. *Hypertension.* 2014;63(2):316–323.

206. Li W, Sullivan MN, Zhang S, et al. Intracerebroventricular infusion of the (Pro)renin receptor antagonist PRO20 attenuates deoxycorticosterone acetate-salt-induced hypertension. *Hypertension.* 2015;65(2):352–361.

207. Trebak F, Li W, Feng Y. Neuron specific (Pro)renin receptor knockout reduces sodium appetite and attenuates the development of DOCA-salt induced hypertension. *Hypertension.* 2017;70:AP284.

208. Hunyadi L, Catt KJ. Pleiotropic AT1 receptor signaling pathways mediating physiological and pathogenic actions of Ang II. *Mol Endocrinol.* 2006;20(5):953–970.

209. Garvin JL. Angiotensin stimulates glucose and fluid absorption by rat proximal straight tubules. *J Am Soc Nephrol.* 1990;1(3):272–277.

11

210. Xu L, Dixit MP, Chen R, et al. Effects of angiotensin II on NaPi-IIa co-transporter expression and activity in rat renal cortex. *Biochim Biophys Acta.* 2004;1667(2):114–121.

211. Yingst DR, Massey KJ, Rossi NF, et al. Angiotensin II directly stimulates activity and alters the phosphorylation of Na-K-ATPase in rat proximal tubule with a rapid time course. *Am J Physiol Renal Physiol.* 2004;287(4):F713–F721.

212. Shah S, Hussain T. Enhanced angiotensin II-induced activation of Na+-K+-ATPase in the proximal tubules of obese Zucker rats. *Clin Exp Hypertens.* 2006;28(1):29–40.

213. Horita S, Zheng Y, Hara C. Biphasic regulation of Na+HCO3– cotransporter by angiotensin II type 1A receptor. *Hypertension.* 2002;40(5):707–712.

214. Noonan WT, Woo AL, Nieman ML, et al. Blood pressure maintenance in NHE3-deficient mice with transgenic expression of NHE3 in small intestine. *Am J Physiol Regul Integr Comp Physiol.* 2005;288(3):R685–R691.

215. Kolb RJ, Woost PG, Hopfer U, et al. Membrane trafficking of angiotensin receptor type-1 and mechanochemical signal transduction in proximal tubule cells. *Hypertension.* 2004;44(3):352–359.

216. Quan A, Chakravarty S, Chen JK, et al. Androgens augment proximal tubule transport. *Am J Physiol Renal Physiol.* 2004;287(3):F452–F459.

217. Dixit MP, Xu L, Xu H, et al. Effect of angiotensin II on renal Na+/H+ exchanger-NHE3 and NHE2. *Biochim Biophys Acta.* 2004;1664(1):38–44.

218. Good DW, George T, Wang DH, et al. Angiotensin II inhibits HCO3 absorption via a cytochrome P450 dependent pathway in MTAL. *Am J Physiol.* 1999;276(5pt2):F726–F736.

219. Han HJ, Park SH, Koh HJ, et al. Mechanism of regulation of Na+ transport by angiotensin II in primary renal cells. *Kidney Int.* 2000;57(6):2457–2467.

220. Romero MF, Madhun ZT, Hopfer U, et al. An epoxygenase metabolite of arachidonic acid 5,6 epoxy-eicosatrienoic acid mediates angiotensin-induced natriuresis in proximal tubular epithelium. *Adv Prostaglandin Thromboxane Leukot Res.* 1991;21A:205–208.

221. Romero MF, Hopfer U, Madhun ZT, et al. Angiotensin II actions in the rabbit proximal tubule. Angiotensin II mediated signaling mechanisms and electrolyte transport in the rabbit proximal tubule. *Ren Physiol Biochem.* 1991;14(4–5):191–207.

222. Houillier P, Chambrey R, Achard JM, et al. Signaling pathways in the biphasic effect of angiotensin II on apical Na/H antiport activity in proximal tubule. *Kidney Int.* 1996;50(5):1496–1505.

223. Kwon TH, Nielsen J, Kim H, et al. Regulation of sodium transporters in the thick ascending limb of rat kidney: response to angiotensin II. *Am J Physiol Renal Physiol.* 2003;285(1):F152–F165.

224. He P, Klein J, Yun CC. Activation of Na+/H+ exchanger NHE3 by angiotensin II is mediated by inositol 1,4,5-triphosphate (IP3) receptor-binding protein released with IP3 (IRBIT) and Ca2+/calmodulin-dependent protein kinase II. *J Biol Chem.* 2010;285(36):27869–27878.

225. Bell PD, Peti-Peterdi J. Angiotensin II stimulates macula densa basolateral sodium/hydrogen exchange via type 1 angiotensin II receptors. *J Am Soc Nephrol.* 1999;10(suppl 11):S225–S229.

226. Wang T, Geibisch G. Effects of angiotensin II on electrolyte transport in the early and late distal tubule in rat kidney. *Am J Physiol.* 1996;271(1 Pt 2):F143–F149.

227. Beutler KT, Masilamani S, Turban S, et al. Long-term regulation of ENaC expression in kidney by angiotensin II. *Hypertension.* 2003;41(5):1143–1150.

228. Peti-Peterdi J, Warnock DG, Bell PD. Angiotensin II directly stimulates ENaC activity in the cortical collecting duct via AT(1) receptors. *J Am Soc Nephrol.* 2002;13(5):1131–1135.

229. Stegbauer J, Gurley SB, Sparks MA, et al. AT1 receptors in the collecting duct directly modulate the concentration of urine. *J Am Soc Nephrol.* 2011;22(12):2237–2246.

230. Pulakat L, Cooper S, Knowle D, et al. Ligand-dependent complex formation between the Angiotensin II receptor subtype AT2 and Na+/H+ exchanger NHE6 in mammalian cells. *Peptides.* 2005;26(5):863–873.

231. Bobulescu IA, Di Sole F, Moe OW. Na+/H+ exchangers; physiology and link to hypertension and organ ischemia. *Curr Opin Nephrol Hypertens.* 2005;14(5):485–494.

232. Lara Lda S, Cavalcante F, Axelband F, et al. Involvement of Gi/o/cGMP/PKG pathway in the AT2-mediated inhibition of outer cortex proximal tubule Na+-ATPase by Ang-(1-7). *Biochem J.* 2006;395(1):183–190.

233. Haithcock D, Jiao H, Cui XL, et al. Renal proximal tubular AT2 receptor: signaling and transport. *J Am Soc Nephrol.* 1999;10(suppl 11):S69–S74.

234. Quan A, Baum M. Effect of luminal angiotensin II receptor antagonists on proximal tubule transport. *Am J Hypertens.* 1999;12(5):499–503.

235. Hakam AC, Hussain T. Angiotensin II type 2 receptor agonist directly inhibits proximal tubule sodium pump activity in obese but not in lean Zucker rats. *Hypertension.* 2006;47(6):1117–1124.

236. Padia SH, Howell NL, Siragy HM, et al. Renal angiotensin type 2 receptors mediate natriuresis via angiotensin III in the angiotensin II type 1 receptor-blocked rat. *Hypertension.* 2006;47(3):537–544.

237. Gildea JJ, Wang X, Shah N, et al. Dopamine and angiotensin type 2 receptors cooperatively inhibit sodium transport in human renal proximal tubule cells. *Hypertension.* 2012;60(2):396–403.

238. Hong NJ, Garvin JL. Angiotensin II type 2 receptor-mediated inhibition of NaCl absorption is blunted in thick ascending limbs from Dahl salt-sensitive rats. *Hypertension.* 2012;60(3):765–769.

239. Yang J, Chen C, Ren H, et al. Angiotensin II AT(2) receptor decreases AT(1) receptor expression and function via nitric oxide/cGMP/Sp1 in renal proximal tubule cells from Wistar-Kyoto rats. *J Hypertens.* 2012;30(6):1176–1184.

240. Beutler KT, Masilamani S, Turban S, et al. Long-term regulation of ENaC expression in kidney by angiotensin II. *Hypertension.* 2003;41(5):1143–1150.

241. Davies E, McKenzie SM. Extra adrenal production of corticosteroids. *Clin Exp Pharmacol Physiol.* 2003;30(7):437–445.

242. Kurdi M, De Mello WC, Booz GW. Working outside the system: an update on the unconventional behavior of the renin-angiotensin system components. *Int J Biochem Cell Biol.* 2005;37(7):1357–1367.

243. Zou Y, Akazawa H, Qin Y, et al. Mechanical stress activates angiotensin II type 1 receptor without the involvement of angiotensin II. *Nat Cell Biol.* 2004;6(6):499–506.

244. Yatabe J, Sanada H, Yatabe MS, et al. Angiotensin II type 1 receptor blocker attenuates the activation of ERK and NADPH oxidase by mechanical strain in mesangial cells in the absence of angiotensin II. *Am J Physiol Renal Physiol.* 2009;296(5):F1052–F1060.

245. Baker KM, Kumar R, Intracellular Ang II. induces cell proliferation independent of AT1 receptor. *Am J Physiol Cell Physiol.* 2006;291(5):C995–C1001.

246. Schütz S, Le Moullec JM, Corvol P, et al. Early expression of all the components of the renin-angiotensin system in human development. *Am J Pathol.* 1996;149(6):2067–2079.

247. Niimura F, Kon V, Ichikawa I. The renin-angiotensin system in the development of congenital anomalies of the kidney and urinary tract. *Curr Opin Pediatr.* 2006;18(2):161–166.

248. Tabacova S, Little R, Tsong Y, et al. Adverse pregnancy outcomes associated with maternal enalapril antihypertensive treatment. *Pharmacoepidemiol Drug Saf.* 2003;12(8):633–646.

249. Buttar HS. An overview of the influence of ACE inhibitors on fetal-placental circulation and perinatal development. *Mol Cell Biochem.* 1997;176(1–2):61–67.

250. Cooper WO, Harnandez-Diaz S, Arbogast PG, et al. Major congenital malformations after first-trimester exposure to ACE inhibitors. *N Engl J Med.* 2006;354(23):2443–2451.

251. Schaefer C. Angiotensin II-receptor-antagonists: further evidence of fetotoxicity but not teratogenicity. *Birth Defects Res A Clin Mol Teratol.* 2003;67(8):591–594.

252. Niimura F, Okubo S, Fogo A, et al. Temporal and spatial expression pattern of the angiotensinogen gene in mice and rats. *Am J Physiol.* 1997;272(1 Pt 2):R142–R147.

253. Kumar D, Moss G, Primhak R, et al. Congenital renal tubular dysplasia and skull ossification defects similar to teratogenic effects of angiotensin converting enzyme (ACE) inhibitors. *J Med Genet.* 1997;34(7):541–545.

254. Gribouval O, Gonzales M, Neuhaus T, et al. Mutations in genes in the renin-angiotensin system are associated with autosomal recessive renal tubular dysgenesis. *Nat Genet.* 2005;37(9):964–968.

255. Lacoste M, Cai Y, Guicharnaud L, et al. Renal tubular dysgenesis, a not uncommon autosomal recessive disorder leading to oligohydramnios: role of the renin-angiotensin system. *J Am Soc Nephrol.* 2006;17(8):2253–2263.

256. Nishimura H, Yerkes E, Hohenfellner K, et al. Role of the angiotensin type 2 receptor gene in congenital anomalies of the kidney and urinary tract, CAKUT, of mice and men. *Mol Cell.* 1999;3(1):1–10.

257. Gubler MC, Antignac C. Renin-angiotensin system in kidney development: renal tubular dysgenesis. *Kidney Int.* 2010;77(5):400–406.

258. Yosypiv IV, El-Dahr SS. Role of the renin-angiotensin system in the development of the ureteric bud and renal collecting system. *Pediatr Nephrol.* 2005;20(9):1219–1229.

259. Fiselier T, Monnens L, van Munster P, et al. The renin-angiotensin-aldosterone system in infancy and childhood in basal conditions and after stimulation. *Eur J Pediatr.* 1984;143(1):18–24.

260. Sulyok E, Nemeth M, Tenyi I, et al. Relationship between the postnatal development of the renin-angiotensin-aldosterone system and electrolyte and acid-base status of the NaCl-supplemented premature infants. In: Spitzer A, ed. *The Kidney during Development Morphogenesis and Function.* New York: Masson Publishing USA Inc; 1982:273–281.

261. Peleg E, Peleg D, Yaron A, et al. Perinatal development of angiotensin-converting enzyme in the rat's blood. *Gynecol Obstet Invest.* 1988;25(1):12–15.

262. Walther T, Faber R, Maul B, et al. Fetal, neonatal cord and maternal plasma concentrations of angiotensin converting enzyme (ACE). *Prenat Diagn.* 2002;22(2):111–113.

263. Bender JW, Davitt MK, Jose P. Angiotensin-1-converting enzyme activity in term and premature infants. *Biol Neonate.* 1978;34(1–2):19–23.

264. Forhead AJ, Melvin R, Balouzet V, et al. Developmental changes in plasma angiotensin—converting enzyme concentration in fetal and neonatal lambs. *Reprod Fertil Dev.* 1998;10(5):393–398.

265. Raimbach SJ, Thomas AL. Renin and angiotensin converting enzyme concentrations in the fetal and neonatal guinea-pig. *J Physiol.* 1990;423-441-451.

266. Forhead AJ, Gulati V, Poore KR, et al. Ontogeny of pulmonary and renal angiotensin-converting enzyme in pigs. *Mol Cell Endocrinol.* 2001;185(1–2):127–133.

267. O'Connor SJ, Fowden AL, Holdstock N, et al. Developmental changes in pulmonary and renal angiotensin-converting enzyme concentration in fetal and neonatal horses. *Reprod Fertil Dev.* 2002;14(7–8):413–417.

268. Hattori MA, Del Ben GL, Carmona AK, et al. Angiotensin I-converting enzyme isoforms (high and low molecular weight) in urine of premature and full-term infants. *Hypertension.* 2000;35(6):1284–1290.

269. Miyawaki M, Okutani T, Higuchi R, et al. Plasma angiotensin II levels in the early neonatal period. *Arch Dis Child Fetal Neonatal Ed.* 2006;91(5):F359–F362.

270. Franco MC, Casarini DE, Carneiro-Ramos MS, et al. Circulating renin-angiotensin system and catecholamines in childhood: is there a role for birthweight? *Clin Sci.* 2008;114(5):375–380.

271. Sippell WG, Dörr HG, Bidlingmaier F, et al. Plasma levels of aldosterone, corticosterone, 11-deoxycorticosterone, progesterone, 17-hydroxyprogesterone, cortisol, and cortisone during infancy and childhood. *Pediatr Res.* 1980;14(1):39–46.

272. Kohlstedt K, Brandis RP, Muller-Esterl W, et al. Angiotensin-converting enzyme is involved in outside-in signaling in endothelial cells. *Circ Res.* 2002;94(1):60–67.

11

273. Zeng C, Wang Z, Hopfer U, et al. Rat strain effects of AT1 receptor activation on D1 dopamine receptors in immortalized renal proximal tubule cells. *Hypertension.* 2005;46(4):799–805.
274. Zeng C, Hopfer U, Asico LD, et al. Altered AT1 receptor regulation of ETB receptors in renal proximal tubule cells of spontaneously hypertensive rats. *Hypertension.* 2005;46(4):926–931.
275. AbdAlla S, Lother H, Quitterer U. AT1-receptor heterodimers show enhanced G-protein activation and altered receptor sequestration. *Nature.* 2000;407(6800):94–98.
276. Abadir PM, Periasamy A, Carey RM, et al. Angiotensin II type 2 receptor-bradykinin B2 receptor functional heterodimerization. *Hypertension.* 2006;48(2):316–322.
277. Takezako T, Unal H, Karnik SS, et al. Current topics in angiotensin II type 1 receptor research: Focus on inverse agonism, receptor dimerization and biased agonism. *Pharmacol Res.* 2017;123:40–50.
278. Zha D, Cheng H, Li W, et al. High glucose instigates tubulointerstitial injury by stimulating hetero-dimerization of adiponectin and angiotensin II receptors. *Biochem Biophys Res Commun.* 2017;493:840–846.
279. Zhuo JL. Intracrine renin and angiotensin II: a novel role in cardiovascular and renal cellular regulation. *J Hypertens.* 2006;24(6):1017–1020.
280. Barker DJ, Osmond C, Golding J, et al. Growth in utero, blood pressure in childhood and adult life, and mortality from cardiovascular disease. *BMJ.* 1989;298(6673):564–567.
281. Alexander BT. Fetal programming of hypertension. *Am J Physiol Regul Integr Comp Physiol.* 2006;290(1):R1–R10.
282. Woods LL, Rasch R. Perinatal ANG II programs adult blood pressure, glomerular number, and renal function in rats. *Am J Physiol.* 1998;275(5 Pt 2):R1593–R1599.
283. Gilbert JS, Lang AL, Grant AR, et al. Maternal nutrient restriction in sheep: hypertension and decreased nephron number in offspring at 9 months of age. *J Physiol.* 2005;565(Pt 1):137–147.
284. Leduc L, Levy E, Bouity-Voubou M, et al. Fetal programming of atherosclerosis: possible role of the mitochondria. *Eur J Obstet Gynecol Reprod Biol.* 2010;149(2):127–130.
285. Ojeda NB, Intapad S, Alexander BT. Sex differences in the developmental programming of hypertension. *Acta Physiol (Oxf).* 2014;210(2):307–316.
286. Tain YL, Lee WC, Wu KL, et al. Targeting arachidonic acid pathway to prevent programmed hypertension in maternal fructose-fed male adult rat offspring. *J Nutr Biochem.* 2016;38:86–92.
287. Tain YL, Lee WC, Leu S, et al. High salt exacerbates programmed hypertension in maternal fructose-fed male offspring. *Nutr Metab Cardiovasc Dis.* 2015;25(12):1146–1151.
288. Tiu AC, Bishop MD, Asico LD, et al. Primary pediatric hypertension: current understanding and emerging concepts. *Curr Hypertens Rep.* 2017;19(9):70.
289. Drukker A, Guignard JP. Renal aspects of the term and preterm infant: a selective update. *Current Opin Pediatr.* 2002;14(2):175–182.
290. Pezzati M, Vangi V, Biagiotti R, et al. Effects of indomethacin and ibuprofen on mesenteric and renal blood flow in preterm infants with patent ductus arteriosus. *J Pediatr.* 1999;135(6):733–738.
291. Olsson A, Walia R, Shah SS. Ibuprofen for the treatment of patent ductus arteriosus in preterm or low birth weight (or both) infants. *Cochrane Database Syst Rev.* 2015;(2):CD003481.
292. Merke DP, Bornstein SR. Congenital adrenal hyperplasia. *Lancet.* 2005;365(9477):2125–2136.
293. Chang SS, Grunder S, Hanukoglu A, et al. Mutations in subunits of the epithelial sodium channel cause salt wasting with hyperkalemic acidosis, pseudohypoaldosteronism type 1. *Nat Genet.* 1996;12(3):248–533.
294. Stipsanelli A, Daskalakis G, Koutra P, et al. Renin-angiotensin system dysregulation in fetuses with hydronephrosis. *Eur J Obstet Gynecol Reprod Biol.* 2010;150(1):39–41.
295. Bertagnolli M. Preterm birth and renin-angiotensin-aldosterone system: evidences of activation and impact on developmental cardiovascular disease risks. *Protein Pept Lett.* 2017;24:793–798.
296. Danilczyk U, Penninger JM. Angiotensin-converting enzyme II in the heart and the kidney. *Circ Res.* 2006;98(4):463–471.

CHAPTER 12

Renal Modulation: Arginine Vasopressin and Atrial Natriuretic Peptide

Nilka de Jesús-González, MD, MSc, Melvin Bonilla-Felix, MD

- Arginine Vasopressin
- Atrial Natriuretic Peptide

Introduction

Total body fluid homeostasis is vital for human survival. Before birth, fetal mechanisms to conserve fluid are not essential because the placenta has a major role maintaining fluid homeostasis. At birth, the newborn becomes responsible for keeping homeostasis while facing dramatic environmental changes; therefore, the kidneys assume a central role maintaining fluid homeostasis. Despite having completed nephrogenesis by 36 weeks of postmenstrual age, renal tubular function is still immature at birth, limiting the newborn's ability to handle water and sodium.[1,2]

Understanding the developmental changes and mechanisms involved in fluid homeostasis events is crucial to manage newborns and infants. We review the role and development of two hormonal pathways that regulate the body fluid composition during the prenatal and perinatal periods: (1) arginine vasopressin (AVP) system, which has a major role modulating water homeostasis, and (2) atrial natriuretic peptide (ANP) system, which has a major role in sodium excretion.

Arginine Vasopressin

Arginine Vasopressin Synthesis and Secretion

Arginine vasopressin is synthesized in the cell bodies of magnocellular neurons that originate in the supraoptic and paraventricular nuclei of the hypothalamus and is stored in neurosecretory granules in their posterior pituitary nerve terminals (Table 12.1).

When the AVP stimuli-secretion arises, voltage-gated calcium channels in the magnocellular nerve terminals open, transient calcium influx occurs, neurosecretory granules fuse with magnocellular neuron membranes, and AVP is released into the systemic circulation.[3-6] This secretion is triggered by multiple physiologic and pathophysiologic stimuli. Changes in plasma osmolality and changes in effective circulating blood volume are the main triggers for AVP secretion (see Table 12.1). Under normal physiologic conditions, a rise in plasma osmolality, as minimal as 2 to 5 mOsm/kg H_2O, is sensed by the osmoreceptors in the hypothalamus and is the main stimulus of AVP secretion.[4,7] Conversely, changes in effective circulating volume become important stimuli for AVP secretion when the decrease in the effective circulating blood volume is greater than 8% to 10%.[8,9] Dunn et al. displayed this relationship in their experiments where male Sprague-Dawley rats were exposed to three different experimental scenarios: (1) fluid restriction (hypertonic hypovolemia—leading to both a rise in plasma osmolality and a decrease in blood volume), (2) intraperitoneal injections of hypertonic saline (hypertonic isovolemia—leading to only a rise in plasma osmolality), and (3) intraperitoneal injections of polyethylene glycol (isotonic hypovolemia—leading to a decrease in effective circulating volume only).[9] When

Table 12.1   SUMMARY OF ARGININE VASOPRESSIN AND ATRIAL NATRIURETIC PEPTIDE KIDNEY-RELATED HORMONAL PATHWAYS

	Arginine Vasopressin	Atrial Natriuretic Peptide

Stimuli	• Increased plasma osmolality
	• Decreased effective blood volume
	• Thermic stress
	• Pain
	• Hypoxia
	• Hypoglycemia
	• Intracranial hemorrhage
	• Hydrocephalus
	• Drugs
	  • Nonsteroidal antiinflammatory agents
	  • Opiates
	  • Thiazides, furosemide
	  • Mannitol
	  • Contrast dye
		• Atrial wall stretch
		• Hypoxia
		• Endothelin 1
		• Glucocorticoids
		• Mineralocorticoids
		• Prostaglandins
		• Angiotensin II
		• Arginine vasopressin

Hormone Synthesis Site	Magnocellular cells at the supraoptic and paraventricular nuclei of the hypothalamus	Atrial cardiomyocyte
Hormone Storage and Secretion	Neurosecretory granules at the posterior pituitary	Atrial cardiomyocyte
Hormone Receptor	Vasopressin 2 receptor (V_2R)	Type A natriuretic peptide (NPR-A)
Effector Cells	Principal cell at the collecting duct (V_2R locates on the basolateral membrane)	• Podocytes • Mesangial cells • Proximal tubular cells • Thick ascending loop of Henle cells • Medullary collecting duct cells
Intracellular Signaling	• Adenylate cyclase second messenger system • cAMP activates protein kinase A (PKA) which then phosphorylates AQP2	• Guanylyl cyclase second messenger system • cGMP activates cGMP-gated channels, cGMP-dependent phosphodiesterases, and c-GMP dependent kinases cGKI and cGKII
Final Effect	Insertion of AQP2 into the apical membrane of principal cells, increasing water permeability	• Podocytes—F-actin reorganization leading to cellular relaxation and modulation of cellular characteristics. • Mesangial cells—hyperpolarization, cellular relaxation, and increased ultrafiltration • Proximal tubular cells—inhibits Na reabsorption by inhibiting Na-dependent transport systems • Thick ascending limb of Henle—inhibits chloride transport in a cGMP-dependent manner by directly inhibiting Na-K-2Cl (NKCC) cotransporter activity, leads to decreased urine concentrating capacity and increased urine flow • Medullary collecting duct cells—inhibits cyclic nucleotide-gated (CNG) cation channels, by a PKG-dependent channel phosphorylation and allosteric changes; ENaC, by decreasing the probability of keeping ENaC open; and heterodimeric channel complex in cilia, transient potential vanilloid 4 (TRPV4) and polycystin-2 (TRPP2), by inhibiting flow-activated calcium entry into the cells via PKG
Hormone Degradation	Phosphodiesterases	Type C natriuretic peptide (NPR-C)—"clearance receptors"

rats were exposed to intraperitoneal injections of hypertonic saline, a positive linear correlation was observed between a rise in plasma osmolality and a rise in AVP ($r > 0.9$). Conversely, when rats were exposed to intraperitoneal polyethylene glycol an exponential, rather than linear, rise in AVP became apparent when volume had fallen by 8% to 10%. When rats were exposed to fluid restriction, an initial twofold to threefold linear rise in plasma AVP levels was observed, similar to the hypertonic isovolemia scenario, which was later followed by a 10-fold rise when additional blood volume had been lost, similar to the hypertonic hypovolemia scenario.[9] Earlier experiments by Johnson et al. reported similar results in sheep models.[10]

Other stimuli for AVP secretion in newborns include pain, thermic stress, hypoxia, hypoglycemia, hydrocephalus, intracranial hemorrhage, and drugs (see Table 12.1).[4,11]

Development

During fetal life, AVP is detectable in the human pituitary as early as at 11 to 12 weeks of gestational age, rapidly increasing thereafter until the second trimester of pregnancy (Table 12.2).[12] Vasopressin neurons in an adultlike organization are observed early during fetal life, with an increase in number of vasopressin neurons until the 26th week of gestational age, along with vasopressin gene expression.[13–18]

Similarly, during fetal life, a rise in plasma maternal and fetal osmolality leads to AVP secretion. In chronically catheterized sheep model, Weitzman et al. showed that pituitary AVP secretion is stimulated by hypertonic saline infusion during fetal life.[19] Likewise, in fetal ewes, increasing maternal plasma osmolality either by water deprivation or by mannitol infusion resulted in higher fetal AVP serum concentrations. Angiotensin II is another stimulator of AVP secretion. In ovine fetuses, angiotensin II-induced fetal AVP secretion has been shown to be mediated through stimulation of angiotensin receptor 1.[20]

In the perinatal period, the response to the hypoxia and increased intracranial pressure induced by labor has been proposed as another stimulus of AVP release (see Table 12.2).[21,22] This is supported by studies demonstrating higher AVP levels in the human umbilical cord of infants delivered vaginally than infants delivered without labor.[23]

Table 12.2 KIDNEY-RELATED DEVELOPMENTAL HIGHLIGHTS OF ARGININE VASOPRESSIN AND ATRIAL NATRIURETIC PEPTIDE HORMONAL PATHWAYS

	Arginine Vasopressin	Atrial Natriuretic Peptide
Is hormone secreted during fetal period?	Yes	Yes
Is there a main renal role of this hormone during fetal period?	No	No
What are the main stimuli for hormone secretion in the perinatal period?	Hypoxia and increased intracranial pressure	Atrial wall stretch due to decreased pulmonary vascular resistance and increased left atrial venous return
Reasons for immature renal response to hormone at birth	• Inhibition of AVP-stimulated cAMP generation by prostaglandins via EP3 receptors • Increased cAMP phosphodiesterase activity • Low medullary tonicity due to immature salt reabsorption machinery at the thick ascending limb of Henle and urea concentration and shorter loops of Henle	• Lower ANP levels due to increase circulating ANP clearance • Attenuated renal response to ANP

Vasopressin Signal Transduction

Arginine vasopressin exerts its antidiuretic action by binding to the V_2 vasopressin receptor (V_2R), a G-stimulatory (G_s) protein coupled receptor on the basolateral membrane of renal collecting duct principal epithelial cells (see Table 12.1).[24,25] The V_2R has seven transmembrane domains, with a groove for antidiuretic hormone (ADH) binding in the extracellular region and a binding site for a G_s protein in its intracellular domain.[26] Once AVP binds to V_2R, an intracellular adenylate cyclase second messenger system gets activated.[24,25] Intracellular cyclic adenosine monophosphate (cAMP) increases and activates protein kinase A, which then phosphorylates the cytoplasmic carboxy-terminal end of water channel aquaporin 2 (AQP2), resulting in the insertion of this water channel into the apical membrane of the principal cell and subsequent increased water permeability.[27-31] Once cAMP is generated, it is promptly degraded by phosphodiesterase (see Table 12.1).

Development

Despite the documented presence of AVP during fetal life, the immature kidneys have poor response to AVP.[32] In ovine models, AVP infusion did not change fetal plasma osmolality.[33,34] In humans, Heller administered pituitary extract containing AVP to newborn infants and adult controls.[35] In adults, a rapid increment in urine osmolality was observed, while in infants, urine concentration remained unchanged.[35] These findings support poor response of AVP by immature kidneys.

Multiple lines of evidence suggest that this poor response of immature kidneys to AVP is related to resistance to AVP rather than to lack of receptors (see Table 12.2). Otrowski et al. showed that V_2R is expressed in rats at 16 days of gestation in the developing medullary and cortical collecting duct cells.[36] After birth, V_2R was also observed in the cells of thick ascending limbs of loop of Henle, papillary epithelium, macula densa, and short distal nephron segments.[36] Similarly, Rajerison and coworkers also demonstrated that AVP binding sites are present on medullopapillary membranes harvested from neonatal rat kidneys.[37] These data suggest that V_2R is present early in gestation, making lack of V_2R a less likely cause of poor response of immature kidneys to AVP.

On the other hand, an immature intracellular secondary messenger system has been implicated in the AVP resistance and, consequently, a reduced urine concentrating ability in neonates compared to adults (see Table 12.2). With regard to the development of the intracellular secondary messenger system, studies have shown that adenylyl cyclase response and cAMP generation are both markedly reduced in the neonatal period and that AVP-stimulated urine concentrating ability develops in parallel with cAMP generation.[37-43] To characterize the mechanisms contributing to this low cAMP generation, we measured V_2R-independent stimulation of adenylyl cyclase in the immature cortical collecting ducts of rabbits using direct adenylyl cyclase stimulators (NaF and foskolin).[39] Interestingly, maximal cAMP generation was not elicited.[39] At the same time, when isolated microperfused immature cortical collecting ducts of rabbits were exposed to a cAMP analog, 8-chlorophenylthiol-cAMP, water permeability was not increased to the levels observed with AVP in mature cortical collecting ducts.[40] These findings suggest that the diminished AVP response is due, at least in part, to factors distal to cAMP generation.[40]

Degradation of cAMP has a prominent role in the blunted response of immature collecting duct to AVP (see Table 12.2). In newborn rat renal homogenates, high levels of cAMP phosphodiesterase activity have been reported.[41] In neonatal cortical collecting ducts, the administration of rolipram, a phosphodiesterase intravenous (IV) inhibitor, not only diminished phosphodiesterase activity, but most importantly, eliminated the blunted AVP-stimulated water permeability usually observed in immature cortical collecting ducts.[44] Taken together, these findings suggest that phosphodiesterases have an important role inhibiting AVP response in the immature collecting duct.

High prostaglandin activity has also been implicated in the diminished response of immature collecting duct to AVP (see Table 12.2). In fetal lambs, high urinary levels of prostaglandin have been reported, and in piglets, inhibition of prostaglandin activity with indomethacin led to increased urine osmolality and cAMP excretion.[19,45] Urinary excretion of prostaglandin E_2 (PGE$_2$) has been inconsistent in human newborns. Sulyok and colleagues reported low urinary PGE$_2$ levels in preterms that increase during first weeks of life, while Joppich and colleagues reported higher levels of PGE$_2$ in preterm than in full-term neonates.[46,47] Joppich and colleagues also observed increasing urine osmolality and cAMP excretion with decreasing PGE$_2$ in full-terms.[47]

However, prostaglandin interactions with AVP and cAMP are complex and may lead to both stimulatory and inhibitory water reabsorption responses by the collecting duct. PGE$_2$ alone stimulates cAMP generation and leads to enhanced water permeability. Conversely, in the presence of AVP, PGE$_2$ blunts AVP-stimulated cAMP generation and water reabsorption.[48] Notably, in the presence of a direct adenylyl cyclase stimulator or cAMP analog, no inhibitory effect was observed.[48] These findings suggest that PGE$_2$ decreases AVP-stimulated water reabsorption by blunting cAMP generation. Pretreatment of cortical collecting ducts with indomethacin, a cyclooxygenase inhibitor, resulted in AVP-mediated cAMP generation in neonatal cortical collecting ducts to levels similar to mature cortical collecting ducts. Notably, when cortical collecting ducts were incubated in pertussis toxin, an inhibitor of G inhibitor protein (G$_i$), similar results were reported. Finally, when immature collecting ducts were incubated with indomethacin and pertussis toxin, no additive effect was observed.[39] Altogether, these findings suggest that prostaglandin may contribute, at least in part, to diminished AVP-stimulated water reabsorption via the activation of G$_i$ and subsequent blunting of cAMP generation on an immature cortical collecting duct.

Prostaglandin EP$_3$ subtype receptor has been proposed as the major site for prostaglandin inhibitory effects on cAMP generation. EP$_3$ receptor has been localized in the cortical collecting ducts and is coupled to G$_i$, with PGE$_2$ inhibiting cAMP generation via EP$_3$ receptor/G$_i$ activation.[49,50] EP$_3$ receptor expression is developmentally regulated with higher levels in the first 2 weeks of life in immature collecting ducts followed by a rapid decrease to adult levels afterwards.[51] This could explain the observation in newborn rats that renal cortex has higher affinity for PGE$_2$ than the adult cortex.[52]

In contrast, studies in chronically catheterized fetal sheep failed to show increased urine osmolality after indomethacin administration.[53] Similarly, in vitro microperfusion of isolated rabbit tubules did not lead to maximal AVP-stimulated water reabsorption when tubules were preincubated with indomethacin.[40] Steps distal to cAMP generation in the AVP signaling pathway, which are not mediated by prostaglandins, contributing to this diminished AVP-stimulated water reabsorption (i.e., cAMP degradation by phosphodiesterases) could potentially explain these results.

Aquaporins: Water Channels

Aquaporins are 26 to 34 kD glycosylated proteins sharing 50% to 85% homology containing six transmembrane-spanning domains organized in homotetramers. There are several aquaporin isoforms that differ in their water transport properties, solute selectivity, and tissue expression; and at least seven AQP isoforms are expressed at different sites in the kidney.[54] AQP2 is expressed in the principal cells of the collecting tubules. It is the main target for AVP-mediated water transport (see Table 12.1).[54] AQP3 and AQP4 are expressed in the basolateral membrane of collecting duct principal cells in the cortical and medullary collecting duct, respectively, and have a role in the movement of water from the principal cell to the plasma.[55] Water enters the principal cell via apical AQP2 and leaves through AQP3 and AQP4 located on the basolateral membrane.[56] AQP1 is constitutively expressed on the apical and basolateral membranes of water-permeable proximal tubular cell and descending loop of Henle.[54,57,58] It is also expressed in the descending vasa recta capillaries.[54,58] Lack of AQP1 in the collecting duct suggests that it does not participate in the AVP-mediated water reabsorption.[57] AQP7 is expressed on the apical membrane of the distal portion of the proximal tubule (the S3 segment), suggesting that AQP7 has a role in proximal tubule water absorption.[59] AQP6 is expressed in the type A intercalated cells of the collecting duct, exclusively in the intracellular space with no expression on the plasma membrane.[60] Yasui and colleagues proposed that AQP6 may have a role in vesicle acidification; however, studies are required to further elucidate its role.[60] AQP8 is expressed in low amounts in proximal tubules and collecting duct principal cells, but its functions remain to be elucidated.[61]

Development

AQP2 expression has also been implicated as a contributor to the limited urine concentration ability during the first year of life (see Table 12.2). In rats, AQP2 expression was low at birth but steadily increased to maximal expression at 10 weeks of age in parallel with increased urine concentrating ability.[62] When immature rats were water deprived, AQP2 expression increased to adult levels, but this was not accompanied by a proportional increase in urine osmolality. In preterm and full-term newborns, urinary excretion of AQP2, a marker of AVP activation in the collecting duct, was similar to adults' levels and was not correlated with changes in urine concentrating ability.[63–66] These findings suggest that although AQP2 expression may contribute to the reduced urine concentrating ability in the neonate, it is probably not a major limiting factor. The expression of AQP1, AQP3, and AQP4 increases progressively during fetal life, but they do not have major changes in expression after birth; thus, these AQPs do not seem to limit water reabsorption by the neonatal kidneys.[67–69]

Aquaporins also seem to play an important role in the transcellular solute-free water flow through the placenta. Four different types of AQPs have been identified (AQPs 1, 3, 8, and 9) in the placenta. Aquaporin 3, primarily expressed in the apical membranes of syncytiotrophoblasts,[70] appears to have an important role regulating placental water flux during gestation, with its expression changing throughout gestation. This is supported by studies in mouse models showing increased AQP3 expression along with placental permeability to water early in fetal life followed by a decrease in AQP3 expression and placental water permeability at the end of gestation.[71,72] Aquaporin 1, primarily expressed in the fetal chorioamnion,[73] has been implicated in the water flux between the fetus and the amniotic fluid. Supporting this role is the observation that there is significant polyhydramnios in AQP1 knockout mouse models.[74] Aquaporin 1 also has a variable expression during gestation with higher expression early in fetal life, followed by a decrease and rise again near term.[75] Aquaporin 8 is expressed in trophoblast epithelial cells,[75] and AQP9 is expressed in the amnion and allantoin; their roles in placental water exchange remain to be elucidated.[70,76,77]

Medullary Interstitium Tonicity

Finally, relatively low interstitial sodium chloride and urea concentration and anatomically shorter loops of Henle have been implicated in the reduced urinary concentrating ability observed in immature kidneys (see Table 12.2).[78] Immature salt reabsorption machinery in the thick ascending limb of Henle and urea recycling mechanisms lead to low medullary tonicity, which limits water movement across collecting ducts.[79,80] Likewise, low dietary protein intake may have a limiting role in urea generation.[81,82] Shorter loops of Henle limit the performance of the countercurrent system. With renal growth after birth, loop length increases progressively.[80]

Atrial Natriuretic Peptide

Atrial Natriuretic Peptide Synthesis and Secretion

Atrial natriuretic peptide (ANP) is mostly synthesized in the atrial cardiomyocytes as a 151-amino acid pre-pro-hormone (pre-pro-ANP) and stored as a 126-amino acid prohormone in secretory granules.[83,84] ANP is also synthesized in cardiac ventricles and hypothalamus but at lower levels than in atrial cardiomyocytes.[85] To become active ANP, pro-ANP undergoes a proteolytic cleavage by corin, a transmembrane trypsinlike serine protease, which is also very abundant in myocytes.[86]

Atrial natriuretic peptide is continuously secreted in the atria, but its synthesis and secretion are modulated by stretch-mediated and neurohumoral-mediated factors (see Table 12.1). Atrial wall stretching, caused by changes in central venous return and atrial chamber dilation, is the main stimulus for ANP secretion.[87-89] This is supported by early studies by Lang and coworkers showing that increasing atrial pressure of isolated rat heart led to ANP secretion.[90] Similarly, they showed that ANP plasma levels increased in anesthetized rats exposed to volume expansion.[90] Likewise, anesthetized dogs with atrial distention secondary to mitral valve obstruction also had increased ANP levels.[91] In humans, a rise in central venous pressure (i.e., right atrial pressure) of 1 mm Hg leads to a 10 to 15 pg/mL increase in circulating ANP.

Hypoxia is another potent stimulus for ANP secretion (see Table 12.1). In isolated hearts from rabbits and rats exposed to hypoxia, increased ANP has been documented, with longer hypoxia periods leading to higher ANP levels.[92] Once tissues are reoxygenated, ANP levels return to baseline.[92] In healthy humans exposed to moderate acute hypoxemia by being exposed to a gas mixture containing 10% oxygen, 4.5% CO_2, and 85.5% N_2 resulted in an increase in ANP from 17.7 +/− 3.4 to 27.2 +/− 1.7 pg/mL.[93] Also, in animal models and humans, myocardial infarction induced cardiac ischemia leads to significant increment in ANP release.[94,95] The mechanisms implicated in this hypoxia-induced response include alpha- and beta-adrenergic as well as endothelin stimulation. Studies in Langendorff-perfused rat hearts exposed to hypoxia showed that treatment with phentolamine and propranolol reduced atrial natriuretic factor (ANF) release by half, suggesting a partial contribution of alpha- and beta-adrenergic stimulation to hypoxia-induced ANP release.[96] On the other hand, supporting endothelin-mediated ANP release in the setting of ischemia, Skvorak and coworkers showed that isolated rat atria exposed to anoxia present significant increments in ANP secretion, fully reversible after normal oxygen levels are achieved.[97] Moreover, treatment with an endothelin-1 receptor agonist, BQ123, blocks ANP secretion in this scenario.[97]

Vasoconstrictor hormones such as angiotensin II and vasopressin have also been implicated as stimuli for ANP secretion (see Table 12.1). However, it is yet unclear whether they directly affect ANP secretion or indirectly affect it by causing vasoconstriction and increased venous return. ANP secretion is stimulated by angiotensin II in isolated rabbit hearts and in atrial appendages excised from fresh rat hearts but not in rat heart-lung circuits.[98-100] In vivo experiments in anesthetized rats that received angiotensin II led to changes in cardiac atrial pressure and increments in ANP release.[101] In addition, other experiments in rats exposed to angiotensin at doses that do not affect atrial pressures also led to increased ANP levels.[102] Experiments with AVP in vitro have shown contradictory results. Rat atria incubated in AVP showed ANP secretion.[103] However, in isolated rat hearts, ANP secretion was inhibited by AVP.[102] In isolated rat heart-lung circuit, no increments in ANP secretion were observed when exposed to AVP or angiotensin.[99]

As with other hormonal secretory processes, the ANP secretory process involves four steps: (1) signal transduction at the cell membrane, (2) integration of several intracellular messengers, (3) hormone packing, trafficking, and release, and (4) extracellular fluid transport.

Once atrial cardiomyocytes receive the initial stimuli by atrial stretch or endothelin 1 (or other potential neurohumoral factors) via the stretch activated ion channels and/or endothelin receptor (other neuroendocrine hormone receptors), respectively, G proteins serve as transducers of ANP secretion (see Table 12.1). There are two different G proteins serving as transducers in the atrial myocytes: (1) Gi/o-mediated, pertussis toxin sensitive and (2) Gq-mediated, pertussis toxin insensitive. Atrial stretch caused by central venous return changes, as seen with extracellular fluid volume expansion, is regulated by Gi/o-mediated stretch-stimulated, pertussis toxin sensitive mechanism, while ANP secretion at basal state and stimulated by neuroendocrine factors is regulated by the Gq-mediated, pertussis toxin insensitive protein.[104,105]

Calcium and cyclic nucleotides play important roles in the secretion processes of multiple hormones. For ANP secretion, the role of calcium seems to be complex. Calcium channel agonists increase ANP secretion in atrial myocyte cultures, but they inhibit ANP secretion in isolated rat hearts and rabbit atria.[106-108] Inhibition of calcium release from the sarcoplasmic reticulum, either with ryanodine or thapsigargin, inhibited stretch-stimulated ANP secretion in atrial myocyte cultures and isolated rat atria, but not the ANP basal secretion.[109–111] Calcium depletion decreases endothelin-mediated ANP secretion in myocytes cultures.[112] Taken together, these findings suggest that calcium may have a positive modulatory role under conditions of stretch-mediated or neurohumoral-mediated stimulation. The cyclic nucleotides (cAMP and cGMP) seem to have an inhibitory effect on ANP secretion. This is supported by evidence showing that cAMP stimulators, such as forskolin, phosphodiesterase inhibitors, and adrenomedullin, as well as cGMP generation inhibit ANP secretion.[113–117]

Glucocorticoids, mineralocorticoids, and prostaglandins have also been implicated in the stimulus of ANP secretion (see Table 12.1). Glucocorticoids and mineralocorticoids upregulate ANP gene expression in rat myocytes increasing ANP production.[118,119] On the other hand, PGF2 alpha stimulates synthesis and secretion of ANP, which is mediated by stretch-induced ANP secretion. This is supported by experiments in rats and rat atrial myocyte cultures showing that atrial stretch and PGF2 alpha led to ANP secretion, but the effect of the two together was not greater than the effect of the individual stimuli. Also, prostaglandin synthesis inhibition with indomethacin led to reduction of basal ANP secretion as well as hypoxia/endothelin-1 stimulated ANP secretion. Taken together, these findings suggest an important role of prostaglandins, glucocorticoids, and mineralocorticoids mediating ANP synthesis and secretion.

Development

During pregnancy, ANP has been proposed to play a major role in the regulation of vascular tone, with maternal ANP levels steadily increasing at 12 weeks of gestation followed by a decline postpartum.[120] In the human placenta, significant ANP expression has been demonstrated in extravillous trophoblasts and, to a lesser degree, in decidual cells, suggesting local placental synthesis.[121] However, in mouse placenta, ANP synthesis remains controversial.[122–124] Importantly, ANP does not seem to cross placenta, as evidenced by experiments in pregnant rats, where no active or passive transport of radiolabeled ANP across the placenta was observed.[125]

Atrial natriuretic peptide is secreted during fetal life, with ANP mRNA being detected as early as 8.5 days of gestation in rat embryos (see Table 12.2).[126] Importantly, in humans and rats, ANP is synthesized in the ventricular cardiomyocytes, while it is synthesized in the atrial cardiomyocytes in ovine fetus.[127–129] These findings are important when extrapolating animal data to humans where ANP release stimulating mechanisms may not be the same in different species. ANP secretion does not seem to be related to maternal ANP concentrations. Another important aspect of fetal ANP secretion is that fetal ANP levels during pregnancy are higher than maternal levels.[127,130–132] The cause for higher fetal than maternal ANP levels is not clear.[127,130–132]

Mid- and late-gestation animals can increase ANP levels in response to various stimuli, including angiotensin II infusion, AVP infusion, indomethacin treatment, acute fetal volume expansion, hypertonicity, and fetal hypoxia.[127,132–134] However, ANP probably has a small role in renal homeostasis and fluid balance during intrauterine life, which is chiefly ensured by the placenta. In general, supraphysiologic ANP doses infused to fetal animals leads to lower arterial blood pressure and a moderate diuretic effect, but there is not a significant increase in natriuresis.[128,134]

At birth, loss of the placental circulation produces dramatic hemodynamic changes such as decreased pulmonary vascular resistance and increased left atrial venous return, leading to atrial distension stimulating ANP secretion from myocardial cells (see Table 12.2).[135] In humans, plasma ANP levels are elevated during the first days of life, with peak levels on days 1 to 2 of life, which then decrease by the second week of life.[136,137] This pattern parallels the postnatal diuresis period, leading to extracellular space contraction seen in infants, which is then followed by the sodium retention period for somatic growth.[138]

Atrial Natriuretic Peptide Signal Transduction

Atrial natriuretic peptide exerts its action in the kidney via activation of a type A natriuretic peptide receptor (NPR-A) (see Table 12.1). This receptor has (a) on the extracellular aspect: a glycosylated domain where ANP binds, (b) single transmembrane segment, (c) on the intracellular aspect: a noncatalytic, kinaselike, ATP-binding domain, a hinge region, and a guanylyl cyclase domain (the latter is the catalytic effector of the receptor). Two peptide receptor chains, dimerized via a disulfide bridge, are required to activate the function of NPR-A.[139] When ANP binds the extracellular domain, the intracellular kinaselike domain undergoes a conformational change leading to relaxation of guanylyl cyclase tonic inhibition, increasing cytosolic cyclic guanosine monophosphate (cGMP) production.[85] cGMP in turn activates cGMP-gated channels, cGMP-dependent phosphodiesterases, and the cGMP-dependent protein kinases cGKI and cGKII, as will be discussed below (see Table 12.1).[140,141]

In addition to the kidneys, NPR-A is also expressed in the heart, lungs, adrenal glands, adipose tissue, and eyes.[142] In the kidneys, the NPR-A receptor is expressed throughout the nephron (glomerular cells and tubular epithelial cells).[143,144] In the glomerulus, NPR-A receptors are located on the surface of the podocytes and mesangial cells. Glomerular podocytes respond to ANP stimulation by upregulating their cGMP synthesis (see Table 12.1). However, the role of ANP-induced cGMP production in podocytes remains unclear. Experiments in isolated rat glomeruli suggest that F-actin filaments may be reorganized, leading to cellular relaxation and modulation in filtration characteristics.[145] In mesangial cells, ANP-induced cGMP production, via NPR-A, increases hyperpolarization leading to cellular relaxation and increases ultrafiltration associated with increased glomerular hydrostatic pressure and filtration rate (see Table 12.1).[146] ANP also increases glomerular filtration rate and glomerular permeability by promoting vasodilatation of the afferent arteriole and vasoconstriction of the efferent arteriole and by causing a direct, reversible increment of the radius and number of large pores, respectively.[147,148]

In tubular cells, ANP inhibits the basolateral Na-K ATPase through type II cGMP-dependent protein kinase (PKGII) induced phosphorylation.[149,150] In proximal tubule cells, ANP inhibits Na reabsorption without altering glomerular filtration rate (GFR) by inhibiting Na-dependent transport systems (see Table 12.1). Potassium, chloride, and organic acid transporters in the proximal tubule are also regulated by ANP.[151–153] In the thick ascending loop cells, ANP inhibits chloride transport in a cGMP-dependent manner by directly inhibiting Na-K-2Cl (NKCC) cotransporter activity, and this, in turn, leads to decreased urine concentrating capacity and increased urine flow (see Table 12.1).[154,155] Medullary collecting duct cells are the main site of ANP action. In these cells, ANP promotes sodium excretion by inhibiting cyclic nucleotide-gated (CNG) cation channels including the epithelial sodium channel designated ENaC (see Table 12.1).[156–162] Furthermore, ANP has been shown to inhibit water permeability by 40% to 50% in non–AVP-stimulated renal collecting ducts.[163]

NPR-A stimulation also regulates blood pressure by inducing vasodilatation, increased endothelial permeability, and inhibition of the sympathetic system.[164] This is supported by evidence showing that targeted deletions of ANP or NPR-A gene in transgenic animals induce severe arterial hypertension, while hypotension is observed with overexpression of these genes.[87]

ANP is also ligand for NPR-C, "clearance receptor." This receptor has (1) on the extracellular aspect, a domain where ANP binds, (2) a single transmembrane segment, and (3) on the intracellular aspect, a 37-amino acid long domain.[164] NPR-C is expressed in kidneys, heart, brain, endothelium, adrenal glands, and smooth muscle cells similar or greater than NPR-A.[164,165] However, unlike NPR-A, NPR-C has no guanyl cyclase activity. On the contrary, NPR-C activation leads to decreased cAMP levels.[166] As a "clearance receptor," NPR-C's main function is to internalize and degrade ANP, as well as other natriuretic peptides, to modulate their activity in various tissues (see Table 12.1).[164,167] This is supported by evidence in the NPR-C knockout mouse which has hypotension and reduced urinary concentration ability as a result of increased bioavailability of ANP.[168]

Development

Natriuretic peptide receptors are present in the placenta as evidenced by expression of NPR-A in human uterine tissues, including decidua, chorion, and myometrium, and in the placenta.[125] Notably, natriuretic peptide receptors in the human placenta are more significantly expressed on its fetal components than on the maternal microvillous membranes.[169] NPR-C is downregulated in fetoplacental artery endothelial cells by the end of gestation, which is mediated, at least in part, by increased placental basic fibroblast growth factor secretion.[170] This concerted downregulation by the end of gestation leads to increases in local ANP and cGMP concentrations, which may be critical for maintaining adequate blood flow in the placental and uterine tissues.

Renal response to ANP is still largely immature at birth. This is supported by evidence showing that natriuresis after ANP infusion is less efficient in young than adult sheep and rats.[131,171] Two proposed mechanisms for this immature response are (1) lower ANP levels due to increased circulating ANP clearance and (2) attenuated renal response to ANP (see Table 12.2). In young and adult rats, ANP infusion leads to dose-dependent increments in urine sodium and cGMP excretion.[171] However, in young rats, ANP levels after infusion are lower than in adults, implying that ANP gets cleared faster in immature rats.[171] Enhanced NPR-C and neutral endopeptidase activity have been proposed as main contributors of ANP clearance in young rats, after experiments demonstrating that ANP levels in young rats doubled those of adult rats following NPR-C and neutral endopeptidases inhibition.[172] On the other hand, attenuated renal response to ANP has been demonstrated by multiple experiments. In rats, expression of renal ANP receptors is low at birth, increasing thereafter to reach adult levels at the end of the fifth week of life.[173] In addition, although intracellular cGMP production has been found to be higher in immature rats, active extracellular transport of cGMP is attenuated in immature rats.[174] This correlates with a parallel maturation of the signal transduction pathways, as demonstrated by a progressive increase in ANP-induced renal cGMP synthesis during the first weeks of life.[175]

REFERENCES

1. McCance RA, Young WF. The secretion of urine by newborn infants. *J Physiol*. 1941;99(3):265–282.
2. Hinchliffe SA, Sargent PH, Howard CV, et al. Human intrauterine renal growth expressed in absolute number of glomeruli assessed by the disector method and Cavalieri principle. *Lab Invest*. 1991;64(6):777–784.
3. Hatton GI. Emerging concepts of structure-function dynamics in adult brain: the hypothalamo-neurohypophysial system. *Prog Neurobiol*. 1990;34(6):437–504.
4. Robertson GL. Antidiuretic hormone: normal and disordered function. *Endocrinol Metab Clin North Am*. 2001;30(3):671–694.
5. Pow DV, Morris JF. Dendrites of hypothalamic magnocellular neurons release neurohypophysial peptides by exocytosis. *Neuroscience*. 1989;32(2):435–439.
6. Grant FD, Reventos J, Kawabata S, et al. Transgenic mouse models of vasopressin expression. *Hypertension*. 1993;22(4):640–645.
7. Verney EB. The antidiuretic hormone and the factors which determine its release. *Proc R Soc Lond B Biol Sci*. 1947;135(878):25–106.
8. Gauer OH, Henry JP. Circulatory basis of fluid volume control. *Physiol Rev*. 1963;43:423–481.
9. Dunn FL, Brennan TJ, Nelson AE, Robertson GL. The role of blood osmolality and volume in regulating vasopressin secretion in the rat. *J Clin Invest*. 1973;52(12):3212–3219.
10. Johnson JA, Zehr JE, Moore WW. Effects of separate and concurrent osmotic and volume stimuli on plasma ADH in sheep. *Am J Physiol*. 1970;218(5):1273–1280.
11. Roberts MM, Robinson AG, Hoffman GE, Fitzsimmons MD. Vasopressin transport regulation is coupled to the synthesis rate. *Neuroendocrinology*. 1991;53(4):416–422.
12. Mastorakos G, Ilias I. Maternal and fetal hypothalamic-pituitary-adrenal axes during pregnancy and postpartum. *Ann N Y Acad Sci*. 2003;997:136–149.
13. Goudsmit E, Neijmeijer-Leloux A, Swaab DF. The human hypothalamo-neurohypophyseal system in relation to development, aging and Alzheimer's disease. *Prog Brain Res*. 1992;93:237–247.
14. Murayama K, Meeker RB, Murayama S, Greenwood RS. Developmental expression of vasopressin in the human hypothalamus: double-labeling with in situ hybridization and immunocytochemistry. *Pediatr Res*. 1993;33(2):152–158.
15. Altman J, Bayer SA. The development of the rat hypothalamus. *Adv Anat Embryol Cell Biol*. 1986;100:1–178.
16. Okamura H, Fukui K, Koyama E, et al. Time of vasopressin neuron origin in the mouse hypothalamus: examination by combined technique of immunocytochemistry and [3H]thymidine autoradiography. *Brain Res*. 1983;285(2):223–226.
17. Hyodo S, Yamada C, Takezawa T, Urano A. Expression of provasopressin gene during ontogeny in the hypothalamus of developing mice. *Neuroscience*. 1992;46(1):241–250.
18. Laurent FM, Hindelang C, Klein MJ, et al. Expression of the oxytocin and vasopressin genes in the rat hypothalamus during development: an in situ hybridization study. *Brain Res Dev Brain Res*. 1989;46(1):145–154.

19. Weitzman RE, Fisher DA, Robillard J, et al. Arginine vasopressin response to an osmotic stimulus in the fetal sheep. *Pediatr Res.* 1978;12(1):35–38.
20. Shi L, Mao C, Wu J, et al. Effects of i.c.v. losartan on the angiotensin II-mediated vasopressin release and hypothalamic fos expression in near-term ovine fetuses. *Peptides.* 2006;27(9):2230–2238.
21. Hadeed AJ, Leake RD, Weitzman RE, Fisher DA. Possible mechanisms of high blood levels of vasopressin during the neonatal period. *J Pediatr.* 1979;94(5):805–808.
22. Rees L, Forsling ML, Brook CG. Vasopressin concentrations in the neonatal period. *Clin Endocrinol (Oxf).* 1980;12(4):357–362.
23. Ramin SM, Porter JC, Gilstrap LC, Rosenfeld CR. Stress hormones and acid-base status of human fetuses at delivery. *J Clin Endocrinol Metab.* 1991;73(1):182–186.
24. Grantham JJ, Burg MB. Effect of vasopressin and cyclic AMP on permeability of isolated collecting tubules. *Am J Physiol.* 1966;211(1):255–259.
25. Sands JM, Nonoguchi H, Knepper MA. Vasopressin effects on urea and H2O transport in inner medullary collecting duct subsegments. *Am J Physiol.* 1987;253(5 Pt 2):F823–F832.
26. Ruiz-Opazo N, Akimoto K, Herrera VL. Identification of a novel dual angiotensin II/vasopressin receptor on the basis of molecular recognition theory. *Nat Med.* 1995;1(10):1074–1081.
27. Fushimi K, Uchida S, Hara Y, et al. Cloning and expression of apical membrane water channel of rat kidney collecting tubule. *Nature.* 1993;361(6412):549–552.
28. Fushimi K, Sasaki S, Marumo F. Phosphorylation of serine 256 is required for cAMP-dependent regulatory exocytosis of the aquaporin-2 water channel. *J Biol Chem.* 1997;272(23):14800–14804.
29. Nielsen S, Chou CL, Marples D, et al. Vasopressin increases water permeability of kidney collecting duct by inducing translocation of aquaporin-CD water channels to plasma membrane. *Proc Natl Acad Sci USA.* 1995;92(4):1013–1017.
30. Valenti G, Procino G, Tamma G, et al. Minireview: aquaporin 2 trafficking. *Endocrinology.* 2005;146(12):5063–5070.
31. Kuwahara M, Fushimi K, Terada Y, et al. cAMP-dependent phosphorylation stimulates water permeability of aquaporin-collecting duct water channel protein expressed in Xenopus oocytes. *J Biol Chem.* 1995;270(18):10384–10387.
32. Robillard JE, Weitzman RE. Developmental aspects of the fetal renal response to exogenous arginine vasopressin. *Am J Physiol.* 1980;238(5):F407–F414.
33. Herin P, Kim JK, Schrier RW, et al. Ovine fetal response to water deprivation: aspects on the role of vasopressin. *Q J Exp Physiol.* 1988;73(6):931–940.
34. Towstoless MK, Congiu M, Coghlan JP, Wintour EM. Placental and renal control of plasma osmolality in chronically cannulated ovine fetus. *Am J Physiol.* 1987;253(3 Pt 2):R389–R395.
35. Heller H. The renal function of newborn infants. *J Physiol.* 1944;102(4):429–440.
36. Ostrowski NL, Young WS, Knepper MA, Lolait SJ. Expression of vasopressin V1a and V2 receptor messenger ribonucleic acid in the liver and kidney of embryonic, developing, and adult rats. *Endocrinology.* 1993;133(4):1849–1859.
37. Rajerison RM, Butlen D, Jard S. Ontogenic development of antidiuretic hormone receptors in rat kidney: comparison of hormonal binding and adenylate cyclase activation. *Mol Cell Endocrinol.* 1976;4(4):271–285.
38. Bonilla-Felix M. Development of water transport in the collecting duct. *Am J Physiol.* 2004;287(6):F1093–F1101.
39. Bonilla-Felix M, John-Phillip C. Prostaglandins mediate the defect in AVP-stimulated cAMP generation in immature collecting duct. *Am J Physiol.* 1994;267(1 Pt 2):F44–F48.
40. Bonilla-Felix M, Vehaskari VM, Hamm LL. Water transport in the immature rabbit collecting duct. *Pediatr Nephrol.* 1999;13(2):103–107.
41. Gengler WR, Forte LR. Neonatal development of rat kidney adenyl cyclase and phosphodiesterase. *Biochim Biophys Acta.* 1972;279(2):367–372.
42. Schlondorff D, Weber H, Trizna W, Fine LG. Vasopressin responsiveness of renal adenylate cyclase in newborn rats and rabbits. *Am J Physiol.* 1978;234(1):F16–F21.
43. Forrest JN, Stanier MW. Kidney composition and renal concentration ability in young rabbits. *J Physiol.* 1966;187(1):1–4.
44. Quigley R, Chakravarty S, Baum M. Antidiuretic hormone resistance in the neonatal cortical collecting tubule is mediated in part by elevated phosphodiesterase activity. *Am J Physiol Renal Physiol.* 2004;286(2):F317–F322.
45. Joppich R, Häberle DA, Weber PC. Studies of the immaturity of the ADH-dependent cAMP system in conscious newborn piglets—possible impairing effects of renal prostaglandins. *Pediatr Res.* 1981;15(3):278–281.
46. Sulyok E, Ertl T, Csaba IF, Varga F. Postnatal changes in urinary prostaglandin E excretion in premature infants. *Biol Neonate.* 1980;37(3–4):192–196.
47. Joppich R, Scherer B, Weber PC. Renal prostaglandins: relationship to the development of blood pressure and concentrating capacity in pre-term and full term healthy infants. *Eur J Pediatr.* 1979;132(4):253–259.
48. Nadler SP, Hebert SC, Brenner BM. PGE2, forskolin, and cholera toxin interactions in rabbit cortical collecting tubule. *Am J Physiol.* 1986;250(1 Pt 2):F127–F135.
49. Takeuchi K, Abe T, Takahashi N, Abe K. Molecular cloning and intrarenal localization of rat prostaglandin E2 receptor EP3 subtype. *Biochem Biophys Res Commun.* 1993;194(2):885–891.
50. Negishi M, Sugimoto Y, Hayashi Y, et al. Functional interaction of prostaglandin E receptor EP3 subtype with guanine nucleotide-binding proteins, showing low-affinity ligand binding. *Biochim Biophys Acta.* 1993;1175(3):343–350.

12

51. Bonilla-Felix M, Jiang W. Expression and localization of prostaglandin EP3 receptor mRNA in the immature rabbit kidney. *Am J Physiol*. 1996;271(1 Pt 2):F30–F36.
52. Meléndez E, Reyes JL, Escalante BA, Meléndez MA. Development of the receptors to prostaglandin E2 in the rat kidney and neonatal renal functions. *Dev Pharmacol Ther*. 1989;14(2):125–134.
53. Matson JR, Stokes JB, Robillard JE. Effects of inhibition of prostaglandin synthesis on fetal renal function. *Kidney Int*. 1981;20(5):621–627.
54. Nielsen S, Frøkiær J, Marples D, et al. Aquaporins in the kidney: from molecules to medicine. *Physiol Rev*. 2002;82(1):205–244.
55. Knepper MA, Nielsen S, Chou CL, DiGiovanni SR. Mechanism of vasopressin action in the renal collecting duct. *Semin Nephrol*. 1994;14(4):302–321.
56. Liu H, Wintour EM. Aquaporins in development—a review. *Reprod Biol Endocrinol*. 2005;3(1):18.
57. Nielsen S, Smith BL, Christensen EI, et al. CHIP28 water channels are localized in constitutively water-permeable segments of the nephron. *J Cell Biol*. 1993;120(2):371–383.
58. Nielsen S, Pallone T, Smith BL, et al. Aquaporin-1 water channels in short and long loop descending thin limbs and in descending vasa recta in rat kidney. *Am J Physiol*. 1995;268(6 Pt 2):F1023–F1037.
59. Nejsum LN, Elkjær M-L, Hager H, et al. Localization of aquaporin-7 in rat and mouse kidney using RT-PCR, immunoblotting, and immunocytochemistry. *Biochem Biophys Res Commun*. 2000;277(1):164–170.
60. Yasui M, Kwon TH, Knepper MA, et al. Aquaporin-6: an intracellular vesicle water channel protein in renal epithelia. *Proc Natl Acad Sci USA*. 1999;96(10):5808–5813.
61. Elkjaer ML, Nejsum LN, Gresz V, et al. Immunolocalization of aquaporin-8 in rat kidney, gastrointestinal tract, testis, and airways. *Am J Physiol Renal Physiol*. 2001;281(6):F1047–F1057.
62. Bonilla-Felix M, Jiang W. Aquaporin-2 in the immature rat: expression, regulation, and trafficking. *J Am Soc Nephrol*. 1997;8(10):1502–1509.
63. Elliot S, Goldsmith P, Knepper M, et al. Urinary excretion of aquaporin-2 in humans: a potential marker of collecting duct responsiveness to vasopressin. *J Am Soc Nephrol*. 1996;7(3):403–409.
64. Tsukahara H, Hata I, Sekine K, et al. Renal water channel expression in newborns: measurement of urinary excretion of aquaporin-2. *Metabolism*. 1998;47(11):1344–1347.
65. Walker DW, Mitchell MD. Prostaglandins in urine of foetal lambs. *Nature*. 1978;271(5641):161–162.
66. Nyul Z, Vajda Z, Vida G, et al. Urinary aquaporin-2 excretion in preterm and full-term neonates. *Biol Neonate*. 2002;82(1):17–21.
67. Bonilla-Felix M. Development of water transport in the collecting duct. *Am J Physiol Renal Physiol*. 2004;287(6):F1093–F1101.
68. Yasui M, Serlachius E, Löfgren M, et al. Perinatal changes in expression of aquaporin-4 and other water and ion transporters in rat lung. *J Physiol*. 1997;505:3–11.
69. Yamamoto T, Sasaki S, Fushimi K, et al. Expression of AQP family in rat kidneys during development and maturation. *Am J Physiol*. 1997;272(2 Pt 2):F198–F204.
70. Damiano A, Zotta E, Goldstein J, et al. Water channel proteins AQP3 and AQP9 are present in syncytiotrophoblast of human term placenta. *Placenta*. 2001;22(8–9):776–781.
71. Beall MH, Wang S, Yang B, et al. Placental and membrane aquaporin water channels: correlation with amniotic fluid volume and composition. *Placenta*. 2007;28(5–6):421–428.
72. Jansson T, Powell TL, Illsley NP. Gestational development of water and non-electrolyte permeability of human syncytiotrophoblast plasma membranes. *Placenta*. 1999;20(2–3):155–160.
73. Mann SE, Ricke EA, Yang BA, et al. Expression and localization of aquaporin 1 and 3 in human fetal membranes. *Am J Obstet Gynecol*. 2002;187(4):902–907.
74. Mann SE, Ricke EA, Torres EA, Taylor RN. A novel model of polyhydramnios: amniotic fluid volume is increased in aquaporin 1 knockout mice. *Am J Obstet Gynecol*. 2005;192(6):2041–2044.
75. Liu H, Koukoulas I, Ross MC, et al. Quantitative comparison of placental expression of three aquaporin genes. *Placenta*. 2004;25(6):475–478.
76. Wang S, Chen J, Beall M, et al. Expression of aquaporin 9 in human chorioamniotic membranes and placenta. *Am J Obstet Gynecol*. 2004;191(6):2160–2167.
77. Wang S, Kallichanda N, Song W, et al. Expression of aquaporin-8 in human placenta and chorioamniotic membranes: evidence of molecular mechanism for intramembranous amniotic fluid resorption. *Am J Obstet Gynecol*. 2001;185(5):1226–1231.
78. Michael H. Principles of nephron differentiation. *Am J Physiol*. 1978;235(5):F387–F393.
79. Horster M. Loop of Henle functional differentiation: in vitro perfusion of the isolated thick ascending segment. *Pflugers Arch*. 1978;378(1):15–24.
80. Horster MF, Gilg A, Lory P. Determinants of axial osmotic gradients in the differentiating countercurrent system. *Am J Physiol*. 1984;246(2 Pt 2):F124–F132.
81. Edelmann CM, Barnett HL, Stark H. Effect of urea on concentration of urinary nonurea solute in premature infants. *J Appl Physiol*. 1966;21(3):1021–1025.
82. Edelmann CM. BarnettHL, Troupkou V. Renal concentrating mechanisms in newborn infants. Effect of dietary protein and water content, role of urea, and responsiveness to antidiuretic hormone. *J Clin Invest*. 1960;39(7):1062–1069.
83. Yandle TG. Biochemistry of natriuretic peptides. *J Intern Med*. 1994;235(6):561–576.
84. de Bold AJ. Atrial natriuretic factor: a hormone produced by the heart. *Science*. 1985;230(4727):767–770.
85. Gardner DG, Chen S, Glenn DJ, Grigsby CL. Molecular biology of the natriuretic peptide system: implications for physiology and hypertension. *Hypertension*. 2007;49(3):419–426.
86. Yan W, Wu F, Morser J, Wu Q. Corin, a transmembrane cardiac serine protease, acts as a pro-atrial natriuretic peptide-converting enzyme. *Proc Natl Acad Sci U S A*. 2000;97(15):8525–8529.

87. de Bold AJ, Ma KK, Zhang Y, et al. The physiological and pathophysiological modulation of the endocrine function of the heart. *Can J Physiol Pharmacol.* 2001;79(8):705–714.

88. de Bold AJ, Borenstein HB, Veress AT, Sonnenberg H. A rapid and potent natriuretic response to intravenous injection of atrial myocardial extract in rats. Reprinted from Life Sci. 28:89-94, 1981. *J Am Soc Nephrol.* 2001;12(2):403–409, 408–409.

89. Levin ER, Gardner DG, Samson WK. Natriuretic peptides. *N Engl J Med.* 1998;339(5):321–328.

90. Lang RE, Thölken H, Ganten D, et al. Atrial natriuretic factor—a circulating hormone stimulated by volume loading. *Nature.* 1985;314(6008):264–266.

91. Ledsome JR, Wilson N, Courneya CA, Rankin AJ. Release of atrial natriuretic peptide by atrial distension. *Can J Physiol Pharmacol.* 1985;63(6):739–742.

92. Baertschi AJ, Hausmaninger C, Walsh RS, et al. Hypoxia-induced release of atrial natriuretic factor (ANF) from the isolated rat and rabbit heart. *Biochem Biophys Res Commun.* 1986;140(1):427–433.

93. du Souich P, Saunier C, Hartemann D, et al. Effect of moderate hypoxemia on atrial natriuretic factor and arginine vasopressin in normal man. *Biochem Biophys Res Commun.* 1987;148(3):906–912.

94. Tikkanen T, Tikkanen I, Fyhrquist F. Elevated plasma atrial natriuretic peptide in rats with myocardial infarcts. *Life Sci.* 1987;40(7):659–663.

95. Tan AC, van Loenhout TT, Lamfers EJ, et al. Atrial natriuretic peptide after myocardial infarction. *Am Heart J.* 1989;118(3):490–494.

96. Lew RA, Baertschi AJ. Mechanisms of hypoxia-induced atrial natriuretic factor release from rat hearts. *Am J Physiol.* 1989;257(1 Pt 2):H147–H156.

97. Skvorak JP, Sutton ET, Rao PS, Dietz JR. Mechanism of anoxia-induced atrial natriuretic peptide release in the isolated rat atria. *Am J Physiol.* 1996;271(1 Pt 2):R237–R243.

98. Focaccio A, Volpe M, Ambrosio G, et al. Angiotensin II directly stimulates release of atrial natriuretic factor in isolated rabbit hearts. *Circulation.* 1993;87(1):192–198.

99. Dietz JR. The effect of angiotensin II and ADH on the secretion of atrial natriuretic factor. *Proc Soc Exp Biol Med.* 1988;187(3):366–369.

100. Veress AT, Milojevic S, Yip C, et al. In vitro secretion of atrial natriuretic factor: receptor-mediated release of prohormone. *Am J Physiol.* 1988;254(5 Pt 2):R809–R814.

101. Katsube N, Schwartz D, Needleman P. Release of atriopeptin in the rat by vasoconstrictors or water immersion correlates with changes in right atrial pressure. *Biochem Biophys Res Commun.* 1985;133(3):937–944.

102. Lachance D, Garcia R. Atrial natriuretic factor release by angiotensin II in the conscious rat. *Hypertension.* 1988;11(6 Pt 1):502–508.

103. Sonnenberg H, Veress AT. Cellular mechanism of release of atrial natriuretic factor. *Biochem Biophys Res Commun.* 1984;124(2):443–449.

104. McGrath MF, de Bold AJ. Determinants of natriuretic peptide gene expression. *Peptides.* 2005;26(6):933–943.

105. Bensimon M, Chang AI, de Bold MLK, et al. Participation of G proteins in natriuretic peptide hormone secretion from heart atria. *Endocrinology.* 2004;145(11):5313–5321.

106. Irons CE, Sei CA, Hidaka H, Glembotski CC. Protein kinase C and calmodulin kinase are required for endothelin-stimulated atrial natriuretic factor secretion from primary atrial myocytes. *J Biol Chem.* 1992;267(8):5211–5216.

107. Ruskoaho H, Toth M, Ganten D, et al. The phorbol ester induced atrial natriuretic peptide secretion is stimulated by forskolin and Bay K8644 and inhibited by 8-bromo-cyclic GMP. *Biochem Biophys Res Commun.* 1986;139(1):266–274.

108. Wen JF, Cui X, Ahn JS, et al. Distinct roles for L- and T-type Ca(2+) channels in regulation of atrial ANP release. *Am J Physiol Heart Circ Physiol.* 2000;279(6):H2879–H2888.

109. Laine M, Arjamaa O, Vuolteenaho O, et al. Block of stretch-activated atrial natriuretic peptide secretion by gadolinium in isolated rat atrium. *J Physiol.* 1994;553–561.

110. Kuroski-de Bold ML, de Bold AJ. Stretch-secretion coupling in atrial cardiocytes. Dissociation between atrial natriuretic factor release and mechanical activity. *Hypertension.* 1991;18(5 suppl):III169–III178.

111. Taskinen P, Ruskoaho H. Stretch-induced increase in atrial natriuretic peptide secretion is blocked by thapsigargin. *Eur J Pharmacol.* 1996;308(3):295–300.

112. Sei CA, Glembotski CC. Calcium dependence of phenylephrine-, endothelin-, and potassium chloride-stimulated atrial natriuretic factor secretion from long term primary neonatal rat atrial cardiocytes. *J Biol Chem.* 1990;265(13):7166–7172.

113. Sato A, Canny BJ, Autelitano DJ. Adrenomedullin stimulates cAMP accumulation and inhibits atrial natriuretic peptide gene expression in cardiomyocytes. *Biochem Biophys Res Commun.* 1997;230(2):311–314.

114. Iida H, Page E. Inhibition of atrial natriuretic peptide secretion by forskolin in noncontracting cultured atrial myocytes. *Biochem Biophys Res Commun.* 1988;157(1):330–336.

115. Muir TM, Hair J, Inglis GC, et al. Hormonal control of atrial natriuretic peptide synthesis and secretion from cultured atrial myocytes. *J Mol Cell Cardiol.* 1993;25(5):509–518.

116. Cui X, Wen JF, Jin H, et al. Subtype-specific roles of cAMP phosphodiesterases in regulation of atrial natriuretic peptide release. *Eur J Pharmacol.* 2002;451(3):295–302.

117. Lee SJ, Kim SZ, Cui X, et al. C-type natriuretic peptide inhibits ANP secretion and atrial dynamics in perfused atria: NPR-B-cGMP signaling. *Am J Physiol Heart Circ Physiol.* 2000;278(1):H208–H221.

118. Shields PP, Dixon JE, Glembotski CC. The secretion of atrial natriuretic factor-(99-126) by cultured cardiac myocytes is regulated by glucocorticoids. *J Biol Chem.* 1988;263(25):12619–12628.

12

119. Dananberg J, Grekin RJ. Corticoid regulation of atrial natriuretic factor secretion and gene expression. *Am J Physiol*. 1992;263(5 Pt 2):H1377–H1381.

120. Yoshimura T, Yoshimura M, Yasue H, et al. Plasma concentration of atrial natriuretic peptide and brain natriuretic peptide during normal human pregnancy and the postpartum period. *J Endocrinol*. 1994;140(3):393–397.

121. Graham CH, Watson JD, Blumenfeld AJ, Pang SC. Expression of atrial natriuretic peptide by third-trimester placental cytotrophoblasts in women. *Biol Reprod*. 1996;54(4):834–840.

122. Cameron VA, Aitken GD, Ellmers LJ, et al. The sites of gene expression of atrial, brain, and C-type natriuretic peptides in mouse fetal development: temporal changes in embryos and placenta. *Endocrinology*. 1996;137(3):817–824.

123. Huang W, Lee D, Yang Z, et al. Evidence for atrial natriuretic peptide-(5-28) production by rat placental cytotrophoblasts. *Endocrinology*. 1992;131(2):919–924.

124. Inglis GC, Kingdom JC, Nelson DM, et al. Atrial natriuretic hormone: a paracrine or endocrine role within the human placenta? *J Clin Endocrinol Metab*. 1993;76(4):1014–1018.

125. Mulay S, Varma DR. Placental barrier to atrial natriuretic peptide in rats. *Can J Physiol Pharmacol*. 1989;67(1):1–4.

126. Zeller R, Bloch KD, Williams BS, et al. Localized expression of the atrial natriuretic factor gene during cardiac embryogenesis. *Genes Dev*. 1987;1(7):693–698.

127. Wei YF, Rodi CP, Day ML, et al. Developmental changes in the rat atriopeptin hormonal system. *J Clin Invest*. 1987;79(5):1325–1329.

128. Cameron VA, Ellmers LJ. Minireview: natriuretic peptides during development of the fetal heart and circulation. *Endocrinology*. 2003;144(6):2191–2194.

129. Cheung CY, Roberts VJ. Developmental changes in atrial natriuretic factor content and localization of its messenger ribonucleic acid in ovine fetal heart. *Am J Obstet Gynecol*. 1993;169(5):1345–1351.

130. Cheung CY, Gibbs DM, Brace RA. Atrial natriuretic factor in maternal and fetal sheep. *Am J Physiol*. 1987;252(2 Pt 1):E279–E282.

131. Robillard JE, Nakamura KT, Varille VA, et al. Ontogeny of the renal response to natriuretic peptide in sheep. *Am J Physiol*. 1988;254(5 Pt 2):F634–F641.

132. Deloof S, Chatelain A. Effect of blood volume expansion on basal plasma atrial natriuretic factor and adrenocorticotropic hormone secretions in the fetal rat at term. *Biol Neonate*. 1994;65(6):390–395.

133. Rosenfeld CR, Samson WK, Roy TA, et al. Vasoconstrictor-induced secretion of ANP in fetal sheep. *Am J Physiol*. 1992;263(3 Pt 1):E526–E533.

134. Cheung CY. Regulation of atrial natriuretic factor secretion and expression in the ovine fetus. *Neurosci Biobehav Rev*. 1995;19(2):159–164.

135. Tulassay T, Seri I, Rascher W. Atrial natriuretic peptide and extracellular volume contraction after birth. *Acta Paediatr Scand*. 1987;76(3):444–446.

136. Weil J, Bidlingmaier F, Döhlemann C, et al. Comparison of plasma atrial natriuretic peptide levels in healthy children from birth to adolescence and in children with cardiac diseases. *Pediatr Res*. 1986;20(12):1328–1331.

137. Mir TS, Laux R, Hellwege HH, et al. Plasma concentrations of aminoterminal pro atrial natriuretic peptide and aminoterminal pro brain natriuretic peptide in healthy neonates: marked and rapid increase after birth. *Pediatrics*. 2003;112(4):896–899.

138. Bierd TM, Kattwinkel J, Chevalier RL, et al. Interrelationship of atrial natriuretic peptide, atrial volume, and renal function in premature infants. *J Pediatr*. 1990;116(5):753–759.

139. Labrecque J, Mc Nicoll N, Marquis M, De Léan A. A disulfide-bridged mutant of natriuretic peptide receptor-A displays constitutive activity. Role of receptor dimerization in signal transduction. *J Biol Chem*. 1999;274(14):9752–9759.

140. Kuhn M. Cardiac and intestinal natriuretic peptides: insights from genetically modified mice. *Peptides*. 2005;26(6):1078–1085.

141. Inoue T, Nonoguchi H, Tomita K. Physiological effects of vasopressin and atrial natriuretic peptide in the collecting duct. *Cardiovasc Res*. 2001;51(3):470–480.

142. Nakao K, Ogawa Y, Suga S, Imura H. Molecular biology and biochemistry of the natriuretic peptide system. II: natriuretic peptide receptors. *J Hypertens*. 1992;10(10):1111–1114.

143. Nonoguchi H, Knepper MA, Manganiello VC. Effects of atrial natriuretic factor on cyclic guanosine monophosphate and cyclic adenosine monophosphate accumulation in microdissected nephron segments from rats. *J Clin Invest*. 1987;79(2):500–507.

144. Terada Y, Moriyama T, Martin BM, et al. RT-PCR microlocalization of mRNA for guanylyl cyclase-coupled ANF receptor in rat kidney. *Am J Physiol*. 1991;261(6 Pt 2):F1080–F1087.

145. Sharma R, Lovell HB, Wiegmann TB, Savin VJ. Vasoactive substances induce cytoskeletal changes in cultured rat glomerular epithelial cells. *J Am Soc Nephrol*. 1992;3(5):1131–1138.

146. Ballermann BJ, Hoover RL, Karnovsky MJ, Brenner BM. Physiologic regulation of atrial natriuretic peptide receptors in rat renal glomeruli. *J Clin Invest*. 1985;76(6):2049–2056.

147. Gunning ME, Brenner BM. Natriuretic peptides and the kidney: current concepts. *Kidney Int Suppl*. 1992;38:S127–S133.

148. Axelsson J, Rippe A, Rippe B. Transient and sustained increases in glomerular permeability following ANP infusion in rats. *Am J Physiol Renal Physiol*. 2011;300(1):F24–F30.

149. Aperia A, Holtbäck U, Syrén ML, et al. Activation/deactivation of renal Na+,K(+)-ATPase: a final common pathway for regulation of natriuresis. *FASEB J*. 1994;8(6):436–439.

150. Brismar H, Holtbäck U, Aperia A. Mechanisms by which intrarenal dopamine and ANP interact to regulate sodium metabolism. *Clin Exp Hypertens*. 2000;22(3):303–307.

151. Darvish N, Winaver J, Dagan D. A novel cGMP-activated Cl– channel in renal proximal tubules. *Am J Physiol*. 1995;268(2 Pt 2):F323–F329.

152. Hirsch JR, Meyer M, Mägert HJ, et al. cGMP-dependent and -independent inhibition of a K+ conductance by natriuretic peptides: molecular and functional studies in human proximal tubule cells. *J Am Soc Nephrol*. 1999;10(3):472–480.

153. Hirsch JR, Weber G, Kleta I, Schlatter E. A novel cGMP-regulated K+ channel in immortalized human kidney epitheliall cells (IHKE-1). *J Physiol*. 1999;519(Pt 3):645–655.

154. Bailly C. Effect of luminal atrial natriuretic peptide on chloride reabsorption in mouse cortical thick ascending limb: inhibition by endothelin. *J Am Soc Nephrol*. 2000;11(10):1791–1797.

155. Nonoguchi H, Tomita K, Marumo F. Effects of atrial natriuretic peptide and vasopressin on chloride transport in long- and short-looped medullary thick ascending limbs. *J Clin Invest*. 1992;90(2):349–357.

156. Zhao D, Pandey KN, Navar LG. ANP-mediated inhibition of distal nephron fractional sodium reabsorption in wild-type and mice overexpressing natriuretic peptide receptor. *Am J Physiol Renal Physiol*. 2010;298(1):F103–F108.

157. Light DB, Corbin JD, Stanton BA. Dual ion-channel regulation by cyclic GMP and cyclic GMP-dependent protein kinase. *Nature*. 1990;344(6264):336–339.

158. Guo L-J, Alli AA, Eaton DC, Bao H-F. ENaC is regulated by natriuretic peptide receptor-dependent cGMP signaling. *Am J Physiol Renal Physiol*. 2013;304(7):F930–F937.

159. Zeidel ML, Kikeri D, Silva P, et al. Atrial natriuretic peptides inhibit conductive sodium uptake by rabbit inner medullary collecting duct cells. *J Clin Invest*. 1988;82(3):1067–1074.

160. Du J, Wong W-Y, Sun L, et al. Protein kinase G inhibits flow-induced Ca2+ entry into collecting duct cells. *J Am Soc Nephrol*. 2012;23(7):1172–1180.

161. Zeidel ML, Silva P, Brenner BM, Seifter JL. cGMP mediates effects of atrial peptides on medullary collecting duct cells. *Am J Physiol*. 1987;252(3 Pt 2):F551–F559.

162. Sonnenberg H, Honrath U, Chong CK, Wilson DR. Atrial natriuretic factor inhibits sodium transport in medullary collecting duct. *Am J Physiol*. 1986;250(6 Pt 2):F963–F966.

163. Nonoguchi H, Sands JM, Knepper MA. Atrial natriuretic factor inhibits vasopressin-stimulated osmotic water permeability in rat inner medullary collecting duct. *J Clin Invest*. 1988;82(4):1383–1390.

164. Brenner BM, Ballermann BJ, Gunning ME, Zeidel ML. Diverse biological actions of atrial natriuretic peptide. *Physiol Rev*. 1990;70(3):665–699.

165. Espiner EA, Richards AM, Yandle TG, Nicholls MG. Natriuretic hormones. *Endocrinol Metab Clin North Am*. 1995;24(3):481–509.

166. Fuller F, Porter JG, Arfsten AE, et al. Atrial natriuretic peptide clearance receptor. Complete sequence and functional expression of cDNA clones. *J Biol Chem*. 1988;263(19):9395–9401.

167. Maack T, Suzuki M, Almeida FA, et al. Physiological role of silent receptors of atrial natriuretic factor. *Science*. 1987;238(4827):675–678.

168. Matsukawa N, Grzesik WJ, Takahashi N, et al. The natriuretic peptide clearance receptor locally modulates the physiological effects of the natriuretic peptide system. *Proc Natl Acad Sci USA*. 1999;96(13):7403–7408.

169. Zhang LC, Liang GD, Zhang YH, et al. Distribution and characteristics of placental ANP receptors in normal and hypertensive pregnancy. *Chin Med J*. 1992;105(1):39–43.

170. Itoh H, Zheng J, Bird IM, et al. Basic FGF decreases clearance receptor of natriuretic peptides in fetoplacental artery endothelium. *Am J Physiol*. 1999;277(2 Pt 2):R541–R547.

171. Chevalier RL, Ariel Gomez R, Carey RM, et al. Renal effects of atrial natriuretic peptide infusion in young and adult rats. *Pediatr Res*. 1988;24(3):333–337.

172. Chevalier RL, Garmey M, Scarborough RM, et al. Inhibition of ANP clearance receptors and endopeptidase 24.11 in maturing rats. *Am J Physiol*. 1991;260(6 Pt 2):R1218–R1228.

173. Semmekrot B, Roseau S, Vassent G, Butlen D. Developmental patterns of renal atrial natriuretic peptide receptors: [125I]alpha-rat atrial natriuretic peptide binding in glomeruli and inner medullary collecting tubules microdissected from kidneys of young rats. *Mol Cell Endocrinol*. 1990;68(1):35–43.

174. Norling LL, Vaughan CA, Chevalier RL. Maturation of cGMP response to ANP by isolated glomeruli. *Am J Physiol*. 1992;262(1 Pt 2):F138–F143.

175. Chevalier RL, Fern RJ, Garmey M, et al. Localization of cGMP after infusion of ANP or nitroprusside in the maturing rat. *Am J Physiol*. 1992;262(3 Pt 2):F417–F424.

12

CHAPTER 13

Acute Problems of Prematurity: Balancing Fluid Volume and Electrolyte Replacements in Very Low Birth Weight and Extremely Low Birth Weight Neonates

Stephen Baumgart, MD, FAAP

- **Immature Epidermal Barrier Function and the Extremely Low Birth Weight Habitus**
- **Transcutaneous (Insensible) Water Loss**
- **Water Loss and Pathogenesis of Transcutaneous Dehydration**
- **Salt Restriction Prophylaxis**
- **Nonoliguric Hyperkalemia in Extremely Low Birth Weight Babies**
- **The Epidermal Barrier: Reducing Transcutaneous Evaporation**
- **Pulmonary Edema Formation**
- **Electrolyte Imbalances and Neurodevelopment**
- **Areas for Further Investigation**
- **Between a Rock and a Hard Place: Suggestions for Vigilant Fluid Balance Therapy in Extremely Low Birth Weight Babies**

Introduction

In this chapter, we will discuss three problem areas for achieving fluid and electrolyte balance in the extremely low birth weight (ELBW) infant (<1000 g at birth), and for his/her historical predecessor, the very low birth weight (VLBW) infant (<1500 g at birth). The most recent clinical research on fluid and electrolyte therapy addresses these groups as separate; however, the principles for achieving fluid balance in each group represent the same physiology at different phases of fetal development.

The first of these problems is poor epidermal barrier function. Especially in ELBW infants, thin, gelatinous skin promotes rapid transcutaneous evaporation, producing severe electrolyte disturbances in the first few days of life as well as presenting a poor barrier to infectious agents, and is also subject to trauma from tape/adhesive injury and from routine contact with bedclothes and handling.

A second area of major concern is pulmonary edema formation. Increased lung water (pulmonary edema) has been suggested in the pathogenesis of several conditions (including patent ductus arteriosus [PDA], with congestive heart failure, and bronchopulmonary dysplasia [BPD]), leading to the controversy of fluid restriction versus fluid replenishment in preventing chronic lung disease in both VLBW and ELBW infants. Equally controversial is the routine use of diuretics and steroids for the treatment of infants with pulmonary edema with acute respiratory distress syndrome (RDS) and chronic lung disease.

Finally, a relatively new area of concern is the neurodevelopmental outcome of those infants manifesting severe electrolyte imbalances early in life, particularly in those who develop hyponatremia or hypernatremia/hyperosmolality in the first few weeks.

Immature Epidermal Barrier Function and the Extremely Low Birth Weight Habitus

The tiny baby (ELBW) experiences large transepidermal water losses immediately upon birth.[1,2] The ELBW baby has little in the way of skin keratin content, and the skin appears translucent, gelatinous, and shiny (Fig. 13.1). In addition, these infants have a proportionally larger extracellular pool (with a nearly normal saline content in equilibrium with the plasma compartment)[3] from which the evaporation of body water leaves the sodium behind (Fig. 13.2).[4,5] During early fetal life, more than 85% of body mass may be composed of water, two-thirds of which resides in the extracellular space; and only one-third of this water resides in the intracellular space. In contrast, by term gestation, the infant is comprised of about 75% water, with approximately one-half in the extracellular and intracellular spaces, respectively. By 3 months postnatal age, only 60% of body mass is water, with two-thirds residing in the intracellular compartment and only one-third in the extracellular space. Finally, the ELBW neonate has a geometrically larger skin surface area than in more mature infants and adults (Fig. 13.3).[6]

The ELBW baby proportionally has over 6 times the skin surface area exposed per kilogram of body weight, with at least 3 times the mass of water content vulnerable to evaporation.[5,6] A 500-g infant has as much as 1400 cm^2 skin exposed per kilogram compared with about 750 cm^2/kg in a term infant and 240 cm^2/kg in the adult. It is important to remember this exposed body mass is largely comprised of extracellular, sodium-rich water available for evaporation.

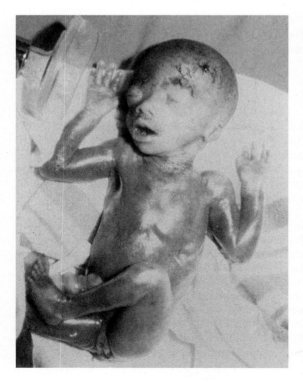

Fig. 13.1 Photograph at birth of a 23-3/7–week gestation 530-g birth weight extremely low birth weight infant born in 1980 showing that the extremely immature skin has little in the way of skin keratin content, and appears translucent, gelatinous, and shiny as if moist with body water rapidly evaporating into the cool-dry delivery-room air. Her eyelids are fused; she is pink, well perfused, and making breathing efforts. She is moving all extremities with apparently good postural tone and spontaneous activity. She went on to survive relatively intact.

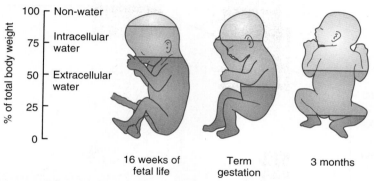

Fig. 13.2 Note the sizable extracellular water compartment (an extension of the amniotic fluid space) during fetal life shown at the left. (With permission W.B. Saunders Co. from Costarino AT, Baumgart S. Modern fluid and electrolyte management of the critically ill premature infant. *Pediatr Clin North Am.* 1986;33:153-178. Derived from summary by Friis-Hansen B. Body water compartments in children. *Pediatrics.* 1961;28:169-181.[45])

Fig. 13.3 Compared to adult physiology, the extremely low birth weight baby proportionally has over 6 times the skin surface area exposed per kilogram of body weight, with at least 3 times the mass of water content vulnerable to evaporation. (See references 5 and 6; Modified with permission Cambridge University Press, Cambridge, UK from Sridhar S, Baumgart S: Chapter 9—Water and electrolyte balance in newborn infants. In, *Neonatal Nutrition and Metabolism*, 2nd Edition, Hay WW and Thureen PJ (Eds), Cambridge University Press, Cambridge, UK, pp 104-14, 2006.)

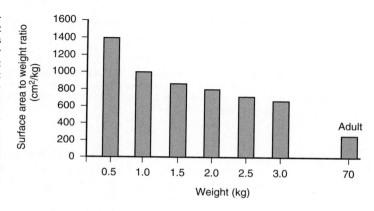

Fig. 13.4 1981, concept of a geometric model for estimating insensible water loss in extremely low birth weight infants, using a metabolic balance for the continuous measurement of body weight loss over a 90 minute period. (With permission, J.B. Lippincott Co. from Baumgart S, Langman CB, Sosulski R, Fox WW, Polin RA: Fluid, electrolyte and glucose maintenance in the very low birthweight infant. *Clin Pediatr.* 1982;21:199-206.)

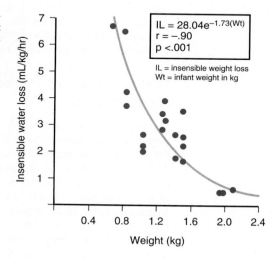

$$IL = 28.04e^{-1.73(Wt)}$$
$$r = -.90$$
$$p < .001$$

IL = insensible weight loss
Wt = infant weight in kg

Transcutaneous (Insensible) Water Loss

In 1981, we proposed a geometric model (Fig. 13.4) for estimating *insensible water loss (IWL)* in extremely low birth weight infants, using a metabolic balance (Potter Baby Scale, Hartford, Connecticut) for the continuous measurement of body weight loss *(insensible weight loss [IL])* over a 1- to 3-hour period.[1,7] Although not widely

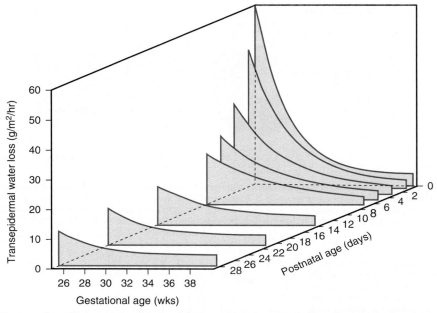

Fig. 13.5 Transepidermal water loss measured for gestational age at birth and postnatal age. (Modified with permission Scandinavian University Press, Stockholm, Sweden from Hammarlund K, Sedin G. Transepidermal water loss in newborn infants. VIII. Relation to gestational age and post-natal age in appropriate and small for gestational age infants. *Acta Paediatr Scand.* 1983;72:721.)

accepted at the time (IWL estimates in ELBW infants ≤700 g were as high as 7.0 mL/kg per hour approaching 170 mL/kg per day), these findings were exactly reproduced by Hammarlund and Sedin in 1983,[2] using an entirely different method to measure water evaporation directly from the skin *(transcutaneous water loss [TEWL])* by measuring vapor gradients (Transcutaneous Evaporimeter, Servomed, Stockholm) measured over the immature skin surface of ELBW and VLBW premature neonates during the first weeks of life. These investigators reported similar estimations of transcutaneous evaporation, yielding rates of 50 to 60 g/m^2 per hour, or approximately 170 to 200 mL/kg per day in the first 1 to 3 days of life (Fig. 13.5).[2]

Water Loss and Pathogenesis of Transcutaneous Dehydration

In 1982, we reported a small series of extremely low birth weight infants, who, despite fluid replenishment to as much as 250 mL/kg per day, nevertheless developed hypernatremic serum sodium concentrations by day 3 of life, with values averaging 155 mEq/L (Fig. 13.6) and peaking in the smallest infants at a serum sodium of nearly 180 mEq/L.[1] These observations led to our first description of the pathogenesis of water depletion, with the "iatrogenic" development of hypernatremia, hyperglycemia, hyperosmolarity, and a hyperkalemic state peculiar to the extremely low birth weight baby, and developing in the first 72 hours of life (Fig. 13.7).[8] In the figure, large free-water losses through transcutaneous evaporation were balanced by clinicians increasing the rates of fluid replacement, usually adding sodium in the second day of life to match anticipated urinary sodium losses. These influxes contributed to an immense sodium load presented to an immature kidney. Added to this exogenous sodium load, the large fluid reservoir in the extracellular space was subjected to transcutaneous evaporation of sodium-free water; the low glomerular filtration rate (GFR) of the fetal kidney compensated by retaining sodium. Furthermore, immature renal tubular function with poor concentrating ability tended to waste additional free water. An osmolar diuresis commonly resulted from dextrose overload and

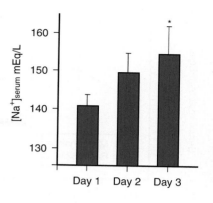

Fig. 13.6 Extremely low birth weight infants are prone to develop hypernatremic serum sodium concentrations by day 3 of life, with values averaging 155 mEq/L and peaking in the smallest infants at a serum sodium of nearly 180 mEq/L (2 standard deviations). (With permission, J.B. Lippincott Co. from Baumgart S, Langman CB, Sosulski R, Fox WW, Polin RA. Fluid, electrolyte and glucose maintenance in the very low birthweight infant. *Clin Pediatr.* 1982;21:199-206.)

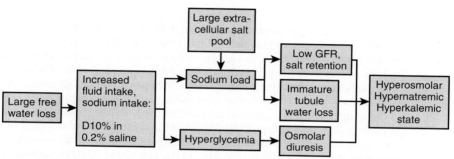

Fig. 13.7 Large free water loss through transcutaneous evaporation is balanced by clinicians increasing the rates of fluid replacement, usually adding sodium in the second day of life to match anticipated urinary sodium losses. These influxes contribute to an immense sodium load presented to an immature kidney glomerular apparatus. Added to this exogenous sodium load, the large salt reservoir in the extracellular space is subjected to rapid transcutaneous dehydration, and the low glomerular filtration rate (GFR) of the fetal kidney leads to salt retention. Immature renal tubules with poor concentrating ability tended to waste additional free water, and an osmolar diuresis may also result from dextrose overload and hyperglycemia. The result is that by 48 to 72 hours of life, a hyperosmolar, hypernatremic state evolves, and hyperkalemia is likely to occur as well. (Modified with permission W.B. Saunders Co. from Baumgart S. Fluid and electrolyte therapy in the premature infant: case management. In: Burg F, Polin RA, eds. *Workbook in Practical Neonatology.* Philadelphia: WB Saunders; 1983:25-39.)

hyperglycemia. These physiologic disturbances ultimately led to a hyperosmolar, hypernatremic state. This state contributed to the development of life-threatening hyperkalemia.

Salt Restriction Prophylaxis

To prevent this syndrome, Costarino et al. conducted a randomized and blinded control trial of sodium restriction versus maintenance sodium administration during the first 5 days of life in infants born less than 1000 g and less than 28 weeks' gestation.[9] Infants were randomly assigned to either a low-sodium group who received no maintenance sodium additive with their parenteral nutrition or to a high-sodium replenishment group who received 3 to 4 mEq/kg per day added to their daily maintenance fluids and administered beginning on day 2 of life.

A safety committee analyzed data at half-enrollment and stopped the study. Two out of the nine infants in the sodium-restricted group became hyponatremic with serum sodium concentrations of 130 mEq/L or less by day 5 of life and were taken out of the study. Conversely, two of the eight infants in the sodium replenishment group became hypernatremic with a serum sodium of 150 mEq/L or more by day 4 and were also removed from the study. Daily assessments of serum sodium concentrations were significantly and consistently higher in the sodium-supplemented infants after day 1 of life (Fig. 13.8).[9]

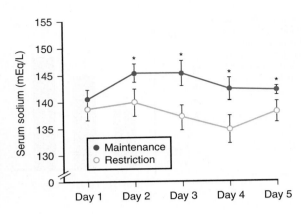

Fig. 13.8 Infants randomly assigned to either a low-sodium group who received no maintenance sodium additive with their parenteral nutrition or to a high-sodium replenishment group who received 3 to 4 mEq/kg per day added to their daily maintenance fluids and administered beginning on day 2 of life. Daily assessments of serum sodium concentrations were significantly and consistently higher in the sodium-supplemented infants after day 1 of life. (Modified with permission Elsevier, Inc. from Costarino AT, Gruskay JA, Corcoran L, Polin RA, Baumgart S. Sodium restriction vs. daily maintenance replacement in very low birthweight premature neonates, a randomized and blinded therapeutic trial. *J Pediatr.* 1992;120:99-106.)

By study design, sodium intake (seen in the *top graph,* Fig. 13.9) ranged between 4 and 6 mEq/kg per day in the sodium-supplemented maintenance group *(shaded bars).*[9] Infants in the restricted group received between 1 and 1¾ mEq/kg per day of sodium as additives (shown as *lightly shaded bars vs. dark shaded bars* in the graph) with medications containing sodium (sodium heparin, sodium ampicillin, and sodium citrated transfusions, etc.). It was impossible to eliminate sodium intake entirely due to these unrecognized sources of exogenously applied salt. Sodium excretion (shown in the *middle graph* of Fig. 13.9) remained the same for the first 3 days of the study, but began to increase after day 4 in infants in the sodium-supplemented group. And shown in the *bottom graph* (see Fig. 13.9), calculated sodium balance was nearly zero in the sodium-supplemented group *(shaded bars)* where intake matched urinary sodium excretion, but remained markedly negative in the sodium-restricted group by as much as 6 mEq/kg per day net sodium loss *(light shaded bars).*

Fluid intakes prescribed independent of the study by the physicians (who did not know the group assignment) were similar in both groups of infants, ranging between 90 and 130 mL/kg per day throughout the first 3 days of life (Fig. 13.10, *top graph*). However, after 3 days, fluid volume exceeded 130 mL/kg per day in the sodium-supplemented infants (indicated by *dark shaded circles*) and was significantly higher than in the salt-restricted infants who only received approximately 90 mL/kg per day (shown by *light shaded circles*). These results suggest that infants in the sodium-supplemented group were prescribed increasing amounts of fluid to compensate for their rising serum sodium. Conversely, infants in the sodium-restricted group required relative fluid restrictions, probably in response to falling serum sodium concentrations. Failure to restrict fluid intake volume after 5 days of age may result in clinically significant hyponatremia.

Of interest (as seen in the *bottom graph,* Fig. 13.10), urine output was fixed throughout the study in both groups, at between 2 and 4 mL/kg per hour (or about 50–100 mL/kg per day), and was not dependent on either the volume of fluid administered or the amount of sodium intake.

Survival was similar in both groups, and the comorbidities of intraventricular hemorrhage (IVH) and patent ductus arteriosum were also similar. There was a trend, however, towards infants developing BPD in the high sodium/high fluid intake group: 7 of 7 infants versus 4 of 8 infants in the low sodium/low fluid intake group ($P = .08$). However, this safety analysis was underpowered to detect the impact of fluid volume administration on these secondary outcomes.

Nonoliguric Hyperkalemia in Extremely Low Birth Weight Infants

During these studies, we encountered an additional electrolyte disturbance, hyperkalemia, in the absence of renal failure ("nonoliguric hyperkalemia") that we further investigated.[10] Gruskay et al. identified eight ELBW infants with serum potassium

Fig. 13.9 Sodium intake (the top graph) ranged between 4 and 6 mEq/kg per day in the sodium-supplemented maintenance group (2–4 mEq/kg per day *shaded bars*). Infants in the restricted group received between 1 and 1¾ mEq/kg per day of sodium as additives (shown as *lightly shaded bars* in the graph) with medications containing sodium (see text). It was impossible to eliminate sodium intake entirely due to these often unrecognized sources of exogenously applied salt. In the bottom graph, calculated sodium balance was nearly zero in the sodium-supplemented group (*shaded bars*) where intake matched urinary sodium excretion, but remained markedly negative in the sodium-restricted group by as much as 6 mEq/kg per day net sodium loss (2 standard deviations, *lightly shaded bars*). (Modified with permission Elsevier, Inc. from Costarino AT, Gruskay JA, Corcoran L, Polin RA, Baumgart S. Sodium restriction vs. daily maintenance replacement in very low birthweight premature neonates, a randomized and blinded therapeutic trial. *J Pediatr.* 1992;120:99-106.)

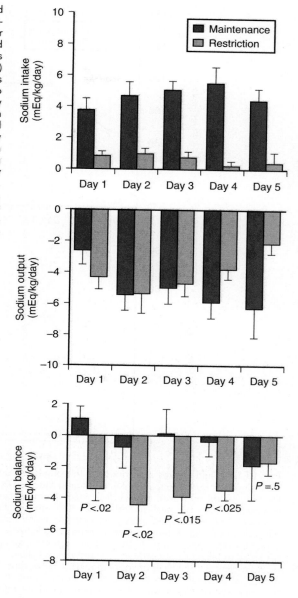

levels 6.8 mEq or more and compared them to 10 comparable ELBW infants who remained normokalemic. Peak serum potassium values averaged 8.0 ± 0.3 mEq/L in the hyperkalemic infants, and all of these infants developed electrocardiographic abnormalities requiring treatment.

Renal testing in these two groups of infants demonstrated similar serum creatinine values and GFRs (Fig. 13.11). In contrast, urine sodium excretion was markedly increased in the hyperkalemic infants, with urine concentrations of sodium exceeding 140 mEq/L (Fig. 13.12); the fractional excretion of sodium was nearly 15% in the hyperkalemic group, compared to only 5% in the normokalemic infants. Both of these observations suggest a profoundly immature tubular conservation of filtered sodium. The hyperkalemic infants revealed significantly less potassium excretion than the normokalemic infants (Fig. 13.13). These authors suggested an immaturity in renal tubular response to aldosterone resulting in these electrolyte disturbances.

Stefano et al. reported a similar investigation of 12 ELBW infants developing nonoliguric hyperkalemia and compared them to 27 infants of similar gestation who

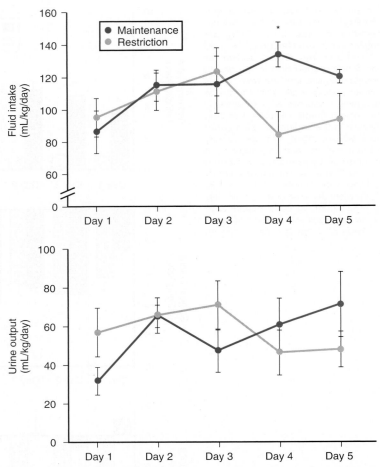

Fig. 13.10 Fluid intakes prescribed by the physicians unaware of the sodium supplemental group assignment were similar in both groups of infants, ranging between 90 and 130 mL/kg per day throughout the first 3 days of life *(top graph)*. However, after 3 days, fluid volume exceeded 130 mL/kg per day in the sodium-supplemented infants (indicated by *dark shaded circles*) and was significantly higher than the salt-restricted infants who only received approximately 90 mL/kg per day (shown by *light shaded circles*). These results suggest that infants in the sodium-supplemented group were prescribed increasing amounts of fluid to compensate for their rising serum sodium. Conversely, infants in the sodium-restricted group required relative fluid volume restriction, probably in response to falling serum sodium concentrations. Failure to restrict fluid intake volume after 5 days, however, may result in clinically significant hyponatremia. Urine output *(bottom graph)* was fixed throughout the study in both groups, at between 2 and 4 mL/kg per hour (or about 50–100 mL/kg per day), and was not dependent on either the volume of fluid administered or the amount sodium intake. (Modified with permission Elsevier, Inc. from Costarino AT, Gruskay JA, Corcoran L, Polin RA, Baumgart S. Sodium restriction vs. daily maintenance replacement in very low birthweight premature neonates, a randomized and blinded therapeutic trial. *J Pediatr.* 1992;120:99-106.)

remained normokalemic.[11] In addition to renal function studies, these authors measured erythrocyte Na⁺/K⁺ ATPase activity and found higher levels in the normokalemic infants, suggesting that the cellular maturation of this enzyme was markedly more immature in the hyperkalemic infants and contributed towards the exudation of potassium from the intracellular compartment. Potassium leak can be exacerbated by high serum sodium levels; when sodium leaks into cells and competitively exceeds the Na⁺/K⁺ ATPase pump capacity to exclude sodium, it further promotes intracellular potassium leak into the extracellular compartment. These authors concluded that hyperkalemia was due to an intracellular-to-extracellular potassium shift with diminished Na⁺/K⁺ ATPase, and that glomerular-tubular imbalance in the kidney did not completely explain why hyperkalemia was developing in these infants. Subsequent observational studies by Lorenz et al. and others have confirmed their findings.[12]

Fig. 13.11 Eight hyperkalemic extremely low birth weight (ELBW) infants compared to 10 comparable ELBW infants who remained normokalemic. Renal functions for these two groups of infants demonstrated similar serum creatinine and glomerular filtration rates. (With permission Elsevier, Inc. from Gruskay J, Costarino AT, Polin RA, Baumgart S. Non-oliguric hyperkalemia in the premature infant less than 1000 grams. *J Pediatr.* 1988;113:381-386.)

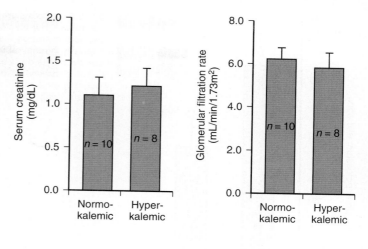

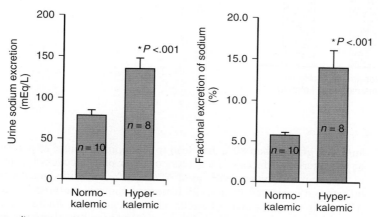

Fig. 13.12 Urine sodium excretion was markedly increased in hyperkalemic infants, with urine concentrations of urine sodium sometimes exceeding 140 mEq/L (standard deviation), and mean fractional excretion of sodium was nearly 15% in the hyperkalemic group, compared to only 5% in the normokalemic infants. Both of these observations suggest a profoundly immature tubular conservation of filtered sodium. (Modified with permission Elsevier, Inc. from Gruskay J, Costarino AT, Polin RA, Baumgart S. Non-oliguric hyperkalemia in the premature infant less than 1000 grams. *J Pediatr.* 1988;113:381-386, 1988.)

The Epidermal Barrier: Reducing Transcutaneous Evaporation

Other than manipulating water and electrolyte administration to ELBW infants, an alternative strategy for preventing these disturbances is to reduce the large transepidermal water losses. Several techniques have been proposed to accomplish this, including incubator humidification, "swamping" infants in mist either within incubators or within plastic body chambers under radiant warmers, application of petroleum-based ointments used on the skin as an emollient, polyvinyl-chloride plastic blankets or body bags, and nonocclusive semi-adherent polyurethane artificial skins. Native transepidermal water evaporation gradually lessens as spontaneous keratinization of the epidermis develops over a 1- to 4-week period after birth in these infants, probably too late to prevent the acute dehydration syndrome described above.[13]

Environmental Humidification

Incubator humidification for premature infants is recommended by the American Academy of Pediatrics and the American College of Obstetricians guidelines.[14] Levels ranging between 50% and 80% relative humidity are recommended. Using a relative

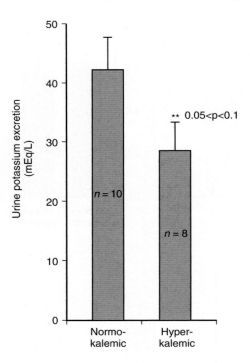

Fig. 13.13 Potassium excess is normally *secreted* from the distal tubule. Hyperkalemic infants' urines had significantly less potassium excretion than normokalemic infants, suggesting an immaturity in renal tubular response to aldosterone resulting in these electrolyte disturbances. (Modified with permission Elsevier, Inc. from Gruskay J, Costarino AT, Polin RA, Baumgart S. Non-oliguric hyperkalemia in the premature infant less than 1000 grams. *J Pediatr.* 1988;113:381-386.)

humidity greater than 80% may lead to "rain-out" because of condensation of water on the interior surfaces of incubators or other plastic covers for tiny infants.

Harpin and Rutter (1985) used 80% to 90% humidified incubators for 33 VLBW infants and compared them to 29 historical controls nurtured in "dry" incubators.[15] All infants were less than 30 weeks' gestation and were studied for the first 2 weeks of life. These authors concluded that saturated humidification was effective but may be associated with water-borne nosocomial infection. Newer humidification technologies are not thought to increase the likelihood of infection.

More recently, Gaylord et al. (2001) studied 70 infants in nonhumidified incubators, comparing them to 85 infants nursed in humidified incubators, again using historical controls.[16] Despite similar fluid balance, infants nursed in an environment with a lower relative humidity were significantly more likely to develop hypernatremia, hyperkalemia, azotemia, and oliguria and received more fluid.

Humidification can be servo-regulated by modern incubators (Giraffe OmniBed). Initially a *relative humidity* between 70% and 80% is chosen for ELBW infants to avoid excessive insensible water loss and electrolyte disturbances in the first week of life. Relative humidity is gradually decreased over 1 to 2 weeks.

I do not recommend exceeding 80% relative humidity during incubator care to prevent "rain out."

Skin Emollients

Research on petroleum-based ointments to treat the skin of newborn infants began as early as 1981 when Rutter and Hull first applied paraffin oil to premature infants every 4 to 6 hours, reducing transepidermal water loss, but not significantly altering fluid balance over the first several days of life.[17] In 1996, Nopper et al. at Stanford University conducted a small randomized trial in 16 infants, using Aquaphor, a preservative-free petroleum ointment to reduce transepidermal water loss, bacterial colonization, and sepsis.[18] These authors claimed better skin integrity and many nurseries adopted this treatment as standard practice for ELBW infants. In 2000, however, Campbell et al. reported an increasing occurrence of candidiasis in their nurseries after the introduction of petroleum ointment use.[19] Furthermore, the multicenter

Table 13.1 TRANSEPIDERMAL EVAPORATION (G/M²/H) WITH AND WITHOUT A FLEXIBLE POLYURETHANE PLASTIC, NONOCCLUSIVE SKIN BARRIER[a]

	Day 1	Day 2	Day 3	Day 4	Day 5, Removal
Naked	27.5	31.3	21.4	18.8	20.8
Dressed	8.9[b]	9.5[b]	9.0[b]	10.6[b]	18.8

[a]Opsite, Smith Nephew Inc., Columbia, South Carolina.
[b]Indicates significant reduction in transepidermal evaporation.
From Knauth A, Gordin M, McNelis W, Baumgart S. A semipermeable polyurethane membrane as an artificial skin in the premature neonate. *Pediatrics.* 1989;83:945-950.

13

Vermont Oxford trial observed an increase in coagulase-negative staphylococcal sepsis occurring in infants who were treated with this petroleum preparation.[20] This technique is no longer used in the United States, but similar techniques are used in developing countries with effectiveness.[21]

Plastic Shields, Bags, or Blankets

Alternatively, we have reported the use of a single layer of Saran polyvinyl chloride to reduce insensible water loss during the first few days of life in low birth weight infants nursed under radiant warmers. To date, however, there have been no studies to evaluate the occurrence of infection or bacterial colonization with use of these plastic "blankets."[22] Knauth et al. alternatively suggested the use of a flexible polyurethane plastic, nonocclusive skin barrier (trade names of these barriers are familiar as Tegadermor, OpSite).[23] Some of these barriers are treated with antimicrobial suppressants and are relatively infection neutral when used as total parenteral nutrition (TPN) catheter site dressings. We evaluated transcutaneous evaporation using these materials and demonstrated a two-thirds reduction in transcutaneous water loss shown during the first 4 days of life (Table 13.1). However, as seen on the right side of this table, after removal on the fifth day, evaporation again increased, either with reexposure of the immature skin or with the exfoliation of the developing keratin underneath this gently adhesive barrier. Israeli scientists have produced a membrane material for this application that is completely adhesive free to avoid such debridement.

Porat et al. recently published their data on the use of polyurethane dressings completely covering low birth weight infants. They demonstrated significant reductions in hypernatremia, excessive fluid volume intake, weight loss, BPD, and mortality with the use of an artificial layer during the first few weeks of life.[24]

Donahue et al., subsequently, conducted a randomized trial of this technique in 61 infants, but did not reveal changes in fluid volume requirements, although improved skin integrity was suggested by these authors.[25] None of these strategies have consistently reduced electrolyte disturbances.

Pulmonary Edema Formation

After the initial first week of life, the risk for dehydration diminishes as the skin barrier matures. Thereafter, and usually during the second or third week of life, water overload may result from overzealous fluid replenishment therapy continued past the first week of life.

Suggested pathogenesis for water overload is depicted in Fig. 13.14.[8] Fluid replenishment, when administered too aggressively, may result in increased lung water and contribute to the pathogenesis of BPD.[26–28] Moreover, high fluid intakes have been associated with the development of a hemodynamically significant PDA and congestive heart failure,[29–31] also contributing to the pathogenesis of BPD.[32] Increased pulsatility and diastolic run-off with a clinically significant PDA may contribute to the development of necrotizing enterocolitis (NEC)[33] and IVH.[34]

Perhaps the root cause of this problem is the premature infant's markedly immature renal development. The fetal kidney at 25 weeks has a lobulated appearance,

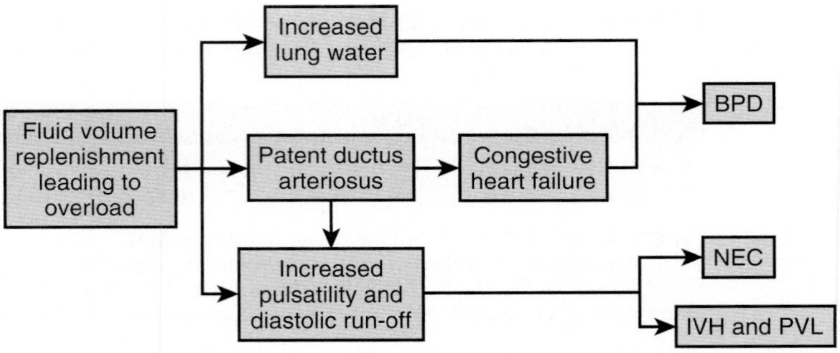

Fig. 13.14 Fluid replenishment volume, when administered too aggressively, may result in increased lung water and contribute to the pathogenesis of bronchopulmonary dysplasia (BPD).[26-28] Moreover, high fluid intakes have been associated with the development of clinically significant patent ductus arteriosus (PDA) and congestive heart failure,[29-31] also contributing to the pathogenesis of BPD.[32] Increased pulsatility and diastolic run-off with a clinically significant PDA may contribute to the development of necrotizing enterocolitis (NEC)[33] and intraventricular hemorrhage (IVH).[34] *PVL,* Periventricular leukomalacia. (Modified with permission W.B. Saunders Co. from Baumgart S. Fluid and electrolyte therapy in the premature infant: case management. In: Burg F, Polin RA, eds. *Workbook in Practical Neonatology.* Philadelphia: WB Saunders; 1983:25-39.)

Table 13.2   META-ANALYSIS OF FOUR STUDIES EVALUATING HIGH VERSUS LOW FLUID VOLUME INTAKE STRATEGIES FOR MAINTENANCE THERAPY IN VERY LOW BIRTH WEIGHT INFANTS

	Study Design	Weights and Gestations	High/Low Fluid Volume Limits	Outcomes
Bell et al. *New Engl J Med.* 1980;302: 598-604	170 sequential matched pairs, 30 days	1.41 kg 31 weeks	122/169 mL/kg/day	PDA, CHF, NEC in high fluid group
Von Stackhauser et al. *Klin Pediatr.* 1980;192:539-546	56 random pairs, 3 days	1.9/2.0 kg 34.6/34.2 weeks	60/150 mL/kg/day	No differences
Lorenz et al. *J Pediatr.* 1982;101: 423-432	88 random matched pairs, 5 days	1.20 kg 29 weeks	60–85 mL/kg/day 80–140 mL/kg/day	No differences
Tammela et al. *Acta Pediatr.* 1992;81: 207-212	100 random pairs, 28 days	1.30 kg 31 weeks	50–150 mL/kg/day 80–200 mL/kg/day	Death, BPD in high fluid group

Patent ductus arteriosus, congestive heart failure, and necrotizing enterocolitis were significantly more common with high fluid volumes administered.
BPD, Bronchopulmonary dysplasia; *CHF,* congestive heart failure; *NEC,* necrotizing enterocolitis; *PDA,* patent ductus arteriosus.
See references 29–32.
Modified from Bell EF, Acarregui MJ. Restricted versus liberal water intake for preventing morbidity and mortality in preterm infants. *Cochrane Database Syst Rev.* 2001;3:CD000503.

with a thin cortex predominated by small, less-well-developed juxta-medullary nephrons and a smaller cortical nephron population. The result of diminutive anatomy is less glomerular surface available for filtration of any fluid volume or salt excess.

Prevention of Iatrogenic Fluid Overload

In testing the prevention strategy of a restricted fluid intake on the development of fluid overload in premature infants, Bell and Acarregui recently reviewed a meta-analysis of four randomized controlled trials comparing low- and high-volume fluid regimens (Table 13.2).[29-33] Of the studies reported, fluid intakes ranged from as low as

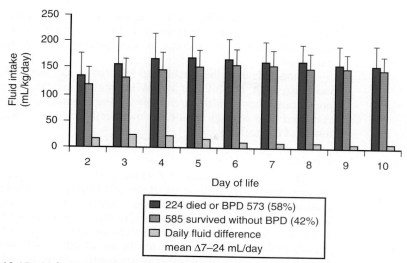

Fig. 13.15 Multivariate logistic regression demonstrated that higher fluid intake volumes with weight retention over the first 10 days of life were significantly associated with higher risk of death or bronchopulmonary dysplasia (BPD) in 1382 extremely low birth weight infants followed prospectively from day 1 of life. Wide ranges of daily fluid volume prescriptions (41–389 mL/kg per day) were observed in this study, with average group differences of as little as 7 to 24 mL/kg per day. (Modified with permission from Elsevier, Inc. from Oh W, Poindexter BB, Perritt R, Lemons JA, Bauer CR, Ehrenkranz RA, Stoll BJ, Poole K, Wright LL, for the Neonatal Research Network. Association between fluid intake and weight loss during the first ten days of life and risk of bronchopulmonary dysplasia in extremely low birth weight infants. *J Pediatr.* 2005;147:786-790.)

50 mL/kg per day to as high as 200 mL/kg per day. All four were conducted primarily in VLBW infants (and not ELBW infants); only two of the studies demonstrated significant differences in the occurrences of PDA, congestive heart failure, BPD, NEC, or death in the high fluid groups. The meta-analysis of all randomized data, however, favored low-fluid-volume infusions, revealing that PDA with congestive heart failure and NEC were more frequently observed in the high fluid group; death was significantly higher as well. More recently, Kavvidia et al. reported the only randomized trial, which included a number of extremely low birth weight infants.[35] No beneficial or adverse effects could be demonstrated in the low- and high-volume groups.

Finally, Oh et al., for the Neonatal Research Network, summarized a cohort of 1382 ELBW infants born at between 401 and 1000 g who were followed prospectively at Network centers to characterize their daily fluid volume intakes prescribed (both parenteral and enteral, net intake mL/kg per day; Fig. 13.15) and percent of birth weight loss daily over the first 10 days of life. The adverse outcomes of BPD and death were analyzed retrospectively.[28] Multivariate logistic regression demonstrated that higher fluid intake volumes with weight retention over the first 10 days of life were significantly associated with higher risk of death or BPD. As in other studies, however, higher birth weight was associated with lower risk for death or BPD, suggesting that even slightly more developmentally mature infants are less likely to require excessive fluid replenishment to maintain electrolyte balance.

More recently, Stephens et al. reported on 204 surviving VLBW infants (<32 weeks and ≤1250 g at birth) ranked into low-, intermediate-, and high-fluid groups. These authors concluded that "High fluid intake (>170 mL/kg/day) in the first days of life was associated with increased risk of PDA."[36,37]

Another recent report by Niwas et al. compared restricted (125 mL/kg per day) versus more liberal fluid administration (155 mL/kg per day) in 113 ELBW infants

(<900 g at birth), finding no association with any mortality or morbidities.[38] This study may have been underpowered to detect such differences and did not combine death and BPD as an outcome as was done for the Neonatal Research Network analysis.[28]

I conclude from these published data that careful fluid volume restriction reduces mortality, PDA, and NEC in VLBW infants and may also be prudent for the ELBW population. There is also a trend toward less chronic lung disease. However, a more restricted fluid strategy should not mean restriction of caloric intake or insufficient intake of electrolytes.

Diuretic Therapy

Diuretic therapy to treat fluid overload and pulmonary edema after it occurs also remains controversial. In 2002, Brion and Primhak reported a meta-analysis of six randomized controlled trials for the combination of spironolactone and thiazide diuretics given for 3 weeks duration or longer, with minor benefits on pulmonary function.[39] A year later, Brion and Soll conducted a second meta-analysis, describing six randomized controlled trials for the use of furosemide in treating lung edema in acute RDS.[40] Oxygenation was only transiently improved with furosemide. However, furosemide is also a vasodilator and was associated with the development of symptomatic PDA. Moreover, in some cases, significant hypovolemia developed, requiring excess fluid administration to recover blood pressure. Brion concluded that furosemide should not be recommended for treating acute RDS. Of note, none of these studies was done in the era of antenatal steroid therapy. Therefore, combinations of therapies effective for treating pulmonary edema and the development of BPD have not been adequately tested or reported in the present era.

Corticosteroid Therapy

Prenatally, the pulmonary epithelium actively secretes chloride ion with water, but the postnatal lung changes over to an active Na^+/K^+ exchange-mediated absorptive mechanism. This transitional change from a secretory organ to one in which lung fluid is reabsorbed may be disrupted by RDS or a clinically significant PDA.[35]

Helve et al. reported the use of postnatal steroids on the epithelial sodium channel and noted that mRNA expression was diminished in very low birth weight infants with RDS, compared with term control infants.[41] Subsequently, when given dexamethasone for the treatment of BPD occurring after 1 month of age in four of these subjects, increased sodium channel mRNA expression was observed, suggesting a potential role for postnatal steroids in resorbing lung edema and diminishing lung water.

In 1999, Omar and Lorenz reported that ELBW infants exposed to antenatal steroids had higher urine output during the first 2 days of life when compared to controls.[41a] The authors speculated that the increased urine output may be due to better mobilization of lung fluid through the augmentation of Na^+/K^+ ATPase in the pulmonary epithelium. These authors also observed a lower calculated insensible water loss during the first 4 days of life and speculated that prenatal steroids may also have improved epidermal barrier function.

Electrolyte Imbalances and Neurodevelopment

Hyponatremia

Bhatty et al. investigated the short- and long-term risks of hyponatremia in a group of extremely low birth weight infants.[42] Clinically significant hyponatremia was defined as a serum sodium concentration less than 125 mEq/L. Thirty-five infants developing hyponatremia during the first few weeks of life were compared retrospectively to 43 nonhyponatremic birth-weight-matched control infants using multivariate regression analysis. Although not statistically significant, hyponatremic infants were generally more ill—all subsequently developed BPD, had longer ventilator and

Table 13.3   PUBLISHED STUDIES SUGGESTING HYPONATREMIA IS ASSOCIATED WITH ADVERSE NEURODEVELOPMENTAL OUTCOMES

	Study Design	Population	Developmental Deficits
Leslie et al. *J Paediatr Child Health*. 1995;31:312-316	Case controls	ELBW	Sensory-neural hearing loss
Murphy et al. *BMJ*. 1997;314:404-408	Case controls	VLBW	Cerebral palsy
Ertl and Sulyok. *Biol Neonate*. 2001;79:109-112	Multivariate analysis, case controls	VLBW	Sensory-neural hearing loss

ELBW, Extremely low birth weight; *VLBW*, very low birth weight.
See references 43–45.

13

oxygen courses, and longer hospital stays. Moreover, more severe IVH (grades 3-and-4) were observed in 23% of the hyponatremic subjects and only 5% of the nonhyponatremic infants. Severe retinopathy (grades 3-and-4) was also more prevalent in the hyponatremic subjects. There was a higher occurrence of spastic cerebral palsy in infants who developed hyponatremia, more hypotonia, and an increased occurrence of sensory-neural hearing loss and behavioral problems in later childhood.

The degree of hyponatremia at onset, the lowest serum sodium concentration, and the duration of hyponatremia did not correlate with subsequent neurodevelopmental outcomes. In contrast, the 11 infants with more rapid correction of serum sodium concentrations (by more than 10 mEq/L in 24 hours) experienced the worst neurodevelopmental outcomes. The authors concluded that rapid correction of hyponatremia, particularly within the first 24 hours of onset of serum sodium concentration less than 125 mEq/L, may be associated with adverse neurodevelopmental sequelae; and that the calculated sodium correction should provide a rate no more than 0.4 mEq/L per hour, or at most 10 mEq/L per day. These data suggest that rapid correction of hyponatremia may have adverse neurodevelopmental consequences, and in most situations, we avoid the use of 3% hypertonic saline acutely for correction of hyponatremia.

Many other studies have suggested an association between hyponatremia and later neurodevelopmental problems (Table 13.3). In a case-control study, Leslie et al. demonstrated a significant increase in sensory-neural hearing deficits in extremely low birth weight infants who had a sodium concentration less than 125 mEq/L.[43] Ertl et al. also found an association between hearing impairment and hyponatremia.[44] Murphy et al. reported an increased incidence of cerebral palsy in very low birth weight infants with hyponatremia.[45] However, none of these studies reported the course of development or treatment of hyponatremia, nor made recommendations for therapy.

In a long-term follow-up study, Al-Dahhana et al. reported that sodium-supplemented VLBW infants less than 32 weeks given 4 to 5 mEq/kg per day in their diets, between 4 and 14 days of life, had better performance IQs, better motor and memory indices, and improved parental behavioral assessments at age 10 years.[46] This report suggests that routine sodium restriction in premature infants, although expedient to prevent hypernatremia, may not be beneficial with respect to long-term outcomes.

Hypernatremia

In contrast (and despite the frequent observation of hypernatremia in extremely low birth weight infants already described), the data associating hypernatremia with central nervous system disruptions have not been as closely examined. Simmons et al. in 1974 suggested that use of hypertonic sodium bicarbonate was associated with the development of IVHs.[47] However, Lupton et al. in 1990 reevaluated serum sodium concentrations during the first 4 days of life in very low birth weight infants, who had developed IVH in that time period, and found no association with hypernatremia.[48] The study by Lupton et al., however, defined hypernatremia at serum sodium levels greater than 145 mEq/L, which may not comprise a critical threshold for evaluating neurologic impairment.[49,50]

None of these reports on hypernatremia directly addresses the occurrences of developmental delays with electrolyte imbalance in the extremely low birth weight population, and further investigation is needed.

Areas for Further Investigation

There are many areas for further investigation. For the extremely low birth weight baby, in whom virtually every therapy is experimental, protocols to standardize care should be developed in each provider's institution along with safety and outcome evaluations.

Epidermal barrier augmentation seems to be a first, natural step in these investigations, to avoid the disruption of fluid and electrolyte balance in the first place. Materials for promoting a temporary artificial skin barrier that is neutral to infection are more elusive than initially appreciated.

Manipulations of both sodium and free water volume intake are also warranted. A more strict and precise definition of fluid balance is needed. Right now, we depend on serial measurements of serum sodium concentrations to evaluate whether ELBW infants need more or less water volume replenishment. The trouble with this approach is that serum sodium concentration must be abnormal before we adjust fluid intake to offset changing losses. Further investigation of sodium channel development, and the promotion of natural lung water resorption through endogenous means, is a more complex area for basic science investigations. Clinical trials of diuretics and steroid administration should be performed before prescribing these therapies routinely.

Sodium requirements and water restriction are hot topics for investigation, given the numerous associations with neurodevelopmental impairments. Randomized controlled trials for routine sodium replacement versus restriction therapy are warranted.

Between a Rock and a Hard Place: Suggestions for Vigilant Fluid Balance Therapy in Extremely Low Birth Weight Infants

Maintenance fluid therapy is at best a moving target that should be addressed by adjusting fluid volumes required at least twice daily. We should try to anticipate and to avoid both extremes of underhydration and overhydration in ELBW infants (Fig. 13.16). On day 1 of life, the primary problem is the high transepidermal water loss (TEWL). We recommend checking serum electrolytes every 8 hours during the first day or 2 of life and adjusting an electrolyte-free solution upwards in 10 to 20 mL increments every 6 to 8 hours, depending on the rate of rise in the measured serum sodium concentration. The key to this strategy is checking serum/urine electrolytes more frequently, because once the serum sodium rises, the infant is already becoming volume depleted. By day 2 the problem of hyperkalemia often emerges; however, nonoliguric hyperkalemia can be ameliorated by adequate provision of protein and calories. On day 3 TEWL begins to diminish as keratin deposition occurs or in response to incubator care with additional humidification. At this juncture, the serum sodium concentration may suddenly decrease because of an increased fractional excretion of sodium. This physiologic transition can be anticipated by diminishing fluid intake when the serum sodium concentrations falls. The occurrence of iatrogenic hyponatremia is most often observed at this time; it may be associated with ductal patency[51] and is best addressed by aggressive fluid restriction.

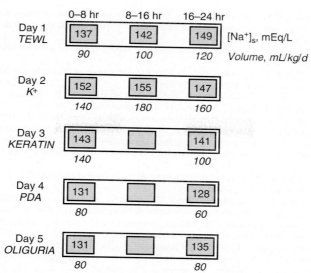

Fig. 13.16 On day 1 of life, the primary problem is the tremendously high transepidermal water loss (TEWL). We recommend checking serum electrolytes every 8 hours during the first day or 2 of life, and adjusting an electrolyte-free solution upwards in 10 to 20 mL increments every 6 to 8 hours, depending on the rate of rise in the measured serum sodium concentration. The key to this strategy is checking serum/urine electrolytes more frequently, because once the serum sodium rises, you are already behind. By day 2, the problem of hyperkalemia often emerges—volume replacement maximizes, as serum sodium concentration peaks, and sodium leaks into the cells displacing potassium outwards from the intracellular compartment. Then on day 3 TEWL begins to diminish as keratin deposition occurs, or in response to incubator care with additional humidification. At this juncture, the serum sodium concentration may suddenly decrease. We should anticipate this change by diminishing water volume *immediately* when we first see the serum sodium concentrations fall, thus anticipating fluid overload and the risk for promoting a hemodynamically significant patent ductus arteriosus (PDA) by day 4 of life; imaging the ductus prospectively may be of consequential benefit. The occurrence of iatrogenic hyponatremia is most often observed at this time and may be associated with patent ductus physiology[51] and is best addressed by aggressive water volume restriction to as little as 60 mL/kg per day, minimizing the *rate* of sodium correction and avoiding entirely the use of hypertonic salt infusions. Oliguria observed while treating for PDA and hyponatremia should not be addressed by liberalizing fluid volume administration, nor by the use of furosemide which may actually dilate the PDA.[39] Rather, maintenance fluid restriction should be continued while the PDA is addressed definitively either with Indocin or by surgical ligation. (Modified with permission Cambridge University Press, Cambridge, UK from Sridhar S, Baumgart S. Water and electrolyte balance in newborn infants. In: Hay WW, Thureen PJ, eds. *Neonatal Nutrition and Metabolism.* 2nd ed. Philadelphia, PA: Elsevier Science; 2006 [in press].)

REFERENCES

1. Baumgart S, Langman CB, Sosulski R, et al. Fluid, electrolyte and glucose maintenance in the very low birthweight infant. *Clin Pediatr.* 1982;21:199–206.
2. Hammarlund K, Sedin G. Transepidermal water loss in newborn infants. VIII. Relation to gestational age and post-natal age in appropriate and small for gestational age infants. *Acta Paediatr Scand.* 1983;72:721.
3. Michel CC. Fluid movements through capillary walls. In: Renkin EM, Michel CC, eds. *Handbook of Physiology, Section II.* Vol. II. Bethesda: American Physiologic Society; 1984:[Chapter 9].
4. Costarino AT, Baumgart S. Modern fluid and electrolyte management of the critically ill premature infant. *Pediatr Clin North Am.* 1986;33:153–178.
5. Friis-Hansen B. Body water compartments in children. *Pediatrics.* 1961;28:169–181.
6. Haycock GB, Schwartz GJ, Wisotsky DH. Geometric method for measuring body surface areas: a height-weight formula validated in infants, children and adults. *J Pediatr.* 1978;93:62–66.
7. Baumgart S, Engle WD, Fox WW, et al. Radiant warmer power and body size as determinants of insensible water loss in the critically ill neonate. *Pediatr Res.* 1981;15:1495–1499.
8. Baumgart S. Fluid and electrolyte therapy in the premature infant: case management. In, Workbook. In: Burg F, Polin RA, eds. *Practical Neonatology.* Philadelphia: WB Saunders; 1983:25–39.
9. Costarino AT, Gruskay JA, Corcoran L, et al. Sodium restriction vs. daily maintenance replacement in very low birthweight premature neonates, a randomized and blinded therapeutic trial. *J Pediatr.* 1992;120:99–106.
10. Gruskay J, Costarino AT, Polin RA, Baumgart S. Non-oliguric hyperkalemia in the premature infant less than 1000 grams. *J Pediatr.* 1988;113:381–386.

11. Stefano JL, Norman ME, Morales MC, et al. Decreased erythrocyte Na+, K+ ATPase activity associated with cellular potassium loss in extremely low birth weight infants with nonoliguric hyperkalemia. *J Pediatr*. 1993;122:276–284.

12. Lorenz JM, Kleinman LI. Nonoliguric hyperkalemia in preterm neonates (Letter). *J Pediatr*. 1989;114:507.

13. Kalia YN, Nonato LB, Lund CH, Guy RH. Development of skin barrier function in premature infants. *J Investig Derm*. 1998;111:320–326.

14. *Guidelines for Perinatal Care*, 2nd ed. Elk Grove Village, IL: American Academy of Pediatrics and American College of Obstetricians and Gynecologists; 1988:278.

15. Harpin VA, Rutter N. Humidification of incubators. *Arch Dis Child*. 1985;60:219.

16. Gaylord MS, Wright K, Lorch K, et al. Improved fluid management utilizing humidified incubators in extremely low birth weight infants. *J Perinatol*. 2001;21:438–443.

17. Rutter N, Hull D. Reduction of skin water loss in the newborn. I. Effect of applying topical agents. *Arch Dis Child*. 1981;56:669.

18. Nopper AJ, Horii KA, Sookdeo-Drost S, et al. Topical ointment therapy benefits premature infants. *J Pediatr*. 1996;128:660.

19. Campbell JR, Zaccaria E, Baker CJ. Systemic candidiasis in extremely low birth weight infants receiving topical petrolatum ointment for skin care: a case-control study. *Pediatrics*. 2000;105:1041–1045.

20. Edwards WH, Conner JM, Soll RF/Vermont Oxford Network Neonatal Skin Care Study Group. The effect of prophylactic ointment therapy on nosocomial sepsis rates and skin integrity in infants with birth weights of 501-1000 g. *Pediatrics*. 2004;113:1195–1203.

21. Salam RA, Darmstadt GL, Bhutta ZA. Effect of emollient therapy on clinical outcomes in preterm neonates in Pakistan: a randomised controlled trial. *Arch Dis Child Fetal Neonatal Ed*. 2015;100(3):F210–F215.

22. Baumgart S. Reduction of oxygen consumption, insensible water loss and radiant heat demand with use of a plastic blanket for low birthweight infants under radiant warmers. *Pediatrics*. 1984;74:1022–1028.

23. Knauth A, Gordin M, McNelis W, Baumgart S. A semipermeable polyurethane membrane as an artificial skin in the premature neonate. *Pediatrics*. 1989;83:945–950.

24. Porat R, Brodsky N. Effect of Tegederm use on outcome of extremely low birth weight (ELBW) infants. *Pediatr Res*. 1993;33:231(A).

25. Donahue ML, Phelps DL, Richter SE, Davis JM. A semipermeable skin dressing for extremely low birth weight infants. *J Perinatol*. 1996;16(1):20–26.

26. Palta M, Babbert D, Weinstein MR, Peters ME. Multivariate assessment of traditional risk factors for chronic lung disease in very low birth weight neonates. *J Pediatr*. 1991;119:285–292.

27. Van Marter LJ, Pagano M, Allred EN, et al. Rate of bronchopulmonary dysplasia as a function of neonatal intensive care practices. *J Pediatr*. 1992;120:938–946.

28. Oh W, Poindexter BB, Perritt R, et al; for the Neonatal Research Network. Association between fluid intake and weight loss during the first ten days of life and risk of bronchopulmonary dysplasia in extremely low birth weight infants. *J Pediatr*. 2005;147:786–790.

29. Bell EF, Warburton D, Stonestreet BS, Oh W. Effect of fluid administration on the development of symptomatic patent ductus arteriosus and congestive heart failure in premature infants. *N Engl J Med*. 1980;302:598–604.

30. von Stockhausen HB, Struve M. Die Auswirkungen einer stark unterschiedlichen parenteral en Flussigkeitszufuhr bei Fruh- und Neugeborenen in den ersten drei Lebenstagen. *Klin Padiatr*. 1980;192:539–546.

31. Lorenz JM, Kleinman LI, Kotagal UR, Reller MD. Water balance in very low-birth weight infants: relationship to water and sodium intake and effect on outcome. *J Pediatr*. 1982;101:423–432.

32. Tammella OKT, Koivisto ME. Fluid restriction for preventing bronchopulmonary dysplasia? Reduced fluid intake during the first weeks of life improves the outcome of low-birth-weight infants. *Acta Paediatr*. 1992;81:207–212.

33. Bell EF, Acarregui MJ. Restricted versus liberal water intake for preventing morbidity and mortality in preterm infants. *Cochrane Database Syst Rev*. 2001;(3):CD000503.

34. Perlman JM, McMenamin JB, Volpe JJ. Fluctuating cerebral blood flow velocity in respiratory distress syndrome: relationship to the development of intraventricular hemorrhage. *N Engl J Med*. 1983;309:209–213.

35. Kavvidia V, Greenough A, Dimitriou G, Forsling ML. Randomized trial of two levels of fluid input in the perinatal period—effect on fluid balance, electrolyte and metabolic disturbances in ventilated VLBW infants. *Acta Paediatr*. 2000;89:237–241.

36. Stephens BE, Gargus FA, Walden RV, et al. Fluid regimens in the first week of life may increase risk of patent ductus arteriosus in extremely low birth weight infants. *J Perinatol*. 2007;28:123–128.

37. Stephens BE, Vohr BR. Fluid regimens and risk of patent ductus arteriosus in extremely low birth weight infants. *J Pernatol*. 2008;28:653.

38. Niwas R, Baumgart S, DeCristofaro JD. Fluid intake in the first week of life: effect on morbidity and mortality in extremely low birth weight infants (less than 900 grams). *J Med Med Sci*. 2010;1(5).

39. Brion LP, Primhak RA, Ambrosio-Perez I. Diuretics acting on the distal renal tubule for preterm infants with (or developing) chronic lung disease. *Cochrane Database Syst Rev*. 2000;(3):CD001817.

40. Brion LP, Soll RF. Diuretics for respiratory distress syndrome in preterm infants. *Cochrane Database Syst Rev*. 2000;2:CD001454.

41. Helve O, Pitkanen OM, Andersson S, et al. Low expression of human epithelial sodium channel in airway epithelium of preterm infants with respiratory distress. *Pediatrics*. 2004;113:1267–1272.

41a. Omar SA, DeCristofaro JD, Agarwal BI, et al. Effects of prenatal steroids on water and sodium homeostasis in extremely low birth weight neonates. *Pediatrics*. 1999;104:482–488.

42. Bhatty SB, Tsirka A, Quinn PB, et al. Rapid correction of hyponatremia in extremely low birth weight (ELBW) premature neonates is associated with long term developmental delay. *Pediatr Res*. 1997;41:140A and Privileged Communication, Dr. DeCristofaro.

43. Leslie GI, Kalaw MB, Bowen JR, Arnold JD. Risk factors for sensorineural hearing loss in extremely premature infants. *J Paediatr Child Health*. 1995;31:312–316.

44. Ertl T, Hadzsiev K, Vincze O, et al. Hyponatremia and sensorineural hearing loss in preterm infants. *Biol Neonate*. 2001;79:109–112.

45. Murphy DJ, Hope PL, Johnson A. Neonatal risk factors for cerebral palsy in very preterm infants: case-control study. *BMJ*. 1997;314:404–408.

46. Al-Dahhana J, Jannoun L, Haycock G. Developmental risks and protective factors for influencing cognitive outcome at 5-1/2 years of age in very low birthweight children. *Dev Med Child Neurol*. 2002;44:508–516.

47. Simmons MA, Adcock EW 3rd, Bard H, Battaglia FC. Hypernatremia and intracranial hemorrhage in neonates. *New Engl J Med*. 1974;291:6–10.

48. Lupton BA, Roland EH, Whitfield MF, Hill A. Serum sodium concentration and intraventricular hemorrhage in premature infants. *Am J Dis Child*. 1990;144:1019–1021.

49. Berg CS, Barnette AR, Myers BJ, et al. Sodium bicarbonate administration and outcome in preterm infants. *J Pediatr*. 2010;157:684–687.

50. Corbet AJ, Adams JM, Kenny JD, et al. Controlled trial of bicarbonate therapy in high-risk premature newborn infants. *J Pediatr*. 1977;91:771–776.

51. Gupta J, Sridhar S, Baumgart S, DeCristofaro JD. Hyponatremia in extremely low birth weight (ELBW) infants may precede the development of a significant patent ductus arteriosus (PDA) in the first week of life. *Pediatric Res*. 2002;51:387A.

13

CHAPTER 14

Lung Fluid Balance in Developing Lungs and Its Role in Neonatal Transition

Sarah D. Keene, MD, Richard D. Bland, MD, Lucky Jain, MD, MBA

Often signaled by a loud cry, the birth of a neonate marks a remarkable transition from its dependence for gas exchange on the placenta to an independent state of air breathing and gas exchange in the lungs. Clearing the fluid-filled lungs is a significant component of this transition. Scientists have long known that fetal lungs are full of fluid, initially presumed to be an extension of the amniotic fluid pool. However, studies have confirmed[1,2] that fetal lungs themselves, rather than the amniotic sac, are the source of the chemically distinct liquid that fills the lungs during development. Through an active process involving chloride secretion by the respiratory epithelium, this liquid forms a slowly expanding structural template that prevents collapse and is essential for growth of fetal lungs.[3,4]

For effective gas exchange to occur, rapid clearance of liquid from potential alveolar airspaces during and soon after birth is essential for establishing the timely switch from placental to pulmonary gas exchange. It is clear now that traditional explanations that relied on mechanical factors and Starling forces can only account for a small fraction of the fluid absorbed[5,6] and that the normal transition from liquid to air inflation is considerably more complex than the characteristic "vaginal squeeze" theory suggests. Physiologic events beginning days before spontaneous delivery are accompanied by changes in the hormonal milieu of the fetus that pave the way for a smooth neonatal transition, including clearance of the large body of lung fluid. Respiratory morbidity resulting from failure to clear the lung fluid is common and can be particularly problematic in some infants delivered prematurely or when delivery occurs operatively before the onset of spontaneous labor. The same pathways are involved in the development of pulmonary edema in acute respiratory distress syndrome (ARDS) that develops in response to infections such as respiratory syncytial virus.[7] This chapter considers some of the experimental work that provides the basis for our current understanding of lung liquid dynamics before, during, and after birth, focusing on the various pathways and mechanisms by which this process occurs.

Fetal Lung Liquid and Its Physiologic Significance

As stated, the lung is a secretory organ during development, displaying breathing-like movements, but without any contribution to respiratory gas exchange. The small fraction of the combined ventricular output of blood from the heart that circulates through the pulmonary circulation[8] allows the delivery to the lung epithelium of the substrates needed to make surfactant and secretion of up to 5 mL/kg per hour lung fluid at term gestation.[9,10] Several studies have shown that the presence of an appropriate

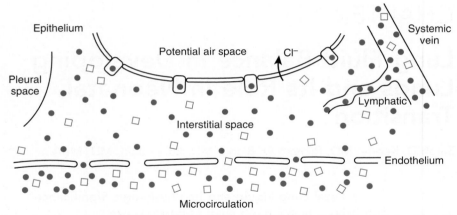

Fig. 14.1 Schematic diagram of the fluid compartments in the fetal lung, showing the tight epithelial barrier to protein and the more permeable vascular endothelium, which restricts the passage of globulins (□) more than it restricts albumin (●). In the fetal mammalian lung, chloride secretion in the respiratory epithelium is responsible for liquid production within potential air spaces. (After Bland RD. Pathogenesis of pulmonary edema after premature birth. *Adv Pediatr*. 1989;34:175-222.)

volume of secreted liquid within the fetal respiratory tract is essential for normal lung growth and development before birth.[1,2,11] Conditions that interfere with normal production of lung liquid, such as pulmonary artery occlusion,[12] diaphragmatic hernia with displacement of abdominal contents into the chest,[13] and uterine compression of the fetal thorax from chronic leak of amniotic fluid,[14] also inhibit lung growth. Conversely, excessive accumulation of lung fluid, such as that after tracheal occlusion, leads to excessive but abnormal lung growth.[1]

Fig. 14.1 is a schematic diagram showing the fluid compartments of the fetal lung. Potential air spaces are filled with liquid that is rich in chloride ($\approx$150 mEq/L) and almost free of protein (<0.03 mg/mL).[15] Whereas the lung epithelium has tight intercellular junctions that provide an effective barrier to macromolecules, including albumin, the vascular endothelium has wider openings that allow passage of large plasma proteins, including globulins and fibrinogen.[16–18] Consequently, liquid in the interstitial space, which was sampled in fetal sheep by collecting lung lymph, has a protein concentration that is about 100 times greater than the protein concentration of liquid contained in the lung lumen.[19] Despite the large transepithelial difference in protein osmotic pressure, which tends to inhibit fluid flow out of the interstitium, active transport of chloride (Cl^-) ions across the fetal lung epithelium generates an electrical potential difference that averages about −5 mV, luminal side negative.[4]

The osmotic force created by this secretory process overcomes that of the protein gradient, pulling liquid from the pulmonary microcirculation through the interstitium into potential air spaces.

In vitro experiments using cultured explants of lung tissue and monolayers of epithelial cells harvested from human fetal lung have indicated that cation-dependent chloride transport, driven by epithelial cell Na^+, K^+-ATPase, is the mechanism responsible for liquid secretion into the lumen of the mammalian lung during fetal life.[20–22] In fetal sheep and lambs, lung epithelial Cl^- transport is inhibited by diuretics that block Na^+, K^+, $2Cl^-$ cotransport.[23–25] This finding supports the concept that the driving force for transepithelial Cl^- movement in the fetal lung is similar to the mechanism described for Cl^- transport across other epithelia, although the specific anion channels responsible have not yet been definitively identified.[26] Accordingly, Cl^- enters the epithelial cell across its basal membrane linked to sodium (Na^+) and potassium (K^+) (Fig. 14.2). Na^+ enters the cell down its electrochemical gradient and is subsequently extruded in exchange for K^+ (three Na^+ ions exchanged for two K^+ ions) by the action of Na^+, K^+-ATPase located on the basolateral surface of the cell.

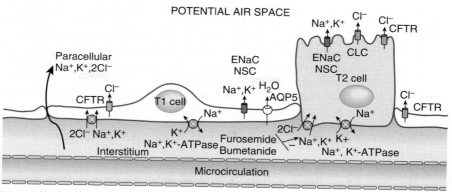

Fig. 14.2 Schematic drawing of the fluid compartments of the fetal lung, highlighting the lung epithelium, consisting of type I cells that occupy most of the surface area of the lung lumen and type II cells that manufacture and secrete surfactant. These cells also secrete Cl by a process that involves Na^+, K^+, $2Cl^-$ cotransport and Na^+, K^+-ATPase (Na pump) activity. This energy-dependent process, which can be blocked by loop diuretics, furosemide, and bumetanide, increases the concentration of Cl within the cell so that it exceeds its electrochemical equilibrium, with resultant extrusion of Cl through anion-selective channels on the apical membrane surface (cystic fibrosis transmembrane conductance regulator [CFTR] or chloride channels [CLCs]). Sodium (Na) and water follow the movement of Cl into the lung lumen. *AQP,* Aquaporin; *ENaC,* epithelial sodium channel; *NSC,* nonselective channel.

This energy-dependent process increases the concentration of Cl^- within the cell so that it exceeds its electrochemical equilibrium. Cl^- then passively exits the epithelial cell through anion-selective channels that are located on the apical membrane surface. Na^+ traverses the epithelium via paracellular pathways or via nonselective cation channels that have been identified in fetal distal airway epithelium; water can flow either between epithelial cells or through water channels, one of which (aquaporin 5) is abundantly expressed in alveolar type I (AT-I) lung epithelial cells.[27,28]

Although the Cl^- concentration of liquid withdrawn from the lung lumen of fetal sheep is about 50% greater than that of plasma, the Na^+ concentration is virtually identical to that of plasma.[3,16] The concentration of bicarbonate in lung liquid of fetal sheep is less than 3 mEq/L, yielding a pH of approximately 6.3 and indicating that the lung epithelium may actively transport bicarbonate out of the lung lumen. The demonstration that acetazolamide, a carbonic anhydrase inhibitor, blocks secretion of lung liquid in fetal sheep supports this view. Both physiologic and immunohistochemical studies have shown that H^+-ATPases are present on the respiratory epithelium of fetal sheep, where they likely provide an important mechanism for acidification of liquid within the lung lumen during development. In vitro electrophysiologic studies using fetal rat lung epithelial cells provided evidence that exposure to an acid pH might activate Cl^- channels and thereby contribute to the production of fetal lung liquid.[29] In fetal dogs and monkeys, however, the bicarbonate concentration of lung luminal liquid is not significantly different from that of fetal plasma.[30] Thus, the importance of lung liquid pH and acidification mechanisms during human lung development in utero remains unclear.

The volume of liquid within the lung lumen of fetal sheep increases from 4 to 6 mL/kg at midgestation[25] to more than 20 mL/kg near term.[18,19] The hourly flow rate of lung liquid increases from approximately 2 mL/kg body weight at midgestation to approximately 5 mL/kg body weight at term.[9,10,31] Increased production of luminal liquid during development reflects a rapidly expanding pulmonary microvascular and epithelial surface area that occurs with proliferation and growth of lung capillaries and respiratory units.[25,32] The observation that unilateral pulmonary artery occlusion decreases lung liquid production in fetal sheep by at least 50%[33] shows that the pulmonary circulation, rather than the bronchial circulation, is the major source of fetal lung liquid. Intravenous infusion of isotonic saline at a rate sufficient to increase lung microvascular pressure and lung lymph flow in fetal lambs had no effect on liquid flow across the pulmonary epithelium.[34] Thus, transepithelial Cl⁻ secretion appears to be the major driving force responsible for the production of liquid in the fetal lung lumen. In vitro studies of epithelial ion transport across the fetal airways indicate that the epithelium of the upper respiratory tract also secretes Cl⁻, thereby contributing to lung liquid production.[35–37] However, most of this liquid forms in the distal portions of the fetal lung, where total surface area is many times greater than it is in the conducting airways.

How Is the Fetal Lung Fluid Cleared?

Several studies have demonstrated that both the rate of lung liquid production and the volume of liquid within the lumen of the fetal lung normally decrease before birth, most notably during labor.[19,31,38–40] Thus, lung water content is about 25% greater after premature delivery than it is at term, and newborn animals that are delivered by cesarean section without prior labor have considerably more liquid in their lungs than do animals that are delivered either vaginally or operatively after the onset of labor (Table 14.1).[41,42] In studies with fetal sheep, extravascular lung water was 45% less in mature fetuses that were in the midst of labor than in fetuses that did not experience labor, and there was a further 38% decrease in extravascular lung water measured in term lambs that were studied 6 hours after a normal vaginal birth.[19]

To achieve this, the lung epithelium is believed to switch from a predominantly Cl⁻-secreting membrane prior to birth to a predominantly Na⁺-absorbing membrane after. Work performed over the past two decades to understand the mechanism(s) responsible for fetal lung fluid clearance have shown that active Na⁺ transport across the pulmonary epithelium drives liquid from lung lumen to the interstitium, with subsequent absorption into the vasculature.[43–46] In the lung, Na⁺ reabsorption is a two-step process (Fig. 14.3).[47] The first step is passive movement of Na⁺ from the lumen across the apical membrane into the cell through Na⁺ permeable ion channels. The second step is active extrusion of Na⁺ from the cell across the basolateral membrane into the serosal space. Several investigators have demonstrated that the initial entry step primarily involves sodium-specific apical channels (epithelial sodium channels [ENaC]) that are particularly sensitive to amiloride, a diuretic. Indeed, cDNAs that encode amiloride-sensitive Na⁺ channels in other Na⁺ transporting epithelia have also been cloned from airway epithelial cells.[48–50] This is consistent with studies by O'Brodovich et al.,[51] who have shown that intraluminal instillation of amiloride in fetal guinea pigs delays lung fluid clearance.

More recent studies using the patch-clamp technique have confirmed the role of ENaC channels in AT-I and AT-II cells in the vectorial transport of Na⁺ from the apical surface.[48,52,53] Increased production of the mRNA for amiloride-sensitive ENaC in the developing lung[54] has been correlated with the transition from a secretory to absorptive state. Much of this information has come from studies using AT-II cells. Recent studies have shown that AT-I cells also express functional Na⁺ channels and other transporters capable of salt and fluid transport.[55–57] Based on work in animals

Table 14.1 FACTORS THAT CAN DELAY CLEARANCE OF FETAL LUNG FLUID

Failure of antenatal decrease in fetal lung fluid	• Delivery without labor • Prematurity
Excessive production of fluid	• Elevated transvascular pressure (e.g., cardiogenic edema) • Increased vascular permeability
Decreased epithelial transport of sodium and water	• Decreased number or function of type I and II cells • Decreased sodium-channel expression and activity • Loss of function mutations of ENaC • Decreased Na⁺, K⁺-ATPase function

ENaC, Epithelial sodium channel.

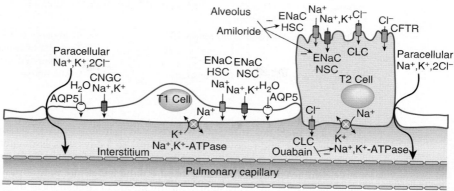

Fig. 14.3 Epithelial sodium absorption in the fetal lung near birth. Na enters the cell through the apical surface of both alveolar type I (AT-I) and AT-II cells via amiloride-sensitive epithelial sodium channels (ENaCs), both highly selective channels (HSCs) and nonselective channels (NSCs), and via cyclic nucleotide gated channels (CNGC) (seen only in AT-I cells). Electroneutrality is conserved with chloride movement through the cystic fibrosis transmembrane conductance regulator (CFTR) or through chloride channels (CLCs) in AT-I and AT-II cells or paracellularly through tight junctions. The increase in cell Na stimulates Na^+, K^+-ATPase activity on the basolateral aspect of the cell membrane, which drives out three Na ions in exchange for two K ions, a process that can be blocked by the cardiac glycoside ouabain. If the net ion movement is from the apical surface to the interstitium, an osmotic gradient would be created, which would in turn direct water transport in the same direction, either through aquaporins (AQPs) or by diffusion.

and humans, ENaC channels are thought to be responsible for 40% to 70% of sodium transport.[58] Nonspecific cation channels and cyclic nucleotide gated channels are also present in alveolar cells and contribute to the amiloride-insensitive sodium and fluid uptake.

Sodium Channel Pathology in the Lung

ENaC channels are primarily composed of three subunit types, α, β, and γ, each with a role in sodium transport but with varied relative importance in mammalian species. A fourth subunit, δ, first identified in the brain and since shown to be coexpressed with the other subunits in lung tissue, is of uncertain significance.[59,60] Hummler et al.[61] have shown that inactivating the α-ENaC (α-subunit of the ENaC) leads to defective lung liquid clearance and premature death in mice. Inactivating β- and γ-ENaC subunits also leads to early death in newborn mice, though this is due to fluid and electrolyte imbalances, suggesting that α-ENaC expression is critical for fetal lung fluid absorption. In later work, Hummler et al.[62] showed that a mouse model of increased α-ENaC activity demonstrated increased alveolar fluid clearance after induction of pulmonary edema. This is direct evidence that in vivo ENaC constitutes the rate-limiting step for Na^+ absorption in epithelial cells of the lung, and thus in the adaptation of newborn lungs to air breathing. It also supports the hypothesis that in many newborns who have difficulty in the transition to air breathing, Na^+ channel activity may be diminished, albeit transiently.

Studies in human neonates have shown that immaturity of Na^+ transport mechanisms contributes to the development of transient tachypnea of the newborn (TTN) and respiratory distress syndrome (RDS; Table 14.2).[63,64] Gowen et al.[64] were the first to show that human neonates with TTN had an immaturity of the lung epithelial transport, measured as an amiloride-induced drop in the potential difference between the nasal epithelium and subcutaneous space. Nasal potential difference is a good measure of the net electrogenic transport of Na^+ and Cl^- across the epithelial layer and has been shown to mirror image ion transport occurring in the lower respiratory

Table 14.2 PATHOLOGIC STATES ASSOCIATED WITH ABNORMAL LUNG ION TRANSPORT

Decreased sodium and water transport	• Respiratory distress syndrome • Transient tachypnea of the newborn • Pulmonary edema
Excessive sodium and water transport	• Cystic fibrosis

tract. The potential difference was reduced in infants with TTN, suggesting deficient Na$^+$ transport, and recovery from TTN in 1 to 3 days was associated with an increase in potential difference to normal level.

Similar studies have now been conducted in premature newborns with RDS, and the results are consistent with impaired Na$^+$ transport in these infants.[63] Barker et al.[63] measured nasal transepithelial potential difference in premature infants less than 30 weeks' gestation. Authors found that maximal nasal epithelial potential difference increased with birth weight and was lower in infants with RDS. Premature infants without RDS had a nasal potential difference similar to normal full-term infants. Furthermore, the ability of amiloride to affect the potential difference was lower in preterm infants with RDS on day 1 of life, reflecting lower amiloride-sensitive Na transport. A clear gender difference is seen in RDS in humans, with male infants at higher risk, though the mechanisms are not clearly identified. Fetal lung cells from male rats have shown impaired sodium transport compared to those from female pups, potentially due to differences in responsiveness to sex hormones.[65,66]

Additional evidence indicates that the ability of various agents to increase lung fluid absorption in fetal lambs is gestational-age dependent.[38,67-72] The mechanism for poor response of immature lungs to agents that stimulate Na$^+$ transport is not known. Deficiencies could exist in one or more of several steps, including β-receptor, GTP-binding proteins, adenyl cyclase, protein kinase A, or the Na$^+$ channel and its regulatory proteins. Studies have shown that the expression of α-subunit of ENaC is developmentally regulated in rats[54] and in humans.[70] Helve et al.[73,74] studied ENaC RNA levels in full-term and preterm infants with and without RDS. Lower α- and β-ENaC levels were noted in preterm infants, correlated with decreasing gestational age. This continues in late preterm (LPT) infants and up to early term, with infants less than 39 and 0/7 weeks having lower α-ENaC mRNA levels just after birth.[75] Together, these studies provide important evidence for the role of Na channel activity in the pathogenesis of RDS and TTN.

Pseudohypoaldosteronism type I (a renal salt-wasting disease) has been reported to be associated with mutations involving the α-subunit of ENaC.[72] Indeed, patients with the autosomal recessive form of the disease have been reported with severe RDS at birth and childhood pulmonary disease of varying degrees, with documented gene abnormalities in alpha ENaC.[76-78] However not all patients have neonatal lung disease, which is unexpected given that the α-subunit is so critical for ENaC function.

A complex and yet incompletely defined relationship exists between Na$^+$ and Cl$^-$ channels. Cystic fibrosis (CF) is a genetic disease caused by mutations of the CF transmembrane conductance regulator (CFTR), which has been identified as a cyclic AMP (cAMP)-dependent Cl channel.[79] In the lungs of CF patients, amiloride-sensitive Na$^+$ absorption is increased, and aerosolized amiloride has been used to reverse this imbalance.[61,80,81] However, despite the absence of functional CFTR activity in fetuses who will go on to develop CF, fetal lung fluid production during gestation is unaffected, and the lungs are normally developed at birth. These findings contrast with recent studies on infants with congenital diaphragmatic hernia (CDH), who do not have a specific deficiency in ENaC or other channels. However, these infants do have respiratory distress at birth and may have this compounded by decreased alveolar fluid clearance. Animal models of term equivalent CDH rats show net lung fluid secretion rather than the absorption seen in control subjects.[82] Animal and human studies have also shown decreased levels of various ENaC subunits (α- and β-subunits in rats; β- and γ-subunits in humans) in term infants with CDH, the cause of which is unknown.[83] Therefore, examining the molecular mechanisms and the cellular regulation of Na$^+$ reabsorption is important in understanding both normal lung development and physiology, but also abnormalities in lung Na and water balance in both fetal and adult lungs.

What Causes the Neonatal Lung Epithelium to Switch to an Absorptive Mode?

Developmental changes in transepithelial ion and fluid movement in the lung can be viewed as occurring in three distinct stages.[84] In the first (fetal) stage, the lung epithelium remains in a secretory mode, relying on active Cl$^-$ secretion via Cl$^-$ channels and relatively low reabsorption activity of Na$^+$ channels. The second (transitional) stage involves a reversal in the direction of ion and water movement. A multitude of factors may be involved in this transition, including exposure of epithelial cells to high concentrations of steroids and cyclic nucleotides and to an air interface. This stage involves not only increased expression of Na$^+$ channels in the lung epithelia but possibly also a switch from nonselective cation channels to highly selective Na$^+$ channels. The net increase in Na$^+$ movement into the cell can also cause a change in resting membrane potential, leading to a slowing and eventually a reversal of the direction of Cl$^-$ movement through Cl$^-$ channels. The third and final (adult) stage represents lung epithelia with predominantly Na$^+$ reabsorption through Na$^+$ channels and possibly Cl$^-$ reabsorption through Cl$^-$ channels, with a fine balance between the activity of ion channels and tight junctions. Such an arrangement can help ensure adequate humidification of alveolar surface while preventing excessive buildup of fluid. There is also recent evidence to show that fetal lung fluid clearance is facilitated by ciliary function[85] and that term neonates with genetic defects of cilia structure or function (primary ciliary dyskinesia) have a high prevalence of neonatal respiratory disease.[85]

A considerable amount of research effort in this area has focused on physiologic changes that trigger the change in lung epithelia from a Cl$^-$ secretory to a Na$^+$ reabsorption mode.[23,45,52,84,86–88] Although several endogenous mediators (Box 14.1), including catecholamines, vasopressin, and prolactin, have been proposed to increase lung fluid absorption, none explains this switch convincingly.[71,89,90] Mechanical factors, such as stretch and exposure of the epithelial cells to air interface, are other probable candidates that have not been well studied. Jain et al.[52] have shown that alveolar expression of highly selective Na$^+$ channels in the lung epithelia is regulated by the lung microenvironment, especially the presence of glucocorticoids, air interface, and oxygen concentration.[91] Furthermore, regulation of Na$^+$ channels is mediated through these factors in a tissue-specific manner.[92,93] For example, aldosterone is a major factor in the kidneys and colon, but probably not in the lungs.[94] In the kidneys, it works by activating transcription of genes for ENaC subunits.[94] In ovine lung, the

---

Box 14.1   ENDOGENOUS FACTORS THAT CAN ENHANCE LUNG FLUID CLEARANCE

β-Adrenergics and catecholamines
Dopamine
Arginine vasopressin
Prostaglandin E$_2$
Prolactin
Surfactant
Oxygen
Tumor necrosis factor α
Epidermal growth factor
Steroids
Alveolar expansion (stretch)

glucocorticoid betamethasone has been shown to increase the production ENaC subunit mRNAs, but aldosterone does not show this effect.[95] Of the several factors that have been proposed to have a lung-specific effect on Na$^+$ reabsorption, some have been investigated, including glucocorticoids, oxygen, β-adrenergics, and surfactant.[87,89,96]

High doses of glucocorticoids, acting through serum and glucocorticoid regulated kinase,[26] have been shown to stimulate transcription of ENaC in several Na$^+$-transporting epithelia as well as in the lung.[70] In the alveolar epithelia, glucocorticoids were found to induce lung Na$^+$ reabsorption in the late gestation fetal lung.[71] In addition to increasing transcription of Na$^+$ channel subunits, steroids increase the number of available channels by decreasing the rate at which membrane-associated channels are degraded and increase the activity of existing channels. Glucocorticoids have also been shown to enhance the responsiveness of lungs to β-adrenergic agents and thyroid hormones.[97] The enhanced Na$^+$ reabsorption induced by glucocorticoids can be blocked by amiloride, suggesting a role for ENaC. This effect was not observed with triiodothyronine (T$_3$) or with cAMP. Cord blood cortisol levels, which are higher in infants delivered vaginally and at term, have been shown to be associated with ENaC levels measured by mRNA in the first hours of life.[75] Glucocorticoid induction was found to be receptor-mediated and primarily transcriptional. This observation is important because it provides an additional explanation for the beneficial effect of antenatal steroids on the lung.

In the rat fetal lung, O'Brodovich et al.[51,54] have previously shown that the expression of α-ENaC is markedly increased at about 20 days' gestation (corresponding to the saccular stage of lung development) and can be accelerated by exposure to dexamethasone and increased levels of thyroid hormone. Such an effect would translate into accelerated fetal lung fluid reabsorption at birth. Jain et al.[52] have shown that steroids are highly effective in enhancing the expression of highly selective Na$^+$ channels in lung epithelial cells. Under conditions of steroid deprivation, alveolar cells express predominantly a nonselective cation channel that is unlikely to transport the large load of Na$^+$ and alveolar fluid clearance imposed at birth. However, when these steroid-deprived (both fetal and adult) cells are exposed to dexamethasone, there is a rapid transition to highly selective Na$^+$ channels, which are readily seen in other Na$^+$ and fluid transporting systems such as the kidneys and colon.[52] In addition, steroids have been shown to have beneficial effects on the surfactant system as well as pulmonary mechanics.[97–102]

Considerable evidence shows that high levels of endogenous catecholamines at birth may be important for accelerating alveolar fluid clearance.[103–105] It would be logical to conclude that in the absence of an endogenous surge in fetal catecholamines, exogenous catecholamines would be effective in initiating fetal lung fluid clearance. However, recent studies show that exogenous addition of epinephrine in guinea pigs failed to stimulate fluid clearance in the newborn lungs.[105] There are several possible explanations for this finding. First, catecholamines work on the fetal Na$^+$ channel (mostly nonselective) by increasing its activity, not by increasing the gene transcription or translation of the proteins required to assemble the channel.[84,89] Thus, if the developmentally regulated ENaC channels are not available in adequate numbers at birth, no amount of extra catecholamines will make a difference. Steroids, on the other hand, increase the transcription of the ENaC genes and, through another mechanism involving proteosomal degradation, increase the total number of ENaC channels available at birth; however, a longer duration (4–24 hours) of exposure is required for such an effect. Indeed, if these in vitro findings were to hold true in vivo, then neonates exposed to antenatal steroids would be more responsive to other exogenous agents that enhance Na$^+$ channel activity (i.e., catecholamines).

Indeed, several recent trials have aimed to test the benefit of antenatal steroids on two groups at risk for postnatal respiratory distress and not currently treated with antenatal steroids: LPT infants (34 and 0/7 weeks to 36 and 6/7 weeks) and term infants delivered by elective cesarean section.[106] LPT infants are at risk for both RDS and TTN and a recent large trial of prenatal betamethasone found a reduction in overall respiratory distress and TTN specifically,[107] though widespread adoption has been slow due to concerns about hypoglycemia. Similarly in term infants, treatment with prenatal steroids has demonstrated a decrease in TTN and respiratory distress, especially in those delivered at 37 weeks, early term.[108,109] Postnatal steroids have less promise, because a significant ($\cong$40%) reduction in fetal lung fluid occurs before spontaneous delivery and rapid clearance of the remaining fluid has to occur within hours after birth. Thus it is doubtful that postnatal steroid treatment initiated after the infant has become symptomatic would be a successful alternate strategy. Other pathways, such as catecholamines, will need to be explored. Helms et al.[55,110] have recently shown that dopamine can greatly enhance Na^+ channel activity working via a non–cAMP-dependent posttranslational mechanism. In adult ARDS, clinical trials of β-agonist and steroid therapy have shown improvement in lung fluid clearance or ventilator-free days but not definitively in mortality.[111] A small pilot study of the beta agonist salbutamol in neonates with TTN shows promise,[112] but no standard treatment for TTN has been clearly identified.

Summary

The transition from placental gas exchange to air breathing is a complex process that requires adequate removal of fetal lung fluid and a concomitant increase in perfusion of the newly ventilated alveoli. In neonates who are unable to make this transition, varying degrees of respiratory distress and impairment of gas exchange are common. Therapeutic approaches that can facilitate fetal lung fluid clearance are likely to reduce pulmonary morbidity in the neonatal period and help in designing therapies to combat lung edema formation in postnatal life.

REFERENCES

1. Alcorn D, Adamson TM, Lambert TF, et al. Morphological effects of chronic tracheal ligation and drainage in the fetal lamb lung. *J Anat*. 1977;123:649–660.
2. Moessinger AC, Singh M, Donnelly DF, et al. The effect of prolonged oligohydramnios on fetal lung development, maturation and ventilatory patterns in the newborn guinea pig. *J Dev Physiol*. 1987;9:419–427.
3. Adams FH, Fujiwara T, Rowshan G. The nature and origin of the fluid in the fetal lamb lung. *J Pediatr*. 1963;63:881–888.
4. Olver RE, Strang LB. Ion fluxes across the pulmonary epithelium and the secretion of lung liquid in the foetal lamb. *J Physiol*. 1974;241:327–357.
5. Karlberg P, Adams FH, Geubelle F, Wallgren G. Alteration of the infant's thorax during vaginal delivery. *Acta Obstet Gynecol Scand*. 1962;41:223–229.
6. Olver RE, Walters DV, Wilson SM. Developmental regulation of lung liquid transport. *Annu Rev Physiol*. 2004;66:77–101.
7. Song W, Wei S, Matalon S. Inhibition of epithelia sodium channels by respiratory syncytial virus in vitro and in vivo. *Ann N Y Acad Sci*. 2010;1203:79–84.
8. Rudolph AM, Heymann MA. Circulatory changes during growth in the fetal lamb. *Circ Res*. 1970;26:289–299.
9. Adamson TM, Brodecky V, Lambert TF, et al. Lung liquid production and composition in the 'in utero' foetal lamb. *Aust J Exp Biol Med Sci*. 1975;53:65–75.
10. Mescher EJ, Platzker AC, Ballard PL, et al. Ontogeny of tracheal fluid, pulmonary surfactant, and plasma corticoids in the fetal lamb. *J Appl Physiol*. 1975;39:1017–1021.
11. Harding R, Hooper SB. Regulation of lung expansion and lung growth before birth. *J Appl Physiol*. 1996;81:209–224.
12. Wallen LD, Kulisz E, Maloney JE. Main pulmonary artery ligation reduces lung fluid production in fetal sheep. *J Dev Physiol*. 1991;16:173–179.
13. Harrison MR, Bressack MA, Churg AM, de Lorimier AA. Correction of congenital diaphragmatic hernia in utero. II. Simulated correction permits fetal lung growth with survival at birth. *Surgery*. 1980;88:260–268.
14. Walters DV, Ramsden CA, Olver RE. Dibutyryl cAMP induces a gestation-dependent absorption of fetal lung liquid. *J Appl Physiol*. 1990;68:2054–2059.
15. Adamson TM, Boyd RD, Platt HS, Strang LB. Composition of alveolar liquid in the foetal lamb. *J Physiol*. 1969;204:159–168.
16. Body RD, Hill JR, Humphreys PW, et al. Permeability of lung capillaries to macromolecules in foetal and new-born lambs and sheep. *J Physiol*. 1969;201:567–588.
17. Normand IC, Olver RE, Reynolds EO, Strang LB. Permeability of lung capillaries and alveoli to non-electrolytes in the foetal lamb. *J Physiol*. 1971;219:303–330.
18. Normand IC, Reynolds EO, Strang LB. Passage of macromolecules between alveolar and interstitial spaces in foetal and newly ventilated lungs of the lamb. *J Physiol*. 1970;210:151–164.

19. Bland RD, Hansen TN, Haberkern CM, et al. Lung fluid balance in lambs before and after birth. *J Appl Physiol.* 1982;53:992–1004.

20. Barker PM, Boucher RC, Yankaskas JR. Bioelectric properties of cultured monolayers from epithelium of distal human fetal lung. *Am J Physiol.* 1995;268:L270–L277.

21. McCray PB, Bettencourt JD, Bastacky J. Developing bronchopulmonary epithelium of the human fetus secretes fluid. *Am J Physiol.* 1992;262:L270–L279.

22. McCray PB, Bettencourt JD, Bastacky J. Secretion of lung fluid by the developing fetal rat alveolar epithelium in organ culture. *Am J Respir Cell Mol Biol.* 1992;6:609–616.

23. Carlton DP, Cummings JJ, Chapman DL, et al. Ion transport regulation of lung liquid secretion in foetal lambs. *J Dev Physiol.* 1992;17:99–107.

24. Cassin S, Gause G, Perks AM. The effects of bumetanide and furosemide on lung liquid secretion in fetal sheep. *Proc Soc Exp Biol Med.* 1986;181:427–431.

25. Olver RE, Schneeberger EE, Walters DV. Epithelial solute permeability, ion transport and tight junction morphology in the developing lung of the fetal lamb. *J Physiol.* 1981;315:395–412.

26. Wilson SM, Olver RE, Walters DV. Developmental regulation of lumenal lung fluid and electrolyte transport. *Respir Physiol Neurobiol.* 2007;159:247–255.

27. Borok Z, Lubman RL, Danto SI, et al. Keratinocyte growth factor modulates alveolar epithelial cell phenotype in vitro: expression of aquaporin 5. *Am J Respir Cell Mol Biol.* 1998;18:554–561.

28. Dobbs LG, Gonzalez R, Matthay MA, et al. Highly water-permeable type I alveolar epithelial cells confer high water permeability between the airspace and vasculature in rat lung. *Proc Natl Acad Sci USA.* 1998;95:2991–2996.

29. Blaisdell CJ, Edmonds RD, Wang XT, et al. pH-regulated chloride secretion in fetal lung epithelia. *Am J Physiol Lung Cell Mol Physiol.* 2000;278:L1248–L1255.

30. O'Brodovich H, Merritt TA. Bicarbonate concentration in rhesus monkey and guinea pig fetal lung liquid. *Am Rev Respir Dis.* 1992;146:1613–1614.

31. Kitterman JA, Ballard PL, Clements JA, et al. Tracheal fluid in fetal lambs: spontaneous decrease prior to birth. *J Appl Physiol.* 1979;47:985–989.

32. Schneeberger EE. Plasmalemmal vesicles in pulmonary capillary endothelium of developing fetal lamb lungs. *Microvasc Res.* 1983;25:40–55.

33. Shermeta DW, Oesch I. Characteristics of fetal lung fluid production. *J Pediatr Surg.* 1981;16:943–946.

34. Carlton DP, Cummings JJ, Poulain FR, Bland RD. Increased pulmonary vascular filtration pressure does not alter lung liquid secretion in fetal sheep. *J Appl Physiol.* 1992;72:650–655.

35. Cotton CU, Lawson EE, Boucher RC, Gatzy JT. Bioelectric properties and ion transport of airways excised from adult and fetal sheep. *J Appl Physiol.* 1983;55:1542–1549.

36. Krochmal EM, Ballard ST, Yankaskas JR, et al. Volume and ion transport by fetal rat alveolar and tracheal epithelia in submersion culture. *Am J Physiol.* 1989;256:F397–F407.

37. Zeitlin PL, Loughlin GM, Guggino WB. Ion transport in cultured fetal and adult rabbit tracheal epithelia. *Am J Physiol.* 1988;254:C691–C698.

38. Brown MJ, Olver RE, Ramsden CA, et al. Effects of adrenaline and of spontaneous labour on the secretion and absorption of lung liquid in the fetal lamb. *J Physiol.* 1983;344:137–152.

39. Chapman DL, Carlton DP, Nielson DW, et al. Changes in lung lipid during spontaneous labor in fetal sheep. *J Appl Physiol.* 1994;76:523–530.

40. Dickson KA, Maloney JE, Berger PJ. Decline in lung liquid volume before labor in fetal lambs. *J Appl Physiol.* 1986;61:2266–2272.

41. Bland RD. Dynamics of pulmonary water before and after birth. *Acta Paediatr Scand Suppl.* 1983;305:12–20.

42. Bland RD, Bressack MA, McMillan DD. Labor decreases the lung water content of newborn rabbits. *Am J Obstet Gynecol.* 1979;135:364–367.

43. Bland RD. Loss of liquid from the lung lumen in labor: more than a simple "squeeze". *Am J Physiol Lung Cell Mol Physiol.* 2001;280:L602–L605.

44. Guidot DM, Folkesson HG, Jain L, et al. Integrating acute lung injury and regulation of alveolar fluid clearance. *Am J Physiol Lung Cell Mol Physiol.* 2006;291:L301–L306.

45. Jain L, Eaton DC. Alveolar fluid transport: a changing paradigm. *Am J Physiol Lung Cell Mol Physiol.* 2006;290:L646–L648.

46. Uchiyama M, Konno N. Hormonal regulation of ion and water transport in anuran amphibians. *Gen Comp Endocrinol.* 2006;147:54–61.

47. Matthay MA, Folkesson HG, Verkman AS. Salt and water transport across alveolar and distal airway epithelia in the adult lung. *Am J Physiol.* 1996;270:L487–L503.

48. Voilley N, Lingueglia E, Champigny G, et al. The lung amiloride-sensitive Na^+ channel: biophysical properties, pharmacology, ontogenesis, and molecular cloning. *Proc Natl Acad Sci USA.* 1994;91:247–251.

49. Canessa CM, Horisberger JD, Rossier BC. Epithelial sodium channel related to proteins involved in neurodegeneration. *Nature.* 1993;361:467–470.

50. Canessa CM, Schild L, Buell G, et al. Amiloride-sensitive epithelial Na^+ channel is made of three homologous subunits. *Nature.* 1994;367:463–467.

51. O'Brodovich H, Hannam V, Seear M, Mullen JB. Amiloride impairs lung water clearance in newborn guinea pigs. *J Appl Physiol.* 1990;68:1758–1762.

52. Jain L, Chen XJ, Ramosevac S, et al. Expression of highly selective sodium channels in alveolar type II cells is determined by culture conditions. *Am J Physiol Lung Cell Mol Physiol.* 2001;280:L646–L658.

14

53. O'Brodovich H. Epithelial ion transport in the fetal and perinatal lung. *Am J Physiol.* 1991;261: C555–C564.

54. O'Brodovich H, Canessa C, Ueda J, et al. Expression of the epithelial Na+ channel in the developing rat lung. *Am J Physiol.* 1993;265:C491–C496.

55. Helms MN, Self J, Bao HF, et al. Dopamine activates amiloride-sensitive sodium channels in alveolar type 1 cells in a lung slice preparation. *Am J Physiol Lung Cell Mol Physiol.* 2006;291:L610–L618.

56. Johnson MD, Bao HF, Helms MN, et al. Functional ion channels in pulmonary alveolar type I cells support a role for type I cells in lung ion transport. *Proc Natl Acad Sci USA.* 2006;103: 4964–4969.

57. Johnson MD, Widdicombe JH, Allen L, et al. Alveolar epithelial type I cells contain transport proteins and transport sodium, supporting an active role for type I cells in regulation of lung liquid homeostasis. *Proc Natl Acad Sci USA.* 2002;99:1966–1971.

58. Matthay MA, Folkesson HG, Clerici C. Lung epithelial fluid transport and the resolution of pulmonary edema. *Physiol Rev.* 2002;82:569–600.

59. Ji HL, Su XF, Kedar S, et al. Delta-subunit confers novel biophysical features to alpha beta gamma-human epithelial sodium channel (ENaC) via a physical interaction. *J Biol Chem.* 2006;281:8233–8241.

60. Bangel-Ruland N, Sobczak K, Christmann T, et al. Characterization of the epithelial sodium channel delta-subunit in human nasal epithelium. *Am J Respir Cell Mol Biol.* 2010;42:498–505.

61. Hummler E, Barker P, Gatzy J, et al. Early death due to defective neonatal lung liquid clearance in alpha-ENaC-deficient mice. *Nat Genet.* 1996;12:325–328.

62. Hummler E, Planès C. Importance of ENaC-mediated sodium transport in alveolar fluid clearance using genetically-engineered mice. *Cell Physiol Biochem.* 2010;25:63–70.

63. Barker PM, Gowen CW, Lawson EE, Knowles MR. Decreased sodium ion absorption across nasal epithelium of very premature infants with respiratory distress syndrome. *J Pediatr.* 1997;130: 373–377.

64. Gowen CW, Lawson EE, Gingras J, et al. Electrical potential difference and ion transport across nasal epithelium of term neonates: correlation with mode of delivery, transient tachypnea of the newborn, and respiratory rate. *J Pediatr.* 1988;113:121–127.

65. Haase M, Laube M, Thome UH. Sex-specific effects of sex steroids on alveolar epithelial Na+ transport. *Am J Physiol Lung Cell Mol Physiol.* 2017;312:L405–L414.

66. Kaltofen T, Haase M, Thome UH, Laube M. Male Sex is Associated with a Reduced Alveolar Epithelial Sodium Transport. *PLoS ONE.* 2015;10(8).

67. Barker PM, Brown MJ, Ramsden CA, et al. The effect of thyroidectomy in the fetal sheep on lung liquid reabsorption induced by adrenaline or cyclic AMP. *J Physiol.* 1988;407:373–383.

68. Barker PM, Gowen CW, Lawson EE, Knowles MR. Decreased sodium ion absorption across nasal epithelium of very premature infants with respiratory distress syndrome. *J Pediatr.* 1997;130:373–377.

69. Perks AM, Cassin S. The effects of arginine vasopressin and epinephrine on lung liquid production in fetal goats. *Can J Physiol Pharmacol.* 1989;67:491–498.

70. Venkatesh VC, Katzberg HD. Glucocorticoid regulation of epithelial sodium channel genes in human fetal lung. *Am J Physiol.* 1997;273:L227–L233.

71. Wallace MJ, Hooper SB, Harding R. Regulation of lung liquid secretion by arginine vasopressin in fetal sheep. *Am J Physiol.* 1990;258:R104–R111.

72. Chang SS, Grunder S, Hanukoglu A, et al. Mutations in subunits of the epithelial sodium channel cause salt wasting with hyperkalaemic acidosis, pseudohypoaldosteronism type 1. *Nat Genet.* 1996;12:248–253.

73. Helve O, Pitkänen O, Janér C, Andersson S. Pulmonary fluid balance in the human newborn infant. *Neonatology.* 2009;95:347–352.

74. Helve O, Janér C, Pitkänen O, Andersson S. Expression of the epithelial sodium channel in airway epithelium of newborn infants depends on gestational age. *Pediatrics.* 2007;120:1311–1316.

75. Janér C, Pitkänen OM, Süvari L, et al. Duration of gestation and mode of delivery affect the genes of transepithelial sodium transport in pulmonary adaptation. *Neonatology.* 2015;107:27–33.

76. Milla CE, Zirbes J. Pulmonary complications of endocrine and metabolic disorders. *Paediatr Respir Rev.* 2012;13(1):23–28.

77. Akçay A, Yavuz T, Semiz S, et al. Pseudohypoaldosteronism type 1 and respiratory distress syndrome. *J Pediatr Endocrinol Metab.* 2002;15(9):1557–1561.

78. Schaedel C, Marthinsen L, Kristoffersson AC, et al. Lung symptoms in pseudohypoaldosteronism type 1 are associated with deficiency of the alpha-subunit of the epithelial sodium channel. *J Pediatr.* 1999;135(6):739–745.

79. Liedtke CM. Electrolyte transport in the epithelium of pulmonary segments of normal and cystic fibrosis lung. *FASEB J.* 1992;6:3076–3084.

80. Knowles MR, Olivier K, Noone P, Boucher RC. Pharmacologic modulation of salt and water in the airway epithelium in cystic fibrosis. *Am J Respir Crit Care Med.* 1995;151:S65–S69.

81. Mall M, Grubb BR, Harkema JR, et al. Increased airway epithelial Na+ absorption produces cystic fibrosis-like lung disease in mice. *Nat Med.* 2004;10:487–493.

82. Folkesson HG, Chapin CJ, Beard LL, et al. Congenital diaphragmatic hernia prevents absorption of distal air space fluid in late-gestation rat fetuses. *Am J Physiol Lung Cell Mol Physiol.* 2006;290:L478–L484.

83. Ringman Uggla A, von Schewelov K, Zelenina M, et al. Low pulmonary expression of epithelial Na(+) channel and Na(+), K(+)-ATPase in newborn infants with congenital diaphragmatic hernia. *Neonatology.* 2010;99:14–22.

84. Jain L, Eaton DC. Physiology of fetal lung fluid clearance and the effect of labor. *Semin Perinatol.* 2006;30:34–43.
85. Noone PG, Leigh MW, Sannuti A, et al. Primary ciliary dyskinesia: diagnostic and phenotypic features. *Am J Respir Crit Care Med.* 2004;169:459–467.
86. Jain L. Alveolar fluid clearance in developing lungs and its role in neonatal transition. *Clin Perinatol.* 1999;26:585–599.
87. Jain L, Chen XJ, Brown LA, Eaton DC. Nitric oxide inhibits lung sodium transport through a cGMP-mediated inhibition of epithelial cation channels. *Am J Physiol.* 1998;274:L475–L484.
88. Jain L, Chen XJ, Malik B, et al. Antisense oligonucleotides against the alpha-subunit of ENaC decrease lung epithelial cation-channel activity. *Am J Physiol.* 1999;276:L1046–L1051.
89. Chen XJ, Eaton DC, Jain L. Beta-adrenergic regulation of amiloride-sensitive lung sodium channels. *Am J Physiol Lung Cell Mol Physiol.* 2002;282:L609–L620.
90. Cummings JJ, Carlton DP, Poulain FR, et al. Vasopressin effects on lung liquid volume in fetal sheep. *Pediatr Res.* 1995;38:30–35.
91. Bouvry D, Planes C, Malbert-Colas L, et al. Hypoxia-induced cytoskeleton disruption in alveolar epithelial cells. *Am J Respir Cell Mol Biol.* 2006;35:519–527.
92. Anantharam A, Tian Y, Palmer LG. Open probability of the epithelial sodium channel is regulated by intracellular sodium. *J Physiol.* 2006;574:333–347.
93. Renard S, Voilley N, Bassilana F, et al. Localization and regulation by steroids of the alpha, beta and gamma subunits of the amiloride-sensitive Na^+ channel in colon, lung and kidney. *Pflugers Arch.* 1995;430:299–307.
94. Eaton D, Ohara A, Ling BN. Cellular regulation of amiloride blockable Na^+ channels. *Biomed Res.* 1991;12:31–35.
95. McCartney J, Richards EM, Wood CE, Keller-Wood M. Mineralocorticoid effects in the late gestation ovine fetal lung. *Physiol Rep.* 2014;2(7).
96. Guidot DM, Modelska K, Lois M, et al. Ethanol ingestion via glutathione depletion impairs alveolar epithelial barrier function in rats. *Am J Physiol Lung Cell Mol Physiol.* 2000;279:L127–L135.
97. Jobe AH, Ikegami M, Padbury J, et al. Combined effects of fetal beta agonist stimulation and glucocorticoids on lung function of preterm lambs. *Biol Neonate.* 1997;72:305–313.
98. Ervin MG, Berry LM, Ikegami M, et al. Single dose fetal betamethasone administration stabilizes postnatal glomerular filtration rate and alters endocrine function in premature lambs. *Pediatr Res.* 1996;40:645–651.
99. Pillow JJ, Hall GL, Willet KE, et al. Effects of gestation and antenatal steroid on airway and tissue mechanics in newborn lambs. *Am J Respir Crit Care Med.* 2001;163:1158–1163.
100. Smith LM, Ervin MG, Wada N, et al. Antenatal glucocorticoids alter postnatal preterm lamb renal and cardiovascular responses to intravascular volume expansion. *Pediatr Res.* 2000;47:622–627.
101. Willet KE, Jobe AH, Ikegami M, et al. Lung morphometry after repetitive antenatal glucocorticoid treatment in preterm sheep. *Am J Respir Crit Care Med.* 2001;163:1437–1443.
102. Willet KE, Jobe AH, Ikegami M, et al. Antenatal endotoxin and glucocorticoid effects on lung morphometry in preterm lambs. *Pediatr Res.* 2000;48:782–788.
103. Baines DL, Folkesson HG, Norlin A, et al. The influence of mode of delivery, hormonal status and postnatal O_2 environment on epithelial sodium channel (ENaC) expression in perinatal guinea-pig lung. *J Physiol.* 2000;522(Pt 1):147–157.
104. Berthiaume Y, Staub NC, Matthay MA. Beta-adrenergic agonists increase lung liquid clearance in anesthetized sheep. *J Clin Invest.* 1987;79:335–343.
105. Finley N, Norlin A, Baines DL, Folkesson HG. Alveolar epithelial fluid clearance is mediated by endogenous catecholamines at birth in guinea pigs. *J Clin Invest.* 1998;101:972–981.
106. Tutdibi E, Gries K, Bücheler M, et al. Impact of labor on outcomes in transient tachypnea of the newborn: population-based study. *Pediatrics.* 2010;125:e577–e583.
107. Gyamfi-Bannerman C, Thom EA, Blackwell SC, Jain L, et al; NICHD Maternal–Fetal Medicine Units Network. Antenatal Betamethasone for Women at Risk for Late Preterm Delivery. *N Engl J Med.* 2016;374(14):1311–1320.
108. Ahmed M, Sayed Ahmed W, Mohammed T. Antenatal steroids at 37 weeks, does it reduce neonatal respiratory morbidity? A randomized trial. *J Matern Fetal Neonatal Med.* 2015;28:1486–1490.
109. Stutchfield P, Whitaker R, Russell I. Antenatal betamethasone and incidence of neonatal respiratory distress after elective caesarean section: pragmatic randomized trial. *BMJ.* 2005;331:662.
110. Helms MN, Chen XJ, Ramosevac S, et al. Dopamine regulation of amiloride-sensitive sodium channels in lung cells. *Am J Physiol Lung Cell Mol Physiol.* 2006;290:L710–L722.
111. Morty RE, Eickelberg O, Seeger W. Alveolar fluid clearance in acute lung injury: what have we learned from animal models and clinical studies? *Intensive Care Med.* 2007;33:1229–1240.
112. Armangil D, Yurdakök M, Korkmaz A, et al. Inhaled beta-2 agonist salbutamol for the treatment of transient tachypnea of the newborn. *J Pediatr.* 2011;159:398–403.

CHAPTER 15

Use of Diuretics in the Newborn

Jean-Pierre Guignard, MD

- Body Fluid Homeostasis
- Mechanisms and Sites of Action of Diuretics
- Clinical Use of Diuretics
- Adverse Effects of Diuretics

Introduction

Diuretics are pharmacologic agents that increase the excretion of water and electrolytes. They are primarily used in states of inappropriate salt and water retention. Such states can be the consequence of congestive heart failure (CHF), renal diseases, or liver disease. Diuretics are also used in various conditions not evidently associated with salt retention. Such conditions include oliguric states, respiratory disorders, electrolyte disorders, and nephrogenic diabetes insipidus. Diuretics can also be valuable tools in the laboratory differential diagnosis of congenital tubulopathies.

The rationale use of diuretics in newborn infants requires a clear understanding of the physiology and physiopathology of immature kidneys.[1,2]

Body Fluid Homeostasis

The kidney is responsible for maintaining the extracellular fluid (ECF) volume and osmolality constant despite large variations in salt and water intake.

Extracellular Fluid Volume

NaCl, the major osmotically active solute in ECF, determines its volume. The overall balance between sodium intake and its urinary excretion thus regulates ECF volume and consequently cardiac output and blood pressure. Volume receptors are distributed in the low-pressure capacitance vessels (great veins and atria), as well as in the high-pressure resistance vessels (arterial vascular tree). Arterial sensors perceive the adequacy of blood flow in the arterial circuit, a parameter coined as *effective arterial circulating volume*. This volume is also monitored by baroreceptors located in the juxtaglomerular apparatus of the kidney. When sensed by these receptors, a decrease in renal perfusion pressure leads to the activation of the renin-angiotensin-aldosterone system (RAAS). Aldosterone stimulates sodium reabsorption and potassium excretion. Although aldosterone is the main hormone regulating long-term changes in sodium excretion, other hormones and paracrine factors, including angiotensin II, the prostaglandins, dopamine, the catecholamines, and atrial natriuretic peptide (ANP), also modulate sodium renal handling. The release of the latter, a potent vasodilator and natriuretic agent, is modulated by sensors (the stretch receptors) that sense the atrial filling volume.[3]

Plasma Osmolality

The plasma osmolality is maintained within narrow limits.[3] Small (2%–3%) changes in plasma osmolality are sensed by osmoreceptors located in the hypothalamus, which by stimulating or inhibiting the release of vasopressin lead to increases or decreases in the excretion of free water. By acting on the baroreceptors, the effective circulating volume also influences the release of vasopressin. Dilution of urine depends on sodium delivery to the distal nephron diluting site; concentration of urine, modulated by vasopressin, requires the presence of a hypertonic renal medullary interstitium.[3]

Clinical Use of Diuretics

Sodium-Retaining States

Sodium retention is the primary target of diuretics. Salt and water retention with or without edema formation can occur as a primary event or as a consequence of reduced effective circulating volume with secondary hyperaldosteronism. CHF is the main neonatal condition associated with sodium retention.[4] The increased pressure in the venous circulation and capillaries favors the movement of fluid into the interstitium and leads to the formation of edema. Failure of the heart to provide normal tissue perfusion is sensed as a decrease in effective circulating volume by the kidney, which retains sodium and water. Treatment of the condition consists in restoring normal cardiac output. By mobilizing the edematous fluid, diuretics improve the symptoms of CHF. The pulmonary edema secondary to heart failure requires the urgent use of diuretics to reduce the life-threatening pulmonary congestion.[5,6] The use of diuretics can be lifesaving when the ECF volume is expanded.

Diuretics may on the contrary further compromise the patient's condition when sodium retention occurs in response to homeostatic mechanisms mobilized to defend the circulating volume. The same reasoning applies to states of nephrotic or liver cirrhosis edemas.[7,8] The use of diuretics (loop diuretics, thiazides, and potassium-sparing diuretics) in these conditions requires a clear understanding of the patient's underlying pathophysiologic condition and careful monitoring of the hemodynamic state.[5,6]

Oliguric States

Loop diuretics are often administered to patients with oliguric renal insufficiency in the hope of promoting diuresis and improving renal perfusion and glomerular filtration rate (GFR). When present, the diuretic response may actually worsen the renal hypoperfusion.[9,10]

Respiratory Disorders

Interstitial and alveolar edema is present in idiopathic respiratory distress syndrome (RDS) of preterm babies, as well as in transient tachypnea of term neonates. Inadequate fetal lung fluid clearance is partly responsible for the edema. Administration of diuretics (loop diuretics) could accelerate the reabsorption of lung fluid and pulmonary recovery in these patients with lung edema.[11]

Central Nervous System Disorders

Large hemorrhages into the brain ventricles may result in fluid retention and dilatation of the fluid-producing brain cavities. Diuretics (acetazolamide, furosemide) are sometimes used to prevent or reduce the accumulation of fluid in the ventricles.[12]

Electrolyte Disorders

Diuretics can be used in various situations associated with dyselectrolytemia. They can increase potassium excretion in hyperkalemic states (loop diuretics, thiazides), increase calcium excretion in hypercalcemia (loop diuretics), or decrease the rate of calcium excretion in hypercalciuric states (thiazides). Increased bicarbonate excretion can be achieved by acetazolamide, and increased excretion of hydrogen ions can be stimulated by loop diuretics.[5,13,14]

Nephrogenic Diabetes Insipidus

Diuretics (thiazides) can paradoxically decrease urine output in nephrogenic diabetes insipidus.[15]

Arterial Hypertension

Arterial hypertension may be a consequence of, or aggravated by, sodium retention and consecutive expansion of the ECF volume. This type of hypertension responds to diuretic-induced natriuresis.[16]

Differential Diagnosis of Congenital Tubulopathies

Diuretics such as acetazolamide, furosemide, and hydrochlorothiazide can be used to test distal tubular acidification or distal sodium reabsorption defects in patients with congenital tubulopathies.

Classification of Diuretics According to the Site of Action

Diuretics can be classified according to their site and mode of action (Fig. 15.1 and Table 15.1). They all increase sodium and water excretion and variably modify the excretion of other electrolytes (Table 15.2). *Filtration diuretics* increase salt and water excretion by primarily increasing GFR. *Osmotic diuretics* depress salt and electrolyte reabsorption in the proximal tubule and in Henle loop. *Carbonic anhydrase inhibitors* act primarily on the proximal tubule. *Loop diuretics,* the most potent diuretics, inhibit Na$^+$ reabsorption in the ascending limb of Henle loop. *The thiazide and thiazide-like diuretics* act in the distal convoluted tubule and *potassium-sparing diuretics* in the late distal tubule and collecting duct.[13,14] New diuretics with different modes of action (*vasopressin antagonists, adenosine antagonists, natriuretic peptides,* etc.) are being developed and tested. All diuretics share adverse effects that are actually extensions of their primary effects on electrolyte excretion (Table 15.3), as well as nonelectrolyte adverse effects (Table 15.4).

Although diuretics are very widely used in neonatal intensive care units (NICUs), the extent of and expectations for diuretic therapy by neonatologists caring for low

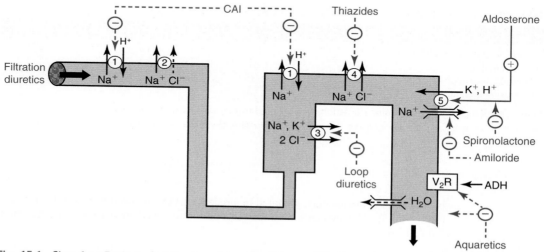

Fig. 15.1 Sites 1 to 5: sites of sodium transport along the nephron. Numbers 1 to 5 represent the sites and mechanisms of Na$^+$ transport. The group of diuretics acting at the different sites is indicated. *1,* Na/H exchanger 1 (NHE1). *2,* Na-glucose cotransporter 2 (SLGT2). *3,* Na-K-2Cl cotransporter (NKCC2) (furosemide receptor). *4,* Na-Cl cotransporter (NCC) (thiazides receptor). 5, H$^+$,K$^+$-ATPase and epithelial sodium channel (amiloride receptor): ENaC (potassium-sparing diuretics). The aquaretics act on the collecting duct vasopressin type 2 receptor (V$_2$R). *CAI,* Carbonic anhydrase inhibitor; *ENaC,* sodium epithelium channel.

Table 15.1   CLINICAL USE OF DIURETICS IN NEONATES

Filtration Diuretics
- Oliguric prerenal failure

Osmotic Diuretics
- Oliguric prerenal failure
- Elevated intracranial pressure

Carbonic Anhydrase Inhibitors
- Production of alkaline diuresis
- Posthemorrhagic ventricular dilatation
- Assessment of distal urinary acidification

Loop Diuretics
- Edematous states (congestive heart failure, renal and liver diseases)
- Respiratory disorders (transient tachypnea, respiratory distress syndrome, chronic lung disease in preterm neonates, compromised lung mechanics)
- Prerenal failure (asphyxia)
- Posthemorrhagic ventricular dilatation
- Indomethacin-induced oliguria
- Electrolyte disorders (hyperkalemia, hypercalcemia, severe hyponatremia)
- Assessment of distal urinary acidification

Thiazides
- Edematous states (congestive heart failure, renal and liver diseases)
- Respiratory disorders (chronic lung diseases in preterm neonates)
- Hypercalciuria
- Proximal renal tubular acidosis
- Nephrogenic diabetes insipidus
- Diagnosis of renal tubular hypokalemic disorders

Potassium-Sparing Diuretics
- Adjunctive therapy with loop or thiazide diuretics
- Prevention of hypokalemia
- Nephrogenic diabetes insipidus
- Cystic fibrosis

Table 15.2   ACUTE EFFECTS OF DIURETICS ON ELECTROLYTE EXCRETION

	Na^+	K^+	Ca^{2+}	Mg^{2+}	H^+	Cl^-	HCO_3^-	$H_2PO_4^-$
Carbonic anhydrase inhibitors	↑	↑↑	=	~	↓	(↑)	↑↑	↑↑
Loop diuretics	↑↑	↑↑	↑↑	↑↑	↑	↑↑	↑	↑
Thiazide diuretics	↑	↑↑	~	(↑)	↑	↑	↑	↑
K^+-sparing diuretics	↑	↓	↓	↓	↓	↑	(↑)	=

In the absence of significant volume depletion, which would trigger complex adjustments.
(↑), Slight increase; ↑, moderate increase; ↑↑, marked increase; ↓, decrease; =, no change; ~, variable effects.

birth weight neonates may, as stated in a recent survey,[17] exceed evidence for efficacy (Table 15.5). The dosages of diuretics commonly used in neonates are given in Table 15.6.

Filtration Diuretics

Agents that increase diuresis by increasing GFR are called *filtration diuretics*. These agents include the glucocorticoids; theophylline; and inotropic agents such as isoproterenol, dopamine, and dobutamine. By increasing GFR, these drugs only moderately increase Na^+ excretion. Dopamine and theophylline are sometimes used in neonates

Table 15.3 ELECTROLYTE DISTURBANCES INDUCED BY DIURETICS COMMONLY USED IN NEONATES

	Loop	Thiazides	K+-Sparing
Hypovolemia	+++	+	+
Hyponatremia	++	+++	−
Hypokalemia	+++	++	−
Hyperkalemia	−	−	++
Hypercalciuria	++	−	−
Hypercalcemia	−	+	−
Hypomagnesemia	+	+	−
Hypophosphatemia	+	+	−
Hyperuricemia	++	++	−
Metabolic acidosis	−	−	+
Metabolic alkalosis	++	++	−

+++, Marked increase in electrolyte disturbances; ++, moderate increase in electrolyte disturbances; +, mild increase in electrolyte disturbances; − indicates no effects.
Adapted from Chemtob S, Kaplan BS, Sherbotie JR, Aranda JV. Pharmacology of diuretics in the newborn. *Pediatr Clin North Am.* 1989;36:1231-1250.

Table 15.4 GENERAL NONELECTROLYTE SIDE EFFECTS OF DIURETICS

Diuretic		Nonelectrolyte Side Effects
Carbonic anhydrase inhibitors	—	CNS depression, paresthesia, calculus formation
Loop diuretics	—	Ototoxicity (usually reversible), nephrocalcinosis in neonates, PDA in neonates, hyperuricemia, hyperglycemia, hyperlipidemia, hypersensitivity
Thiazides	—	Hyperglycemia, insulin resistance, hyperlipidemia, hypersensitivity (fever, rash, purpura, anaphylaxis, interstitial nephritis), hyperuricemia
K+-sparing	Amiloride	Diarrhea, headache
	Triamterene	Glucose intolerance, interstitial nephritis, blood dyscrasias
	Spironolactone	Gynecomastia, hirsutism, peptic ulcers, ataxia, headache

CNS, Central nervous system; *PDA,* patent ductus arteriosus.

Table 15.5 SPECIFIC INDICATIONS WITH QUESTIONABLE BENEFITS IN CLINICAL TRIALS

Condition	Diuretic(s)	Reference
Oliguric prerenal failure	Mannitol	Better et al.,[18] Rigden et al.[19]
	Furosemide	Kellum,[9] Dubourg et al.[40]
Respiratory distress syndrome	Furosemide	Jain and Eaton[42]
Transient tachypnea of the newborn	Furosemide	Wiswell et al.,[43] Kassab M.[44]
Chronic lung disease	Furosemide	Brion and Primhak,[45] Brion et al.[46]
	Thiazides	Brion et al.[76]
	Thiazides + spironolactone	Brion et al.[76]
	Furosemide + thiazides	Brion et al.[76]
	Furosemide + metolazone	Segar et al.[47]
	Intratracheal furosemide	Aufricht et al.[60]
Posthemorrhagic ventricular dilatation	Furosemide + acetazolamide	International PHVD Drug Trial Group,[21] Kennedy et al.,[22] International PHVD Drug Trial Group,[53] Whitelaw et al.[54]
Indomethacin-induced oliguria	Furosemide	Eades and Christensen,[24] Brion et al.,[76]
	Dopamine	Andriessen et al.,[56] Lee et al.[57] Barrington and Brion[59]
Furosemide-induced nephrocalcinosis	Thiazides	Campfield et al.[65]
Nephrocalcinosis secondary to the use of vitamin D in hypophosphatemic rickets	Thiazides	Seikaly and Baum[72]
Compromised lung mechanics after cardiac surgery	Intratracheal furosemide	Aufricht et al.[60]
Cystic fibrosis	Aerolized amiloride	Pons et al.,[81] Ratjen and Bush[82]
Asthma	Intratracheal furosemide	Aufricht et al.[60]

PHVD, Posthemorrhagic ventricular dilatation.

Table 15.6 DOSAGES OF DIURETICS COMMONLY USED IN NEONATES

Drug	Route/Interval (qh)	Dosage (mg/kg/day)	Half-Life (h)	Comments
Furosemide	PO: 12–24	1–2	≈1.5	Effective at GFR <10
	IV: 12–24	0.5–1.5	idem	Doses may be increased up to 5 mg/kg in CRF
	CIVI	100–200 µg/kg/h		Hypokalemia; Mg, Ca depletion Ototoxicity; metabolic alkalosis
Torasemide	PO	0.5–1	≈3.5	Longer half-life and larger duration than furosemide Effective at GFR <10 Idem furosemide
Ethacrynic acid	PO: 12–24	1–2	≈1	Effective at GFR <10 Idem furosemide
Bumetanide	PO: 12–24	0.01–0.10	≈1	Effective at GFR <10
	IV: 12–24	0.01–0.05	idem	Idem furosemide
	CIVI	5–10 µg/kg/h		
Hydrochlorothiazide	PO: 12–24	1–3	≈2.5	Not effective at GFR <20 Hypokalemia metabolic alkalosis
Chlorthalidone	PO: 24–48	0.5–2.0	45	Not effective at GFR <20 Hypokalemia metabolic alkalosis
Metolazone	PO: 12–24	0.2–0.4	8–10	Effective at GFR <20 Hypokalemia
Spironolactone	PO: 6–12	1–3	≈1.6	Delayed effect. Cave CRF or K suppl. Hyperkalemia, acidosis
Canrenoate-K	IV: 24	4–10	≈16	Single IV dose Hyperkalemia, acidosis
Triamterene	PO: 12–24	2–4	≈4.2	Cave RF or K suppl. Hyperkalemia, acidosis
Amiloride	PO: 24	0.5	≈21	Cave RF or K suppl. Hyperkalemia, acidosis

CIVI, Constant IV infusion; *CRF*, chronic renal failure; *GFR*, glomerular filtration rate (mL/min per 1.73 m²); *IV*, intravenous; *PO*, oral; *RF*, renal failure.
Adapted from Guignard JP. Diuretics. In: Yaffe S, Aranda J, eds. *Neonatal and Pediatric Pharmacology—Therapeutic Principles in Practice*. 4th ed. Philadelphia: Lippincott Williams & Wilkins, Wolters Kluwer; 2011:629-645.

in the hope of improving renal perfusion and GFR rather than for their natriuretic and diuretic effect. They are discussed in Chapter 7.

Osmotic Diuretics

Osmotic diuretics are agents that inhibit the reabsorption of solute and water by altering osmotic driving forces along the nephron.

Chemistry

Mannitol, a hexahydric alcohol related to mannose with a molecular weight of 182 d, is the main representative of this class of agents.[18]

Mechanisms and Sites of Action

Freely filtered and (mostly) not reabsorbed, osmotic diuretics increase the tubular fluid osmolality, thus impairing the diffusion of water out of the tubular lumen, as well as that of NaCl by a solvent drag effect. The osmotic diuretics act in the proximal tubule and in the loop of Henle. By attracting water from the intracellular compartment, osmotic diuretics increase ECF volume and renal blood flow. Increased medullary blood flow washes out the hypertonic medulla, thus impairing the concentrating mechanism. By inhibiting NaCl reabsorption out of the water-impermeable thick ascending limb, osmotic diuretics also impair the dilution of urine. Osmotic diuretics increase nonspecifically the excretion of all electrolytes. The natriuresis induced by osmotic diuretics is only approximately 10% of the filtered load.

Efficacy and Therapeutic Uses

Osmotic diuretics increase the excretion of Na^+, K^+, Cl^-, Mg^{++}, Ca^{++}, Cl^-, and HCO_3^-. They improve renal perfusion without significantly affecting GFR. Mannitol has been used to increase urine flow rate in patients with prerenal failure,[18,19] promote the excretion of toxic substances by forced diuresis, and reduce elevated intracranial and intraocular pressures.

Adverse Effects: Interactions

Circulatory overload, acute renal tubular necrosis, intracranial hemorrhage, and CHF have been described in patients given intravenous (IV) mannitol. Mannitol is presently not recommended in neonates.

Carbonic Anhydrase Inhibitors

Agents in this group act by inhibiting the carbonic anhydrase in renal tubular cells and in the brush border of proximal tubular cells.

Chemistry

Acetazolamide, a sulfonamide derivative, is the main inhibitor of carbonic anhydrase used in humans.

Mechanisms and Sites of Action

Inhibition of carbonic anhydrase results in depressed cellular formation and subsequent secretion of H^+. As a consequence, the HCO_3^- ions that are normally reabsorbed by combining to H^+ in the tubular lumen are excreted in the urine. Acetazolamide is a weak diuretic agent, at best producing the excretion of 5% of the Na^+ and water filtered load.

Pharmacokinetic Properties

Acetazolamide is readily absorbed and is eliminated in the urine. It crosses the placental barrier and is secreted in breast milk.

Efficacy and Therapeutic Uses

Acetazolamide increases the urinary excretion of HCO_3^-, Na^+, and K^+, promoting alkaline diuresis with consequent systemic metabolic acidosis. Acetazolamide may be useful to alkalinize the urine when necessary, such as when chemotherapy is given. Acetazolamide can also be used to assess reliably the distal acidification ability by measuring the urine minus blood PCO_2 in alkaline urine.[20]

Specific Indications With Questionable Benefits (See Table 15.5)

Posthemorrhagic Ventricular Dilatation. Acetazolamide has been used alone or in association with furosemide in the treatment of posthemorrhagic ventricular dilatation (PHVD) in the hope of avoiding the need for surgical management. Randomized controlled studies have led to the conclusion that this treatment was ineffective in decreasing the rate of shunt placement and that it was associated with increased neurologic morbidity. The use of diuretics in PHVD is thus not recommended.[21,22]

Adverse Effects: Interactions

The occurrence of metabolic acidosis is common if the urinary losses of HCO_3^- are not substituted. Side effects include paresthesias, drowsiness, rash, fever, and the formation of renal calculi. Blood dyscrasias and hepatic failure are occasionally seen.

Loop Diuretics: Inhibition of Na^+-K^+-$2Cl^-$ Cotransport

Loop diuretics induce natriuresis by inhibiting the active reabsorption of NaCl in the loop of Henle.

Chemistry

Loop diuretics have diverse chemical structures.[23,24] Furosemide and bumetanide are sulfonamide derivatives, torsemide is a sulfonylurea, and ethacrynic acid is a phenoxyacetic acid derivative.

Mechanisms and Sites of Action

Loop diuretics block the Na^+-K^+-$2Cl^-$ cotransporter in the thick ascending limb of Henle loop, where 25% of the NaCl filtered load is usually reabsorbed. They are consequently highly effective because only a small proportion of the filtered Na^+ that escapes reabsorption in the loop can be reabsorbed downstream. Loop diuretics act from within the tubular lumen, where they are actively secreted by the organic acid pump. The effect of loop diuretics is more closely related to their urinary excretion rate than to their plasma concentration. By inhibiting NaCl reabsorption in Henle loop, loop diuretics abolish the lumen-positive voltage and thus the driving force for Ca^{2+} and Mg^{2+} reabsorption. They consequently increase Ca^{2+} and Mg^{2+} excretion. Inhibition of NaCl transport upstream of the distal tubule results in increased Na^+ delivery to the later portion of the distal tubule and cortical collecting duct. This part of the nephron responds by increasing the tubular secretion of K^+ and H^+, thus decreasing urine pH and increasing the urinary excretion of K^+. This secretion is also stimulated by the state of secondary hyperaldosteronism usually present as a consequence of diuretic-induced decrease in ECF volume.[3] By inhibiting NaCl reabsorption in the water-impermeable thick ascending limb of Henle loop, loop diuretics interfere with both the diluting and the concentrating mechanism.

Pharmacokinetic Properties

Furosemide is rapidly reabsorbed from the gastrointestinal (GI) tract and is mainly excreted unchanged in the urine. It is 99% bound to plasma albumin and has a bioavailability close to 60% to 70%. Furosemide and ethacrynic acid displace bilirubin from albumin-binding sites.[13] Loop diuretics cross the placental barrier and are secreted in breast milk. The diuretic response to loop diuretics appears within a few minutes after IV administration and within 30 to 60 minutes after oral administration. The effect does not last more than 2 hours after IV injection and 6 hours after oral administration. Compared with furosemide, torsemide release and half-life are prolonged.[25-27] The nonrenal clearance of loop diuretics is increased in patients with chronic renal failure. The half-life is prolonged in patients with renal and liver insufficiency and in premature and term neonates in whom half-lives as long as 45 hours have been observed.[28] Although the pharmacology of furosemide has been well studied in children[29] and neonates,[28] that of other loop diuretics is not as well defined. The pharmacokinetics and pharmacodynamics of bumetanide have been studied in critically ill children[30] and infants.[31]

Efficacy and Therapeutic Uses

Loop diuretics are the most potent natriuretic agents, also markedly increasing Cl^-, K^+, Ca^{2+}, and Mg^{2+} excretion.[23] They have steep dose-response curves. They remain active in patients with advanced renal failure. Loop diuretics are the most frequently used diuretics in neonates, infants, and children.[32]

Continuous Intravenous Infusion of Loop Diuretics

Clinical trials in infants indicate that continuous infusion therapy can produce more efficient and better-controlled diuresis with less fluid shifts and greater hemodynamic stability.[33] Administration of a small loading dose of the diuretic before starting the continuous infusion accelerates the diuretic response.[24] Alternatively, starting with a relatively high continuous infusion dose (0.2 mg/kg/h) of furosemide has been claimed to be optimal.[34] In hemodynamically stable postoperative cardiac patients, intermittent furosemide has been shown to be more efficacious than continuous infusion of furosemide.[35]

Indications

Edematous States. CHF is the most common indication to the use of loop diuretics in neonates and infants. In infants with severe CHF, the diuretic effect of furosemide is inversely related to the serum aldosterone level. The concomitant administration of a K^+-sparing diuretic improves the response to loop diuretics.[36] Furosemide increases the peripheral venous capacitance and can thus be useful independently from its diuretic effect. In adults, torsemide has been shown to be at least as effective as furosemide in reducing salt and water retention,[37] to have a longer duration of action, and to reduce the overall treatment costs of CHF compared with furosemide.[38]

Nephrotic Syndrome. In hypovolemic infants with massive nephrotic edema, IV furosemide can be used to promote sodium and water excretion. Furosemide (1–2 mg/kg) should be given only after careful expansion of the extracellular space with IV albumin (5 mL/kg of 20% albumin in 60 min). The dose can be repeated. The effect is transient but may be useful in patients with severe ascites or pulmonary edema. The therapy may be associated with potentially serious complications such as CHF or RDS.[39]

Specific Indications With Questionable Benefits (See Table 15.5)

Oliguric States. Furosemide is frequently used in oliguric states secondary to prerenal or renal failure in the hope of promoting diuresis and improving renal function. Although furosemide may increase urine output and facilitate the clinical management of the patient, it is unlikely to improve GFR. By inducing diuresis and possibly hypovolemia, loop diuretics carry the risk of further stressing the oliguric kidney. There is as yet no clinical or experimental evidence that loop diuretics can prevent acute renal failure or improve the outcome of patients with acute renal failure.[9,40]

Respiratory Distress Syndrome. Furosemide administration has produced conflicting results in preterm neonates with RDS. Although furosemide usually acutely induces diuresis and a transient improvement in pulmonary function, a recent critical review of the literature failed to find evidence for long-term benefits of routine administration of furosemide (or any diuretic) in preterm infants with RDS.[41] The review also concluded that elective administration of furosemide should be weighed against the risk of precipitating hypovolemia or of developing a symptomatic patent ductus arteriosus (PDA) by stimulating prostaglandin synthesis.

Transient Tachypnea of the Newborn. Transient tachypnea of the newborn (TTN), sometimes called *wet lungs,* is a common self-limited disease of term newborns that results from delayed lung fluid clearance.[42] This deficit is probably secondary to immature sodium epithelium channel (ENaC). Furosemide has been proposed to hasten fluid lung clearance and thus improve the pulmonary condition. In a randomized study, the oral administration of 2 mg/kg followed by 1 mg/kg 12 hours later increased weight loss but did not improve the severity or duration of symptoms.[43] A recent survey by the Cochrane Neonatal Group indicated that furosemide was not effective in promoting reabsorption of lung fluid and concluded that diuretics could not be recommended for the treatment of TTN.[44] The possibility that furosemide given to the mother before cesarean section might shorten the duration of the illness remains to be investigated.

Preterm Infants With or Developing Chronic Lung Disease. Loop diuretics have been given to preterm infants with chronic lung disease (CLD) in the hope of decreasing the need for oxygen or ventilatory support. A critical review of the available literature has concluded that (1) furosemide has very inconstant effects in preterm infants younger than 3 weeks of age developing CLD and (2) that in infants older than 3 weeks of age with CLD, the acute IV administration of furosemide (1 mg/kg) improved lung compliance and airway resistance for only 1 hour. The chronic administration of furosemide improved both oxygenation and lung compliance.[45] The overall conclusion of the authors of the Cochrane review was that the routine use of loop diuretics in infants with or developing CLD, whether administered IV or enterally, cannot be recommended until randomized trials assessing their effects on survival, duration of oxygen administration and ventilatory support, and long-term outcome are available.[45]

A similar conclusion was drawn by the thorough analysis of studies on the effect of aerosolized furosemide in preterm infants with CLD.[46] Although data in preterm infants older than 3 weeks of age with CLD showed that a single dose of aerosolized furosemide improved pulmonary mechanics, the data in premature infants younger than 3 weeks of age were too scarce to confirm this effect. Based on current available evidence, the routine or sustained use of IV or aerolized furosemide cannot be recommended.[45,46] The suggestion that adding metazolone to furosemide would overcome tolerance to the latter awaits confirmation.[47] Despite the lack of evidence for benefit of diuretic therapy in neonates with CLD, furosemide remains the seventh most commonly reported medication in the NICU.[48] As stated in a recent paper[49] and in an editorial comment,[50] it is surprising that neonatologists are still willing to routinely prescribe diuretics in spite of the lack of evidence for benefit from randomized controlled trials, as well as for the lack of information on long-term complications of diuretic therapy. A large randomized controlled trial is clearly needed, using current standards of care including prenatal steroids, surfactant, and caffeine.[51]

Posthemorrhagic Ventricular Dilatation. PHVD is a common complication of intraventricular hemorrhage in preterm infants. It carries a high risk of long-term disability. Combined furosemide-acetazolamide treatment has been used in the hope of avoiding the need for placing a ventriculoperitoneal shunt. A large trial in 177 infants showed that acetazolamide and furosemide treatment resulted in a borderline increase in the risk for motor impairment at 1 year and in an increased risk for nephrocalcinosis without evidently decreasing the risk for disability, chronic motor impairment, or death.[52] A critical review of the three available randomized trials in newborn infants with PHVD concluded that combined furosemide-acetazolamide therapy is neither effective nor safe in treating preterm infants with PHVD.[53,54]

Indomethacin-Induced Oliguria. Oliguria occurs frequently after administration of indomethacin for medical closure of symptomatic PDA in preterm infants. Inhibition of prostaglandin synthesis by indomethacin is responsible for the oliguria. Because furosemide increases the production of prostaglandins, it could potentially help prevent the indomethacin-related toxicity while at the same time decreasing the ductal response to indomethacin. A Cochrane analysis of studies available in 2001 demonstrated that furosemide increased urine output in all patients, leading to a 5% weight loss during a three-dose course. This diuretic response was considered as being risky in dehydrated neonates.[55] The review concluded that there was as yet not enough evidence to support the administration of furosemide to preterm infants with PDA treated with indomethacin.[55] This conclusion has been confirmed by more recent studies showing that (1) furosemide given before each indomethacin dose resulted in a significant increase in serum creatinine and worsening of hyponatremia without increasing urine output[56] and (2) furosemide increased the incidence of acute renal failure without, however, affecting the PDA closure rate.[57] A delay in ductus arteriosus closure has recently been demonstrated in neonatal rats given furosemide.[58] Noteworthy is the conclusion that there is as yet no evidence from randomized trials to support the use of dopamine to prevent renal dysfunction in indomethacin-treated preterm infants.[59] The same conclusion probably applies to the premature infants presenting with ibuprofen-induced oliguria.

Hypercalcemic States. Loop diuretics can promote calcium excretion and decrease hypercalcemia. Isotonic saline must be infused concomitantly to prevent volume depletion.

Severe Hyponatremia. Severe hyponatremia can be treated by loop diuretics and the concomitant isovolumetric infusion of hypertonic saline.

Asthma and Compromised Lung Mechanics. Direct intratracheal administration of furosemide has been claimed to produce beneficial effects in patients with asthma, in infants with bronchopulmonary dysplasia, and in toddlers with compromised lung mechanics after cardiac surgery. In the latter study, a systemic effect was observed within 15 minutes after intratracheal instillation of the agent.[60] This technique has not yet been validated.

Laboratory Investigation: Assessment of Distal Tubular Acidification. The simultaneous administration of furosemide and fludrocortisone has been shown to be an easy, effective, and well-tolerated alternative to standard ammonium chloride loading to assess distal tubular urine acidification and confirm the diagnosis of distal renal tubular acidosis.[61]

Drug Dosage

See Table 15.6.

Adverse Effects: Interactions

Adverse effects, including volume depletion, postural hypotension, dizziness and syncope, hyponatremia, and hypokalemia, are commonly observed when using loop diuretics. These effects are dose dependent and often occur after overzealous use of large doses of diuretics or chronic administration.

Hypochloremic Metabolic Alkalosis

This occurs frequently as a consequence of direct stimulation by loop diuretics of H^+ secretion in the collecting tubule.

Hypercalciuria and Nephrocalcinosis

Elevated Ca^{2+} urinary losses after chronic furosemide administration may lead to *nephrocalcinosis* in term[62] and premature infants[63] with secondary hyperparathyroidism, bone resorption, and rickets. When prolonged, hypercalciuria may lead to renal impairment.[64] Although thiazide diuretics decrease calcium and oxalate excretion, adding thiazides to loop diuretics does not appear beneficial.[65]

Patent Ductus Arteriosus

The beneficial renal effect of combining furosemide and indomethacin is still controversial.[24] The suggestion that stimulating prostaglandin synthesis by furosemide could promote closure of PDA has not been confirmed (see earlier discussion).

Ototoxicity

The use of furosemide has been identified as an independent risk factor for sensorineural hearing loss in preterm infants.[66] Hearing loss may be transient or permanent. It is usually associated with elevated blood concentrations of loop diuretics. The coadministration of loop diuretics and aminoglycosides increases the risk of ototoxicity. By avoiding elevated peak concentrations of furosemide, the continuous infusion may decrease this risk.[24]

Necrotizing Enterocolitis

A survey in very low birth weight infants suggests that loop diuretics do not increase the risk of NEC but that in affected neonates with mild forms of NEC, they might stimulate the progression to more severe forms of NEC.[67]

Extrarenal Effects of Loop Diuretics

The effects of loop diuretics are usually ascribed to their diuretic properties mediated by the inhibition of the renal Na^+-K^+-$2Cl^-$ cotransporter. However, as described in an excellent review by Cotton et al.,[68] loop diuretics also present with nondiuretic effects such as promotion and release of prostanoids; vascular smooth muscle relaxation; direct ductus arteriosus relaxation; improvement in lung compliance, pulmonary resistance, and tidal volume independently from the diuretic response. This paper should be consulted for interesting data and hypotheses on the nondiuretics effects of loop diuretics.

Miscellaneous

Pancreatitis, jaundice, impaired glucose tolerance, thrombocytopenia, and serious skin disorders are occasionally observed. The majority of adverse effects occur with the use of high doses of the diuretics.

Interactions

Drug interactions may occur with the coadministration of nephrotoxic antibiotics, nonsteroidal antiinflammatory drugs, anticoagulants, and cisplatin.

Distal Convoluted Tubule: Inhibitors of Na^+Cl^- Cotransport

The thiazides inhibit NaCl reabsorption in the distal convoluted tubule.

Chemistry

The benzothiadiazide derivatives are sulfonamides. They are weak diuretics that inhibit the reabsorption of NaCl at the diluting site in the early distal tubule. The main thiazides include chlorothiazide and hydrochlorothiazide. Thiazide-like agents such as chlorthalidone and metolazone belong to this group.

Mechanisms and Sites of Action

The thiazide diuretics are organic anions. They gain access to the tubular lumen by filtration and by secretion in the proximal tubule. They decrease NaCl reabsorption in the distal convoluted tubule by inhibiting the Na^+-Cl^- apical cotransporter. This cotransporter, sometimes called "thiazide-sensitive sodium chloride cotransporter (TSC)," is predominantly expressed in the epithelial cells of the distal convoluted tubule. Its expression is upregulated by aldosterone.[3] To reach their site of action on the luminal side of the tubular cells, the thiazides must be secreted by the anionic organic acid pathway in the proximal tubule. Approximately 4% to 5% of the Na^+ filtered load is being reabsorbed in the distal tubule, and inhibition of Na^+ reabsorption at this site can only modestly increase NaCl excretion. Some of the thiazides also slightly increase the excretion of HCO_3^- by weakly inhibiting the carbonic anhydrase. By increasing Na^+ delivery to the late distal tubule, the thiazides lead to increased reabsorption of Na^+ at this site in exchange for K^+ and H^+, which are then excreted in the urine.[13,14] By inhibiting NaCl reabsorption in the early distal tubule, the thiazides blunt the ability to dilute the urine. They do not interfere with the concentrating mechanism. The thiazides stimulate Ca^{2+} reabsorption in the distal tubule, probably by opening the apical membrane Ca^{2+} channels. The thiazides (but not metolazone) are ineffective at GFRs less than 30 mL/min per 1.73 m^2.

Pharmacokinetic Properties

The thiazides are rapidly absorbed after oral administration. They variably bind to plasma proteins. They are eliminated unchanged, exclusively (chlorothiazide, hydrochlorothiazide, chlorthalidone) or in great part (approximately 80%) (metolazone) in the urine. Administration of thiazides initiates diuresis in 2 hours, an effect that lasts for 12 hours. The response to metolazone is somewhat more rapid (1 hour) and lasts longer (12–24 hours). The thiazides cross the placental barrier and are secreted in breast milk.

Efficacy and Therapeutic Uses

Thiazide diuretics moderately increase the excretion of Na^+, Cl^-, and water. All thiazides (chlorothiazide, hydrochlorothiazide) and thiazide-like diuretics have overall similar effects when used in maximal doses. When administered chronically, they decrease the excretion of Ca^{2+}, as well as that of uric acid, probably as a consequence of increased proximal reabsorption secondary to volume depletion. The excretion of Mg^{2+} is somewhat increased, as is the excretion of K^+ and fixed acids. The prophylactic coadministration of K^+-sparing diuretics can prevent the occurrence of severe hypokalemia. Alternatively, potassium and magnesium supplementation may be useful in patients at risk of symptomatic hypokalemia. The thiazides (but not metolazone) increase the excretion of HCO_3^-. In the absence of significant volume depletion, the thiazides do not normally influence renal hemodynamics and GFR. In contrast with the thiazides and chlorthalidone, metolazone remains effective at GFRs less than 30 mL/min per 1.73 m^2.

Indications

The main indications for the administration of thiazide diuretics include edematous states, hypertension, and a few specific indications.

Specific Indications With Questionable Benefits (See Table 15.5)

Hypercalciuria

The thiazides decrease calcium excretion, and this effect may be useful in states of idiopathic hypercalciuria, as well as to prevent calcium losses in patients receiving glucocorticoids.[69] They have been associated to loop diuretics in the hope of decreasing the risk of hypercalciuria and nephrocalcinosis in very low birth weight infants; disappointing results have been observed.[70] In young rats with established furosemide-induced nephrocalcinosis, thiazides failed to improve the calcinosis.[71] The use of thiazides has been associated with an increase in total serum cholesterol and in the ratio of low-density lipoprotein (LDL) to high-density lipoprotein (HDL).[71] In children with X-linked hypophosphatemia on renal phosphate and vitamin D therapy, hydrochlorothiazide decreased the urinary excretion of calcium but did not reverse the nephrocalcinosis.[72]

Proximal Renal Tubular Acidosis

The thiazides have been used to raise the plasma bicarbonate concentration in proximal renal tubular acidosis. This effect on bicarbonate reabsorption is the consequence of the chronic volume contraction induced by the thiazides, a condition that is deleterious for body growth.[73]

Nephrogenic Diabetes Insipidus

The thiazides have been successfully used in children with nephrogenic diabetes insipidus. By inducing volume contraction, they enhance the proximal tubular reabsorption of water and electrolytes, thus significantly decreasing urine output. Although usefully decreasing urine output, volume contraction may inhibit growth in young children with nephrogenic diabetes insipidus. The concomitant use of hydrochlorothiazide and amiloride obviates the need for the K^+ supplementation and has been shown as useful as the standard treatment with hydrochlorothiazide and indomethacin in reducing urine output.[74,75]

Chronic Lung Disease

The thiazide and thiazide-like diuretics have been used in the hope of improving pulmonary mechanisms and clinical outcome in preterm infants with CLD. A critical analysis of available well-planned studies led to the conclusion that in preterm infants older than 8 weeks with CLD, a 4-week treatment with thiazides and spironolactone reduced the need for furosemide, improved lung compliance, decreased the risk of death, and tended to decrease the risk for lack of extubation after 8 weeks in intubated infants without access to corticosteroids, bronchodilators, or aminophylline.[76] There was little evidence to support any benefit on the need for ventilatory support, length of hospital stay, or long-term outcome in infants receiving current therapy. There was also no evidence to support the hypothesis that adding spironolactone to thiazides or metolazone to furosemide improved the outcome of preterm infants.[76] However, the addition of K^+-sparing diuretics to thiazide did decrease the risk of hypokalemia.

Laboratory Investigation: Diagnosis of Renal Hypokalemic Tubulopathies

Assessment of the maximal diuretic response induced by the administration of hydrochlorothiazide (1 mg/kg orally) allows us to differentiate Bartter from Gitelman syndrome, the former presenting with a blunted response to the diuretic agent.[77]

Drug Dosage

See Table 15.6.

Adverse Effects: Interactions

The thiazides may adversely affect water balance and induce electrolyte imbalances (see Table 15.3). They induce an increase in total serum cholesterol and in the LDL-to-HDL ratio.[71] Other side effects include GI disturbances, hypersensitivity reactions, cholestatic jaundice, pancreatitis, thrombocytopenia, hyperlipidemia, and hyperglycemia in diabetic and prediabetic patients. Precipitation of hepatic encephalopathy has been observed in patients with hepatic cirrhosis. The thiazides displace bilirubin from albumin and should be cautiously administered to patients with jaundice.

Cortical Collecting Duct: K⁺-Sparing Drugs

Diuretics that inhibit Na^+ reabsorption in the cortical collecting duct decrease the urinary excretion of K^+ and H^+ and can produce hypokalemia and metabolic acidosis.[14]

Chemistry

Two types of diuretics form the group of K^+-sparing diuretics: the inhibitors of a renal epithelial Na^+ channels (ENaC) and the antagonists of mineralocorticoid receptors. The overall effects of these two groups of diuretics differ only in their mode of action.

Mechanisms and Sites of Action

The antagonists of the action of aldosterone on the principal cells of the collecting duct increase Na^+ excretion and decrease K^+ and H^+ secretion. Spironolactone, the main agent in this group, competitively inhibits the binding of aldosterone to the mineralocorticoid receptor, thus decreasing the synthesis of aldosterone-induced proteins. The aldosterone antagonists have greater effects in situations of hyperaldosteronism. They do not modify the renal hemodynamics. Highly selective antagonists of the mineralocorticoid receptor are currently under investigation.[78]

The K^+-sparing diuretics amiloride and triamterene block the entry of Na^+ into the cell through the ENaC in the apical membrane. Because of changes in electrical profile across the apical membrane, the diffusion of both H^+ and K^+ from cells into tubular fluid decreases. Activation of the RAAS by the diuretics also impairs the excretion of K^+, H^+, Ca^{2+}, and Mg^{2+}. The ENaC blockers do not affect renal hemodynamics.

Pharmacokinetic Properties

Spironolactone is rapidly absorbed from the GI tract, with a bioavailability close to 90%. It is 90% bound to plasma proteins and is excreted mainly in the urine and to a lesser extent in the feces. Spironolactone has a slow onset of action, requiring 2 to 3 days for maximum effect.[79] Canrenoate potassium has actions similar to those of spironolactone. It is available for IV administration.

Amiloride is incompletely absorbed from the GI tract, with a bioavailability of only 50%. It is not bound to plasma proteins and is excreted unchanged in the urine. Its half-life is 6 to 9 hours. It is prolonged in patients with hepatic or renal failure. Triamterene is unreliably absorbed. It is metabolized by hepatic conjugation. One-fifth of the dose is excreted unchanged in the urine. Its half-life is 1 to 3 hours.

All K^+-sparing diuretics cross the placental barrier and are secreted in breast milk.

Efficacy and Therapeutic Uses

The overall effects on electrolyte excretion are similar for spironolactone, amiloride, and triamterene. They are weak natriuretic agents that reduce the excretion of potassium and hydrogen ions. K^+-sparing diuretics are mainly used in Na^+-retaining states in association with loop or thiazide diuretics. They enhance the natriuretic effect while at the same time limiting K^+ losses. Refractory edema secondary to CHF, cirrhosis of the liver, and the nephrotic syndrome represent the most common indications for the use of K-sparing diuretics. In these conditions associated with secondary hyperaldosteronism, spironolactone is the first choice agent provided renal function is not impaired. Because they induce K^+ retention, K^+-sparing diuretics should not be used in patients with impaired renal function or in those receiving K^+ supplementation. They should also be avoided in patients prone to developing metabolic acidosis. Amiloride has been successfully used in association with hydrochlorothiazide in patients with nephrogenic diabetes insipidus, obviating the need for using indomethacin.[74]

Specific Indications With Questionable Benefits (See Table 15.5)

K^+-sparing diuretics are often used in association with thiazide diuretics in the management of preterm infants with CLD. Although they certainly decrease the risk of hypokalemia and facilitate the clinical management of the infants, there is as yet no definite proof that their association to thiazides improves the long-term outcome of preterm infants with CLD.[76]

The respiratory function of patients with cystic fibrosis has been claimed to be improved by the inhalation of amiloride,[80] possibly by the blocking effect of ENaC in pulmonary tissue. Such a beneficial effect has not been confirmed in placebo-controlled trials.[81,82]

Drug Dosage

See Table 15.6.

Adverse Effects: Interactions

The main adverse effect of K^+-sparing diuretics is the increase of plasma K+ concentration to harmful levels. Close monitoring of K^+ concentration is thus mandatory. GI disturbances, dizziness, photosensitivity, and blood dyscrasias have been reported after the use of triamterene.

Significant adverse effects have been observed with spironolactone: gynecomastia, hirsutism, impotence, and menstrual irregularities can occur. Gynecomastia in men is related to both the dose and duration of treatment. Breast enlargement and tenderness occur in women. The pathogenesis of the adverse effects of spironolactone on the endocrine system is probably related to an antiadrenergic action and to reduced 17-hydroxylase activity.

Interactions

K^+-sparing diuretics should not be used in patients receiving angiotensin-converting enzyme inhibitors because the association can worsen the risk of hyperkalemia.

New Developments in Diuretic Therapy

Three categories of diuretics are under investigation: the adenosine A_1 receptor antagonists, the natriuretic peptides, and the arginine-vasopressin antagonists.[83]

Adenosine A_1 Receptor Antagonists

Theophylline, an A_1 adenosine nonspecific receptor antagonist, has natriuretic and diuretic properties. It has been shown, both in experimental studies and clinical trials, to protect newborn kidneys in conditions of asphyxia and RDS. The effect and the use of theophylline are described in Chapter 7.

Natriuretic Peptides

ANP and B-type natriuretic peptide (BNP) are two peptides with natriuretic and diuretic properties.[83] Both are released by cardiac cells in the atria in response to increased blood volume. ANP (28 amino acids) and BNP (32 amino acids) act via the natriuretic peptide receptor A (NPR-A). In addition to increasing the excretion of Na^+, both peptides inhibit the sympathetic system and the RAAS. They also relax vascular smooth muscle. ANP and BNP are degraded by the metalloproteinase neutral endopeptidase 24.11 (NEP). Urodilatin is a noncirculating natriuretic peptide (32 amino acids) secreted by distal tubular cells that is not degraded by the NEP located in the proximal tubular cells.[84] ANP favors filtration by relaxing the afferent artery and the mesangial cells.[85] The natriuretic peptides inhibit Na^+ proximal reabsorption and decrease distal Na^+ reabsorption indirectly by blunting angiotensin II and aldosterone synthesis and directly by inhibiting the thiazide-sensitive Na^+ channel. ANP increases diuresis by inhibiting the V_2 receptor-mediated action of arginine vasopressin (AVP) on water permeability.

The natriuretic peptides have not yet been used as diuretic agents in neonates but may have interesting properties in patients presenting with inappropriate salt and water retention.

Arginine Vasopressin Antagonists

AVP acts on three type of receptors: (1) the V_{1A} receptors mediating vasoconstriction, (2) the V_{1B} mediating the release of adreno-cortico-tropic-hormone (ACTH), and (3) the V_2 receptors mediating free-water reabsorption in the collecting duct. AVP also stimulates Na^+-K^+-$2Cl^-$ cotranspoort in the ascending limb of Henle loop via V_2 receptors. By selectively increasing the excretion of free-water, the AVP antagonists may prove useful in the treatment of severe hyponatremic states.[83,86,87]

REFERENCES

1. Guignard JP, John EG. Renal function in the tiny, premature infant. *Clin Perinatol*. 1986;13:377–401.
2. Guignard JP. Renal morphogenesis and development of renal function. In: Taeusch HW, Ballard RA, Gleason CA, eds. *Avery's Diseases of the Newborn*. 8th ed. Philadelphia, PA: WB Saunders Co; 2005:1257–1266.
3. Giebisch G, Windhager E. The urinary system. Part VI. In: Boron WF, Boulpaep EL, eds. *Medical Physiology*. Philadelphia, PA: Saunders; 2003:735–876.
4. Guignard JP, Gouyon JB. Body fluid homeostasis in the newborn infant with congestive heart failure: effects of diuretics. *Clin Perinatol*. 1988;15:447–466.
5. Lowrie L. Diuretic therapy of heart failure in infants and children. *Prog Pediatr Cardiol*. 2000;12:45–55.
6. Morrison RT. Edema and principles of diuretic use. *Med Clin North Am*. 1997;81:689–704.
7. Schrier RW, Fassett RG. A critique of the overfill hypothesis of sodium and water retention in the nephrotic syndrome. *Kidney Int*. 1998;53:1111–1117.
8. Vande Walle JG, Donckerwolcke RA. Pathogenesis of edema formation in the nephrotic syndrome. *Pediatr Nephrol*. 2001;16:283–293.
9. Kellum JA. Use of diuretics in the acute care setting. *Kidney Int Suppl*. 1998;66:S67–S70.
10. Gouyon JB, Guignard JP. Drugs and acute renal insufficiency in the neonate. *Biol Neonate*. 1986; 50:177–181.
11. Brion LP, Yong SC, Perez IA, et al. Diuretics and chronic lung disease of prematurity. *J Perinatol*. 2001;21:269–271.
12. Whitelaw A, Aquilina K. Management of posthaemorrhagic ventricular dilatation. *Arch Dis Child Fetal Neonatal Ed*. 2012;97:F229–233.
13. Chemtob S, Kaplan BS, Sherbotie JR, et al. Pharmacology of diuretics in the newborn. *Pediatr Clin North Am*. 1989;36:1231–1250.
14. Wells TG. The pharmacology and therapeutics of diuretics in the pediatric patient. *Pediatr Clin North Am*. 1990;37:463–504.
15. Knoers N, Monnens LA. Amiloride-hydrochlorothiazide versus indomethacin-hydrochlorothiazide in the treatment of nephrogenic diabetes insipidus. *J Pediatr*. 1990;117:499–502.
16. Ong WH, Guignard JP, Sharma A, et al. Pharmacological approach to the management of neonatal hypertension. *Semin Neonatol*. 1998;3:149–163.
17. Hagadorn JL, Sanders MR, Staves C, et al. Diuretics for very low birth weight infants in the first 28 days: a survey of the US neonatologists. *J Perinatol*. 2011;31:677–681.
18. Better OS, Rubinstein I, Winaver JM, et al. Mannitol therapy revisited (1940–1997). *Kidney Int*. 1997;52:886–894.
19. Rigden SP, Dillon MJ, Kind PR, et al. The beneficial effect of mannitol on post-operative renal function in children undergoing cardiopulmonary bypass surgery. *Clin Nephrol*. 1984;21:148–151.
20. Alon U, Hellerstein S, Warady BA. Oral acetazolamide in the assessment of (urine-blood) PCO2. *Pediatr Nephrol*. 1991;5:307–311.
21. International PHVD Drug Trial Group. International randomized controlled trial of acetazolamide and furosemide in posthaemorrhagic ventricular dilatation in infancy. *Lancet*. 1998;352:433–440.
22. Kennedy CR, Ayers S, Campbell MJ, et al. Randomized, controlled trial of acetazolamide and furosemide in posthemorrhagic ventricular dilatation in infancy: follow-up at 1 year. *Pediatrics*. 2001;198:597–607.
23. Brater DC. Diuretic therapy. *N Engl J Med*. 1998;339:387–395.
24. Eades SK, Christensen ML. The clinical pharmacology of loop diuretics in the pediatric patient. *Pediatr Nephrol*. 1998;12:603–616.
25. Dubourg L, Mosig D, Drukker A, et al. Torasemide is an effective diuretic in the newborn rabbit. *Pediatr Nephrol*. 2000;14:476–479.
26. Wargo KA. A comprehensive review of the loop diuretics. *Ann Pharmacother*. 2009;43:1836–1847.
27. Lyseng-Williamson KA. Torasemide prolonged release. *Drugs*. 2009;1363–1372.

28. Mirochnick MH, Miceli JJ, Kramer PA, et al. Furosemide pharmacokinetics in very low birth weight infants. *J Pediatr.* 1988;112:653–657.
29. Prandota J. Clinical pharmacology of furosemide in children: a supplement. *Am J Ther.* 2001;8:275–289.
30. Marshall JD, Wells TG, Letzig L, et al. Pharmacokinetics and pharmacodynamics of bumetanide in critically ill pediatric patients. *J Clin Pharmacol.* 1998;38:994–1002.
31. Sullivan JE, Witte MK, Yamashita TS, et al. Pharmacokinetics of bumetanide in critically ill infants. *Clin Pharmacol Ther.* 1996;60:405–413.
32. Hagadorn JL, Sanders MR, Staves C, et al. Diuretics for very low birth weight infants in the first 28 days: a survey of the US neonatologists. *J Perinatol.* 2011;31:677–681.
33. Luciani GB, Nichani S, Chang AC, et al. Continuous versus intermittent furosemide infusion in critically ill infants after open heart operations. *Ann Thorac Surg.* 1997;64:1133–1139.
34. van der Vorst MM, Ruys-Dudok van Heel I, Kist-van Holthe JE, et al. Continuous intravenous furosemide in haemodynamically unstable children after cardiac surgery. *Intensive Care Med.* 2001;27:711–715.
35. Klinge JM, Scharf J, Hofbeck M, et al. Intermittent administration of furosemide versus continuous infusion in the postoperative management of children following open heart surgery. *Intensive Care Med.* 1997;23:693–697.
36. Baylen BG, Johnson G, Tsang R, et al. The occurrence of hyperaldosteronism in infants with congestive heart failure. *Am J Cardiol.* 1980;45:305–310.
37. Knauf H, Mutschler E. Clinical pharmacokinetics and pharmacodynamics of torasemide. *Clin Pharmacokinet.* 1998;34:1–24.
38. Young M, Plosker GL. Torasemide: a pharmacoeconomic review of its use in chronic heart failure. *Pharmacoeconomics.* 2001;19:679–703.
39. Haws RM, Baum M. Efficacy of albumin and diuretic therapy in children with nephrotic syndrome. *Pediatrics.* 1993;91:1142–1146.
40. Dubourg L, Drukker A, Guignard J-P. Failure of the loop diuretic torasemide to improve renal function of hypoxemic vasomotor nephropathy in the newborn rabbit. *Pediatr Res.* 2000;47:504–508.
41. Brion LP, Soll RF. Diuretics for respiratory distress syndrome in preterm infants. *Cochrane Database Syst Rev.* 2008;(1):CD001454.
42. Jain L, Eaton DC. Physiology of fetal lung fluid clearance and the effect of labor. *Semin Perinatol.* 2006;30:34–43.
43. Wiswell MC, Rawings JS, Smith FR, et al. Effect of furosemide on the clinical course of transient tachypnea of the newborn. *Pediatrics.* 1985;75:908–910.
44. Kassab M, Khriesat WM, Anabrees J. Diuretics for transient tachypnea of the newborn. *Cocharane Database St Rev.* 2015;(3):CD003064.
45. Brion LP, Primhak RA. Intravenous or enteral loop diuretics for preterm infants with (or developing) chronic lung disease. *Cochrane Database Syst Rev.* 2002;(1):CD001453.
46. Brion LP, Primhak RA, Yong W. Aerosolized diuretics for preterm infants with (or developing) chronic lung disease. *Cochrane Database Syst Rev.* 2006;(3):CD001694.
47. Segar JL, Robillard JE, Jonason KJ, et al. Addition of metolazone to overcome tolerance to furosemide in infants with bronchopulmonary dysplasia. *J Pediatr.* 1992;120:966–973.
48. Segar JL. Neonatal diuretic therapy: furosemide, thiazides, and spironolactone. *Clin Perinatol.* 2012;209–220.
49. Slaughter JL, Stenger MR, Reagan PB. Variation in the use of diuretics therapy for infants with bronchopulmonary dysplasia. *Pediatrics.* 2013;131:716–723.
50. Stewart AL, Brion LP. Routine use of diuretics in very-low-birth-weight infants in the absence of supporting evidence. *J Perinatol.* 2011;31:633–634.
51. Schmidt B, Roberts R, Millar D, et al. Evidence-based neonatal drug therapy for prevention of bronchopulmonary dysplasia in very-low-birth-weight infants. *Neonatology.* 2008;93:284–287.
52. Kennedy CR, Ayers S, Campbell MJ, et al. Randomized, controlled trial of acetazolamide and furosemide in posthemorhagic ventricular dilatation in infancy: follow-up at 1 year. *Pediatrics.* 2001;198:597–607.
53. International PHVD Drug Trial Group. International randomized controlled trial of acetazolamide and furosemide in posthaemorrhagic ventricular dilatation in infancy. *Lancet.* 1998;352:433–440.
54. Whitelaw A, Kennedy CR, Brion LP. Diuretic therapy for newborn infants with posthemorrhagic ventricular dilatation. *Cochrane Database Syst Rev.* 2001;(2):CD002270.
55. Brion LP, Campbell DE. Furosemide for symptomatic patent ductus arteriosus in indomethacin-treated infants. *Cochrane Database Syst Rev.* 2001;(3):CD001148.
56. Andriessen P, Struis NC, Niemarkt J, et al. Furosemide in preterm infants treated with indomethacin for patent ductus arteriosus. *Acta Paediatr.* 2009;98:797–803.
57. Lee BS, Byun SY, Chung ML, et al. Effect of furosemide on ductal closure and renal function in indomethacin-treated preterm infants during the early neonatal period. *Neonatology.* 2010;98:191–199.
58. Toyoshima K, Momma K, Nakanishi T. In vivo dilatation of the ductus arteriosus induced by furosemide in the rat. *Pediatr Res.* 2010;67:173–176.
59. Barrington K, Brion LP. Dopamine versus no treatment to prevent renal dysfunction in indomethacin-treated preterm newborn infants. *Cochrane Database Syst Rev.* 2002;(3):CD003213.
60. Aufricht C, Votava F, Marx M, et al. Intratracheal furosemide in infants after cardiac surgery: its effects on lung mechanics and urinary output, and its levels in plasma and tracheal aspirate. *Intensive Care Med.* 1997;23:992–997.
61. Walsh SB, Shirley DG, Wrong OM, et al. Urinary acidification assessed by simultaneous furosemide and fludrocortisone treatment: an alternative to ammonium chloride. *Kidney Int.* 2007;71:1310–1316.

15

62. Saarela T, Laning P, Koivisto M, et al. Nephrocalcinosis in full-term infants receiving furosemide treatment for congestive heart failure: a study of the incidence and 2-year follow up. *Eur J Pediatr.* 1999;158:668–672.

63. Gimpel C, Krause A, Franck P, et al. Exposure to furosemide as the strongest risk factor for nephrocalcinosis in preterm infants. *Pediatr Int.* 2010;52:51–56.

64. Downing GJ, Egelhoff JC, Daily DK, et al. Kidney function in very low birth weight infants with furosemide-related renal calcifications at ages 1 to 2 years. *J Pediatr.* 1992;120:599–604.

65. Campfield T, Braden G, Flynn-Valone P, et al. Effect of diuretics on urinary oxalate, calcium, and sodium excretion in very low birth weight infants. *Pediatrics.* 1997;99:814–818.

66. Borradori C, Fawer CL, Buclin T, et al. Risk factors of sensorineural hearing loss in preterm infants. *Biol Neonate.* 1997;71:1–10.

67. Cole MA, DeRienzo C, Kutchibhatia M, et al. Necrotizing enterocolitis and the use of loop diuretics in very low birth weight neonates. *Am J Surg.* 2016;211:645–648.

68. Cotton R, Suarez S, Reese J. Unexpected extra-renal effects of loop diuretics in the preterm neonate. *Acta Paediatr.* 2012;101:835–845.

69. Lukert BP, Raisz LG. Glucocorticoid-induced osteoporosis: pathogenesis and management. *Ann Intern Med.* 1990;112:352–364.

70. Knoll S, Alon US. Effect of thiazide on established furosemide-induced nephrocalcinosis in the young rat. *Pediatr Nephrol.* 2000;14:32–35.

71. Reusz GS, Dobos M, Tulassay T. Hydrochlorothiazide treatment of children with hypercalciuria: effects and side effects. *Pediatr Nephrol.* 1993;7:699–702.

72. Seikaly MG, Baum M. Thiazide diuretics arrest the progression of nephrocalcinosis in children with X-linked hypophosphatemia. *Pediatrics.* 2001;108:E6.

73. Kahlhoff H, Manz F. Nutrition, acid-base status and growth in early childhood. *Eur J Nutr.* 2001;40:221–230.

74. Kirchlechner V, Koller DY, Seidl R, et al. Treatment of nephrogenic diabetes insipidus with hydrochlorothiazide and amiloride. *Arch Dis Child.* 1999;80:548–552.

75. Knoers N, Monnens LA. Amiloride-hydrochlorothiazide versus indomethacin-hydrochlorothiazide in the treatment of nephrogenic diabetes insipidus. *J Pediatr.* 1990;117:499–502.

76. Brion LP, Primhak RA, Ambrosio-Perez I. Diuretics acting on the distal renal tubule for preterm infants with (or developing) chronic lung disease. *Cochrane Database Syst Rev.* 2002;(1):CD001817.

77. Colussi G, Bettinelli A, Tedeschi S, et al. A thiazide test for the diagnosis of renal tubular hypokalemic disorders. *Clin J Am Soc Nephrol.* 2007;2:454–460.

78. Delyani JA. Mineralocorticoid receptor antagonists: the evolution of utility and pharmacology. *Kidney Int.* 2000;57:1408–1411.

79. Buck ML. Clinical experience with spironolactone in pediatrics. *Ann Pharmacother.* 2005;39:823–828.

80. Hofmann T, Senier I, Bittner P, et al. Aerosolized amiloride: dose effect on nasal bioelectric properties, pharmacokinetics, and effect on sputum expectoration in patients with cystic fibrosis. *J Aerosol Med.* 1997;10:147–158.

81. Pons G, Marchand MC, d'Athis P, et al. French multicenter randomized double-blind placebo-controlled trial on nebulized amiloride in cystic fibrosis patients. The amiloride-AFLM Collaborative Study Group. *Pediatr Pulmonol.* 2000;30:25–31.

82. Ratjen F, Bush A. Amiloride: still a viable treatment option in cystic fibrosis? *Am J Respir Crit Care Med.* 2008;178:1191–1192.

83. Costello-Boerrigter LC, Boerrigter G, Burnett JC Jr. Revisiting salt and water retention: new diuretics, aquaretics, and natriuretics. *Med Clin North Am.* 2003;87:475–491.

84. Forssmann W, Meyer M, Forssmann K. The renal urodilatin system: clinical implications. *Cardiovasc Res.* 2001;51:450–462.

85. Semmekrot B, Guignard J-P. Atrial natriuretic peptide during early human development. *Biol Neonate.* 1991;60:341–349.

86. Costello-Boerrigter LC, Boerrigter G, Burnett JC. Pharmacology of vasopressin antagonists. *Heart Fail Rev.* 2009;14:75–82.

87. Kumar S, Berl T. Vasopressin antagonists in the treatment of water-retaining disorders. *Semin Nephrol.* 2008;28:279–288.

CHAPTER 16

Neonatal Hypertension: Diagnosis and Management

Joseph Flynn, MD, MS

- Outcome
- Incidence
- Differential Diagnosis
- Clinical Presentation
- Diagnostic Evaluation
- Treatment
- Normative Values for Neonatal Blood Pressure

Introduction

First described in the 1970s,[1,2] awareness of neonatal hypertension has increased over the past several decades. However, there is still uncertainty over which neonates require treatment for hypertension primarily because of conflicting data on normative blood pressure values in neonates. This chapter reviews the existing data on normal neonatal blood pressure and presents a reasonable approach to evaluation and management based upon likely causes and pathophysiology. Finally, research needs, especially those related to late-onset hypertension and long-term outcome, are reviewed.

Normative Values for Neonatal Blood Pressure

Factors Affecting Blood Pressure at Birth

There are many complexities to the changing patterns of blood pressure (BP) in the newborn period. Infant characteristics such as gestational age at birth, postnatal and postmenstrual (formerly termed postconceptual [AAP 2004]) age, as well as appropriateness of size for gestational age all influence BP. Maternal illnesses such as diabetes and other prenatal factors may also affect BP levels following delivery. As in older children, BP values in neonates may vary according to the method of BP assessment (e.g., intraarterial, Doppler, oscillometric) and according to the infant's state (e.g., sleeping, crying, feeding). All these factors need to be taken into account when reviewing the literature on BP standards as well as in clinical practice. Despite the fact that neonatal BPs have been measured for decades, we are still in the early phase of identifying the normal patterns of infant BPs, and there are still many physiologic changes that need further investigation.

Data on BP on the first day of life was published in 1995 by Zubrow and coworkers.[3] From data on 329 infants on day 1 of life, they were able to define the mean plus upper and lower 95% confidence limits for BP; their data clearly demonstrated increases in BP with increasing gestational age and birth weight (Fig. 16.1A and B). A more recent study by Pejovic and coworkers,[4] limiting their analysis to hemodynamically stable premature and term infants admitted to the neonatal intensive care unit (NICU), also showed that BPs on day 1 of life correlated with gestational

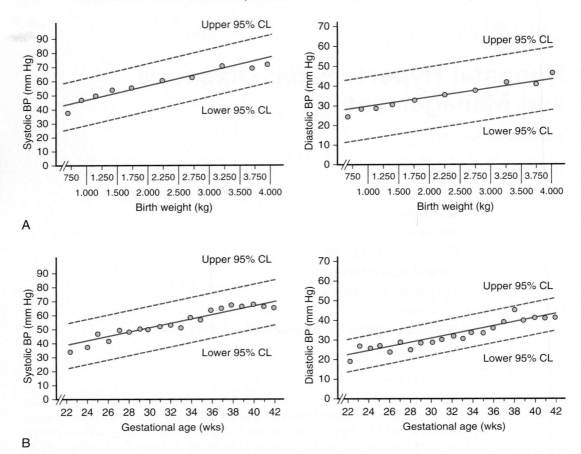

Fig. 16.1 (A and B) Linear regression of systolic and diastolic blood pressures by birth weight (A) and gestational age (B), with 95% confidence limits (CLs; upper and lower *dashed lines*). (Reproduced from Zubrow AB, Hulman S, Kushner H, et al. Determinants of blood pressure in infants admitted to neonatal intensive care units: a prospective multicenter study. *J Perinatol.* 1995;15:470-479, with permission from Nature Publishing Group.)

age and birth weight. Healthy term infants do not seem to demonstrate this same pattern.[5]

After the first day of life, it appears that BPs in premature newborns increase more rapidly over the first week or two of life followed by a slowing of the rate of increase. The previously mentioned Philadelphia study categorized over 600 infants in the NICU into gestational age groups and showed a similar rate of BP increase over the first 5 days of life, regardless of gestational age.[3] The more recent study by Pejovic and colleagues on stable NICU infants showed a similar pattern with BPs in each gestational age category of premature infants increasing at a faster rate over the first week of life with subsequent slowing.[4] In these infants, they determined that the rate of rise was more rapid in the preterm than full-term infants (Fig. 16.2). As premature neonates mature, the strongest predictor of BP is postmenstrual age. Fig. 16.3 from Zubrow and coworkers[3] shows the regression lines between postmenstrual age and systolic and diastolic BP along with the upper and lower 95th confidence limits for systolic and diastolic BP for each week of postmenstrual age.

In term infants, appropriateness for gestational age seems to be an important influence on BP. In an Australian study of healthy term infants,[5] BPs were higher on day 2 of life compared to day 1 but not thereafter. In addition, a correlation between birth weight and BP on day 3 of life was recently demonstrated in a large Japanese study of term infants[6]; this study also showed an increase in BP from days 2 through 4 of life, which is consistent with studies mentioned previously. A Spanish study demonstrated that small for gestational age infants had the lowest BP at birth

Fig. 16.2 Increase in systolic (A), diastolic (B), and mean (C) blood pressure during the first month of life in infants classified by estimated gestational age: *A,* ≤28 weeks; *B,* 29–32 weeks; *C,* 33–36 weeks; *D,* ≥37 weeks. (Reproduced from Pejovic B, Peco-Antic A, Marinkovic-Eric J. Blood pressure in non-critically ill preterm and full-term neonates. *Pediatr Nephrol.* 2007; 22:249-257, with permission from Springer Science + Business Media.)

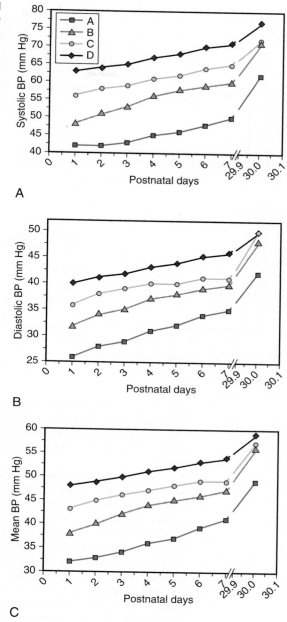

A

B

C

but subsequently had the fastest rate of rise, so by 1 month of age, all term infants had similar BPs.[7] Genetic factors likely also play a role in determining BP, although only limited studies have been completed to date. One study identified the cytochrome P450 (CYP2D6) CC genotype as being associated with higher BPs in preterm infants during hospitalization and at neonatal follow-up.[8] It is likely that additional genetic mutations with an effect on neonatal BP will be identified in the future.

Maternal factors, including medications, underlying illnesses, and adequacy of nutrition during pregnancy, can also influence a neonate's BP.[9] Higher infant BPs have correlated with maternal body mass index greater than 30 kg/m² and low socioeconomic status in Nigerian infants[10] and in an Australian study to premature infants born to mothers with diabetes or neonates with abnormal uteroplacental perfusion by placental pathology.[11] There is some suggestion in the literature that

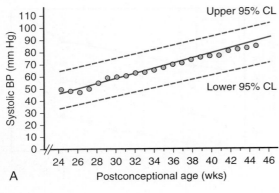

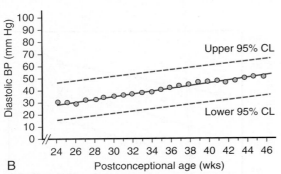

A

B

Fig. 16.3 Linear regression of mean systolic (A) and diastolic (B) blood pressures by postmenstrual (post-conceptual) age in weeks, with 95% confidence limits (CLs; upper and lower *dashed lines*). (Reproduced from Zubrow AB, Hulman S, Kushner H, et al. Determinants of blood pressure in infants admitted to neonatal intensive care units: a prospective multicenter study. *J Perinatol.* 1995;15:470-479, with permission from Nature Publishing Group.)

chorioamnionitis and HELLP (hemolysis, elevated liver enzymes, low platelets) syndrome may be related to lower infant BPs. While these factors may not have caused hypotension or hypertension by definition in all infants, it is clear that many antenatal and postnatal processes combine to influence BP values in the newborn period.

Normal BPs in infants older than 1 month have not been extensively studied recently. The percentile curves reported by the Second Task Force of the National High Blood Pressure Education Program (NHBPEP) (Fig. 16.4)[12] remain the most widely available reference values. These curves allow BP to be characterized as normal or elevated not only by age and gender, but also by length (provided in the legend below the curves). Unfortunately, these BP values were determined by a single measurement on awake infants by the Doppler method, which reduced the number of diastolic BP readings by more than half. Comparison with the more recently published values for 1-year-olds in the Fourth Report from the NHBPEP[13] reveals significant differences that further question the validity of the 1987 curves. Additionally, a recent study of 406 healthy term infants with BPs measured by the oscillometric method on day 2 of life and then at 6 and 12 months of age demonstrated BPs that are slightly higher than the Task Force values.[14] These issues highlight that there is clearly a pressing need for new normative BP data on infants during the first year of life.

What Level of BP Should Be Considered Hypertensive?

In older children, the definition of hypertension is persistent systolic and/or diastolic BP equal to or greater than the 95th percentile for age, gender, and height.[13] As can be deduced from the preceding discussion, there is considerable variation in neonatal BP, and no generally agreed upon reference values are available. For term infants and infants between 1 and 12 months of age, the best available reference data would be those from the Second Task Force Report[12] (see Fig. 16.4). In this age group, the diagnosis of hypertension is made if the infant's BP is repeatedly greater than or equal to the 95th percentile for an infant of comparable age (also note that weight

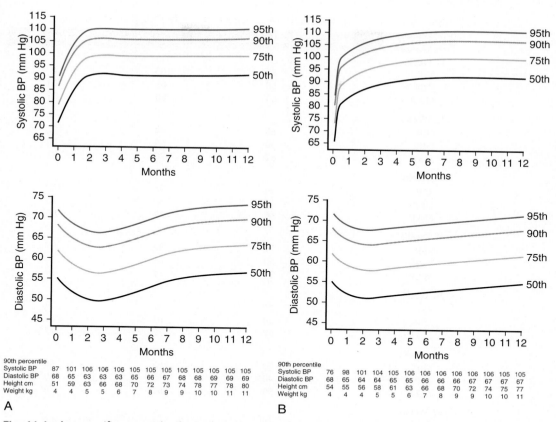

90th percentile (A)

Systolic BP	87	101	106	106	106	105	105	105	105	105	105	105	105
Diastolic BP	68	65	63	63	63	65	66	67	68	68	69	69	69
Height cm	51	59	63	66	68	70	72	73	74	78	77	78	80
Weight kg	4	4	5	5	6	7	8	9	9	10	10	11	11

90th percentile (B)

Systolic BP	76	98	101	104	105	106	106	106	106	106	106	105	105
Diastolic BP	68	65	64	64	65	65	66	66	66	67	67	67	67
Height cm	54	55	56	58	61	63	66	68	70	72	74	75	77
Weight kg	4	4	4	5	5	6	7	8	9	9	10	10	11

A   B

Fig. 16.4 Age-specific percentiles for blood pressure in boys (A) and girls (B) from birth to 12 months of age. (Reprinted from Task Force on Blood Pressure Control in Children. Report of the Second Task Force on Blood Pressure Control in Children—1987. National Heart, Lung and Blood Institute, National Institutes of Health, Bethesda, MD, January 1987.)

and length are given below the curves, and could also be used to help determine if an infant's BP is normal or elevated).

The major unresolved question is what BP values to use in diagnosing hypertension in preterm infants. From the limited published data,[3–6,14,15] it is possible to derive systolic and diastolic BP percentiles, as well as mean arterial pressure percentiles according to postmenstrual age (Table 16.1).[16] Although not derived from a large-scale study (which is sorely needed), these values may be useful clinically. Specifically, infants with BP values persistently at or above the 95th percentile may warrant closer monitoring, and those with BP values above the 99th percentile would clearly merit investigation, and possibly initiation of antihypertensive drug therapy. Although it is tempting to use these values to diagnose hypertension in a similar manner as in older infants and children, such decisions need to be tempered by clinical circumstances and personal experience.

Incidence

Hypertension is so unusual in otherwise healthy term infants that routine BP determination is not advocated for this group.[17] For preterm and otherwise high-risk newborns admitted to modern NICUs, reported incidences of hypertension range from 0.2% to 3%.[1,2,16,18,19] In an Australian study of approximately 2500 infants followed for over 4 years, the prevalence of hypertension was 1.3%.[20] Antenatal steroids, maternal hypertension, umbilical arterial catheter placement, postnatal acute renal failure, and chronic lung disease were among the most common concurrent conditions in babies with elevated BP. A more recent single-center case series from Texas demonstrated

Table 16.1   NEONATAL BLOOD PRESSURE PERCENTILES

Postconceptual Age	50th Percentile	95th Percentile	99th Percentile
44 Weeks			
SBP	88	105	110
DBP	50	68	73
MAP	**63**	**80**	**85**
42 Weeks			
SBP	85	98	102
DBP	50	65	70
MAP	**62**	**76**	**81**
40 Weeks			
SBP	80	95	100
DBP	50	65	70
MAP	**60**	**75**	**80**
38 Weeks			
SBP	77	92	97
DBP	50	65	70
MAP	**59**	**74**	**79**
36 Weeks			
SBP	72	87	92
DBP	50	65	70
MAP	**57**	**72**	**77**
34 Weeks			
SBP	70	85	90
DBP	40	55	60
MAP	**50**	**65**	**70**
32 Weeks			
SBP	68	83	88
DBP	40	55	60
MAP	**49**	**64**	**69**
30 Weeks			
SBP	65	80	85
DBP	40	55	60
MAP	**48**	**63**	**68**
28 Weeks			
SBP	60	75	80
DBP	38	50	54
MAP	**45**	**58**	**63**
26 Weeks			
SBP	55	72	77
DBP	30	50	56
MAP	**38**	**57**	**63**

DBP, Diastolic blood pressure; *MAP*, mean arterial pressure; *SBP*, systolic blood pressure.

a nearly identical incidence of hypertension, although the focus was on treated patients.[21] Prenatal factors such as antenatal steroid administration, maternal hypertension, and maternal substance abuse were associated with the diagnosis of hypertension in that study.

Larger, multicenter studies examining neonatal hypertension have been rare. An incidence of around 1% was found in a study using administrative data from a consortium of pediatric hospitals.[22] The most common factors associated with hypertension in that study were extracorporeal membrane oxygenation (ECMO) treatment and either congenital or acquired renal disease.

Hypertension may also be detected long after discharge from the NICU. In a retrospective review of over 650 infants seen in follow-up after discharge from a tertiary level NICU, Friedman and Hustead found an incidence of hypertension (defined as a systolic BP of greater than 113 mm Hg on three consecutive visits over 6 weeks) of 2.6%.[23] Hypertension in this study was detected at a mean age of approximately 2 months postterm when corrected for prematurity. Infants in this study who developed hypertension tended to have lower initial Apgar scores and slightly longer NICU stays than infants who remained normotensive, indicating a somewhat greater likelihood of developing hypertension in sicker babies. Unfortunately, this study has not been replicated, so the current prevalence of hypertension in high-risk infants remains unclear. However, these data do support routine BP monitoring following NICU discharge, as advocated by the NHBPEP.[13]

Differential Diagnosis

In older infants and children, the potential causes of hypertension in neonates are numerous (Table 16.2), with the largest number of cases probably accounted for by umbilical artery catheter-associated thromboembolism affecting either the aorta and/or the renal arteries. This was first demonstrated in the early 1970s by Neal and colleagues[24] and later confirmed by other investigators. Hypertension was reported to develop in infants who had undergone umbilical arterial catheterization even when thrombi were unable to be demonstrated in the renal arteries. Reported rates of thrombus formation have generally been about 25%.[25]

Although there have been several studies that have examined duration of line placement and line position as factors involved in thrombus formation, these data

Table 16.2 CAUSES OF NEONATAL HYPERTENSION

Renovascular	**Medications/Intoxications**
Thromboembolism	Infant
Renal artery stenosis	Dexamethasone
Mid-aortic coarctation	Adrenergic agents
Renal venous thrombosis	Vitamin D intoxication
Compression of renal artery	Theophylline
Idiopathic arterial calcification	Caffeine
Congenital rubella syndrome	Pancuronium
Renal Parenchymal Disease	Phenylephrine
Congenital	Maternal
Polycystic kidney disease	Cocaine
Multicystic-dysplastic kidney disease	Heroin
Tuberous sclerosis	Antenatal steroids
Ureteropelvic junction obstruction	**Neoplasia**
Unilateral renal hypoplasia	Wilms tumor
Congenital nephrotic syndrome	Mesoblastic nephroma
ACE inhibitor fetopathy	Neuroblastoma
Acquired	Pheochromocytoma
Acute kidney injury	**Neurologic**
Cortical necrosis	Pain
Interstitial nephritis	Intracranial hypertension
Hemolytic-uremic syndrome	Seizures
Obstruction (stones, tumors)	Familial dysautonomia
Pulmonary	Subdural hematoma
Bronchopulmonary dysplasia	**Miscellaneous**
Pneumothorax	Volume overload
Cardiac	Closure of abdominal wall defect
Aortic coarctation	Adrenal hemorrhage
Endocrine	Hypercalcemia
Congenital adrenal hyperplasia	Traction
Hyperaldosteronism	Extracorporeal membrane oxygenation
Hyperthyroidism	Birth asphyxia
Pseudohypoaldosteronism type II	
Glucocorticoid remediable aldosteronism	

have not been conclusive.[26] Longer duration of umbilical catheter placement has been associated with higher rates of thrombus formation.[27] A Cochrane review comparing "low" versus "high" umbilical artery catheters determined that the "high" catheter placement was associated with fewer ischemic events such as necrotizing enterocolitis but that hypertension occurred at equal frequency with either position.[28] Thus, it is assumed that catheter-related hypertension is related to thrombus formation at the time of line placement because of disruption of the vascular endothelium of the umbilical artery, particularly in preterm infants.

Fibromuscular dysplasia leading to renal arterial stenosis is an extremely important cause of renovascular hypertension in the neonate. Many of these infants may have main renal arteries that appear normal on angiography but demonstrate significant branch vessel disease that can cause severe hypertension.[29] In addition, renal arterial stenosis may also be accompanied by mid-aortic coarctation and cerebral vascular stenoses.[29,30] Several other vascular problems may also lead to neonatal hypertension, including renal venous thrombosis, idiopathic arterial calcification, and compression of the renal arteries by tumors.

After renovascular causes, the next largest group of infants with hypertension are those with congenital renal abnormalities. While both autosomal dominant and autosomal recessive polycystic kidney disease (PKD) may present in the newborn period with severe nephromegaly and hypertension, recessive PKD more commonly leads to hypertension early, sometimes in the first month of life.[31–33] Hypertension has also been reported in infants with unilateral multicystic dysplastic kidneys (MCDK),[34] possibly due to renin production by the MCDK itself.[35] Renal obstruction may be accompanied by hypertension, for example, in infants with congenital ureteropelvic-junction obstruction.[36] The importance of congenital urologic malformations as a cause of neonatal hypertension was demonstrated in a referral series from Brazil,[37] in which 13 of 15 hypertensive infants had urologic causes. In addition, the median age at diagnosis of hypertension was 20 days (range 5–70 days), emphasizing the need for regular BP measurement in infants with urologic malformations to detect hypertension.

The other important group of hypertensive neonates are those with bronchopulmonary dysplasia (BPD). BPD-associated hypertension was first described in the mid-1980s by Abman and colleagues,[38] who found that the incidence of hypertension in infants with BPD was 43% versus an incidence of 4.5% in infants without BPD. Over half of the infants with BPD who developed hypertension did not display it until after discharge from the NICU, again highlighting the need for measurement of blood pressure in NICU "graduates."

Other studies have subsequently confirmed that hypertension occurs more commonly in infants with BPD compared to infants of similar gestational age or birth weight without BPD. Factors such as hypoxemia and increased severity of BPD appear to be correlated with the development of hypertension.[39] Since many of these infants will have had an umbilical line placed, it is also possible that BPD is a comorbidity for line-associated thromboembolic disease (see first two paragraphs above). Although updated studies are sorely needed, these observations reinforce the impression that infants with severe BPD are clearly at increased risk and need close monitoring for the development of hypertension. This is especially true in infants who require ongoing treatment with theophylline preparations, diuretics, and/or corticosteroids.

Hypertension may also be secondary to disorders of several other organ systems or may develop as a consequence of treatment with various pharmacologic agents (see Table 16.2). The interested reader is encouraged to consult more comprehensive reviews for a full discussion of these causes.[16]

Clinical Presentation

Except in critically ill infants with severely elevated BP, in many infants in the NICU, elevated BP will be detected on routine monitoring of vital signs, making it difficult to identify infants with true hypertension that warrants further evaluation and/or treatment. This is primarily a consequence of the changing nature of BP in neonates and the difficulty in knowing what BP level should be considered elevated (see preceding sections). However, some classic presentations of neonatal hypertension have been described, including congestive heart failure and cardiogenic shock.[40,41] In the less acutely ill infant, feeding difficulties, unexplained tachypnea, apnea, lethargy, irritability, or seizures may constitute symptoms of unsuspected hypertension. In older infants who have been discharged from the nursery, unexplained irritability or failure to thrive may be the only manifestations of hypertension.

Diagnostic Evaluation

Blood Pressure Measurement

As in older children, accurate BP measurement is crucial so that hypertension will be correctly identified. The gold standard for BP measurement in neonates remains direct intraarterial measurement. There is reasonable correlation between umbilical artery and peripheral artery catheter BPs in neonates,[42] so no specific site is preferred. Indirect methods of measuring the BP such as palpation and auscultation are not practical in neonates, especially in the NICU setting, and ultrasonic Doppler assessment has largely been replaced by oscillometric devices.[43]

Oscillometric devices are easy to use and provide the ability to follow BP trends over time. Studies have shown reasonably good correlation between oscillometric and umbilical or radial artery BP in neonates and young children.[16] They are especially useful for infants who require BP monitoring after discharge from the NICU.[44] However, not all oscillometric devices are equal. A few studies have compared different oscillometric BP monitors to direct arterial measurements in neonates and have shown that accuracy varied depending on the size of the infant[45] with a higher likelihood of oscillometric methods to over-read BP compared to direct measurement.[46]

Many factors can influence the accuracy of BP measurements in neonates. BP will obviously be higher in infants who are crying versus those who are resting (Fig. 16.5), and even in a quiet infant, activities such as feeding or sucking on a pacifier may increase the BP.[6,47] Given this, consistent measurement technique becomes of paramount importance in obtaining accurate BP values. A standard protocol as suggested by Nwankwo and colleagues[48] may result in decreased variability of BP readings, ensuring that accurate BP values will be available to guide clinical decision-making. Elements of this protocol include the following:

- Infant should be either prone or supine, and resting quietly
- Delay BP measurements until 1.5 hours or longer after a medical procedure or feeding
- Use appropriately sized cuff and measure BP in right upper arm
- Obtain several BP measurements in succession using an oscillometric device

Finally, it is important to recognize that calf BP values are equivalent to BP values obtained in the upper arm until about 6 months of age,[49] so it is acceptable to measure BP in the lower extremity—although efforts should be made to use the same extremity for sequential measurements.

Fig. 16.5 Effect of infant state on systolic (*dark bars*) and diastolic (*light bars*) blood pressure. (Data from Satoh M, Inoue R, Tada H, et al. Reference values and associated factors for Japanese newborns' blood pressure and pulse rate: the babies' and their parents' longitudinal observation in Suzuki Memorial Hospital on intrauterine period [BOSHI] study. *J Hypertens.* 2016;34:1578–1585.)

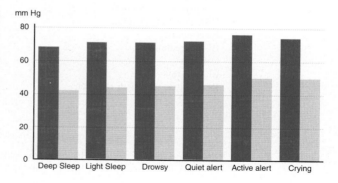

Diagnostic Approach

Diagnosing the cause of the elevated BP should be fairly straightforward in most neonates. A relatively focused history should be obtained, paying attention to determining whether there were any pertinent prenatal exposures, as well as to the details of the infant's clinical course and any concurrent conditions. The procedures that the infant has undergone (e.g., umbilical catheter placement) should be reviewed, and his or her current medication list should be scrutinized for substances that can elevate BP.

The physical examination should be focused on obtaining information to assist in narrowing the differential diagnosis. BP readings should be obtained in all four extremities at least once to rule out aortic coarctation. However, as mentioned above, since lower extremity BP readings may be similar to upper extremity readings, an echocardiogram is required to confirm this diagnosis.[49] The general appearance of the infant should be assessed, with particular attention paid to the presence of any dysmorphic features that may indicate an obvious diagnosis such as congenital adrenal hyperplasia.[50] Careful cardiac and abdominal examinations should be performed. The presence of a flank mass or of an epigastric bruit may point the clinician towards diagnosis of either ureteropelvic junction obstruction or renal artery stenosis, respectively.

Since the correct diagnosis is usually suggested by the history and physical examination, and since there are typically ample prior laboratory data available for review, few additional studies will be needed in most instances. It is important to assess renal function, as well as to examine a specimen of the urine, to ascertain the presence of renal parenchymal disease. Chest x-ray may be useful in infants with signs of congestive heart failure or in those with a murmur on physical examination. Other diagnostic studies, such as cortisol, aldosterone, or thyroxine levels, should be obtained when there is pertinent history (Table 16.3). Plasma renin activity is typically quite high in infancy, particularly in premature infants,[51] making renin values difficult to interpret. Given this, assessment of plasma renin activity in the initial evaluation of hypertension in infants may be deferred. An exception to this would be infants with hypokalemia that might suggest a monogenic form of hypertension.[52]

The role of imaging in the evaluation of hypertensive neonates has been reviewed extensively elsewhere,[53] so only a few comments will be made here. Renal ultrasound with Doppler should be obtained in all hypertensive infants, as it can help uncover potentially correctable causes of hypertension such as renal venous thrombosis,[54] may detect aortic and/or renal arterial thrombi,[26] and can identify anatomic renal abnormalities or other congenital renal diseases. Although nuclear scanning has been shown in some studies to demonstrate abnormalities of renal perfusion caused by thromboembolic phenomenon,[51] in our experience it has had little role in the assessment of hypertensive infants, primarily due to the difficulties in obtaining accurate,

Table 16.3 DIAGNOSTIC TESTING IN NEONATAL HYPERTENSION

Generally Useful	Useful in Selected Infants
Urinalysis (+/− culture)	Thyroid studies
CBC and platelet count	Urine VMA/HVA
Electrolytes	Plasma renin activity
BUN, creatinine	Aldosterone
Calcium	Cortisol
Chest x-ray	Echocardiogram
Renal ultrasound with Doppler	Abdominal/pelvic ultrasound
	VCUG
	Aortography
	Renal angiography
	Nuclear scan (DTPA/Mag-3)

BUN, Blood urea nitrogen; *CBC,* complete blood count; *DTPA,* diethylenetriaminepentaacetic acid; *HVA,* homovanillic acid; *VCUG,* voiding cystourethrogram; *VMA,* vanillylmandelic acid.

interpretable results in this age group. Other studies, including echocardiograms and voiding cystourethrograms, should be obtained as indicated.

For infants with extremely severe BP elevation, renal artery stenosis rises to the top of the differential, making vascular imaging necessary. In our experience, a formal arteriogram utilizing the traditional femoral approach offers the only accurate method of diagnosing renal artery stenosis, particularly given the high incidence of branch vessel disease in children with fibromuscular dysplasia.[30,55] Neither computed tomographic or magnetic resonance angiography has sufficient resolution to detect most cases of renal artery stenosis in neonates and should not be ordered, unless deemed necessary in preparation for arteriography. Although cases of successful angiography with angioplasty have been reported in young infants,[56] most centers lack both the equipment and expertise to perform this safely in newborns. Given these considerations, in most infants with suspected renal artery stenosis, angiography should be deferred, and the hypertension should be managed medically until the baby is large enough for an arteriogram to be performed safely.

Treatment

The first step in treatment should be correction of any iatrogenic causes of hypertension, such as excessive or unnecessary inotrope administration, dexamethasone or other corticosteroids, hypercalcemia, volume overload, or pain. Hypoxemia should be treated in infants with BPD, and appropriate hormonal replacement should be initiated in those with endocrine disorders.

Surgery is indicated for treatment of neonatal hypertension in a limited set of circumstances, most notably in infants with ureteral obstruction or aortic coarctation.[36,57] For infants with renal artery stenosis, it may be necessary to manage the infant medically until it has grown sufficiently to undergo definitive repair of the vascular abnormalities.[58] However, unilateral nephrectomy may be needed in rare cases.[59] Infants with hypertension secondary to Wilms tumor or neuroblastoma will require surgical tumor removal, possibly following chemotherapy. Hypertensive infants with MCDK may also benefit from nephrectomy.[36] Infants with malignant hypertension secondary to autosomal recessive PKD may require bilateral nephrectomy. Fortunately, such severely affected infants are rare.

At some point, a decision will need to be made as to whether antihypertensive medications are indicated. Except in severely hypertensive infants with obvious end-organ manifestations (e.g., congestive heart failure or seizures), this can be a difficult decision. No data exist on the adverse effects of chronic BP elevation in infancy, and few if any antihypertensive medications have ever been studied in neonates. Of note, the recent studies mentioned[22,23,36] demonstrate that despite the lack of such data, a wide variety of antihypertensive medications do get prescribed to hypertensive neonates. Additionally, as noted earlier, determining what BP threshold at which to consider treatment can be difficult due to the lack of robust normative BP data. Therefore, clinical expertise and expert opinion must be relied upon to guide decision-making.

Oral antihypertensive agents (Table 16.4) are best reserved for infants with less severe hypertension or infants whose acute hypertension has been controlled with intravenous infusions and are ready to be transitioned to chronic therapy. We typically start with the calcium channel blocker isradipine[60,61] as it can be compounded into a stable 1 mg/mL suspension,[62] facilitating dosing in small infants. Amlodipine may also be used, but its slow onset of action and prolonged duration of effect may be problematic in the acute setting. Other potentially useful vasodilators include hydralazine and minoxidil. Beta blockers may need to be avoided in infants with chronic lung disease. In such infants, diuretics may have a beneficial effect not only in controlling BP but also in improving pulmonary function.[63] On the other hand, propranolol is available commercially as a suspension, which makes it convenient to use when beta blockade is not contraindicated.

Use of angiotensin-converting enzyme inhibitors (ACEI) in neonates is controversial. Captopril is one of the only antihypertensive agents that has actually been

Table 16.4 RECOMMENDED DOSES FOR SELECTED ANTIHYPERTENSIVE AGENTS FOR
TREATMENT OF HYPERTENSIVE INFANTS

Class	Drug	Route	Dose	Interval	Comments
ACE inhibitors	Captopril	Oral	<3 m: 0.01–0.5 mg/kg/dose Max 2 mg/kg/day >3 m: 0.15–0.3 mg/kg/dose Max 6 mg/kg/day	TID	1. First dose may cause rapid drop in BP, especially if receiving diuretics 2. Monitor serum creatinine and K+ 3. Intravenous enalaprilat NOT recommended— see text 4. Limited experience with Lisinopril in infants
	Enalapril[a]	Oral	0.08–0.6 mg/kg/day	QD-BID	
	Lisinopril[a]	Oral	0.07–0.6 mg/kg/day	QD	
α and β-antagonists	Labetalol	Oral	0.5–1.0 mg/kg/dose Max 10 mg/kg/day	BID-TID	Heart failure, BPD relative contraindications
		IV	0.20–1.0 mg/kg/dose 0.25–3.0 mg/kg/hr	Q4–6 h infusion	
	Carvedilol	Oral	0.1 mg/kg/dose up to 0.5 mg/kg/dose	BID	May be useful in heart failure
β-antagonists	Esmolol	IV	100–500 mcg/kg/min	Infusion	Very short-acting— constant infusion necessary
	Propranolol[a]	Oral	0.5–1.0 mg/kg/dose Max 8–10 mg/kg/day	TID	Monitor heart rate; avoid in BPD
Calcium channel blockers	Amlodipine	Oral	0.05–0.3 mg/kg/dose Max 0.6 mg/kg/day	QD-BID	All may cause reflex tachycardia
	Isradipine	Oral	0.05–0.15 mg/kg/dose Max 0.8 mg/kg/day	QID	
	Nicardipine	IV	1–4 mcg/kg/min	Infusion	
Central α-agonist	Clonidine	Oral	5–10 mcg/kg/day Max 25 mcg/kg/day	TID	May cause mild sedation
Diuretics	Chlorothiazide[a]	Oral	5–15 mg/kg/dose	BID	Monitor electrolytes
	Hydrochlorothiazide	Oral	1–3 mg/kg/dose	QD	
	Spironolactone	Oral	0.5–1.5 mg/kg/dose	BID	
Direct vasodilators	Hydralazine	Oral	0.25–1.0 mg/kg/dose Max 7.5 mg/kg/day	TID-QID	Tachycardia and fluid retention are common side effects
		IV	0.15–0.6 mg/kg/dose	Q4 h	
	Minoxidil	Oral	0.1–0.2 mg/kg/dose	BID-TID	Tachycardia and fluid retention common side effects; prolonged use causes hypertrichosis
	Sodium nitroprusside	IV	0.5–10 mcg/kg/min	Infusion	Thiocyanate toxicity can occur with prolonged (>72 h) use or in renal failure

ACE, Angiotensin converting enzyme; *BID*, twice daily; *BPD*, bronchopulmonary dysplasia; *IV*, intravenous; *QD*, once daily; *QID*, four times daily; *TID*, three times daily.
[a]Commercially marketed suspension available.

demonstrated to be effective in infants,[64] but it is well known to cause an exaggerated fall in BP in premature infants.[65] Hyperkalemia, acute kidney injury, and severe hypotension have also been reported in infants treated with enalapril.[66] These effects are related to the activation of the renin-angiotensin-aldosterone system (RAAS) in neonates, which is a reflection of the importance of the RAAS in nephron development.[67] Although few data exist on this topic, the concern over use of ACEI in infants is that they may impair the final stages of renal maturation. Based on this concern, we typically avoid use of captopril (and other ACEI) until the preterm infant has reached a corrected postmenstrual age of 44 weeks.

Intermittently administered intravenous agents have a role in therapy in selected hypertensive infants. Hydralazine and labetalol in particular may be useful in infants with mild to moderate hypertension that are not yet candidates for oral therapy because of necrotizing enterocolitis or other forms of gastrointestinal dysfunction. Enalaprilat, the intravenous angiotensin converting enzyme inhibitor, has also been used in the treatment of neonatal renovascular hypertension.[68,69] However, even doses at the lower end of published ranges may lead to significant, prolonged hypotension and oliguric acute kidney injury. It should also be noted that all available pediatric dosing recommendations for enalaprilat are based on the previously mentioned, uncontrolled case series. For these reasons, I do not recommend its use in hypertensive neonates.

In infants with acute severe hypertension, continuous intravenous infusions of antihypertensive agents should be utilized. The advantages of intravenous infusions are numerous, most importantly including the ability to quickly titrate the infusion rate to achieve the desired level of BP control. As in patients of any age with malignant hypertension, care should be taken to avoid too rapid a reduction in BP[70] to avoid cerebral ischemia and hemorrhage, a problem that premature infants, in particular, are already at increased risk of due to the immaturity of their periventricular circulation. Here again, continuous infusions of intravenous antihypertensives offer a distinct advantage. Published experience[71,72] suggests that the calcium channel blocker nicardipine may be particularly useful in infants with acute severe hypertension. Other drugs that have been successfully used in neonates include esmolol,[73] labetalol,[74] and nitroprusside.[75] Oral agents in general are probably not appropriate given their variable onset and duration of effect and unpredictable antihypertensive response. Whatever agent is used, BP should be monitored continuously via an indwelling arterial catheter or by frequently repeated (every 10–15 min) cuff readings with an oscillometric device so that the dose can be titrated to achieve the desired degree of BP control.

Outcome

While the underlying cause of hypertension clearly plays a role in determining long-term outcome, for most hypertensive infants, the long-term prognosis should be good. For infants with hypertension related to an umbilical artery catheter, available information suggests that the hypertension will usually resolve over time.[21,76,77] These infants may require increases in their antihypertensive medications over the first several months following discharge from the nursery as they undergo rapid growth. Following this, it is usually possible to wean their antihypertensives by making no further dose increases as the infant continues to grow. While long-term follow-up data on hypertensive neonates are sparse, at least one study indicates that most infants will be off medication by 6 months of age.[21] For infants discharged on antihypertensive medications, some method of following home BPs and adjusting medication doses between office visits can be useful. This could include BP monitoring by the primary care provider, or use of home BP equipment such as a Dinamap.

Some forms of neonatal hypertension may persist beyond infancy, usually hypertension related to PKD and other forms of renal parenchymal disease.[22,23,26,71] Infants with renal venous thrombosis may also remain hypertensive,[78] and some of these children will ultimately benefit from removal of the affected kidney. Persistent or late hypertension may also be seen in children who have undergone repair of renal artery stenosis or thoracic aortic coarctation.[79] Reappearance of hypertension in these situations should prompt a search for restenosis by the appropriate imaging studies.

Better long-term outcome studies of infants with neonatal hypertension are needed. Since many of these infants are delivered prior to the completion of nephron development, it is possible that they may not develop the full complement of glomeruli normally seen in term infants. Reduced nephron mass is hypothesized to be a risk factor for the development of adult hypertension.[80,81] Thus, it may be possible that hypertensive neonates (and possibly also normotensive premature neonates) are at increased risk compared to term infants for the development of hypertension in late adolescence or early adulthood.[82] A high incidence of prematurity in children with otherwise unexplained hypertension was recently demonstrated in a single-center case series.[83] Given the improvements in survival of the most premature infants, it is imperative that appropriately designed studies be conducted to address these questions.

Conclusion

Although there are many areas in which better data are needed, particularly with respect to pathophysiology, diagnostic thresholds, and antihypertensive medications, much has been learned about neonatal hypertension over the past decades. Normal BP in neonates depends on a variety of factors, including birth weight, gestational age, postnatal age, and maternal factors. Hypertension is more often seen in infants with concurrent conditions such as BPD or in those who have undergone umbilical arterial catheterization. A careful diagnostic evaluation should lead to determination of the underlying cause of hypertension in most infants. Treatment decisions should be tailored to the severity of the hypertension and may include intravenous and/or oral therapy. In addition, most infants will resolve their hypertension over time, although a small number may have persistent BP elevation throughout childhood.

REFERENCES

1. Adelman RD. Neonatal hypertension. *Ped Clin North Am.* 1978;25:99–110.
2. Watkinson M. Hypertension in the newborn baby. *Arch Dis Child Fetal Neonatal Ed.* 2002;86:F78–F88.
3. Zubrow AB, Hulman S, Kushner H, et al. Determinants of blood pressure in infants admitted to neonatal intensive care units: A prospective multicenter study. *J Perinatol.* 1995;15:470–479.
4. Pejovic B, Peco-Antic A, Marinkovic-Eric J. Blood pressure in non-critically ill preterm and full-term neonates. *Pediatr Nephrol.* 2007;22:249–257.
5. Kent A, Kecskes Z, Shadbolt B, et al. Normative blood pressure data in the early neonatal period. *Pediatr Nephrol.* 2007;22:1335–1341.
6. Satoh M, Inoue R, Tada H, et al. Reference values and associated factors for Japanese newborns' blood pressure and pulse rate: the babies' and their parents' longitudinal observation in Suzuki Memorial Hospital on intrauterine period (BOSHI) study. *J Hypertens.* 2016;34:1578–1585.
7. Lurbe E, Garcia-Vicent C, Torro I, et al. First-year blood pressure increase steepest in low birthweight newborns. *J Hypertens.* 2007;25:81–86.
8. Dagle JM, Fisher TJ, Haynes SE, et al. Cytochrome P450 (CYP2D6) genotype is associated with elevated systolic blood pressure in preterm infants after discharge from the neonatal intensive care unit. *J Pediatr.* 2011;159:104–109.
9. Kent AL, Chaudhari T. Determinants of neonatal blood pressure. *Curr Hypertens Rep.* 2013;15:426–432.
10. Sadoh WE, Ibhanesehbor SE, Monguno AM, Gubler DJ. Predictors of newborn systolic blood pressure. *West Afr J Med.* 2010;29:86–90.
11. Kent AL, Shadbolt B, Hu E, et al. Do maternal- or pregnancy-associated disease states affect blood pressure in the early neonatal period? *Aust N Z J Obstet Gynaecol.* 2009;49:364–370.
12. Task Force on Blood Pressure Control in Children. Report of the Second Task Force on Blood Pressure Control in Children—1987. National Heart, Lung and Blood Institute, National Institutes of Health, Bethesda, MD, January 1987.
13. National High Blood Pressure Education Program Working Group on High Blood Pressure in Children and Adolescents. The fourth report on the diagnosis, evaluation, and treatment of high blood pressure in children and adolescents. *Pediatrics.* 2004;114(2 suppl 4th Report):555–576.
14. Kent A, Kecskes Z, Shadbolt B, et al. Blood pressure in the first year of life in healthy infants born at term. *Pediatr Nephrol.* 2007;22:1743–1749.
15. Kent A, Meskell S, Falk M, et al. Normative blood pressure data in non-ventilated premature neonates from 28-36 weeks gestation. *Pediatr Nephrol.* 2009;24:141–146.
16. Dionne JM, Abitbol CL, Flynn JT. Hypertension in infancy: diagnosis, management and outcome. *Pediatr Nephrol.* 2012;27(1):17–32. Erratum in: *Pediatr Nephrol.* 2012 Jan;27(1):159–160.

17. American Academy of Pediatrics Committee on Fetus and Newborn. Routine evaluation of blood pressure, hematocrit and glucose in newborns. *Pediatrics*. 1993;92:474–476.
18. Buchi KF, Siegler RL. Hypertension in the first month of life. *J Hypertens*. 1986;4:525–528.
19. Singh HP, Hurley RM, Myers TF. Neonatal hypertension: incidence and risk factors. *Am J Hypertens*. 1992;5:51–55.
20. Seliem WA, Falk MC, Shadbolt B, et al. Antenatal and postnatal risk factors for neonatal hypertension and infant follow-up. *Pediatr Nephrol*. 2007;22:2081–2087.
21. Sahu R, Pannu H, Yu R, et al. Systemic hypertension requiring treatment in the neonatal intensive care unit. *J Pediatr*. 2013;163:84–88.
22. Blowey DL, Duda PJ, Stokes P, Hall M. Incidence and treatment of hypertension in the neonatal intensive care unit. *J Am Soc Hypertens*. 2011;5:478–483.
23. Friedman AL, Hustead VA. Hypertension in babies following discharge from a neonatal intensive care unit. *Pediatr Nephrol*. 1987;1:30–34.
24. Neal WA, Reynolds JW, Jarvis CW, et al. Umbilical artery catheterization: demonstration of arterial thrombosis by aortography. *Pediatrics*. 1972;50:6–13.
25. Seibert JJ, Taylor BJ, Williamson SL, et al. Sonographic detection of neonatal umbilical-artery thrombosis: clinical correlation. *AJR Am J Roentgenol*. 1987;148:965–968.
26. Wesström G, Finnström O, Stenport G. Umbilical artery catheterization in newborns. I. Thrombosis in relation to catheter type and position. *Acta Paediatr Scand*. 1979;68:575–581.
27. Boo NY, Wong NC, Zulkifli SS, et al. Risk factors associated with umbilical vascular catheter-associated thrombosis in newborn infants. *J Paediatr Child Health*. 1999;35:460–465.
28. Barrington KJ. Umbilical artery catheters in the newborn: effects of position of the catheter tip. *Cochrane Database Syst Rev*. 2009;(1):CD000505.
29. Tullus K, Brennan E, Hamilton G, et al. Renovascular hypertension in children. *Lancet*. 2008;371:1453–1663.
30. Das BB, Recto M, Shoemaker L, et al. Midaortic syndrome presenting as neonatal hypertension. *Pediatr Cardiol*. 2008;29:1000–1001.
31. Boyer O, Gagnadoux MF, Guest G, et al. Prognosis of autosomal dominant polycystic kidney disease diagnosed in utero or at birth. *Pediatr Nephrol*. 2007;22:380–388.
32. Dell KM. The spectrum of polycystic kidney disease in children. *Adv Chronic Kidney Dis*. 2011;18:339–347.
33. Guay-Woodford LM, Desmond RA. Autosomal recessive polycystic kidney disease: the clinical experience in North America. *Pediatrics*. 2003;111(5 Pt 1):1072–1080.
34. Moralıoğlu S, Celayir AC, Bosnalı O, et al. Single center experience in patients with unilateral multicystic dysplastic kidney. *J Pediatr Urol*. 2014;10:763–768.
35. Konda R, Sato H, Ito S, et al. Renin containing cells are present predominantly in scarred areas but not in dysplastic regions in multicystic dysplastic kidney. *J Urol*. 2001;166:1910–1914.
36. Murphy JP, Holder TM, Ashcraft KW, et al. Ureteropelvic junction obstruction in the newborn. *J Pediatr Surg*. 1984;19:642–648.
37. Lanzarini VV, Furusawa EA, Sadeck L, et al. Neonatal arterial hypertension in nephro-urological malformations in a tertiary care hospital. *J Hum Hypertens*. 2006;20:679–683.
38. Abman SH, Warady BA, Lum GM, et al. Systemic hypertension in infants with bronchopulmonary dysplasia. *J Pediatr*. 1984;104:929–931.
39. Anderson AH, Warady BA, Daily DK, et al. Systemic hypertension in infants with severe bronchopulmonary dysplasia: associated clinical factors. *Am J Perinatol*. 1993;10:190–193.
40. Hawkins KC, Watson AR, Rutter N. Neonatal hypertension and cardiac failure. *Eur J Pediatr*. 1995;154:148–149.
41. Xiao N, Tandon A, Goldstein S, Lorts A. Cardiogenic shock as the initial presentation of neonatal systemic hypertension. *J Neonatal Perinatal Med*. 2013;6:267–272.
42. Butt W, Whyte H. Blood pressure monitoring in neonates: comparison of umbilical and peripheral artery catheter measurements. *J Pediatr*. 1984;105:630–632.
43. Low JA, Panagiotopoulos C, Smith JT, et al. Validity of newborn oscillometric blood pressure. *Clin Invest Med*. 1995;18:163–167.
44. Park MK, Menard SM. Normative oscillometric blood pressure values in the first 5 years of life in an office setting. *Am J Dis Child*. 1989;143:860–864.
45. Dannevig I, Dale H, Liestol K, et al. Blood pressure in the neonate: three non-invasive oscillometric pressure monitors compared with invasively measure blood pressure. *Acta Pediatrica*. 2005;94:191–196.
46. O'Shea J, Dempsey E. A comparison of blood pressure measurements in newborns. *Am J Perinatol*. 2009;26:113–116.
47. Yiallourou SR, Poole H, Prathivadi P, et al. The effects of dummy/pacifier use on infant blood pressure and autonomic activity during sleep. *Sleep Med*. 2014;15:1508–1516.
48. Nwankwo M, Lorenz J, Gardiner J. A standard protocol for blood pressure measurement in the newborn. *Pediatrics*. 1997;99:E10.
49. Crossland DS, Furness JC, Abu-Harb M, et al. Variability of four limb blood pressure in normal neonates. *Arch Dis Child Fetal Neonatal Ed*. 2004;89:F325–F327.
50. Speiser PW, White PC. Congenital Adrenal Hyperplasia. *N Engl J Med*. 2003;349:776–788.
51. Richer C, Hornych H, Amiel-Tison C, et al. Plasma renin activity and its postnatal development in preterm infants. Preliminary report. *Biol Neonate*. 1977;31:301–304.
52. Vehaskari VM. Heritable forms of hypertension. *Pediatr Nephrol*. 2009;24:1929–1937.
53. Roth CG, Spottswood SE, Chan JC, et al. Evaluation of the hypertensive infant: a rational approach to diagnosis. *Radiol Clin North Am*. 2003;41:931–944.

16

54. Elsaify WM. Neonatal renal vein thrombosis: grey-scale and Doppler ultrasonic features. *Abdom Imaging.* 2009;34:413–418.
55. Vo NJ, Hammelman BD, Racadio JM, et al. Anatomic distribution of renal artery stenosis in children: implications for imaging. *Pediatr Radiol.* 2006;36:1032–1036.
56. Peco-Antic A, Djukic M, Sagic D, et al. Severe renovascular hypertension in an infant with congenital solitary pelvic kidney. *Pediatr Nephrol.* 2006;21:437–440.
57. Rajpoot DK, Duel B, Thayer K, Shanberg A. Medically resistant neonatal hypertension: revisiting the surgical causes. *J Perinatol.* 1999;19(8 Pt 1):582–583.
58. Bendel-Stenzel M, Najarian JS, Sinaiko AR. Renal artery stenosis: long-term medical management before surgery. *Pediatr Nephrol.* 1995;10:147–151.
59. Kiessling SG, Wadhwa N, Kriss VM, et al. An unusual case of severe therapy-resistant hypertension in a newborn. *Pediatrics.* 2007;119:e301–e304.
60. Flynn JT, Warnick SJ. Isradipine treatment of hypertension in children: a single-center experience. *Pediatr Nephrol.* 2002;17:748–753.
61. Miyashita Y, Peterson D, Rees JM, et al. Isradipine treatment of acute hypertension in hospitalized children and adolescents. *J Clin Hypertens (Greenwich).* 2010;12:850–855.
62. MacDonald JL, Johnson CE, Jacobson P. Stability of isradipine in an extemporaneously compounded oral liquid. *Am J Hosp Pharm.* 1994;51:2409–2411.
63. Kao LC, Durand DJ, McCrea RC, et al. Randomized trial of long-term diuretic therapy for infants with oxygen-dependent bronchopulmonary dysplasia. *J Pediatr.* 1994;124(5 Pt 1):772–781.
64. O'Dea RF, Mirkin BL, Alward CT, et al. Treatment of neonatal hypertension with captopril. *J Pediatr.* 1988;113:403–406.
65. Tack ED, Perlman JM. Renal failure in sick hypertensive premature infants receiving captopril therapy. *J Pediatr.* 1988;112:805–810.
66. Ku LC, Zimmerman K, Benjamin DK, et al. Safety of Enalapril in Infants Admitted to the Neonatal Intensive Care Unit. *Pediatr Cardiol.* 2017;38:155–161.
67. Guron G, Friberg P. An intact renin-angiotensin system is a prerequisite for normal renal development. *J Hypertens.* 2000;18:123–137.
68. Wells TG, Bunchman TE, Kearns GL. Treatment of neonatal hypertension with enalaprilat. *J Pediatr.* 1990;117:664–667.
69. Mason T, Polak MJ, Pyles L, et al. Treatment of neonatal renovascular hypertension with intravenous enalapril. *Am J Perinatol.* 1992;9:254–257.
70. Flynn JT, Tullus K. Severe hypertension in children and adolescents: pathophysiology and treatment. *Pediatr Nephrol.* 2009;24:1101–1112.
71. Flynn JT, Mottes TA, Brophy PB, et al. Intravenous nicardipine for treatment of severe hypertension in children. *J Pediatr.* 2001;139:38–43.
72. Gouyon JB, Geneste B, Semama DS, et al. Intravenous nicardipine in hypertensive preterm infants. *Arch Dis Child Fetal Neonatal Ed.* 1997;76:F126–F127.
73. Wiest DB, Garner SS, Uber WE, et al. Esmolol for the management of pediatric hypertension after cardiac operations. *J Thorac Cardiovas Surg.* 1998;115:890–897.
74. Thomas CA, Moffett BS, Wagner JL, et al. Safety and efficacy of intravenous labetalol for hypertensive crisis in infants and small children. *Pediatr Crit Care Med.* 2011;12:28–32.
75. Benitz WE, Malachowski N, Cohen RS, et al. Use of sodium nitroprusside in neonates: efficacy and safety. *J Pediatr.* 1985;106:102–110.
76. Adelman RD. Long-term follow-up of neonatal renovascular hypertension. *Pediatr Nephrol.* 1987;1:35–41.
77. Caplan MS, Cohn RA, Langman CB, et al. Favorable outcome of neonatal aortic thrombosis and renovascular hypertension. *J Pediatr.* 1989;115:291–295.
78. Mocan H, Beattie TJ, Murphy AV. Renal venous thrombosis in infancy: long-term follow-up. *Pediatr Nephrol.* 1991;5:45–49.
79. O'Sullivan JJ, Derrick G, Darnell R. Prevalence of hypertension in children after early repair of coarctation of the aorta: a cohort study using casual and 24 hour blood pressure measurement. *Heart.* 2002;88:163–166.
80. Mackenzie HS, Lawler EV, Brenner BM. Congenital olionephropathy: The fetal flaw in essential hypertension? *Kidney Int.* 2006;55:S30–S34.
81. Keller G, Zimmer G, Mall G, et al. Nephron number in patients with primary hypertension. *N Engl J Med.* 2003;348:101–108.
82. Shankaran S, Das A, Bauer CR, et al. Fetal origin of childhood disease: intrauterine growth restriction in term infants and risk for hypertension at 6 years of age. *Arch Pediatr Adolesc Med.* 2006;160:977–981.
83. Gupta-Malhotra M, Banker A, Shete S, et al. Essential hypertension vs. secondary hypertension among children. *Am J Hypertens.* 2015;28:73–80.

CHAPTER 17

Edema

Yosef Levenbrown, DO, Andrew Thomas Costarino, MD, MSCE

Several systems act in concert to regulate total body water (TBW), allowing homeostasis of the circulating intravascular volume and maintenance of cellular and extracellular electrolytes in the appropriate concentrations. Edema, defined here as an abnormal accumulation of extracellular water (ECW), can result from malfunction of these fluid regulatory systems. This chapter provides an overview of the water regulatory mechanisms and then examines how the dysfunction of these mechanisms can lead to a state of edema. Lastly, the chapter examines some common clinical scenarios of the neonatal population that are associated with edema.

The Basics: Body Water Compartments

The volume and distribution of body water changes significantly during gestation and infancy. TBW is 78% of body weight at birth, but by 1 year of age, the percent of TBW declines to approximately 60%. There is a parallel decline in the ECW volume, which demonstrates a decrease from 45% of the TBW to 27% during the first postnatal year. As a result of the loss of ECW, the percentage of body weight that is intracellular water (ICW) increases during the first 3 months of age from 34% to 43%. This transient increase in ICW volume is followed by a decrease to around 35% at 1 year of age. At around 3 months of age, the ICW overtakes the ECW as the major contributor to TBW. This trend continues until, eventually, the ICW volume doubles that of the ECW.[1]

Between 1 and 3 years of age, a slight increase is found in all three body water components, after which TBW and ECW decrease slightly until around puberty, at which point the adult values are reached. This decline in TBW and ECW that occurs between age 3 years and puberty is likely a result of the increase in both the quantity and size of cells in the major organ systems, especially the cells of the musculoskeletal system, the skin, and central nervous system (CNS). These three organ systems tend to retain more water in the intracellular compartment, leading to the decrease in both TBW and the proportion of ECW. TBW also is inversely proportional to the amount of body fat because of the low content of water in fat cells. During the first year of life, there is a very rapid increase in the amount of body fat. This is followed by a decrease during the preschool years and finally by a slight increase in amount of body fat during the prepubescent years. These changes in body fat composition correlate well with the above-mentioned changes in TBW. Overall, ICW appears to remain relatively constant, likely because the composition of the intracellular content remains constant.[1]

Starling Forces

Water movement across an idealized capillary wall was described qualitatively by Starling[2] in 1896 and can be defined by the following equation:

$$J_v = K_{fc}[(P_c - P_t) - \sigma_d(\pi_p - \pi_t)]$$

where J_v is the volume flow of fluid across the capillary wall, K_{fc} is the filtration coefficient of the capillary wall (volume flow/unit time per 100 g of tissue per unit pressure), P_c is the capillary hydrostatic pressure, P_t is the interstitial fluid or tissue hydrostatic pressure, σ_d is the osmotic reflection coefficient of all plasma proteins, π_p is the colloid osmotic pressure (COP) of the plasma, and π_t is the COP of the tissue fluids. To best understand how the interplay of these forces affects overall fluid balance, it is best to analyze them individually.

Hydrostatic Forces

The hydrostatic pressure in the intravascular space (P_c) is the principle force driving water and electrolytes out of the capillary into the interstitial space. The filtration force of the capillary hydrostatic pressure is opposed by the tissue pressure surrounding the capillaries (P_t). Thus the net difference between capillary and tissue hydrostatic pressure ($P_c - P_t$) is the driving force promoting filtration or absorption of fluid out of or into the capillary lumen.

Under physiologic conditions, the average capillary hydrostatic pressure is estimated to be about 17 mm Hg.[3] An increase in small artery, arteriolar, or venous pressure will increase the capillary hydrostatic pressure favoring filtration. A reduction of these pressures will have the opposite effect. Whereas an increased arteriolar resistance or closure of arteries reduces the downstream capillary hydrostatic pressure, an increase in the venous resistance results in increased upstream capillary hydrostatic pressure. In general, changes in the venous resistance result in a greater effect on the capillary pressure than changes in arteriolar resistance.[4]

In the nonedematous state, P_t in loose tissues is close to zero or even negative (−1 to −4 mm Hg). Negative interstitial pressure often occurs under physiologic conditions when the lymphatic system is pumped from muscle contraction while there is minimal leakage of fluid from the intravascular space.[3] Tissue pressure can change significantly if fluid moves into tissue space.[5]

Osmotic Forces

The plasma COP (π_p) is the primary counterbalancing force to capillary hydrostatic pressure that promotes fluid retention in intravascular space. In his landmark publication, Starling[2] demonstrated that this force is generated from the osmotic pressure associated with the plasma proteins. Total osmotic pressure of plasma approximates 6000 mm Hg, but most of this pressure is generated by the electrolytes, which are present in almost equal concentrations in both the intravascular and extravascular compartments of the ECW. In contrast, the plasma proteins are minimally present in the tissue surrounding the capillary.[2] Therefore, the direct and indirect effect of the charged plasma proteins generates the difference in osmotic pressure, the plasma oncotic pressure. Normally, the plasma oncotic pressure averages 28 mm Hg.[3,4]

Albumin is the primary plasma protein that is responsible for approximately 80% of the total COP. The other 20% is generated by globulins. It is the number of particles rather than the mass of a solute that determines its osmotic pressure. Thus, while albumin compromises only 50% of total plasma protein concentration, it has the greatest number of molecules present in the plasma and therefore makes the greatest contribution to the plasma oncotic pressure.[6]

Another characteristic of albumin plays an important role through its effect on osmotic pressure. The albumin molecule has a net negative charge as the protein binds chloride anions. The charged albumin and its bound chloride attract cations (mainly Na^+). The excess cations within the intravascular space due to the albumin binding increase the osmotic pressure within the plasma significantly more than the albumin particles alone would generate. This is known as the Gibbs-Donnan effect. On average, the normal human COP is 28 mm Hg. Whereas 19 mm Hg is attributable to dissolved proteins, 9 mm Hg is generated by the imbalance of cations associated with the Gibbs-Donnan effect.[3,4]

The interstitial fluid COP (π_t) is generated from smaller size proteins and the minimal amount of albumin that manages to leak out of the pores in the capillary walls. In healthy adults, the percentage of albumin that leaks into the interstitial space each hour is approximately 4% to 5%. This leakage of albumin is known as the transcapillary escape rate (TER), and it varies with capillary permeability, capillary recruitment, and hydrostatic pressure.[6] The concentration of these proteins in the interstitial fluid is approximately 40% of the protein concentration in the plasma. Thus the average colloid osmotic interstitial pressure is about 8 mm Hg, favoring the movement of fluid into the intravascular compartment.

The Osmotic Reflection Coefficient

The reflection coefficient is the relative impediment to the passage of a substance through the capillary wall. The reflection coefficient of water across a capillary wall (fully permeable) is 0, and that of albumin (fully impermeable) is 1. Thus all solutes that can be filtered across a capillary wall will have a reflection coefficient between 0 and 1. The reflection coefficient of a substance depends both on the nature of the solute and the characteristics of the endothelial wall being crossed.

The reflection coefficient is a key component of the COP. True COP (π) is determined by the following equation:

$$\pi = \sigma RT(C_i - C_o)$$

where σ is the reflection coefficient, R is the gas constant, T is the absolute temperature (in degrees Kelvin), C_i is the albumin concentration inside the capillary, and C_o is the albumin concentration outside the capillary.[4,5]

The Filtration Coefficient

The filtration coefficient is an expression that quantifies the ability of a given fluid to cross the capillary wall. The filtration coefficient is proportional to the surface area of the capillaries, to the number of pores per centimeter squared, and to the radius of the pores raised to the fourth power. It is inversely proportional to the thickness of the capillary wall and to the viscosity of the fluid being filtered. Not only does K_{fc} differ among the various organs, it may even increase or decrease within the same organ because of the closure or opening of more capillaries with similar conductance characteristics within a given organ.

Alterations in permeability of fluid or osmotic particles (either K_{fc} or σ_d) may lead to edema formation without changes in either hydrostatic or osmotic pressure.[6]

The Starling Hypothesis

The Starling hypothesis includes the factors previously described to relate direction movement across a capillary membrane. It is expressed mathematically as follows:

$$Q_f = k[(P_c + \pi_i) - (P_i + \pi_p)]$$

where Q_f is the fluid movement across the capillary wall, k is the filtration constant for the capillary membrane, P_c is the capillary hydrostatic pressure, π_i is the interstitial fluid oncotic pressure, P_i is the interstitial fluid hydrostatic pressure, and π_p is the plasma oncotic pressure. When Q_f yields a positive value, it indicates that the sum flow of fluid will be out of the capillaries into the vascular space (filtration). A negative value for Q_f indicates net flow of fluid into the vascular space (absorption). During normal tissue hydration, the values of the elements of this relationship result in a near zero balance across the capillary wall. Some fluid ($\approx 0.5\%$ of the plasma volume) is filtered out of the capillary at the arterial end of the capillary, where the average capillary pressure tends to be 15 to 25 mm Hg greater than at the venous side. Most of this fluid is subsequently reabsorbed at the venous end of the capillaries where the capillary pressure is lower.[3] Over the entire length of the capillary, the small net amount of fluid filtered out and not subsequently reabsorbed is cleared by the lymphatic system, through which it makes its way back into the blood circulation.

Under physiologic conditions, arterial pressure, venous pressure, postcapillary resistance, interstitial fluid hydrostatic and oncotic pressures, and plasma oncotic pressure all remain relatively constant. Therefore, the primary variable that determines net fluid movement across a capillary wall under physiologic conditions is change in the precapillary resistance, which influences the capillary hydrostatic pressure.[4]

The Role of Aquaporins in Regulating Fluid Balance

The Importance of Aquaporins in Maintaining Water Homeostasis

Four pathways appear to be responsible for water transport in mammalian tissues. They include (1) passive diffusion of water across the cell membrane lipid bilayer; (2) movement of water through cotransporter channels, such as the Na–glutamate or the Na–glucose cotransporter; (3) paracellular water transport through tight junctions between cells; and (4) water transport via a family of transmembrane proteins called the aquaporins (AQPs).[7] Predicted to exist in the 1950s, these molecules were characterized in the 1990s as facilitators of water movement across the plasma membrane down osmotic gradients. More than 10 isoforms of these AQPs have been identified, with specific ones isolated in different organ systems (e.g., AQP1 through AQP4, as well as APQ6 and APQ7 are highly expressed in the kidneys). Most of these proteins have a common molecular structure, with six transmembrane domains and intracellular NH_2^- and COOH-terminal. Although all the AQPs facilitate the transport of water, the aquaglyceroporins, a subclass of AQPs, transport both water and small nonpolar molecules such as glycerol and urea.[8]

The AQPs serve to allow water movement to occur much faster than passive diffusion across the lipid bilayer, and they are more efficient than cotransporter-associated water transport. Paracellular transport of water plays a minimal role in water transport within healthy tissues. Thus the AQPs appear to be responsible for the high water permeability and water transport regulation in various tissues, including the erythrocytes and the nephron tubules. Conversely, dysfunction or lack of expression of AQPs likely plays a role in the pathogenesis in diseases such as nephrogenic diabetes insipidus, cataracts, Sjögren syndrome, congestive heart failure, syndrome of inappropriate antidiuretic hormone secretion (SIADH), and traumatic CNS edema.

The Role of Aquaporins in the Kidneys

The majority of water reabsorption that occurs in the nephron is facilitated by the AQPs. Most of the fluid that is filtered at the glomerulus is then reabsorbed in the proximal tubule and the descending limb of the loop of Henle. AQP1, which is expressed in the apical and basolateral segment of the renal tubular epithelial cell plasma membrane, is primarily responsible for this water transport.[8] Additionally, in the outer medullary descending vasa recta, which is rich in AQP1 channels, water resorption occurs despite the existence of hydrostatic forces that favor influx. This observation suggests that in this portion of the vasa recta, water transport involves the water only AQP1 pathway, facilitated by transtubular sodium and urea concentration gradients creating the osmotic driving force for water movement.[9]

In the distal tubule and collecting duct, other AQPs serve to regulate water resorption with a dominant role played by AQP2 and its interaction with arginine vasopressin (AVP). Although only 15% of the filtrate reaches the distal nephron, regulation of water resorption in this segment allows the kidneys to "fine tune" water balance to accommodate the needs of the body. The osmotic driving force for the water movement through the collecting duct epithelia is the hypertonic milieu of the medullary portion of the kidneys created by active transport of sodium and urea from the lumen of the thick ascending loop of Henle into the interstitial space surrounding the collecting ducts. AVP secretion by the pituitary gland, in response to central volume and osmoreceptors, upregulates AQP2 expression to match the fluid needs of the body. This occurs when AVP binds to the V2 receptor in the collecting duct of the nephron, increasing intracellular cyclic adenosine monophosphate (cAMP) production. The cAMP in turn stimulates protein kinase A–dependent phosphorylation of the AQP2 protein. Vesicles carrying the phosphorylated AQP then fuse with the nephron epithelial cells, implanting the AQP in the wall of the apical plasma membrane. This results in dramatically increased water permeability of the collecting duct epithelial cell. After entering the duct cell from the collecting duct lumen through the AQP2 channels, the water exits the cell through the AQP3 and AQP4 channels located in the cell basolateral membrane, causing the water to enter the interstitial space of the nephron. AVP is also responsible for upregulating the AQP4 channels, but not the AQP3 channels.[8,10]

The Role of Aquaporins in the Lungs

Both the presence of AQPs in lung tissue and physiologic studies of lung water permeability indicate a role of these proteins in lung water homeostasis. AQPs 1, 3, 4, and 5 have been isolated in human lungs. AQP1 is expressed in the plasma membrane of the endothelial cells lining the pulmonary capillaries and in some pneumocytes. AQP4 has been isolated in the basolateral membrane of the airway epithelium of the trachea as well as in the large airways, and AQP5 has been identified in the apical membrane of type I alveolar epithelial cells.[11-13] The observation that different AQPs are concentrated in different regions of lung tissue suggests that the different AQPs play different roles within the pulmonary system.[8,14]

The flow of water through a membrane down its osmotic gradient can be quantified as the coefficient of osmotic water permeability (P_f). Studies on whole-lung preparations of sheep and mouse lung tissue have demonstrated a relatively high P_f across the alveolar to epithelial barriers. In other words, water freely flows across the alveolar epithelium. Such high values for P_f are similar to the P_f values in the renal tubular epithelium, suggesting the presence of lung AQPs.[14]

Studies of knockout mice provide further insight into the role of AQPs in the lung. Bai et al.[11] demonstrated that water permeability of lung epithelium was decreased more than 10-fold in AQP1 knockout mice. Ma et al.[12] observed that a similar decrement in osmotic water movement occurs in AQP5 null mice, but a 30% decrease was present in AQP1/AQP5 double knockout mice. In this study, Ma et al.[12] demonstrated that without the benefit of AQP5, the P_f of the type I alveoli epithelia was similar to the water permeability of cells that did not contain water channels at all.[15] The AQPs are likely also critical in the osmotic flow of water in the lung microvasculature because water movement in the pulmonary capillary is greatly decreased by AQP1 deletion.[11,15]

Lung water homeostasis changes dramatically as an infant moves from the intrauterine to the extrauterine environment. By term, human fetal lungs are producing approximately 500 mL of fluid each day. At birth, a volume of water approximately 30 mL/kg body weight must be emptied or resorbed, and the lung epithelium must abruptly switch from net secretion to net absorption of lung water. Most of the lung fluid is emptied mechanically during delivery and as the baby takes its first breath. However, a significant amount of fluid remains to be absorbed during the first postnatal days. Understanding the operative factors in the transition in lung water homeostasis at birth is clinically important because premature infants and critically ill term infants appear to have an impaired ability for the lung to reabsorb water that is associated with the occurrence of acute respiratory distress syndrome (RDS) and chronic bronchopulmonary dysplasia (BPD).

The evidence indicating an important role of AQPs in lung water homeostasis during usual conditions makes these proteins a natural object of study for understanding the sudden birth-associated changes in lung water. However, although the switch from net water secretion to absorption in newborn lungs involves an increased expression of the epithelial membrane sodium channels and of the sodium pump, current evidence for the role of AQPs is conflicting. Yasui et al.[16] observed a transient increase in AQP4 mRNA in rat lungs that occurs just after birth. This increase in AQP4 coincides with the time period when lung water content decreases from prenatal to neonatal values. The increased AQP4 mRNA was specific to the lung and was not found in other organs that express AQP4. Moreover, it was shown by immunocytochemistry that this induction of AQP4 occurred specifically in the bronchial epithelium of newborn rats, the area in the lungs identified as the primary location of postnatal lung liquid absorption.[16] Also, fetal lung AQP4 mRNA was induced by maternal administration of β-agonists and glucocorticoids. This finding is consistent with the observation that both substances have been shown to accelerate the clearance of lung water at birth.[16] These observations led Yasui and colleagues[16] to believe that AQP4 contributes to lung fluid transition shortly after birth.

In contrast, several investigators studying AQP1, AQP4, and APQ5 knockout mice have failed to observe an effect on neonatal alveolar fluid clearance in the absence of these AQPs. The apparent benign nature of these knockout conditions was present even when fluid production was maximally stimulated with β-agonists and upregulation of type II alveoli cells. Furthermore, these findings were consistent whether the alveolar fluid was simply fluid that was not removed postnatally or whether it was fluid that was a result of alveolar injury.[11–13] Conversely, these studies did show that alveolar fluid clearance was significantly impaired by the transport inhibitors of the membrane Na channels and Na/K pumps (amiloride and ouabain, respectively). These studies seem to suggest that alveolar fluid clearance during the neonatal transition occurs through an active process driven by osmolar gradients that are generated by Na channels and Na/K pumps.[11,12]

Factors That Combat the Development of Edema

The Lymphatic System

The lymphatic system plays an important role in preventing accumulation of fluid in the interstitial space. In most organ systems, when the capillary pressure is increased enough to increase fluid filtration into the interstitial space, lymph flow subsequently increases in a linear fashion. The ability of lymph flow to prevent the accumulation of fluid in the interstitial space depends not on the absolute quantity of lymph flow, but on the amount of lymph flow relative to the filtration coefficient (K_{fc}) of a given tissue. Tissues that do not have adequate lymphatic flow to drain the fluid that naturally filters out of the capillaries are often equipped with secondary overflow systems that directly drain this excess fluid. Without a secondary overflow system, the inadequate flow of lymph would lead to edema in these tissues. Examples of such overflow systems include the arachnoid granulations in the brain and the canal of Schlemm in the eye. In the lung and the liver, capillary filtration overflow causes pulmonary edema and ascites. Although these are generally considered pathologic processes, they protect these vital organs from the harmful effects that fluid engorgement would have on the actual parenchyma of these organs.[5]

The lymphatic system also plays an important role in preventing accumulation of proteins that have been filtered out of the capillaries. Removal of these proteins prevents an increase in the tissue oncotic pressure that would tend to draw more fluid into the interstitial space.[5]

Alterations in Starling Forces

The filtration of fluids from the intravascular compartment in response to an elevation of the capillary pressure causes an increase in the surrounding tissue pressure in response to this accumulation of fluid. At first, when fluid begins to accumulate, there is a large increase in the interstitial pressure for a small increase in fluid volume (i.e., low tissue compliance). This increased interstitial pressure further opposes fluid filtration. However, as fluid continues to leak into the interstitial space, the tissue compliance eventually increases, thereby decreasing the effectiveness of this protective mechanism.

Filtration of fluid into the interstitial space causes a decline in the tissue COP by diluting the interstitial proteins. This buffers further fluid filtration by decreasing the tissue COP (π_t), which increases the second term in the Starling relationship ($\sigma_d(\pi_p - \pi_t)$). The ability of these forces to change as needed to protect the tissues from further fluid accumulation, as well as the ability of the lymph flow to increase in response to increased filtration, provides an "edema safety factor" that is able to prevent further translocation of fluids into the interstitial space.[5]

Various tissues within the body have different methods of compensating for changes in interstitial fluid. In the liver, where the sinusoids are extremely porous and permeable to plasma proteins, alteration in the oncotic pressure ($\pi_p - \pi_t$) is not an effective method to prevent increased capillary filtration. Therefore, acceleration of lymph flow and ascites formation (the overflow system) along with elevations in interstitial pressure provide the forces to counteract the increased capillary filtration. Functionally, when fluid leaks from the circulation into the liver stroma, venting fluid from the parenchyma into the peritoneal space is more effective and less harmful to the organ function than if excess fluid were to accumulate in the liver parenchyma. As fluid accumulates in the peritoneal space, the peritoneal pressure increases. This impedes the further accumulation of ascites by reducing the pressure gradient driving surface transudation and by increasing the rate of reabsorption by the peritoneal capillaries and lymphatics.[17]

The lung combats increased capillary filtration by increasing lymphatic flow and by decreasing the colloid osmotic gradient. Erdmann et al.[18] demonstrated that every increase in left atrial pressure caused an elevation in lung lymph flow to a new steady state within 1 to 2 hours. This increase in lymph flow was approximately linear in relation to the increase in microvascular hydrostatic pressure. The lymphatic system of the lungs is extremely efficient in preventing lung water accumulation. The microvascular hydrostatic pressure had to increase to 50 cm H_2O before lung water accumulation rose 25%, with an increase in lung water of 50% to 100% being the typical threshold for developing pulmonary edema.[5,18]

Factors That Promote the Development of Edema

At the most basic level, edema results from any pathologic state that causes an imbalance in the Starling forces. The following discussion reviews the most common categories of conditions that can cause these Starling force disruptions.

The Porous Nature of the Capillary Wall

The first factor that may promote the development of edema is related to the capillary wall itself. With the exception of the capillaries in the brain, which do not contain open junctions, the walls of most capillary beds contain many different openings through which fluid can move from the lumen into the surrounding tissues.[5] Capillaries within organs, such as the intestinal tract, the bronchial system, and the kidney glomeruli, are fenestrated, with thick diaphragms interspaced between the endothelial cells. The capillaries in the liver and spleen contain walls that are described as discontinuous, containing very large openings. Thus, in these capillary beds, fluid has the ability to cross the capillary walls either through junctions between endothelial cells or through larger openings in the microvessel wall.[5]

In addition to the paracellular route, substances can cross the endothelial barrier through caveolae, which are specialized plasmalemmal vesicles containing a protein known as caveolin-1. This mode of molecular transport is the method by which larger molecules such as proteins cross the capillary wall. The cell surface docking protein gp60 binds to plasma proteins greater than 3 nm. After binding to the plasma

17

protein, gp60 interacts with caveolin-1 as well as various signaling intermediaries, including a G protein and an Src family tyrosine kinase. This cascade results in the formation and subsequent release of plasma protein–containing caveolae from the apical side of the cell membrane. These vesicles are transported to the basal membrane and release their contents through exocytosis. In addition, caveolae-like vesiculo-vacuolar organelles similar to caveolae can interconnect to form secondary structures that function as transmembrane channels for molecular trafficking across a cell. Receptors of endogenous permeability-enhancing agents have been identified on the surface of these channels, leaving open the possibility that they play a role in endothelial permeability.[19]

Loss of the "Edema Safety Factor"

Under normal circumstances, when fluid is filtered out of the capillary space into the interstitium, there is both an increase in the tissue hydrostatic pressure and a simultaneous decline in the tissue COP. These changes, which occur in response to fluid accumulation in the tissues, impede further filtration of fluid out of the capillaries. Lymph flow also has the ability to greatly increase in response to enhanced capillary filtration. If fluid continues to accumulate, these protective forces can become overwhelmed and will be unable to counteract additional fluid filtration. At that point, even small changes in capillary pressure will lead to translocation of large amounts of fluid into the interstitial space.

Chen et al.[20] demonstrated, in a study using the hind paw of a dog, that with the protective alterations in tissue Starling forces and increases in lymphatic flow, fluid accumulation in the interstitium was prevented with an increase in capillary hydrostatic pressure up to 12 mm Hg. Although no visible edema was noted at this pressure threshold, there was a 10% increase in interstitial fluid volume. When the capillary pressure was elevated further to 37.9 mm Hg, gross edema developed as the protective system was overwhelmed.[5,20]

Any condition that increases the permeability of the capillary endothelial wall also impairs the protective efforts of the edema safety factor because proteins leak into the interstitial space, raising the tissue COP. The effect of the increased osmotic pressure ($\sigma_d(\pi_p - \pi_t)$) that occurs with the increase in the tissue COP is magnified by the decrease in σ_d that occurs as the capillaries become "leakier." The overall result of these changes is to decrease fluid reabsorption ($\sigma_d(\pi_p - \pi_t)$), which leads to increased accumulation of fluids in the tissues.[5] Drake et al.[21] were able to define the capillary pressure in the dog lung, above which the lung will gain weight because of accumulation of filtered fluid. They termed this the *critical capillary pressure,* and it represents the limits of the total edema safety factor of the lung. Predictably, when the lung capillaries become leaky to plasma proteins, the critical capillary pressure decreases.[21]

As long as there is an appropriate compensatory increase in the flow rate of the lymphatics in response to changes in the Starling forces, edema will not occur. Initially, there is a linear increase in lymph flow in response to increased filtration, but eventually, with continued filtration, lymph flow plateaus. If there is lymphatic dysfunction, as is often present in critically ill patients,[6] edema will develop even at normal capillary filtration flow rates. A seemingly paradoxical decrease in lymphatic flow occurs in the lung and intestine when edema accumulates. This occurs in these two organs because the high fluid states promote translocation of fluid into the alveoli or into the peritoneum (the overflow systems), decreasing the filling pressure of the lymphatics.[5]

Factors That Increase Permeability of the Vascular Endothelium

Under physiologic conditions, the vascular endothelium cells in most blood vessels are linked with tight junctions that are relatively impermeable to proteins and larger molecules. However, under certain conditions, the permeability of these blood vessels to these larger molecules is increased. The vascular reactivity to the mediators of the systemic inflammatory response in sepsis is one model of endothelial dysfunction.

In this model, the vascular endothelium response reacts in a highly coordinated loss of junctional integrity that allows recoil, or active retraction, of cell borders, resulting in an increased width of the endothelial clefts. These changes allow increased junctional leakage of solute.[22] When this occurs, tissue COP increases, promoting fluid accumulation in the extravascular space. The changes in response to the vascular mediators are represented mathematically by a smaller σ_d that lowers the absolute value of the forces that promote absorption ($\sigma_d(\pi_p - \pi_t)$).

Paracellular flux of plasma fluid and proteins at endothelial cell–cell junctions contributes significantly to endothelial dysfunction in inflammation. Under physiologic conditions, adherens junctions maintain the state of vascular integrity in nearly all vascular beds. Its molecular structure is based on vascular endothelial (VE) cadherin, a transmembrane receptor whose extracellular domain binds to the extracellular domain of another VE cadherin molecule from an adjacent cell. The intracellular domain of the VE cadherin is anchored to the cell cytoskeleton via a family of actin-binding proteins called *catenins*. The stability of this complex is able to withstand fluid shear stress and is essential in maintaining endothelial barrier integrity. During inflammation, the humoral proinflammatory mediators disrupt this assembly, leading to endothelial dysfunction and hyperpermeability (Fig. 17.1).[19]

The loss of endothelial integrity that occurs during inflammatory states typically occurs in three stages. In the first stage, inflammatory agents induce transient vascular leakage through the formation of minute gaps between endothelial cells. During the second stage, activated leukocytes prolong the hyperpermeability. Finally, the microvasculature undergoes remodeling under the influence of angiogenic factors that affect the integrity of the cell junctions.[22]

Recently, vascular endothelial growth factor (VEGF) has been identified as a major angiogenic factor that induces the hyperpermeable state, particularly in the microvasculature of the lungs. Within the lung, the mesenchymal cells, alveolar macrophages, and epithelial cells are the primary cells that express VEGF. Therefore, although VEGF is constantly present in the fluid lining the lung epithelium, VEGF overexpression leads to increased permeability to macromolecules within the pulmonary vasculature and subsequently to pulmonary edema.[22,23] It has been demonstrated that patients with acute RDS, as well as patients at risk for developing this syndrome, have elevated levels of VEGF compared with control subjects.[24] This finding suggests a significant role for VEGF in the high-permeability model of pulmonary edema and in acute respiratory distress syndrome (ARDS). The exact mechanism by which VEGF increases endothelial permeability is unclear. Current evidence indicates its action results in fusion of intracellular vesicles, which then form transcellular pathways through vesiculovacuolar organelles, resulting in fenestrations and ultimately transcellular gaps.[22]

The Role of Hypoalbuminemia

Hypoalbuminemia is a common finding in critically ill patients of all ages and is often proportional to the severity of illness. When hypoalbuminemia occurs, it commonly is the result of an altered distribution of albumin between the intravascular and extravascular compartments. This is most often the result of the capillary leak associated with cytokine release in combination with decreased lymphatic flow.[6] Direct measurements of albumin permeability have demonstrated a threefold increase in TER in patients experiencing sepsis. In the presence of increased TER, infusion of exogenous albumin will distribute the protein to both the extravascular as well as the intravascular space. Thus, in conditions associated with increased capillary permeability, albumin supplementation may lead to increased albumin leakage across the capillary membrane and worsening edema without any improvement in outcome.[6,25]

After surgery, it is common for patients to develop hypoalbuminemia. Postoperative hypoalbuminemia is often the result of a redistribution of albumin between the intravascular and extravascular spaces after surgical trauma. Studies in this patient population indicate that although albumin supplementation can result in a higher serum albumin concentration, morbidity, mortality, and glomerular filtration rate

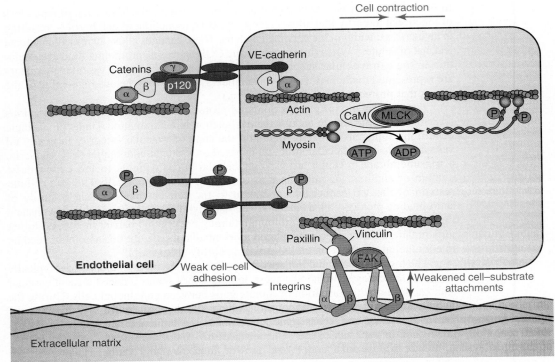

Fig. 17.1 Schematic diagram of microvascular endothelial barrier structure. The barrier is formed by endothelial cells that connect to each other through the junctional adhesive molecule vascular endothelial (VE)–cadherin, which binds to another VE–cadherin molecule from an adjacent cell and connects to the actin cytoskeleton via a family of catenins (α, β, γ, and p120). This endothelial lining is tethered to the extracellular matrix through focal adhesions mediated by transmembrane integrins composed of α and β subunits, focal adhesion kinase (FAK), and cytoskeleton-linking proteins including paxillin and vinculin. The integrity of this barrier is maintained by VE-cadherin–mediated cell–cell adhesions and focal adhesion–supported cell matrix attachment. A dynamic interaction among these structural elements controls the opening and closing of the paracellular pathways for fluid, proteins, and cells to move across the endothelium. In particular, the Ca^{2+}/calmodulin (CaM)–dependent myosin light chain kinase (MLCK) catalyzes phosphorylation of myosin light chains *(small red circles)*, triggering binding of the myosin heavy chain motor domains to actin and their cross-bridge movement. This process utilizes adenosine triphosphate (ATP), converting it into adenosine diphosphate (ADP). This reaction promotes cytoskeleton contraction and cell retraction. In parallel, phosphorylation of VE-cadherin, catenins, or both may cause the junction complex to dissociate from its cytoskeletal anchor, leading to weakened cell–cell adhesion. The cytoskeletal and junctional responses act in concert, causing paracellular hyperpermeability. (Reprinted with permission from Kumar P, Shen Q, Pivetti CD, Lee ES, Wu MH, Yuan SY. Molecular mechanisms of endothelial hyperpermeability: implications in inflammation. *Expert Rev Mol Med.* 2009;11:1-20.)

(used as a marker of intravascular fluid volume) remain unchanged whether or not supplemental albumin is given.[26,27]

In healthy people, albumin is the main determinant of COP. However, in critically ill patients, there is a low correlation between serum albumin concentration and COP. Instead, in critically ill patients, there is a stronger relationship between COP and total protein concentration. This difference in the relative contribution of albumin to COP may be attributable to elevations in acute-phase reactant proteins or immunoglobulins during states of acute illness. Therefore, in critically ill patients, hypoalbuminemia does not necessarily correlate with edema formation[6,28] and may explain why the use of albumin supplementation is ineffective in changing the course of the critically ill state of edema, as well as outcome. Typically, as the acute disease process improves and endothelial dysfunction recovers, patients improve with or without administration of supplemental albumin.[6,29] In fact, in the Cochrane meta-analysis, the subgroup of critically ill patients who received exogenous albumin in states of sepsis, burns, and hypoalbuminemia suggested an increase in mortality in these groups of patients with the use of exogenous albumin. The exceptions to this finding were in clinical settings in which the low albumin was not attributable to redistribution, but occurred after acute blood loss or loss of other protein-rich fluid during surgery.[29]

Unique Features of Water Homeostasis in the Neonatal Population

Changes in Body Water Composition in the Neonate

Neonates must make a transition from the fluid-filled fetal environment to the relatively dry extrauterine world. Remarkably, the majority of this transition occurs over a few minutes in the immediate postnatal life. As a result, there are several challenges to fluid regulation unique to this time of life.

As noted previously, a full-term newborn is 75% TBW with 40% of the TBW contained in the extracellular fluid (ECF) compartment. This proportion is significantly different than in adults, in whom the TBW concentration is reduced to 60% of total body weight and water in the ECF compartment is only 20% of total body weight. The difference between a preterm infant and an adult is even more dramatic. In babies born between 26 and 31 weeks' gestational age, the TBW is approximately 80% to 85% of total body weight, with 65% of body weight from water in the extracellular compartment.

Immediately after birth, the body water mass rapidly declines, mainly because of a decrease in ECF volume as it changes from its postnatal value of 45% of TBW to 30% by 3 months of age. This initial rapid decline in ECF volume is followed by a more gradual decline until age 10 years, when the adult ECF value of 20% total body weight is achieved.[8,30]

In healthy babies, there is a fairly rapid loss of extracellular isotonic fluid. This fluid loss is mainly from the intestinal compartment, and it is evidenced by the expected postnatal weight loss over the first few weeks of life. Infants who do not have an early negative fluid balance often demonstrate RDS. Contraction of the extracellular compartment is facilitated partly by secretion of atrial natriuretic peptide, which is produced by the cells of the myocardium in response to atrial stretch.[31] This occurs in the immediate postnatal period secondary to the dramatic decrease in pulmonary vascular resistance that occurs as the lung is inflated and alveolar gas tensions change. The pulmonary vasculature for the first time accepts the entire cardiac output, delivering it to and stretching the left atria.

Solute Balance in Healthy Neonates

Healthy neonates have an innate ability to excrete sodium. This allows them to maintain an isotonic loss of fluid with the postnatal contraction of the ECF compartment. In addition, neonates have the ability to increase their excretion of sodium in response to the administration of a sodium load. When the contraction of the extracellular compartment is complete, a state of positive sodium balance is reached. This allows neonates to retain the sodium necessary for appropriate growth.[30]

A relatively low albumin concentration in both term and preterm infants is a normal finding in the newborn period, and it does not appear to be associated with the formation of edema.[6,32] Mean values of albumin concentration at birth increase from 1.9 g/dL in infants of gestational ages less than 30 weeks to 3.1 g/dL at term. There is a postnatal increase in serum albumin concentration of approximately 15% in the first 3 weeks of life regardless of the gestational age of the infant. Greenough et al.[33] administered albumen to premature neonates (24–34 weeks' gestational age) at 7 days of age in an attempt to increase serum albumin concentration and promote a diuresis. The investigators' hypothesis was that this therapy would improve pulmonary function by decreasing lung fluid. They observed that compared with the placebo control infants, the albumin-treated infants demonstrated higher serum albumin concentrations, a negative water balance, and weight loss. However, no differences between groups were noted in the amount of ventilator support required.[33] In another study examining the effect of albumin supplementation of parenteral nutrition in preterm infants with RDS, the treatment group demonstrated improved weight gain and blood pressure, but failed to show any benefit in the duration of mechanical ventilation, time of requirement for supplemental oxygen, or time to full enteral feeding. There was also no difference in the incidence of necrotizing enterocolitis or intraventricular hemorrhage between the two groups.[34]

Resistance to the Effect of Arginine Vasopressin in Neonates

Neonatal kidneys demonstrate resistance to the effect of AVP, impairing the ability of this patient population to concentrate urine in response to even very high levels of exogenous vasopressin.[35] The observation of increased urinary excretion of AQP2 (a marker of AQP activity) during the first 2 to 3 postnatal weeks suggested that a deficiency of AQP2 was associated with the impaired ability to concentrate urine during the first few weeks of postnatal life. Subsequent studies, however, have demonstrated that both dehydration and DDAVP (desmopressin) administration appropriately stimulate production of AQP2 in infants' kidneys even during the first 2 to 3 weeks of life.[10]

Current evidence indicates that the inability of immature kidneys to maximally concentrate urine is attributable to multiple deficiencies in several steps in the AVP transduction pathway, including:

- Prostaglandin E_2 (PGE_2)-induced upregulation of a Gi (inhibitory) protein, which results in inhibitory feedback decreasing the production of cAMP. Because cAMP production is a necessary step for AVP-stimulated production of AQP2, enhanced PGE_2 stimulation of inhibiting G proteins will decrease the responsiveness of the kidneys to the effects of the AVP.
- High levels of phosphodiesterase in the cells of the infant collecting duct, which lead to rapid degradation of cAMP.
- Low concentration of urea and sodium in the infant medullary interstitium limit the osmotic gradient available for water reabsorption. This reduced gradient in infants is likely a result of low dietary protein, low expression of urea transporters, and low rates of sodium absorption from the ascending loop of Henle.[10]

The limited ability to concentrate urine in the immediate postnatal period may serve to benefit neonates in making the transition to extrauterine life because it promotes the rapid clearing of the excess extracellular pulmonary fluid.

It is important to note that neonates have intact pituitary production of AVP and only a diminished, not absent, renal response to this hormone. Therefore, even in the neonatal period, an underfilled intravascular compartment is associated with high circulating AVP. This high-AVP state may place hospitalized neonates at risk for water retention. If these patients receive hypotonic intravenous or hypotonic enteral fluids as is typical in this age group, hyponatremia can occur.

True SIADH, although possible in the neonatal population, is uncommon. A low serum sodium concentration during stress states, as in the postoperative period, is often the result of unrecognized intravascular volume depletion with appropriate AVP water retention and hypotonic fluid administration rather than SIADH. These aspects of neonatal water and solute management can be challenging to clinicians because it is difficult to recognize inadequate intravascular volume in this age group. In investigations of acutely ill infants and children, as few as one-third of subjects demonstrated overt signs of dehydration.[30]

Increase in Vascular Endothelial Growth Factor Expression

Vascular endothelial growth factor (VEGF) may be associated with the tendency of neonates to retain water (Fig. 17.2).[32] Newborns and young infants are more likely to retain fluid in response to stimuli such as cardiopulmonary bypass compared with older children and adults. Similarly, the lungs of neonates are more susceptible to alveolar edema in response to infectious and chemical injury. In the first month of life, full-term neonates have higher plasma levels of VEGF, which gradually decrease to the normal values within the first few months after birth.[34,36] The increased baseline serum level of VEGF has been implicated as part of the cause of the edema in

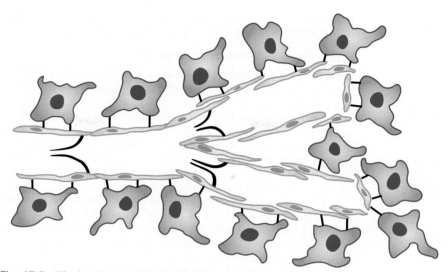

Fig. 17.2   The lymphatic endothelial cells attach directly to the extracellular matrix and surrounding cells via anchoring filaments. Valves prevent lymph reflux to promote unidirectional lymph propulsion. Note the extensive overlap of adjacent endothelial cells in lymphatic capillaries. (Modified with permission from Butler MG, Isogai S, Weinstein BM. Lymphatic development. *Birth Defects Res C Embryo Today.* 2009;87[Part C]: 222-231.)

neonates after cardiopulmonary bypass.[37] Further studies are necessary to delineate the role of VEGF in neonatal edema.

Special Circumstances in the Neonatal Population

Preterm Neonates

Newborn preterm neonates have a limited ability to excrete sodium. Although they can increase sodium excretion in response to a sodium load, they still have a tendency toward a positive sodium balance. Even with "maintenance" sodium intake (1–3 mEq/kg/day), preterm neonates are often in a state of positive sodium balance. When water losses exceed intake, their relative inability to excrete sodium will result in hypernatremia. If water intake is liberalized, the serum osmolality will be maintained at the expense of expansion of the ECF compartment. Expansion of the ECF compartment superimposed on a preexisting state of impaired diuresis may be the reason that in the immediate postnatal period, sodium supplementation of preterm neonates is associated with a worse respiratory outcome with an increased incidence of BPD.[31,38] Early fluid management of these patients should allow isotonic contraction of the extracellular compartment, with a brief period of negative sodium and water balance.

Edema After Indomethacin Closure of Patent Ductus Arteriosus

The use of indomethacin to close patent ductus arteriosus (PDA) has become common in the neonatal population. After indomethacin treatment, infants often go through a state of fluid retention. The mechanism of this effect relates to AQP2 metabolism and its regulation by PGE_2. As discussed previously, the insertion of AQP2 into the apical membrane of the collecting duct within the kidney occurs through a cAMP second messenger system. The absorptive effect of the AVP-stimulated increase in AQP2 insertion into the apical membrane of the collecting duct is regulated and counterbalanced by the effect of PGE_2. PGE_2 binding to the EP3 receptor activates the inhibitory G_i protein, which decreases cAMP generation, thereby decreasing the cAMP-dependent insertion of AQP2 into the collecting duct. This results in an increase excretion of water in the urine. Indomethacin and the other nonsteroidal antiinflammatory drugs decrease PGE production and therefore cause a loss of the counterbalancing inhibitory effect of the PGE$_2$. This leads to an unopposed upregulation of the AQP2 channels with enhanced fluid reabsorption.[8,10]

Pulmonary Edema in Neonates

Compromised lung water clearance is a prominent feature of neonatal RDS and BPD. The pulmonary edema can lead to respiratory failure by impairing respiratory mechanics and causing ventilation–perfusion mismatching.

Similar to all capillary beds, the mechanism of edema formation in the pulmonary vasculature is the result of either increased permeability of the pulmonary vasculature or an increase in the capillary hydrostatic pressure. Clinicians therefore often classify patients based on the primary mechanism associated with the disease. Often, however, it is difficult to make a clear assignment to one of these two categories because each primary mechanism has features of the other.

Of the two primary types, high-permeability edema is frequently more difficult to manage. A breakdown in capillary endothelial tight junctions and the alveolar epithelial barrier leads to the development of protein-rich alveolar edema. High-permeability edema often occurs as the result of an inflammatory insult, and it is typically seen in acute lung injury. Inflammation, the most likely cause of the breakdown in the endothelial–epithelial barrier, very often causes myocardial dysfunction as well.[39]

Cardiogenic pulmonary edema is a result of acute or chronic myocardial or valvular dysfunction, causing increased left ventricular end-diastolic volume and pressure, which then leads to increased pulmonary venous and capillary hydrostatic pressures.[22] Studies of adults have shown that the respiratory gas exchange abnormalities present in the setting of cardiogenic pulmonary edema is worse than predicted simply by the perturbations in the Starling capillary fluid relationship. West and Mathieu-Costello[40] have demonstrated that in the presence of conditions that can increase the pulmonary capillary pressure, the pulmonary capillary walls undergo structural changes. These structural changes result in endothelial and alveolar epithelial disruption as well as increased capillary permeability known as *capillary stress fracture*. The end result of this process is the development of high-permeability pulmonary edema,[40] causing the endothelial permeability to increase. Similar capillary stress fractures can also occur as a result of pulmonary arterial hypertension and in response to elevated alveolar pressures that can sometimes occur during mechanical ventilation. VEGF levels are increased in patients with cardiogenic pulmonary edema and may play a role in its production.[22,41]

Several developmental changes may place neonates at risk for pulmonary edema. For example, in fetuses, the pulmonary endothelial intracellular junctions are fenestrated. By comparison, in adults, the endothelial cells are more tightly joined, creating an intact barrier. The higher endothelial permeability observed in fetuses is likely attributable to the combined actions of lower blood oxygen tensions, as well as a high level of circulating endothelin-1, VEGF, and angiotensin II. Each of these factors creates a tendency to increase vascular permeability. Additionally, nitric oxide (NO), which has been shown to prevent endothelial leakage in the lung, is produced in lower amounts in premature neonates. NO production in the pulmonary vasculature increases as fetuses approach term, subsequently reaching a maximum concentration at age 2 to 3 days.[42,43] Finally, various scaffolding proteins in the pulmonary endothelium, important for endothelial barrier function, change at birth, contributing to the perinatal changes in vascular permeability.[42]

The pulmonary endothelial cells contain microdomains of anionic charge and glycoconjugate specificity located on cell organelles that are responsible for the transport of water, small solutes, and other macromolecules. Mills and Haworth[44] demonstrated that alterations within these domains, rather than the intercellular junctions, have the biggest impact on the change in pulmonary capillary endothelial permeability during the first week of life. Transport of water and small solutes are associated primarily with areas of anionic charge. They demonstrated that in newborn pigs, a greater proportion of the endothelial plasmalemma and its vesicles had anionic charge, suggesting greater transport of fluid into the interstitium. By 1 week of life, the composition of the pulmonary capillary endothelium had altered and was similar to that seen in adults.[44] Neonates are susceptible to pulmonary edema until the maturational changes in these factors that regulate endothelial permeability are complete.

This tendency for neonates to develop pulmonary edema is even greater in preterm neonates. As stated previously, the switch in prenatal ion transport in the fetal airway epithelium from Cl⁻ secretion to Na⁺ absorption plays a significant role in the transition from lung liquid secretion to lung liquid reabsorption. The Na⁺ absorption is facilitated primarily from the amiloride sensitive epithelial sodium channels (ENaCs). This transition is necessary for postnatal adaption to air breathing. Compared with neonates born at gestational ages greater than 30 weeks, the stable maximal baseline nasal potential difference, a surrogate marker for ENaC activity, was lower in infants born at gestational ages less than 30 weeks. Thus, although preterm infants do demonstrate the same transition from Cl⁻ secretion to Na⁺ absorption as full-term infants do, the ENaC activity, which is necessary to facilitate lung fluid clearance, is reduced in preterm neonates compared with term neonates.[45]

Respiratory Distress Syndrome and Bronchopulmonary Dysplasia

Inadequate lung water clearance may cause lung edema in both neonatal RDS and in BPD. At birth, the pulmonary epithelium, which was secreting water into the airway during fetal life, must rapidly begin water absorption. This functional change involves an upregulation of the AQPs, specifically AQP4, and an upregulation of epithelial cell membrane sodium–potassium ATPase and sodium channels. The latter epithelial membrane compounds establish the osmotic gradients needed to drive the water movement through the AQPs. In most healthy infants, the majority of the lung water present before birth is cleared mechanically in the first minutes of life as the baby fills the alveolar sacs with air. The rest of the water remains in the lungs to be cleared over the first several postnatal days. Premature infants often seem to lack the ability to clear this excess fluid from the lungs, which contributes to the pathogenesis RDS and BPD in this patient population. A long-noted clinical observation is that diuresis precedes the improvement in respiratory function from acute RDS, and therapeutic diuretics improve outcome in chronic BPD.[10,16,30]

Several investigators have speculated that impaired clearance of pulmonary fluid in premature infants is attributable to a unique feature of the AQP3 water channel. AQP3, which has been localized to the type II pneumocyte, is pH sensitive. Acidification of the ECF decreases the water permeability of these channels. Thus acidosis caused by impaired oxygen delivery or poor ventilation in a premature infant with RDS leads to an impaired ability to clear the alveolar fluid through AQP3.[8,14]

In addition to the AQPs, other channels play important roles in the clearance of lung fluid in the perinatal period. In fetuses, active secretion of chloride ions (Cl⁻) across the pulmonary epithelium generates the osmotic force that causes water to move from the lung microcirculation into the future airspaces of the lungs. Several days before birth, the Cl⁻ secretion decreases, and Na⁺ uptake by the lung epithelium increases. Lung fluid follows the sodium, causing the fluid from the lung lumen to move into the interstitial space and then into the bloodstream or lymphatic system.[46]

Because the transition within the lungs from the state of secretion to that of absorption takes place a few days before birth, preterm delivery as well as operative delivery without labor are both associated with increased fluid in the pulmonary airspaces. This hypothesis is supported in a rabbit animal model investigation demonstrating that lung water content is 25% greater after preterm delivery compared with term delivery. In addition, the term rabbits born after the onset of labor had less water in their lungs than did rabbits that were delivered operatively without prior onset of labor.[46]

Recent studies have identified amiloride sensitive sodium channels (ENaCs) on the apical surface of the airway epithelium, which appear to be critical in the process of lung fluid clearance. In human fetal lungs, these ENaC subunits are present in the earliest stages of lung development but at lower concentrations than observed in

17

mature fetuses. In preterm infants, there is a significant decrease in the β subunit of the ENaC during the first day of life. The resultant impairment of neonatal lung fluid clearance that results from this decrease in the β subunit may contribute to respiratory distress often seen in these infants.[47] The observation that both term neonates with transient tachypnea of the newborn and older infants with BPD have decreased levels of amiloride-sensitive N-PD (nasal potential difference, a correlate for ENaC activity) support the relationship between ENaC activity and lung fluid clearance.[45,48] Additionally, glucocorticoids, which when given antenatally decrease the incidence of RDS, cause an upregulation of all three ENaC subunits.

Although surfactant deficiency has been implicated as the primary pathology of RDS, it is also likely that the factors that impair fluid clearance from the lung outlined above play a prominent role in the pathogenesis of this condition.[47,49] Fluid management in newborn infants with acute respiratory failure should be undertaken, keeping in mind that these infants are at great risk for expansion of the ECW. Therefore, routine sodium supplementation and excessive parenteral fluid administration should be carefully managed in infants with respiratory distress until postnatal diuresis and natriuresis are observed.[30]

Fluid Retention After Cardiopulmonary Bypass

Cardiopulmonary bypass in infants and children is associated with a generalized disturbance of vascular permeability with significant edema formation as well as effusions. This can lead to a state of extravascular fluid accumulation with severe edema, secondary intravascular volume depletion, and significant organ dysfunction. The basis of this syndrome is thought to be a systemic inflammatory response caused by a mixture of stimuli, including cardiopulmonary bypass circuit–induced complement activation, circulatory shock, and endotoxemia.[37,50] Symptoms of multiple-organ dysfunction such as delayed myocardial recovery, a need for respiratory support, and renal and hepatic abnormalities, are more pronounced in patients with higher degrees of postbypass fluid retention. A longer length of stay postoperatively in the intensive care unit is also associated with a higher fluid retention rate.[51]

In contrast to the generalized edema caused by inflammatory states from other etiologies such as sepsis, the microvascular permeability that occurs after cardiopulmonary bypass may begin to resolve within hours after the surgery.[51] The rapid reversibility of this state suggests that bradykinin, which rapidly and reversibly increases vascular permeability by receptor-mediated endothelial cell contraction and intercellular gap formation, is the primary mediator responsible for this state. In fact, one study demonstrated approximately three times higher plasma concentrations of bradykinin in neonates, infants, and children with higher fluid retention rates after cardiopulmonary bypass. In this context, contact activation of Hageman factor with subsequent formation of prekallikrein and kallikrein, as well as the direct release of bradykinin from kininogens present in mast cells through the activity of proteases such as tryptase, can be implicated as a major cause of the increased bradykinin level. Additionally, bypassing the pulmonary circulation decreases the exposure of the blood to angiotensin-converting enzyme located on the pulmonary endothelium, which typically inactivates bradykinin. The end result is that cardiopulmonary bypass is associated with both an increase in bradykinin production and a decrease in its degradation.[51] In another study, it was found that there was a strong correlation between postcardiopulmonary bypass fluid retention and preoperative elevated levels of VEGF. Although an underlying reason for this elevation in VEGF in this patient population was not identified, the positive correlation with increased fluid retention has been noted.[37]

Although both these studies implicate different mediators as the underlying cause of the increased state of fluid retention, both studies demonstrated a significant association between younger age and greater degrees of postbypass fluid retention. In both studies, almost all patients operated on in the neonatal period demonstrated greater degrees of postbypass fluid retention. Although the underlying cause for this difference based on age is unclear, it is important for clinicians treating neonates after cardiopulmonary bypass to be aware of this increased incidence of postbypass

CHAPTER 18

Kidney Injury in the Neonate

Myda Khalid, MD, Sharon P. Andreoli, MD

Introduction

Acute kidney injury (AKI; previously known as acute renal failure) and chronic kidney disease (CKD; previously known as chronic renal failure) in neonates is a very common problem, and there are many different causes of kidney injury in newborns (Table 18.1). Although many cases of AKI can resolve with return of kidney function to normal, some causes of AKI result in permanent kidney injury that is apparent immediately. Others may result in kidney disease years after the initial insult. It is well known that kidney diseases such as kidney dysplasia, congenital abnormalities of the kidney and genitourinary tract, and cortical necrosis can lead to CKD. In contrast, it has been thought in the past that AKI caused by hypoxic ischemic and nephrotoxic insults was reversible with return of kidney function to normal. However, recent studies have demonstrated that hypoxic and ischemic insults can result in physiologic and morphologic alterations in the kidney that can lead to kidney disease at a later time.[1,2] Thus, as will be discussed in more detail later, AKI in neonates from any cause is a risk factor for later development of CKD.[1-3]

In addition it is becoming well recognized that small-for-gestational-age and premature infants both have a lower nephron mass at birth, which in turn predisposes them to the development of CKD over time.[4,5] In a study evaluating six young adults for proteinuria, renal biopsy revealed focal segmental glomerulosclerosis (FSGS). These patients were all premature infants born between 22 and 30 weeks of gestation

Table 18.1 ETIOLOGY OF ACUTE KIDNEY INJURY IN THE NEONATE

Prerenal Injury
Decreased true intravascular volume
 Dehydration
 Gastrointestinal losses
 Salt wasting kidney or adrenal disease
 Central or nephrogenic diabetes insipidus
 Third space losses (sepsis, traumatized tissue)
Decreased effective intravascular volume blood volume
 Congestive heart failure
 Pericarditis, cardiac tamponade

Intrinsic Kidney Disease
Acute tubular necrosis
 Ischemic/hypoxic insults
 Drug induced
  Aminoglycosides
  Intravascular contrast
  Nonsteroidal antiinflammatory drugs
 Toxin mediated
  Endogenous toxins
   Rhabdomyolysis, hemoglobinuria
Interstitial nephritis
 Drug induced—antibiotics, anticonvulsants
 Idiopathic
Vascular lesions
 Cortical necrosis
 Renal artery thrombosis
 Renal venous thrombosis
Infectious causes
 Sepsis
 Pyelonephritis

Obstructive Uropathy
Obstruction in a solitary kidney
Bilateral ureteral obstruction
Urethral obstruction

Congenital Kidney Diseases
Dysplasia/hypoplasia
Cystic kidney diseases
 Autosomal recessive polycystic kidney disease
 Autosomal dominant polycystic kidney disease
 Cystic dysplasia
In utero exposure to ACEI or ARBs

ACEI, Angiotensin converting enzyme inhibitor; *ARBs,* angiotensin II receptor blockers.

with a mean birth weight of 1054 g and did not have any other risk factors for renal disease.[6] In another study analyzing 5352 children aged 12 to 15, it was found that those born with very low or low birth weight had a higher risk of developing hypertension and a lower glomerular filtration rate (GFR) at later points in time.[7]

AKI is classified into prerenal, intrinsic, and postrenal injury. In addition, the insults may be acquired in the prenatal, perinatal, and/or postnatal period. In newborns, kidney injury may have a prenatal onset in congenital diseases such as kidney dysplasia with or without obstructive uropathy and in genetic diseases such as autosomal recessive polycystic kidney disease. Newborns with congenital and genetic kidney diseases that have a prenatal onset may have stigmata of Potter syndrome caused by in utero oliguria with resultant oligohydramnios. Newborns with Potter syndrome may have life-threatening pulmonary insufficiency, a flattened nasal bridge, low-set ears, joint contractures, and other orthopedic anomalies caused by fetal constraint as a result of the oligohydramnios.

AKI and CKD may also result from the in utero exposure of the developing kidneys to agents that may interfere with nephrogenesis such as angiotensin-converting enzyme (ACE) inhibitors, angiotensin II receptor blockers (ARBs), and perhaps cyclooxygenase (COX) inhibitors.[8-11] Exposure of a developing fetus to ACE inhibitors and ARBs has been associated with kidney dysfunction that is both acute and chronic, undermineralization of the calvarial bones, and in some cases fetal demise.[10,11] Exposure to ACE inhibitors or ARBs is detrimental for kidney development at any point during the pregnancy; however the most damaging effects are noted with exposure during the second and third trimesters[9]; however AKI in newborns is also commonly acquired in the postnatal period because of hypoxic ischemic injury and toxic insults. As in older children, hospital-acquired AKI in newborns is frequently multifactorial in origin.[3,12-18] Given that nephrogenesis proceeds through approximately 34 weeks' gestation, ischemic or hypoxic and toxic insults in the developing kidney in a premature newborn can result not only in AKI, but also in long-term complications secondary to interrupted nephrogenesis. Whether kidney disease is congenital or acquired, it is important to appropriately manage the fluid and electrolyte imbalances and other side effects of kidney injury in newborns.

Definition

Currently, there is no uniform definition of AKI in pediatric or neonatal patients, and AKI is defined in multiple ways, but the majority of definitions of AKI in use involve a change in the serum creatinine level. In neonates, AKI is frequently defined by a change in the serum creatinine according to gestational age. AKI is characterized by an increase in the blood concentration of creatinine and nitrogenous waste products, a decrease in the GFR, and the inability of the kidney to appropriately regulate fluid and electrolyte homeostasis. However, creatinine is an inaccurate marker of kidney function in the neonate for reasons discussed below.

The definition of AKI in pediatric patients has been quite variable. A new classification system called the RIFLE criteria (risk for renal dysfunction, injury to the kidney, failure of kidney function, loss of kidney function, and end-stage kidney disease) has been proposed as a standardized classification of AKI in adults and has been adapted for pediatric patients.[19,20] The pediatric RIFLE (pRIFLE) was found to better classify pediatric AKI and to reflect the course of AKI in children admitted to intensive care units (ICUs).[19] In a study of pediatric patients of whom 36% were neonates, AKI as classified by pRIFLE criteria was shown to correlate with mechanical ventilation, metabolic acidosis, and hypoxia in the neonate.[21] In the pRIFLE criteria, Risk is classified as a reduction in estimated creatinine clearance (eCCl) by 25% or a drop in urine output to less than 0.5 mL/kg per hour for 8 hours. Injury is classified as a drop in eCCl by 50% with urine output reduced by less than 0.5 mL/kg per hour for 16 hours. Failure is when eCCl is reduced by 75% or eCCl is less than 35 mL/min per 1.73 m² with urine output being less than 0.3 mL/kg per hour for 24 hours or anuria for 12 hours. Loss is defined by the failure stage lasting for longer than 4 weeks. End-stage renal disease is when there is persistent failure for longer than 3 months.

Although a decrease in urine output is a common clinical manifestation of AKI, many forms of AKI are associated with normal urine output.[1,3] Whereas newborns with prerenal injury, AKI caused by hypoxic/ischemic insults, or cortical necrosis are more likely to have oligo/anuria (urine output <1.0 mL/kg per hour), newborns with nephrotoxic kidney insults, including aminoglycoside nephrotoxicity and contrast nephropathy, are more likely to have AKI with normal urine output. The morbidity and mortality of nonoliguric AKI are substantially less than oliguric AKI.[12-14,16-18]

Nephron formation in the fetus begins at 5 weeks of gestation with urine production starting at around 10 weeks of gestation.[22] The fetal urine contributes to the development of amniotic fluid, and the production of urine increases with gestational age. Nephrogenesis is complete by approximately 34 to 36 weeks of gestation.[22] Therefore, preterm infants born before 34 weeks of gestation have a

18

D

lower GFR. GFR doubles in the first 2 weeks of life for the term and preterm infant secondary to increased renal blood flow, a higher mean arterial pressure and increased glomerular surface area, and permeability resulting in a subsequent drop in creatinine by about 50%.[22]

Immediately after birth, the serum creatinine in the newborn is a reflection of maternal kidney function due to placental transfer of creatinine and cannot be used as a measure of kidney function.[15,16] In full-term healthy newborns, the GFR rapidly increases and the serum creatinine declines to about 0.4 to 0.6 mg/dL at about 2 weeks of age, while the serum creatinine declines at a slower rate in premature infants.[14–16] In very-low-birth-weight (VLBW) infants with a gestational age around 28 weeks, the renal function improves even more slowly compared to infants born at a gestational age around 32 weeks.[23] It is important to note that creatinine clearance calculated using urine collections in preterm infants typically underestimates the GFR because of low creatinine excretion and tubular reabsorption of creatinine by immature renal tubules.[24] Therefore, caution must be used when using creatinine alone as a marker for kidney injury in preterm infants due to a risk of possible over diagnosis of AKI. It is also important to note that the use of serum creatinine as a determinate of kidney insufficiency requires that the gestational age at time of birth and the postnatal age, as well as maternal factors, are taken into account.

Additional disadvantages of using serum creatinine are that it lags behind changes in GFR and varies with muscle mass, hydration status, and gender.[25] It is clear that a change in the serum creatinine is a rough measure of changes in kidney function and better determinates of real-time kidney renal function are needed. The development, testing, and successful implementation of therapeutic strategies in AKI is going to require the development of sensitive biomarkers so that therapy can be initiated in a timely manner.

This chapter reviews biomarkers of AKI, the epidemiology of kidney injury in newborns, the common causes of AKI and CKD in newborns with a focus on hypoxic ischemic and nephrotoxic insults, management of AKI and CKD in newborns, and long-term follow-up of neonates who have had AKI.

Biomarkers for Acute Kidney Injury

Recent studies have investigated the use of early biomarkers of AKI so that AKI can be recognized before changes in the serum creatinine occur.[17–21] Blood serum and urine biomarkers have been identified and are currently being studied. Some of the biomarkers under investigation include plasma and urine neutrophil gelatinase-associated lipocalin (NGAL) and cystatin C (CysC), interleukin-18 (IL-18), kidney injury molecule-1 (KIM-1), urine osteopontin, urinary epidermal growth factor (EGF), and uromodulin.[18,26] NGAL has shown promise in children undergoing cardiac surgery as an early maker of AKI. Studies in premature and term infants note that urine NGAL is detectable and correlates with birth weight and gestational age; however, levels were increased in neonates with normal renal function.[21,27,28]

Serum CysC is emerging as a promising marker of GFR. CysC is a low-molecular-weight protein that is produced in all human cells with a nucleus, remains independent of muscle mass, is filtered by the glomerulus, and is completely degraded in the tubular walls.[29] CysC production is fairly constant from 1 to 50 years of age.[29] Abitbol et al. found that CysC was a better biomarker than serum Cr in the assessment of GFR in premature infants.[30] In their study, they note that for term infants using a GFR calculation utilizing the combination of CysC and Cr equation by Zappitelli et al. provided a better estimation of GFR compared to Cr or CysC alone.[28,31]

McCaffrey et al. confirmed the correlation of serum CysC and serum NGAL with AKI in children admitted to the pediatric ICU (PICU) without sepsis.[32] Hanna et al. evaluated early urinary biomarkers of AKI in preterm infants less than 32 weeks of gestation and found that infants who went on to develop AKI had higher urinary NGAL, CysC, and osteopontin and a lower urinary EGF and uromodulin. They also noted the urinary biomarkers changed 24 hours prior to the change in serum creatinine.[26] Askenazi et al. also performed a prospective study on 113 VLBW premature infants and had similar findings. In their study, infants with AKI had higher levels of urine NGAL, CysC, osteopontin, clusterin, and alpha glutathione S-transferase and lower urine levels of EGF and uromodulin.[33]

There is also the emerging field of metabolomics in pediatric nephrology which refers to the evaluation of metabolites and their changes in a system due to genetic or environmental stimuli.[34] Metabolites and their patterns can serve as a signature of real-time physiologic and pathophysiologic states in the body, and hence both pattern recognition and metabolite identification can allow them to be used as biomarkers.[35] Metabolomics certainly appears to hold promise for early disease recognition and possibly targeted intervention and treatment in the future.

Epidemiology and Incidence of Kidney Injury in Neonates

AKI in neonates is fairly common and is a major contributor to morbidity and mortality.[25] The precise incidence and prevalence of kidney disease in the newborn are unknown in part due to the lack of a standard definition of AKI and variation in practice patterns when screening for AKI. Studies also vary greatly when assessing AKI based on cut offs for serum creatinine and urine output, making it challenging to compare multiple studies.[36]

Although the precise incidence and prevalence of kidney disease in newborns is unknown, several studies have demonstrated that kidney injury is common in neonatal ICUs (NICUs) and PICUs.[12–21,25,27,28,37–47] The incidence of kidney disease ranged from 6% to 24% of newborns in NICUs and is particularly common in neonates who have undergone cardiac surgery.[14,17,18,42,46] In a prospective study by Askenazi et al., the incidence of AKI in very low birth weight infants within the first 2 weeks of life was found to be 25%.[33]

Neonates with severe asphyxia had a high incidence of AKI; AKI is less common in neonates with moderate asphyxia, and in one study the AKI was nonoliguric, oliguric, and anuric in 60%, 25%, and 15%, respectively.[16] Other studies have demonstrated that a very low birth weight (VLBW; <1500 g), low Apgar score, patent ductus arteriosus (PDA), and maternal administration of antibiotics and nonsteroidal antiinflammatory drugs (NSAIDs) was associated with the development of AKI.[39] Additional studies have also shown that low Apgar score and maternal ingestion of NSAIDs is associated with decreased kidney function in preterm infants.[37,40] A recent study demonstrated that AKI was diagnosed in 56% of infants with perinatal asphyxia.[43]

Several very interesting studies have demonstrated that some newborns may have genetic risk factors for AKI. Polymorphism of the ACE gene or the angiotensin receptor gene with resultant alterations in activity of the renin-angiotensin system might play a role in the development of AKI.[48] In studies in newborns, polymorphisms of tumor necrosis factor α (TNF-α), IL-1b, IL-6, and IL-10 genes were investigated in newborns to determine if polymorphisms of these genes would lead to a more intense inflammatory response and predispose newborns to AKI.[49] The allelic frequency of the individual genes did not differ between newborns with AKI and those without AKI, but the carrier state of being a high TNF-α producer along with a low IL-6 producer was present in 26% of newborns who developed AKI compared with 6% of newborns who did not. The investigators suggested that the combination of these polymorphisms might lead to a greater inflammatory response and the development of AKI in neonates with infection.[49] As described below, future therapies for AKI might involve strategies to interrupt the inflammatory response. In other studies, the incidence of ACE I/D allele genotypes or the variants of the angiotensin I receptor gene did not differ in neonates with AKI compared with neonates without AKI, but they may be associated with PDA and heart failure and indirectly contribute to CKD.[48,50] AKI occurred more commonly in VLBW neonates carrying the heat shock protein 72 (1267) GG genetic variation, which is associated with low inducibility of heat shock protein 72.[51] Given the important role of heat shock proteins in ischemic kidney injury, these findings suggest that some neonates are more susceptible to ischemic injury.[52] Future studies of the genetic background of children at risk for AKI because of medication exposure, toxin exposure, ischemic hypoxic insults, or other insults will likely impact the management of children at risk for AKI and the management of AKI.

To better understand AKI in neonates the National Kidney Collaborative has recently been formed. The Neonatal Kidney Collaborative is a group comprised of neonatologists and nephrologists who have initiated the Assessment of Worldwide Acute Kidney injury Epidemiology in Neonates (AWAKEN) Study.[53] This will be the largest AKI study in neonates to date and will help determine if the Kidney Disease: Improving Global Outcomes (KDIGO) AKI definition in neonates can be used as an appropriate classification tool that could be associated/correlated with length of stay, outcomes, and mortality. The study will also assess the applicability of different definitions of AKI in the neonates. Another goal of the study is to determine how the fluid balance in the neonate relates to outcomes.

Etiology of Kidney Injury in Newborns

There are many different etiologies of AKI and CKD in the neonate (see Table 18.1), and the most common are related to prerenal mechanisms, including hypotension, hypovolemia, hypoxemia, perinatal and postnatal asphyxia, sepsis, and congenital anomalies of the kidney and urinary tract (CAKUT).[54,55]

Prerenal Injury

In prerenal injury, kidney function is decreased because of decreased kidney perfusion, but the kidney is intrinsically normal. Restoration of normal kidney perfusion results in a return of kidney function to normal; acute tubular necrosis (ATN) implies that the kidney has experienced intrinsic damage. However, the evolution of prerenal injury to intrinsic kidney injury is not sudden, and a number of compensatory mechanisms work together to maintain kidney perfusion when kidney perfusion is compromised.[56,57] When kidney perfusion is decreased, the afferent arteriole relaxes its vascular tone to decrease kidney vascular resistance and maintain kidney blood flow. Decreased kidney perfusion results in increased catecholamine secretion, activation of the renin-angiotensin system, and generation of prostaglandins. During kidney hypoperfusion, the intrarenal generation of vasodilatory prostaglandins, including prostacyclin, mediates vasodilatation of the kidney microvasculature to maintain kidney perfusion.[56,57] Administration of aspirin or NSAIDs can inhibit this compensatory mechanism and precipitate acute kidney insufficiency during kidney hypoperfusion. As discussed later, administration of indomethacin for closure of the PDA in premature newborns is associated with a substantial risk of kidney insufficiency.[58–62] It was originally thought that selective COX-2 inhibitors would be kidney-sparing, but it has been recognized that the selective COX-2 inhibitors can adversely affect kidney hemodynamics similar to the effects of nonselective COX inhibitors.[63,64] In addition, clinical use of selective COX-2 inhibitors has been associated with AKI in adult patients.[64] Similarly, when kidney perfusion pressure is low as in renal artery stenosis, the intraglomerular pressure necessary to drive filtration is partly mediated by increased intrarenal generation of angiotensin II to increase efferent arteriolar resistance.[56,65,66] Administration of ACE inhibitors in these conditions can eliminate the pressure gradient needed to drive filtration and precipitate AKI.[65,66] Thus, administration of medications that can interfere with compensatory mechanisms to maintain kidney perfusion can precipitate AKI in certain clinical circumstances.

Prerenal injury results from kidney hypoperfusion caused by true volume contraction or from a decreased effective blood volume.[56] Volume contraction results from hemorrhage, dehydration caused by gastrointestinal losses, salt-wasting kidney or adrenal diseases, central or nephrogenic diabetes insipidus, increased insensible losses, and in disease states associated with third-spaces losses such as sepsis, traumatized tissue, and capillary leak syndrome; decreased effective blood volume occurs when the true blood volume is normal or increased, but kidney perfusion is decreased because of diseases such as congestive heart failure and cardiac tamponade.[56]

Whether prerenal injury is caused by true volume depletion or decreased effective blood volume, correction of the underlying disturbance will return kidney function to normal.

The urine osmolality, urine sodium concentration, the fractional excretion of sodium (FENa), and renal failure index have all been proposed to be used to help differentiate prerenal injury from vasomotor nephropathy or ATN. This differentiation is based on the premise that the tubules are working appropriately in prerenal injury and are, therefore, able to conserve salt and water appropriately. In vasomotor nephropathy, the tubules have progressed to irreversible injury and are unable to appropriately conserve sodium.[42] During prerenal injury, the tubules are able to respond to decreased kidney perfusion by appropriately conserving sodium and water such that the urine osmolality is greater than 400 to 500 mOsm/kg H_2O, the urine sodium is less than 10 to 20 mEq/L, and the FENa is less than 1% in children. It has been noted, however, that there is an inverse correlation of FENa with gestational age.[67] Gallini et al. studied 83 premature infants who were grouped into four categories based on gestational age of less than 27 weeks, 27 to 28 weeks, 29 to 30 weeks, and 31 to 32 weeks and observed that the lower the gestational age the higher the urinary sodium.[67] Due to this phenomenon, it is recommended that for newborns and premature infants the corresponding values suggestive of kidney hypoperfusion are urine osmolality greater than 350 mOsm/kg H_2O, urine sodium less than 20 to 30 mEq/L, and FENa of less than 2.5%.[3,42] However, the use of these numbers to differentiate prerenal injury from ATN requires the patient to have normal tubular function initially. Although this may be the case in some pediatric patients, newborns, particularly premature newborns whose tubules are immature, may have kidney injury with urinary indices showing a higher urine sodium. The interpretation of the elevated urine sodium is challenging because based on the study by Gallini et al., this would be part of normal physiology.[67] Therefore, it is important to consider the state of the function of the tubules before the potential onset that might precipitate vasomotor nephropathy or ATN.

Acute Ischemic Kidney Injury

Ischemic AKI (also known as ATN) can evolve from prerenal injury if the insult is severe and sufficient enough to result in vasoconstriction and ATN. Recent studies suggest that the vasculature of the kidney may play a role in acute injury and chronic injury as well, and the endothelial cell has been identified as a target of injury. Peritubular capillary blood flow has been shown to be abnormal during reperfusion, and there is also loss of normal endothelial cell function in association with distorted peritubular pericapillary morphology and function.[68,69] The mechanism of cellular injury in hypoxic/ischemic AKI is not known, but alterations in endothelin (ET) or nitric oxide (NO) regulation of vascular tone, adenosine triphosphate (ATP) depletion and alterations in the cytoskeleton, changes in heat shock proteins, initiation of the inflammatory response, and the generation of reactive oxygen and nitrogen molecules may each play a role in cell injury.[68-85]

NO is a vasodilator produced from endothelial NO synthase (eNOS) and NO helps regulate vascular tone and blood flow in the kidneys.[73,74] Recent studies suggest that loss of normal eNOS function occurs after ischemic/hypoxic injury, which could precipitate vasoconstriction.[73] In contrast, inducible NO synthase (iNOS) activity increases after hypoxic/ischemic injury, and iNOS can participate in the generation of reactive oxygen and nitrogen molecules. Inducible NO synthase with the generation of toxic NO metabolites, including peroxynitrite, has been shown to mediate tubular injury in animal models of AKI.[74,81] ET peptides are potent vasoconstrictors that have also been shown to play a role in the pathogenesis of AKI in animal models.[84] In animal models of AKI in rats, circulating levels of ET-1 and tissue expression of ET-1 protein levels was substantially increased, and ET(A) and ET(B) receptor gene expression was also increased after ischemic injury.[82] ET receptor agonist for the A receptor has been shown to decrease AKI in animal models.[72] Thus, alterations in the balance of vasoconstrictive and vasostimulatory stimuli are likely to be involved in the pathogenesis of hypoxic/ischemic AKI.

An initial response to hypoxic/ischemic AKI is ATP depletion, which leads to a number of detrimental biochemical and physiologic responses, including disruption of the normal cytoskeletal organization with loss of the apical brush border and loss of polarity with Na^+, K^+-ATPase localized to the apical as well as the basolateral membrane.[85] This has been shown in several animal models of AKI and it has also been shown in human kidney allografts that loss of polarity with mislocation of Na^+, K^+-ATPase to apical membrane contributes to kidney dysfunction in transplanted kidneys.[78] Reactive oxygen molecules are also generated during reperfusion and can contribute to tissue injury.[70] Although tubular cells and endothelial cells are susceptible to injury by reactive oxygen molecules, studies have shown that endothelial cells are more sensitive to oxidant injury than tubular epithelial cells.[71] Other studies have shown an important role for heat shock protein in modifying the kidney response to ischemic injury, as well as playing a role in promoting recovery of the cytoskeleton after AKI.[83]

In children and neonates with multiorgan failure, the systemic inflammatory response is thought to contribute to AKI as well as other organ dysfunction by the activation of the inflammatory response, including increased production of cytokines and reactive oxygen molecules, activation of polymorphonuclear leukocytes (PMNs), and increased expression of leukocyte adhesion molecules.[79] Reactive oxygen molecules can be generated by several mechanisms, including activated PMNs, which may cause injury by the generation of reactive oxygen molecules, including superoxide anion, hydrogen peroxide, hydroxyl radical, hypochlorous acid, peroxynitrite, or by the release of proteolytic enzymes. Myeloperoxidase from activated PMNs converts hydrogen peroxide to hypochloruous acid, which may react with amine groups to form chloramines; each of these can oxidize proteins, DNA, and lipids, resulting in substantial tissue injury.[70,75] Leukocyte endothelial cell adhesion molecules have been shown to be unregulated in ATN, and administration of antiadhesion molecules can substantially decrease kidney injury in animal models of ATN.[77] As described later, several animal models have shown future therapies for hypoxic/ischemic AKI may involve manipulation of the inflammatory response. Studies in humans with AKI have demonstrated an increased evidence of oxidation of proteins, reflecting oxidant stress.[76]

In established ATN, the urinalysis may be unremarkable or demonstrate low-grade proteinuria and granular casts, and urine indices of tubular function demonstrate an inability to conserve sodium and water as described above. The creatinine typically increases by about 0.5 to 1.0 mg/dL (44.2–88.4 μmol/L) per day. Radiographic studies demonstrate kidneys of normal size with loss of corticomedullary differentiation, but a radionucleotide kidney scan with technetium–99-MAG3 (mercapto acetyl triglycine) or technetium–99-DTPA (diethylene-triamine-penta-acetic acid) will demonstrate normal or slightly decreased kidney blood flow with poor function and delayed accumulation of the radioisotope in the kidney parenchyma without excretion of the isotope in the collecting system (Fig. 18.1B).

In the past, it has been thought that the prognosis of ischemic AKI was good except in cases in which the insult was of sufficient severity to lead to vasculature injury and microthrombi formation with the subsequent development of cortical necrosis. However, recent studies demonstrate that chronic changes can occur and that such patients are at risk for later complications.[1,2] As discussed later, AKI before nephrogenesis is complete may also result in disrupted nephrogenesis and reduced nephron number.[86–90]

Hypothermia protocols are now frequently being used in neonates with severe hypoxic-ischemic events and have demonstrated improved neurologic outcomes. Do these protocols improve renal outcomes as well? Selewski et al. retrospectively evaluated 96 neonates who had undergone the hypothermia protocol and noted that 36 out of 96 (38%) infants had AKI.[91] The mortality was noted to be 14% in neonates with AKI vs. 3% in neonates without AKI.[91] In their study, the rate of AKI was the same in infants who received whole body cooling compared to infants who only underwent selective head cooling. Confirming previous studies, they noted that patients with AKI had longer days in the NICU as well as more days on mechanical

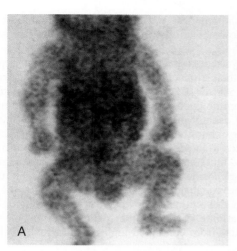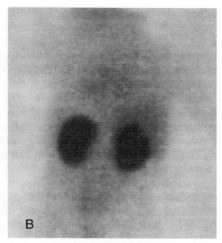

A

B

Fig. 18.1   Mag-3 renal scan in a newborn with (A) cortical necrosis and (B) acute tubular necrosis. Each scan is 4 hours after injection of isotope. (A) demonstrates no kidney parenchymal uptake of isotope in a neonate with cortical necrosis. (B) shows delayed uptake of isotope with parenchymal accumulation of isotope with little to no excretion of isotope into the collecting system. In a normally functioning kidney at 4 hours the isotope should have been excreted in the collecting system.

ventilation.[91] Interestingly, their study reflected a slightly lower rate of AKI compared to infants without the hypothermia protocol; however, given the small sample size, it is difficult to extrapolate these results to a larger cohort. Additional studies in this area will shed more light on the potential nephro-protective effect of the hypothermia protocols.

The recovery of the neonate and the recovery of kidney function depend on the underlying events which precipitated the ischemic/hypoxic insults. Studies also indicate that AKI contributes directly to the morbidity and mortality of neonates and children in the NICUs and PICUs.[25,44] In children who recover from ATN, the kidney function returns to normal, but the length of time before recovery is quite variable. Some children begin to recover kidney function within days of the onset of kidney injury, but recovery may not occur for several weeks in other children. Return of kidney function may be accompanied by a diuretic phase with excessive urine output at a time when the tubules have begun to recover from the insult, but have not recovered sufficiently to appropriately reabsorb solute and water. When the diuretic phase occurs during recovery, close attention to fluid and electrolyte balance is very important to ensure adequate fluid management to promote recovery from ATN and prevent additional kidney injury. As described below, long-term follow-up of newborns with AKI is warranted to evaluate for late complications.

Nephrotoxic Kidney Injury

Nephrotoxic AKI may result from the administration of a number of different medications as well as from indigenous compounds such as hemoglobinuria or myoglobinuria. Nephrotoxic AKI in newborns is commonly associated with aminoglycoside antibiotics, NSAIDs, intravascular contrast media, and amphotericin B; other medications have been implicated less commonly. It is important to note that AKI secondary to nephrotoxic medications is potentially avoidable and at minimum, the degree of AKI is modifiable.[92] While a single nephrotoxic medication increases the risk of AKI, the use of multiple nephrotoxic medications increases the risk exponentially more.[93] In addition, concomitant factors such as neonatal age, acuity of illness, and dosage and duration of medications all play a role in the degree of resulting AKI. In a recent study by Rhone et al. of nephrotoxic medication exposure in very low birth weight infants, the authors found that exposure to one or more nephrotoxic medications occurred in 87% of the infants.[94] The most common exposures were gentamicin (86%), indomethacin (43%), and vancomycin (25%).[94] They also noted that the greatest exposure occurred in the smallest and most immature infants as well as those suffering from AKI.[94] Below we will discuss some of the main drugs causing AKI in the neonate.

Aminoglycosides: Aminoglycosides remain one of the most commonly prescribed antibiotics in the NICU given their efficacy against gram-negative bacteria. They are excreted in the urine and 5% to 10% of the drug accumulates in the renal cortex. High concentrations of aminoglycosides can damage the proximal tubules.[95] Aminoglycoside nephrotoxicity usually presents with nonoliguric AKI with a urinalysis showing minimal urinary abnormalities. The incidence of aminoglycoside antibiotic nephrotoxicity is related to the dose and duration of the antibiotic therapy, as well as the level of kidney function before the initiation of aminoglycoside therapy. The etiology of aminoglycoside nephrotoxicity is thought to be related to the lysosomal dysfunction of proximal tubules and is reversible once the aminoglycoside antibiotics have been discontinued. However, after the aminoglycoside is discontinued, the serum creatinine may continue to increase for several days because of ongoing tubular injury from continued high parenchymal levels of the aminoglycoside.

Angiotensin Converting Enzyme Inhibitors: The renin-angiotensin-system (RAS) plays a significant role in renal development, and infants exposed prenatally to ACE inhibitors and angiotensin receptor blockers have been found to have profound renal function abnormalities.[96,97] Interruption of the RAS can result in abnormal renal development, oligohydramnios, renal failure, and pulmonary hypoplasia.[9,97] Exposure in the second and third trimesters has been found to cause more severe renal abnormalities compared to exposure in the first trimester. Outside of the genitourinary system, ACE inhibitors can also cause central nervous system abnormalities, sensorineural hearing loss, and cardiac abnormalities.[97,98] Typically, prenatal exposure to ACE inhibitors and ARBs tends to happen in women with absent or late prenatal care.[97] Given the harmful effects of these agents on kidney development, it may be prudent to limit the use of ACE inhibitors in neonates less than 34 weeks of gestation when nephron formation may potentially be ongoing. The use of ACE inhibitors in neonates can also result in AKI, which reassuringly is reversible with discontinuation of the medication.[99] Careful monitoring of intravascular volume and avoidance of simultaneous nephrotoxic medications should be done whenever possible to lower the risk of AKI.

NSAIDs: NSAIDs may also precipitate AKI by their effect on intrarenal hemodynamics.[56–64] Neonates have high levels of circulating prostaglandins which are involved in maintaining arteriolar vasodilation, renal blood flow, and renal water clearance.[100] Inhibition of prostaglandins, which occurs with NSAIDs, results in a decrease in renal blood flow and reduction in GFR.[100] Indomethacin therapy to promote closure of PDAs in premature neonates is associated with kidney dysfunction, including a 56% reduction in urinary flow rate, a 27% reduction in GFR, and a 66% reduction in free water clearance.[58,59] Other physiologic alterations after administration of indomethacin and ibuprofen include a decrease in urinary ET-1 and arginine vasopressin, along with a reduction in urinary sodium excretion and FENa.[62] Alterations in kidney function occur in approximately 40% of premature newborns who have received indomethacin, and such alterations are usually reversible.[60] In a large study of more than 2500 premature newborns treated with indomethacin to promote closure of the PDA, infants with preexisting kidney and electrolyte abnormalities and infants whose mothers had received indomethacin tocolysis or who had chorioamnionitis were at significantly increased risk for the development of kidney impairment.[61]

Vancomycin: Vancomycin has been implicated in nephrotoxicity in the neonates; however, some recent studies suggest that monotherapy with appropriate trough levels may not cause AKI.[101] The risk factors for the development of AKI in the setting of vancomycin use appear to be high trough levels, additional nephrotoxin use (such as NSAIDs), positive blood cultures, PDA, low birth weight, and severity of illness.[101,102] The exact mechanism of the injury remains unclear, but is likely related to oxidative injury and stress at the level of the proximal tubule based on animal models.[103]

Vascular Injury

Renal artery thrombosis and renal vein thrombosis will result in AKI if bilateral or if either occurs in a solitary kidney. Renal artery thrombosis is strongly associated with an umbilical artery line and a PDA.[104,105] In the setting of a renal arterial thrombosis, maternal anticardiolipin antibody and maternal lupus anticoagulant levels should be checked, and the neonate should be evaluated further to determine if prothrombotic disorders are present.[106] In addition to AKI, children may demonstrate hypertension, gross or microscopic hematuria, thrombocytopenia, and oliguria. In renal artery thrombosis, the initial ultrasound may appear normal or demonstrate minor abnormalities, but a renal scan will demonstrate little to no blood flow. The risk factors for renal vein thrombosis include birth asphyxia, maternal diabetes, volume contraction, disorders of coagulation, decreased vascular blood flow, increased blood viscosity, and increased serum osmolality.[107] In renal vein thrombosis, the ultrasound demonstrates an enlarged, swollen kidney, but the renal scan typically demonstrates decreased blood flow and function. Therapy should be aimed at limiting extension of the clot by removal of the umbilical arterial catheter, and anticoagulate or fibrinolytic therapy can be considered, particularly if the clot is large.[104,105]

Cortical necrosis is associated with hypoxic/ischemic insults due to perinatal anoxia, placenta abruption, and twin-twin or twin-maternal transfusions with resultant activation of the coagulation cascade.[108,109] Interestingly, intrauterine laser treatment in 18 sets of twins with twin-twin transfusion resulted in no long-term kidney impairment despite severe alterations of kidney function, including anuria and polyuria before the laser treatment.[110] Newborns with cortical necrosis usually have gross or microscopic hematuria and oliguria and may have hypertension as well. In addition to laboratory features of an elevated blood urea nitrogen (BUN) and creatinine, thrombocytopenia may also be present due to the microvascular injury. Radiographic features include a normal kidney ultrasound scan in the early phase, while ultrasound scans in the later phases may show that the kidney has undergone atrophy and has substantially decreased in size. A radionucleotide renal scan will show decreased to no perfusion with delayed or no function (see Fig. 18.1B), in contrast to delayed uptake of the radioisotope, which is observed in ATN (see Fig. 18.1A). The prognosis of cortical necrosis is worse than that of ATN. Children with cortical necrosis may have partial recovery or no recovery at all. Typically, children with cortical necrosis will need short- or long-term dialysis therapy, but children who do recover sufficient renal function are at risk for the late development of CKD as described below.

Congenital Abnormalities of the Kidney and Genitourinary Tract

Obstruction of the urinary tract can cause AKI if the obstruction occurs in a solitary kidney, if it involves the ureters bilaterally, or if there is urethral obstruction. Obstruction can result from congenital malformations such as posterior urethral valves, bilateral ureteropelvic junction (UPJ) obstruction, or bilateral obstructive ureteroceles. Acquired urinary tract obstruction can result from passage of kidney stones or, rarely, tumors. It is important to evaluate for obstruction because the management is to promptly relieve the obstruction.

CAKUT represents the most common cause of CKD in the neonate.[111] Based on the North American Pediatrics Renal Trials and Collaborative Studies report in 2014, the most common cause of underlying end stage renal disease in children receiving a kidney transplant was renal aplasia/hypoplasia/dysplasia accounting for 15.8% of the cases, followed closely by obstructive uropathy being the cause in 15.3% of the children. Renal dysplasia is believed to arise either from defects in the differentiation of the renal parenchyma or due to events secondary to an obstruction of the lower urinary tract as seen in posterior urethral valves, UPJ obstruction, bilateral ureteroceles, or vesicoureteric reflux.[112] The complex array of underlying causes resulting in abnormal kidney formation is not entirely understood and most likely involves genetic, epigenetic, and environmental factors merging together to manifest in a certain phenotype. However, progress is currently being made to identify molecular signals and patterning pathways that contribute to renal dysplasia. Some of the genes that have so far been implicated in renal dysplasia are Pax2 (renal coloboma syndrome), Hnf1beta (renal cysts and diabetes syndrome), Sall1 (Townes-Brocks syndrome), Six2 (CAKUT), Wt1 (Wilms tumor and renal agenesis), Ret (CAKUT), Eya1 (brachio-oto-renal syndrome), miR17~92 (Fiengold syndrome), and Fgf9/Fgf20 (CAKUT).[113–122] In addition, investigators have identified genetic alterations in more than 160 rare kidney diseases.[123]

Medical Management of Acute Kidney Injury in Neonates

Preventive Measures

It is thought that prerenal injury is the most common cause of AKI in neonates in a resource-poor setting, and since dialytic resources were scarce, the mortality rate was high from prerenal failure.[124] Thus, on a global scale, the prevention of AKI in the neonate with adequate hydration is likely to have a larger impact on mortality than other measures.

Intravenous (IV) infusion of theophylline in severely asphyxiated neonates given within the first hour after birth was associated with improved fluid balance, improved creatinine clearance, and reduced serum creatinine levels with no effects on neurologic and respiratory complications.[125] Other studies in asphyxiated neonates also demonstrated improved kidney function and decreased excretion of β-2 microglobulin in the neonates given theophylline within 1 hour of birth.[126,127] However, the clinical significance of the improved kidney function was not clear, and the incidence of persistent pulmonary hypertension was higher in the neonates who had received theophylline group. The beneficial effects of theophylline are likely to be mediated by its adenosine antagonistic properties.[128] Additional studies are needed to determine the significance of these findings and the potential side effects of theophylline.

After intrinsic kidney injury has become established, management of the metabolic complications of AKI involves appropriate monitoring of fluid balance, electrolyte status, acid-base balance, nutrition, and the initiation of renal replacement therapy when appropriate. Diuretic therapy to stimulate urine output eases management of AKI, but the conversion of oliguric to nonoliguric AKI has not been shown to alter the course of AKI.[129] Diuretic therapy has potential theoretical mechanisms to prevent, limit, or improve kidney function. Mannitol (0.5–1.0 g/kg over several minutes) may increase intratubular urine flow to limit tubular obstruction and may limit cell damage by prevention of swelling or by acting as a scavenger of free radicals or reactive oxygen molecules. Lasix (1–5 mg/kg per dose) also increases urine flow rate to decrease intratubular obstruction. When using mannitol in children or neonates with AKI, a lack of response to therapy can precipitate congestive heart failure, particularly if the child's intravascular volume is expanded before mannitol infusion; caution should be used when considering mannitol therapy. In addition, lack of excretion of mannitol may also result in substantial hyperosmolality. Similarly, administration of high doses of furosemide in kidney injury has been associated with ototoxicity.[129] When using diuretic therapy in children with AKI, potential risks and benefits need to be considered. When the neonate is unresponsive to therapy, administering continued high doses of diuretics is not justified and unlikely to be beneficial to the neonate. In neonates who do respond to therapy, continuous infusions may be more effective and may be associated with less toxicity than bolus administration.[129a]

The use of "renal"-dose dopamine (0.5–3.5 μg/kg per minute) to improve kidney perfusion after an ischemic insult in NICUs and PICUs was practiced in the past, but has now fallen out of favor. Although dopamine increases kidney blood flow by promoting vasodilatation and may improve urine output by promoting natriuresis, no definitive studies have demonstrated that low-dose dopamine is effective in decreasing the need for dialysis or improving survival in patients with AKI.[130–135] In fact, a placebo-controlled randomized study of low-dose dopamine in adult patients demonstrated that low-dose dopamine was not beneficial and did not confer clinically significant protection from kidney dysfunction.[130] Other studies have demonstrated that renal-dose dopamine is not effective in the therapy of AKI, and one study demonstrated that low-dose dopamine worsened kidney perfusion and kidney function.[135]

Fenoldopam is a potent short-acting selective dopamine-1 receptor agonist that decreases vascular resistance while increasing kidney blood flow.[136] A meta-analysis of 16 trials of fenoldopam in adults concluded that therapy with fenoldopam decreased the incidence of AKI, decreased the need for renal replacement therapy, decreased the length of ICU stay, and decreased death from any cause.[137] Fenoldopam has been used in a few children with AKI, including two children receiving therapy with a ventricular-assist device as a bridge to cardiac transplantation; therapy with fenoldopam was thought to avoid the need for renal replacement therapy in one child.[138] Yoder et al. retrospectively studied the effect of low dose fenoldopam on urine output, blood pressure, renal function, and electrolyte balance in neonates and found that fenoldopam did not improve urine output or renal function; however no adverse cardiac consequences were noted.[139] Ricci et al. performed a prospective controlled trial in newborn infants on cardiopulmonary bypass to determine if the use of fenoldopam in neonates on conventional diuretics improved renal function. Similar to the findings by Yoder et al., they did not find a reduction in AKI or improvement in urine output.[140] Additional studies utilizing fenoldopam need to be performed in children and neonates with AKI.

Electrolyte Management

Mild hyponatremia is very common in AKI and may be attributable to hyponatremic dehydration, but fluid overload with dilutional hyponatremia is much more common. If the serum sodium is greater than 120 mEq/L, fluid restriction or water removal by dialytic therapy will correct the serum sodium. However, if the serum sodium is less than 120 mEq/L, the neonate is at higher risk for seizures from hyponatremia, and correction to a sodium level of approximately 125 mEq/L with hypertonic saline should be considered.

The kidney tightly regulates potassium balance and excretes approximately 90% of dietary potassium intake, hyperkalemia is a common and potentially life-threatening electrolyte abnormality in AKI in neonates.[141] The serum potassium level may be falsely elevated if the technique of the blood drawing is traumatic or if the specimen is hemolyzed. Hyperkalemia results in disturbances of cardiac rhythm by its depolarizing effect on the cardiac conduction pathways. The concentration of serum potassium that results in arrhythmia is dependent upon the acid-base balance and the other serum electrolytes. Hypocalcemia, which is common in kidney injury, exacerbates the adverse effects of the serum potassium on cardiac conduction pathways. Tall peaked T waves are the first manifestation of cardiotoxicity, and prolongation of the PR interval, flattening of P waves, and widening of QRS complexes are later abnormalities. Severe hyperkalemia will eventually lead to ventricular tachycardia and fibrillation and requires prompt therapy with sodium bicarbonate, IV glucose and insulin, IV calcium gluconate, and albuterol.[142,143] Albuterol infusions of 400 µg given every 2 hours as needed have been shown to rapidly lower serum potassium levels.[143] All of these therapies are temporizing measures and do not remove potassium from the body. Kayexalate given orally per nasogastric tube or per rectum will exchange sodium for potassium in the gastrointestinal tract and result in potassium removal.[141,144] Complications of Kayexalate therapy include possible hypernatremia, sodium retention, and constipation. In addition, Kayexalate therapy has been associated with colonic necrosis.[145] Depending upon the degree of hyperkalemia and the need for correction of other metabolic derangements in AKI, hyperkalemia frequently requires the initiation of dialysis or hemofiltration.

The kidney excretes acids generated in the body by diet and intermediary metabolism; therefore acidosis is very common in AKI. Severe acidosis can be treated with IV or oral sodium bicarbonate, oral sodium citrate solutions, or dialysis therapy. When considering treatment of acidosis, it is important to consider the serum ionized calcium level. Under normal circumstances, approximately half the total calcium is protein bound, and the other half is free and in the ionized form, which is what determines the transmembrane potential and electrochemical gradient. Hypocalcemia is common in AKI, and acidosis increases the fraction of total calcium to the ionized form. Treatment of acidosis can then shift the ionized calcium to the more normal ratio, decreasing the amount of ionized calcium and precipitating tetany or seizures.

The kidney excretes a large amount of ingested phosphorus, therefore hyperphosphatemia is a very common electrolyte abnormality noted during AKI. Hyperphosphatemia should be treated with dietary phosphorus restriction and with oral calcium carbonate or other calcium compounds to bind phosphorus and prevent gastrointestinal absorption of phosphorus.[146] Given that most neonates with AKI have hypocalcemia, the use of calcium-containing phosphate binders provides a source of calcium as well as phosphate-binding capacity.

In many instances AKI is associated with marked catabolism, and malnutrition can develop rapidly, leading to delayed recovery from AKI. Prompt and proper nutrition is essential in the management of the newborn with AKI. If the gastrointestinal tract is intact and functional, enteral feedings with formula (PM 60/40) should be instituted as soon as possible. If the newborn is oligo/anuric and sufficient calories cannot be achieved while maintaining appropriate fluid balance, the earlier initiation of dialysis should be instituted.

Therapies to Decrease Injury and Promote Recovery

Although there is no current specific therapy to prevent kidney injury or promote recovery in human AKI, several potential therapies are being studied, and future management of AKI may also include antioxidant, antiadhesion molecule therapy, the administration of vascular mediators, or mesenchymal stem cells (MSCs) to prevent injury or promote recovery.[147–154] Several different therapies have been shown to prevent, decrease, or promote recovery in animal models of AKI. Melanocyte-stimulating hormone has antiinflammatory activity and has been shown to protect renal tubules from injury.[149] Scavengers of free radicals and reactive oxygen and nitrogen molecules, as well as antiadhesion molecules, have been shown to decrease the degree of injury in animal models of AKI.[148] Recently, very interesting studies have also demonstrated that multipotent MSCs may play a role in promoting recovery from AKI in animal models.[152]

Despite the promise of animal models of intervention in AKI, clinical studies in humans have been largely disappointing, including studies using anaritide (atrial natriuretic peptide) and insulin-like growth factor 1.[147,150] However, because therapy in these studies was initiated when kidney injury was well established, it is likely that the opportunity to intervene and impact the recovery from AKI had been missed.[151,153] As mentioned previously, the development and testing of interventions for AKI will require the development of early biomarkers of injury that are much more sensitive than serum creatinine.

Acute and Chronic Renal Replacement Therapy

Renal replacement therapy is provided to remove endogenous and exogenous toxins and to maintain fluid, electrolyte, and acid-base balance until kidney function returns or to maintain the neonate until kidney transplantation is possible. Renal replacement therapy may be provided by peritoneal dialysis, intermittent hemodialysis, and hemofiltration with or without a dialysis circuit. Each mode of renal replacement therapy has specific advantages and disadvantages (Table 18.2). For AKI, the preferential use of hemofiltration by pediatric nephrologists is increasing, and the use of peritoneal dialysis is decreasing except for neonates and small infants.[155]

No studies in newborns have compared the outcome of AKI or CKD when different renal replacement therapies are used in the treatment of AKI or CKD. Many factors, including the age and size of the child, the cause of kidney injury, the degree of metabolic derangements, blood pressure, and nutritional needs, were considered in deciding when to initiate renal replacement therapy and the modality of therapy.[155]

Table 18.2 COMPARISON OF RENAL REPLACEMENT THERAPIES

	PD	HD	CVVH(D)
Solute removal	+++	++++	+(+++)
Fluid removal	++	+++	+++(+++)
Toxin removal	+	++++	−(+)
Removal of potassium	++	++++	+(++)
Removal of ammonia	+	++++	+(+++)
Need for hemodynamic stability	−	+++	−(−)
Need for anticoagulation	−	++	−/+(−/+)
Ease of access	+++	−	−
Continuous	+++	−	+++(+++)
Respiratory compromise	++	−	−(−)
Peritonitis	++++	−	−
Hypotension	+	+++	+++(+++)
Disequilibrium	−	+++	−(−)
Reverse osmosis water	−	++++	−(−)

CVVH(D), Continuous venovenous hemodiafiltration; *HD,* hemodialysis; *PD,* peritoneal dialysis.

The indications to initiate renal replacement therapy are not absolute and take into consideration a number of factors, including the cause of kidney injury, the rapidity of the onset of kidney injury, the severity of fluid and electrolyte abnormalities, and the nutritional needs of the neonate. Because neonates and infants have less muscle mass than older children, they require initiation of renal replacement therapy at lower levels of serum creatinine and BUN compared with older children. The presence of fluid overload unresponsive to diuretic therapy and the need for enteral feedings or hyperalimentation to support nutritional needs are important factors in considering the initiation of renal replacement therapy.

Peritoneal Dialysis

Peritoneal dialysis has been a major modality of therapy for AKI and CKD in neonates since vascular access is difficult to maintain in neonates. Advantages of peritoneal dialysis are that it is relatively easy to perform and does not require heparinization, and the newborn does not need to be hemodynamically stable to undergo peritoneal dialysis. The disadvantages include a slower correction of metabolic parameters and the potential for peritonitis. To increase the efficiency of peritoneal dialysis, frequent exchanges as often as every hour and use of dialysate with higher glucose concentrations will remove more solute and water, respectively. Relative contraindications include recent abdominal surgery and massive organomegaly or intraabdominal masses as well as ostomies, which may increase the risk of peritonitis.

Access to the peritoneal cavity is usually through a Tenckhoff catheter. Alternately, several VLBW neonates have been successfully dialyzed by using a 14-gauge vascular catheter to access the peritoneal fluid.[156] Commercially available 1.5%, 2.5%, and 4.25% glucose solutions are available for use in peritoneal dialysis. In older children, peritoneal dialysis is usually initiated with volumes of 15 to 20 mL/kg body weight, while neonates usually initiate peritoneal dialysis with slightly lower volumes of 5 to 10 mL/kg body weight; low-volume peritoneal dialysis will have a milder effect on the hemodynamic status of neonates and has been shown to effectively control uremia and promote ultrafiltration in neonates and older children.[157–160] The dialysate volume can be increased depending upon the need for additional solute and fluid removal and the cardiovascular and respiratory status. If the neonate has lactate acidosis, dialysis with the standard solutions will increase the lactate load and aggravate the acidosis. Peritoneal dialysis with a bicarbonate-buffered dialysate solution should be used in neonates with lactate acidosis.

Substantial fluid and electrolyte imbalances can occur during peritoneal dialysis, especially when using frequent exchanges, and prolonged use of hypertonic glucose solutions can result in hyperglycemia, hypernatremia, and hypovolemia. Peritonitis

18

(dialysate white blood count >100/mm³) is another complication of acute peritoneal dialysis and can be treated with intraperitoneal antibiotics. If the neonate develops hypokalemia or hypophosphatemia during the course of dialysis, then 3 to 5 mEq/L of KCl or 2 to 3 mEq/L of potassium phosphate can be added to the dialysate. To avoid hypothermia in neonates, the dialysate should be warmed to body temperature before infusion into the peritoneal cavity.

Although technically challenging, long-term peritoneal dialysis has been carried out in VLBW infants with a weight as low as 930 g,[161] and short-term peritoneal dialysis has been used in smaller premature newborns.[157–160] Peritoneal dialysis has been shown to provide adequate clearance in neonates with AKI after cardiopulmonary bypass.[160] The majority of infants who have undergone long-term peritoneal dialysis were found to have normal developmental milestones or attended regular school and had good growth and development.[159]

Hemodialysis

Hemodialysis has also been used for several years in the treatment of AKI and CKD during childhood.[162,163] Hemodialysis has the advantage that metabolic abnormalities can be corrected rather quickly and hypervolemia can be corrected by rapid ultrafiltration as well. The disadvantages of hemodialysis include the requirement for heparinization, the need for maximally purified water by a reverse osmosis system, and the need for skilled nursing personnel. Hemodialysis is commonly used for treatment of metabolic disorders associated with hyperammonemia from urea cycle defects.[163] Relative contraindications include hemodynamic instability or severe hemorrhage.

During hemodialysis, rapid ultrafiltration may also result in hypotension, which has also been shown to result in additional renal ischemia and potentially prolong the episode of AKI. Rapid removal of BUN and other uremic products can result in dialysis disequilibrium, particularly if the child begins hemodialysis with a high BUN (>120–150 mg/dL [42.8–53.5 mmol/L]). The pathogenesis of this syndrome is complex and multifactorial, but may be related to removal of urea from the blood while brain levels decline slower, such that disequilibrium occurs; symptoms include restlessness, fatigue, headache, nausea, vomiting leading to confusion, seizures, and coma.[164] This severe complication of hemodialysis can be prevented by slowly lowering the BUN during hemodialysis and by the prophylactic infusion of mannitol (0.5–1 g/kg body weight) during hemodialysis to counteract the decline in the serum osmolality that occurs during hemodialysis.

Vascular access in newborns can be provided by umbilical vessels; older infants and children require catheterization of a large vessel to obtain blood flows adequate for hemodialysis. Catheters can be placed in the internal or external jugular veins or in the femoral vein. To avoid hypotension, the total volume of the dialysate circuit, including the dialyzer and tubing, should not exceed 10% of the child blood volume. Blood flow rates to achieve clearances of 1.5 to 3.0 mL/kg per minute are utilized depending upon the indications for dialysis, the initial BUN level and degree of azotemia, and the clinical status of the child. Again, depending upon the clinical status of the child and the degree of azotemia, clearances can be increased to 3 to 5 mL/kg per minute in subsequent dialysis sessions. To maintain adequate control of azotemia and to allow for adequate venovenous nutrition during AKI, frequent hemodialysis (as often as daily) may be needed in neonates.

Hemofiltration

Over the past several years, renal replacement therapy with hemofiltration, including continuous venovenous hemofiltration (CVVH) or with the addition of a dialysis circuit to the hemofilter and continuous venovenous hemodiafiltration (CVVHD), has become increasingly popular in the treatment of AKI during childhood.[165–168] Whereas hemofiltration without dialysis (CVVH) follows the principle of removal of large quantities of ultrafiltrate from plasma with replacement of an isosmotic electrolyte solution, hemofiltration with dialysis (CVVHD) also results in solute removal via the added dialysis circuit. The advantages of hemofiltration (with or without a dialysis circuit) include that it can result in rapid fluid removal; does not require the patient to be hemodynamically stable; and is continuous, avoiding rapid solute and fluid shifts as occurs in hemodialysis. The disadvantages include that hemofiltration may require constant heparinization, and there is a potential for severe fluid and electrolyte abnormalities because of the large volume of fluid removed and subsequently replaced. In neonates at risk of bleeding, regional anticoagulation with citrate can be performed to minimize the risk of bleeding. Hemofiltration and hemodiafiltration were found to allow good control of fluid, electrolyte, and acid-base balance and have been used in newborns with inborn error of metabolism.[165] The survival rate in children weighing up to 10 kg undergoing CVVH is similar to older children and adolescents.[167] As in hemodialysis, catheterization of a large vessel to obtain blood flows are necessary for hemofiltration. Catheters can be placed in the internal or external jugular veins or in the femoral vein. CCVH can also be performed in neonates and children on extracorporeal membrane oxygenation (ECMO) by adding a filter in the ECMO circuit or by inserting a continuous renal replacement therapy machine.[169]

Future Directions

Peritoneal dialysis is the modality of choice for renal replacement therapy in neonates; however, there are circumstances in which peritoneal dialysis is not feasible such as in the setting of gastroschisis, necrotizing enterocolitis, or other intraabdominal pathology. Conventional CVVH machines are typically used off-label when used for children less than 15 kg. There is new and exciting development of dialysis and ultrafiltration machines that have been designed specifically for neonates with the added advantage of having small priming volumes and set ups that are geared towards different patient weights and sizes.[170–172] The Cardio-Renal Pediatric Dialysis Emergency Machine, also known as CARPEDIEM, was designed for use specifically for neonates and was officially approved for use in humans in 2011.[172] In 2013 it was successfully used for CVVH in a 2.9-kg infant for the duration of approximately 20 days.[170] The Newcastle Infant Dialysis and Ultrafiltration System (NIDUS) has also been successfully used in infants weighing 1.8 kg to 5.9 kg. It has advantages similar to CARPEDIEM including a very low blood circuit volume, slower blood flow rates required for the circuit, and very precise fluid removal.[171] The use of the "Aquadex" machine was also described in a single-center experience with 12 children ranging from 4 to 1460 days of age with a weight range of 2.7 to 12.5 kg.[173] The Aquadex machine was originally designed for slow continuous ultrafiltration; however Askenazi et al. were successfully able to use it for convective clearance.[173] Moving forward, such machines have the potential to change the horizons of management in severe AKI and volume overload in critically ill neonates.

Prognosis

In neonates, the prognosis and recovery from AKI is highly dependent upon the underlying etiology of the AKI.[12–14,16–18] Recent studies performed on patients admitted to the PICU also confirm that AKI lends itself to a higher mortality risk independent of all other factors.[174] Factors that are associated with mortality include multiorgan failure, hypotension, a need for pressors, hemodynamic instability, and a need for mechanical ventilation and dialysis.[12–14,16–18] Overall, mortality in newborns with AKI ranges from 10% to 61% and is highest in infants with multiorgan failure.[12–14,16–18] In infants maintained on peritoneal dialysis for AKI, mortality was 64% in oligo/anuric infants compared with 20% in infants with adequate urine output.[16] Other studies have shown that AKI in VLBW infants was independently associated with mortality.[175] Long-term follow-up of children with AKI has shown that death and kidney sequelae are common 3 to 5 years following AKI in pediatric patients, suggesting that the detrimental effects of AKI are long lasting and can manifest as CKD, with early markers being proteinuria, hypertension, and hyperfiltration.[176]

Neonates also appear to be particularly susceptible towards having a higher mortality with AKI as compared to children of other age groups. Sutherland et al. performed a cross-sectional analysis of the 2009 kids database and found the incidence of AKI to be 3.9/1000 admissions.[177] An alarming but not unexpected finding was that inpatient mortality in children with AKI was very high among neonates less than 1 month of age with an incidence of 31.3% vs. 10.1% in children older than 1 month. The other group with a similarly high mortality was children admitted to the ICU with an in-hospital mortality of 32.8% vs. 9.4% in patients not admitted to the ICU, and those on dialysis with a rate of 27.1% vs. 14.2% in children not requiring dialysis.[177]

There is also a correlation between the severity of AKI and the mortality risk. Sanchez-Pinto et al. assessed the correlation between progression and improvement in renal function with mortality in critically ill children.[174] They studied 8260 children age 1 month to 21 years of age in the PICU and found that the degree of severity of AKI independently correlated with a higher mortality. The converse also held true, and improvement in renal function was associated with a decline in mortality.[174] However, in their study they also note that patients with resolved AKI continued to have a higher mortality compared to those who never developed AKI.

AKI in full-term neonates is also associated with kidney disease later in life.[88] In one study of six older children with a history of AKI not requiring dialysis in the neonatal period, only two had normal renal function, three had CKD, and one was on dialysis.[58] Although the number of children studied was small, this study raises concern about the long-term kidney outcome for such children. An inverse relationship between the development of hypertension and proteinuria during adulthood and birth weight has been reported.[87,90]

There is a growing body of evidence confirming the development of CKD in preterm and low birth weight infants, as well as those who suffer from AKI during their neonatal course. Mammen et al. analyzed the long-term risk of CKD in children admitted to the ICU who developed AKI.[178] The number of patients in their study was 126 out of which 30 were neonates.[178] In their prospective cohort study they used the Acute Kidney Injury Network criteria to define stages of AKI and observed an overall incidence of CKD 1 to 3 years after AKI of 10.3%. When broken down by stages, CKD occurred in 4.5% of children with AKI stage 1, 10.6% with stage 2, and 17.1% with stage 3. In addition, 46.8% of the patients were reported to be "at risk for CKD" as defined by having a GFR between 60 and 90 mL/min per 1.73 m^2, hypertension, or hyperfiltration defined by a GFR greater than or equal to 150 mL/min per 1.73 m^2 at the 1-, 2-, or 3-year mark after the episode of AKI.[178] If the "at risk" patients were to be followed for a longer duration of time, it is quite likely that progression towards CKD would be noted.

The long-term effect of AKI in neonates is potentially compounded when the insult occurs before the full complement of nephrons had developed in utero. Because nephrogenesis proceeds until 34 to 35 weeks' gestation, AKI before this time may result in reduced nephron number. Indeed, it has been shown that preterm neonates with AKI have a high incidence of a low GFR and increasing proteinuria several years later,[86] and morphologic studies have shown decreased nephron number and glomerulomegaly.[89] Several studies in animal models and some human studies have documented that hyperfiltration of the remnant nephron may eventually lead to progressive glomerulosclerosis of the remaining nephrons. Typically, the late development of CKD first becomes apparent with the development of hypertension, proteinuria, and eventually an elevated BUN and creatinine. A systemic review and meta-analysis of observational studies performed by White et al. demonstrated that low birth weight is associated with a long-term risk of CKD.[179] Subsequent prospective studies appear to confirm this finding.

The IRENEO study was a single-center, prospective, controlled study in France that was performed to assess complications from AKI in premature infants once they had entered childhood.[180] All children included in the study were born at less than 33 weeks of gestation and were between age 3 and 10 at the time of final evaluation. In this study, no difference was identified between the two groups with regard to eGFR (using serum Cr), urinary microalbumin, or blood pressure. Children with AKI did appear to have a lower renal volume, but this was not found to be statistically significant. However, of all the children included in the study, 10.8% had microalbuminuria and

23% had an eGFR less than 90 mL/min per 1.73 m². Given the small sample size, it is possible that the subgroup analysis did not demonstrate significant differences, but what is particularly notable is that extremely low birth weight infants did have a statistically lower eGFR and lower renal volume as shown in previous studies. A limitation of this study was that follow-up was only until age 3 to 10 years and it is likely that some of the markers of renal injury including proteinuria, hypertension, and a more pronounced reduction in GFR manifest even later in life.

It is well known that neonates with congenital disease such as dysplasia with or without obstructive uropathy, cortical necrosis, or cystic kidney diseases are at risk for later development of CKD. In contrast, it has been thought that ischemic and nephrotoxic kidney injury is reversible with kidney function returning to normal. However, recent studies have shown that hypoxic ischemic and nephrotoxic insults can result in alterations that can lead to kidney disease at a later time.[1–3,86,88–90] Thus, AKI from any cause is a risk factor for subsequent kidney disease.

When premature neonates were investigated during childhood (ages 6.1–12.4 years), defects in tubular reabsorption of phosphorus (TRP) were evident, the TRP was significantly lower, and the urinary excretion of phosphorus was significantly higher compared to control children.[181] Urinary calcium excretion was also higher in children born prematurely compared to control children. Others have found nearly identical findings, and the investigators attributed these alterations to aminoglycoside nephrotoxicity.[182,183] Recent studies have also shown that low birth weight is a risk for FSGS.[6] In addition, extrauterine as well as intrauterine growth retardation was associated with impaired renal function in children who were born preterm.[184] In view of these alterations in kidney function resulting in long-term risk of hypertension, proteinuria, and tubular dysfunction, neonates with AKI and nephrotoxic insults need lifelong monitoring of their kidney function, blood pressure, and urinalysis.[1–3,185]

REFERENCES

1. Goldstein SL, Devarajan P. Acute kidney injury in childhood: should we be worried about progression to CKD? *Pediatr Nephrol*. 2011;26(4):509–522.
2. Basile DP. Rarefaction of peritubular capillaries following ischemic acute renal failure: a potential factor predisposing to progressive nephropathy. *Curr Opin Nephrol Hypertens*. 2004;13(1):1–7.
3. Andreoli SP. Acute kidney injury in children. *Pediatr Nephrol*. 2009;24(2):253–263.
4. Zohdi V, et al. Low Birth Weight due to Intrauterine Growth Restriction and/or Preterm Birth: Effects on Nephron Number and Long-Term Renal Health. *Int J Nephrol*. 2012;2012:136942.
5. Baum M. Neonatal nephrology. *Curr Opin Pediatr*. 2016;28(2):170–172.
6. Hodgin JB, et al. Very low birth weight is a risk factor for secondary focal segmental glomerulosclerosis. *Clin J Am Soc Nephrol*. 2009;4(1):71–76.
7. Khalsa DD, Beydoun HA, Carmody JB. Prevalence of chronic kidney disease risk factors among low birth weight adolescents. *Pediatr Nephrol*. 2016;31(9):1509–1516.
8. Benini D, et al. In utero exposure to nonsteroidal anti-inflammatory drugs: neonatal renal failure. *Pediatr Nephrol*. 2004;19(2):232–234.
9. Cooper WO, et al. Major congenital malformations after first-trimester exposure to ACE inhibitors. *N Engl J Med*. 2006;354(23):2443–2451.
10. Lip GY, et al. Angiotensin-converting-enzyme inhibitors in early pregnancy. *Lancet*. 1997;350(9089): 1446–1447.
11. Martinovic J, et al. Fetal toxic effects and angiotensin-II-receptor antagonists. *Lancet*. 2001;358(9277): 241–242.
12. Andreoli S. Polin RA YM, Berg FD, eds. Renal failure in the newborn unit. In: *Workbook in Practical Neonatology*. Philadelphia, PA: Saunders Company; 2007:329–344.
13. Andreoli SP. Acute renal failure. *Curr Opin Pediatr*. 2002;14(2):183–188.
14. Gouyon JB, Guignard JP. Management of acute renal failure in newborns. *Pediatr Nephrol*. 2000;14(10–11):1037–1044.
15. Hui-Stickle S, Brewer ED, Goldstein SL. Pediatric ARF epidemiology at a tertiary care center from 1999 to 2001. *Am J Kidney Dis*. 2005;45(1):96–101.
16. Karlowicz MG, Adelman RD. Nonoliguric and oliguric acute renal failure in asphyxiated term neonates. *Pediatr Nephrol*. 1995;9(6):718–722.
17. Matthews DE, et al. Peritoneal dialysis in the first 60 days of life. *J Pediatr Surg*. 1990;25(1):110–115, discussion 116.
18. Moghal NE, Brocklebank JT, Meadow SR. A review of acute renal failure in children: incidence, etiology and outcome. *Clin Nephrol*. 1998;49(2):91–95.
19. Akcan-Arikan A, et al. Modified RIFLE criteria in critically ill children with acute kidney injury. *Kidney Int*. 2007;71(10):1028–1035.

20. Bellomo R, et al. Acute renal failure—definition, outcome measures, animal models, fluid therapy and information technology needs: the Second International Consensus Conference of the Acute Dialysis Quality Initiative (ADQI) Group. *Crit Care*. 2004;8(4):R204–R212.
21. Duzova A, et al. Etiology and outcome of acute kidney injury in children. *Pediatr Nephrol*. 2010;25(8):1453–1461.
22. Chevalier RL. Developmental renal physiology of the low birth weight pre-term newborn. *J Urol*. 1996;156(2 Pt 2):714–719.
23. Vanpee M, et al. Postnatal development of renal function in very low birthweight infants. *Acta Paediatr Scand*. 1988;77(2):191–197.
24. Guignard JP, Drukker A. Why do newborn infants have a high plasma creatinine? *Pediatrics*. 1999;103(4):e49.
25. Askenazi DJ, Ambalavanan N, Goldstein SL. Acute kidney injury in critically ill newborns: what do we know? What do we need to learn? *Pediatr Nephrol*. 2009;24(2):265–274.
26. Hanna M, et al. Early urinary biomarkers of acute kidney injury in preterm infants. *Pediatr Res*. 2016;80(2):218–223.
27. Lavery AP, et al. Urinary NGAL in premature infants. *Pediatr Res*. 2008;64(4):423–428.
28. Parravicini E. The clinical utility of urinary neutrophil gelatinase-associated lipocalin in the neonatal ICU. *Curr Opin Pediatr*. 2010;22(2):146–150.
29. Filler G, et al. Cystatin C as a marker of GFR—history, indications, and future research. *Clin Biochem*. 2005;38(1):1–8.
30. Abitbol CL, et al. Neonatal kidney size and function in preterm infants: what is a true estimate of glomerular filtration rate? *J Pediatr*. 2014;164(5):1026–1031, e2.
31. Zappitelli M, et al. Derivation and validation of cystatin C-based prediction equations for GFR in children. *Am J Kidney Dis*. 2006;48(2):221–230.
32. McCaffrey J, et al. Towards a biomarker panel for the assessment of AKI in children receiving intensive care. *Pediatr Nephrol*. 2015;30(10):1861–1871.
33. Askenazi DJ, et al. Acute Kidney Injury Urine Biomarkers in Very Low-Birth-Weight Infants. *Clin J Am Soc Nephrol*. 2016;11(9):1527–1535.
34. Hanna MH, Brophy PD. Metabolomics in pediatric nephrology: emerging concepts. *Pediatr Nephrol*. 2015;30(6):881–887.
35. Weiss RH, Kim K. Metabolomics in the study of kidney diseases. *Nat Rev Nephrol*. 2011;8(1):22–33.
36. Nada A, Bonachea EM, Askenazi DJ. Acute kidney injury in the fetus and neonate. *Semin Fetal Neonatal Med*. 2016.
37. Aggarwal A, et al. Evaluation of renal functions in asphyxiated newborns. *J Trop Pediatr*. 2005;51(5):295–299.
38. Al-Ismaili Z, Palijan A, Zappitelli M. Biomarkers of acute kidney injury in children: discovery, evaluation, and clinical application. *Pediatr Nephrol*. 2011;26(1):29–40.
39. Cataldi L, et al. Potential risk factors for the development of acute renal failure in preterm newborn infants: a case-control study. *Arch Dis Child Fetal Neonatal Ed*. 2005;90(6):F514–F519.
40. Cuzzolin L, et al. Postnatal renal function in preterm newborns: a role of diseases, drugs and therapeutic interventions. *Pediatr Nephrol*. 2006;21(7):931–938.
41. Devarajan P. Emerging biomarkers of acute kidney injury. *Contrib Nephrol*. 2007;156:203–212.
42. Drukker A, Guignard JP. Renal aspects of the term and preterm infant: a selective update. *Curr Opin Pediatr*. 2002;14(2):175–182.
43. Durkan AM, Alexander RT. Acute kidney injury post neonatal asphyxia. *J Pediatr*. 2011;158(2 suppl):e29–e33.
44. Goldstein SL. Pediatric acute kidney injury: it's time for real progress. *Pediatr Nephrol*. 2006;21(7):891–895.
45. Martin-Ancel A, et al. Multiple organ involvement in perinatal asphyxia. *J Pediatr*. 1995;127(5):786–793.
46. Vanpee M, et al. Renal function in very low birth weight infants: normal maturity reached during early childhood. *J Pediatr*. 1992;121(5 Pt 1):784–788.
47. Zaffanello M, et al. Early diagnosis of acute kidney injury with urinary biomarkers in the newborn. *J Matern Fetal Neonatal Med*. 2009;22(suppl 3):62–66.
48. Nobilis A, et al. Variance of ACE and AT1 receptor gene does not influence the risk of neonatal acute renal failure. *Pediatr Nephrol*. 2001;16(12):1063–1066.
49. Vasarhelyi B, et al. Genetic polymorphisms and risk for acute renal failure in preterm neonates. *Pediatr Nephrol*. 2005;20(2):132–135.
50. Treszl A, et al. Interleukin genetic variants and the risk of renal failure in infants with infection. *Pediatr Nephrol*. 2002;17(9):713–717.
51. Fekete A, et al. Association between heat shock protein 72 gene polymorphism and acute renal failure in premature neonates. *Pediatr Res*. 2003;54(4):452–455.
52. Kelly KJ, Baird NR, Greene AL. Induction of stress response proteins and experimental renal ischemia/reperfusion. *Kidney Int*. 2001;59(5):1798–1802.
53. Jetton JG, et al. Assessment of Worldwide Acute Kidney Injury Epidemiology in Neonates: Design of a Retrospective Cohort Study. *Front Pediatr*. 2016;4:68.
54. Andreoli SP. Acute renal failure in the newborn. *Semin Perinatol*. 2004;28(2):112–123.
55. Toth-Heyn P, Drukker A, Guignard JP. The stressed neonatal kidney: from pathophysiology to clinical management of neonatal vasomotor nephropathy. *Pediatr Nephrol*. 2000;14(3):227–239.
56. Badr KF, Ichikawa I. Prerenal failure: a deleterious shift from renal compensation to decompensation. *N Engl J Med*. 1988;319(10):623–629.

57. van Bel F, et al. Indomethacin-induced changes in renal blood flow velocity waveform in premature infants investigated with color Doppler imaging. *J Pediatr*. 1991;118(4 Pt 1):621–626.

58. Allegaert K, et al. Nonselective cyclo-oxygenase inhibitors and glomerular filtration rate in preterm neonates. *Pediatr Nephrol*. 2005;20(11):1557–1561.

59. Cifuentes RF, et al. Indomethacin and renal function in premature infants with persistent patent ductus arteriosus. *J Pediatr*. 1979;95(4):583–587.

60. Gersony WM, et al. Effects of indomethacin in premature infants with patent ductus arteriosus: results of a national collaborative study. *J Pediatr*. 1983;102(6):895–906.

61. Itabashi K, Ohno T, Nishida H. Indomethacin responsiveness of patent ductus arteriosus and renal abnormalities in preterm infants treated with indomethacin. *J Pediatr*. 2003;143(2):203–207.

62. Zanardo V, et al. Urinary ET-1, AVP and sodium in premature infants treated with indomethacin and ibuprofen for patent ductus arteriosus. *Pediatr Nephrol*. 2005;20(11):1552–1556.

63. Guignard JP. The adverse renal effects of prostaglandin-synthesis inhibitors in the newborn rabbit. *Semin Perinatol*. 2002;26(6):398–405.

64. Perazella MA, Eras J. Are selective COX-2 inhibitors nephrotoxic? *Am J Kidney Dis*. 2000;35(5):937–940.

65. Tack ED, Perlman JM. Renal failure in sick hypertensive premature infants receiving captopril therapy. *J Pediatr*. 1988;112(5):805–810.

66. Wood EG, Bunchman TE, Lynch RE. Captopril-induced reversible acute renal failure in an infant with coarctation of the aorta. *Pediatrics*. 1991;88(4):816–818.

67. Gallini F, et al. Progression of renal function in preterm neonates with gestational age < or = 32 weeks. *Pediatr Nephrol*. 2000;15(1–2):119–124.

68. Basile DP. The endothelial cell in ischemic acute kidney injury: implications for acute and chronic function. *Kidney Int*. 2007;72(2):151–156.

69. Sutton TA, Fisher CJ, Molitoris BA. Microvascular endothelial injury and dysfunction during ischemic acute renal failure. *Kidney Int*. 2002;62(5):1539–1549.

70. Andreoli SP. Reactive oxygen molecules, oxidant injury and renal disease. *Pediatr Nephrol*. 1991;5(6):733–742.

71. Andreoli SP, McAteer JA. Reactive oxygen molecule-mediated injury in endothelial and renal tubular epithelial cells in vitro. *Kidney Int*. 1990;38(5):785–794.

72. Forbes JM, et al. Simultaneous blockade of endothelin A and B receptors in ischemic acute renal failure is detrimental to long-term kidney function. *Kidney Int*. 2001;59(4):1333–1341.

73. Goligorsky MS, Brodsky SV, Noiri E. Nitric oxide in acute renal failure: NOS versus NOS. *Kidney Int*. 2002;61(3):855–861.

74. Goligorsky MS, Noiri E. Duality of nitric oxide in acute renal injury. *Semin Nephrol*. 1999;19(3):263–271.

75. Heinzelmann M, Mercer-Jones MA, Passmore JC. Neutrophils and renal failure. *Am J Kidney Dis*. 1999;34(2):384–399.

76. Himmelfarb J, et al. Oxidative stress is increased in critically ill patients with acute renal failure. *J Am Soc Nephrol*. 2004;15(9):2449–2456.

77. Kelly KJ, et al. Antibody to intercellular adhesion molecule 1 protects the kidney against ischemic injury. *Proc Natl Acad Sci USA*. 1994;91(2):812–816.

78. Kwon O, et al. Sodium reabsorption and distribution of Na+/K+-ATPase during postischemic injury to the renal allograft. *Kidney Int*. 1999;55(3):963–975.

79. Luster AD. Chemokines—chemotactic cytokines that mediate inflammation. *N Engl J Med*. 1998;338(7):436–445.

80. Molitoris BA. Putting the actin cytoskeleton into perspective: pathophysiology of ischemic alterations. *Am J Physiol*. 1997;272(4 Pt 2):F430–F433.

81. Radi R, et al. Unraveling peroxynitrite formation in biological systems. *Free Radic Biol Med*. 2001;30(5):463–488.

82. Ruschitzka F, et al. Endothelial dysfunction in acute renal failure: role of circulating and tissue endothelin-1. *J Am Soc Nephrol*. 1999;10(5):953–962.

83. Van Why SK, et al. Hsp27 associates with actin and limits injury in energy depleted renal epithelia. *J Am Soc Nephrol*. 2003;14(1):98–106.

84. Wilhelm SM, et al. Endothelin up-regulation and localization following renal ischemia and reperfusion. *Kidney Int*. 1999;55(3):1011–1018.

85. Zuk A, et al. Polarity, integrin, and extracellular matrix dynamics in the postischemic rat kidney. *Am J Physiol*. 1998;275(3 Pt 1):C711–C731.

86. Abitbol CL, et al. Long-term follow-up of extremely low birth weight infants with neonatal renal failure. *Pediatr Nephrol*. 2003;18(9):887–893.

87. Keijzer-Veen MG, et al. Microalbuminuria and lower glomerular filtration rate at young adult age in subjects born very premature and after intrauterine growth retardation. *J Am Soc Nephrol*. 2005;16(9):2762–2768.

88. Polito C, Papale MR, La Manna A. Long-term prognosis of acute renal failure in the full-term neonate. *Clin Pediatr (Phila)*. 1998;37(6):381–385.

89. Rodriguez MM, et al. Comparative renal histomorphometry: a case study of oligonephropathy of prematurity. *Pediatr Nephrol*. 2005;20(7):945–949.

90. Tulassay T, Vasarhelyi B. Birth weight and renal function. *Curr Opin Nephrol Hypertens*. 2002;11(3):347–352.

91. Selewski DT, et al. Acute kidney injury in asphyxiated newborns treated with therapeutic hypothermia. *J Pediatr*. 2013;162(4):725–729.e1.

92. Goldstein SL, et al. Electronic health record identification of nephrotoxin exposure and associated acute kidney injury. *Pediatrics*. 2013;132(3):e756–e767.

18

93. Moffett BS, Goldstein SL. Acute kidney injury and increasing nephrotoxic-medication exposure in noncritically-ill children. *Clin J Am Soc Nephrol.* 2011;6(4):856–863.
94. Rhone ET, et al. Nephrotoxic medication exposure in very low birth weight infants. *J Matern Fetal Neonatal Med.* 2014;27(14):1485–1490.
95. Kent A, et al. Aminoglycoside toxicity in neonates: something to worry about? *Expert Rev Anti Infect Ther.* 2014;12(3):319–331.
96. Madsen K, et al. Angiotensin II promotes development of the renal microcirculation through AT1 receptors. *J Am Soc Nephrol.* 2010;21(3):448–459.
97. Nadeem S, et al. Renin Angiotensin System Blocker Fetopathy: A Midwest Pediatric Nephrology Consortium Report. *J Pediatr.* 2015;167(4):881–885.
98. Hunseler C, et al. Angiotensin II receptor blocker induced fetopathy: 7 cases. *Klin Padiatr.* 2011;223(1):10–14.
99. Gantenbein MH, et al. Side effects of angiotensin converting enzyme inhibitor (captopril) in newborns and young infants. *J Perinat Med.* 2008;36(5):448–452.
100. Hanna MH, Askenazi DJ, Selewski DT. Drug-induced acute kidney injury in neonates. *Curr Opin Pediatr.* 2016;28(2):180–187.
101. Constance JE, et al. A propensity-matched cohort study of vancomycin-associated nephrotoxicity in neonates. *Arch Dis Child Fetal Neonatal Ed.* 2016;101(3):F236–F243.
102. McKamy S, et al. Incidence and risk factors influencing the development of vancomycin nephrotoxicity in children. *J Pediatr.* 2011;158(3):422–426.
103. Elyasi S, et al. Vancomycin-induced nephrotoxicity: mechanism, incidence, risk factors and special populations. A literature review. *Eur J Clin Pharmacol.* 2012;68(9):1243–1255.
104. Ellis D, Kaye RD, Bontempo FA. Aortic and renal artery thrombosis in a neonate: recovery with thrombolytic therapy. *Pediatr Nephrol.* 1997;11(5):641–644.
105. Payne RM, et al. Management and follow-up of arterial thrombosis in the neonatal period. *J Pediatr.* 1989;114(5):853–858.
106. Resontoc LP, Yap HK. Renal vascular thrombosis in the newborn. *Pediatr Nephrol.* 2016;31(6):907–915.
107. Moudgil A. Renal venous thrombosis in neonates. *Curr Pediatr Rev.* 2014;10(2):101–106.
108. Christensen AM, et al. Postnatal transient renal insufficiency in the feto-fetal transfusion syndrome. *Pediatr Nephrol.* 1999;13(2):117–120.
109. Cincotta RB, et al. Long term outcome of twin-twin transfusion syndrome. *Arch Dis Child Fetal Neonatal Ed.* 2000;83(3):F171–F176.
110. Beck M, et al. Long-term outcome of kidney function after twin-twin transfusion syndrome treated by intrauterine laser coagulation. *Pediatr Nephrol.* 2005;20(11):1657–1659.
111. Phua YL, Ho J. Renal dysplasia in the neonate. *Curr Opin Pediatr.* 2016;28(2):209–215.
112. Ichikawa I, et al. Paradigm shift from classic anatomic theories to contemporary cell biological views of CAKUT. *Kidney Int.* 2002;61(3):889–898.
113. Heliot C, et al. HNF1B controls proximal-intermediate nephron segment identity in vertebrates by regulating Notch signalling components and Irx1/2. *Development.* 2013;140(4):873–885.
114. Massa F, et al. Hepatocyte nuclear factor 1beta controls nephron tubular development. *Development.* 2013;140(4):886–896.
115. Porteous S, et al. Primary renal hypoplasia in humans and mice with PAX2 mutations: evidence of increased apoptosis in fetal kidneys of Pax2(1Neu) +/− mutant mice. *Hum Mol Genet.* 2000;9(1):1–11.
116. Kanda S, et al. Sall1 maintains nephron progenitors and nascent nephrons by acting as both an activator and a repressor. *J Am Soc Nephrol.* 2014;25(11):2584–2595.
117. Self M, et al. Six2 is required for suppression of nephrogenesis and progenitor renewal in the developing kidney. *EMBO J.* 2006;25(21):5214–5228.
118. Gessler M, Konig A, Bruns GA. The genomic organization and expression of the WT1 gene. *Genomics.* 1992;12(4):807–813.
119. Lu BC, et al. Etv4 and Etv5 are required downstream of GDNF and Ret for kidney branching morphogenesis. *Nat Genet.* 2009;41(12):1295–1302.
120. Xu PX, et al. Eya1-deficient mice lack ears and kidneys and show abnormal apoptosis of organ primordia. *Nat Genet.* 1999;23(1):113–117.
121. de Pontual L, et al. Germline deletion of the miR-17 approximately 92 cluster causes skeletal and growth defects in humans. *Nat Genet.* 2011;43(10):1026–1030.
122. Barak H, et al. FGF9 and FGF20 maintain the stemness of nephron progenitors in mice and man. *Dev Cell.* 2012;22(6):1191–1207.
123. Devuyst O, et al. Rare inherited kidney diseases: challenges, opportunities, and perspectives. *Lancet.* 2014;383(9931):1844–1859.
124. Ogunlesi TA, Adekanmbi F. Evaluating and managing neonatal acute renal failure in a resource-poor setting. *Indian J Pediatr.* 2009;76(3):293–296.
125. Jenik AG, et al. A randomized, double-blind, placebo-controlled trial of the effects of prophylactic theophylline on renal function in term neonates with perinatal asphyxia. *Pediatrics.* 2000;105(4):E45.
126. Bakr AF. Prophylactic theophylline to prevent renal dysfunction in newborns exposed to perinatal asphyxia—a study in a developing country. *Pediatr Nephrol.* 2005;20(9):1249–1252.
127. Bhat MA, et al. Theophylline for renal function in term neonates with perinatal asphyxia: a randomized, placebo-controlled trial. *J Pediatr.* 2006;149(2):180–184.
128. Gouyon JB, Guignard JP. Theophylline prevents the hypoxemia-induced renal hemodynamic changes in rabbits. *Kidney Int.* 1988;33(6):1078–1083.
129. Kellum JA. Use of diuretics in the acute care setting. *Kidney Int Suppl.* 1998;66:S67–S70.

129a. Yelton SL, Gaylor MA, Murray KM. The role of continuous infusion loop diuretics. *Ann Pharmacother*. 1995;29(10):1010–1014, quiz 1060–1061.

130. Bellomo R, et al. Low-dose dopamine in patients with early renal dysfunction: a placebo-controlled randomised trial. Australian and New Zealand Intensive Care Society (ANZICS) Clinical Trials Group. *Lancet*. 2000;356(9248):2139–2143.

131. Chertow GM, et al. Is the administration of dopamine associated with adverse or favorable outcomes in acute renal failure? Auriculin Anaritide Acute Renal Failure Study Group. *Am J Med*. 1996;101(1):49–53.

132. Denton MD, Chertow GM, Brady HR. "Renal-dose" dopamine for the treatment of acute renal failure: scientific rationale, experimental studies and clinical trials. *Kidney Int*. 1996;50(1):4–14.

133. Galley HF. Renal-dose dopamine: will the message now get through? *Lancet*. 2000;356(9248):2112–2113.

134. Kellum JA, M Decker J. Use of dopamine in acute renal failure: a meta-analysis. *Crit Care Med*. 2001;29(8):1526–1531.

135. Lauschke A, et al. 'Low-dose' dopamine worsens renal perfusion in patients with acute renal failure. *Kidney Int*. 2006;69(9):1669–1674.

136. Mathur VS, et al. The effects of fenoldopam, a selective dopamine receptor agonist, on systemic and renal hemodynamics in normotensive subjects. *Crit Care Med*. 1999;27(9):1832–1837.

137. Landoni G, et al. Beneficial impact of fenoldopam in critically ill patients with or at risk for acute renal failure: a meta-analysis of randomized clinical trials. *Am J Kidney Dis*. 2007;49(1):56–68.

138. Knoderer CA, et al. Fenoldopam for acute kidney injury in children. *Pediatr Nephrol*. 2008;23(3):495–498.

139. Yoder SE, Yoder BA. An evaluation of off-label fenoldopam use in the neonatal intensive care unit. *Am J Perinatol*. 2009;26(10):745–750.

140. Ricci Z, et al. Fenoldopam in newborn patients undergoing cardiopulmonary bypass: controlled clinical trial. *Interact Cardiovasc Thorac Surg*. 2008;7(6):1049–1053.

141. Rodriguez-Soriano J. Potassium homeostasis and its disturbances in children. *Pediatr Nephrol*. 1995;9(3):364–374.

142. Malone TA. Glucose and insulin versus cation-exchange resin for the treatment of hyperkalemia in very low birth weight infants. *J Pediatr*. 1991;118(1):121–123.

143. Singh BS, et al. Efficacy of albuterol inhalation in treatment of hyperkalemia in premature neonates. *J Pediatr*. 2002;141(1):16–20.

144. Bunchman TE, et al. Pretreatment of formula with sodium polystyrene sulfonate to reduce dietary potassium intake. *Pediatr Nephrol*. 1991;5(1):29–32.

145. Gerstman BB, Kirkman R, Platt R. Intestinal necrosis associated with postoperative orally administered sodium polystyrene sulfonate in sorbitol. *Am J Kidney Dis*. 1992;20(2):159–161.

146. Andreoli SP, Dunson JW, Bergstein JM. Calcium carbonate is an effective phosphorus binder in children with chronic renal failure. *Am J Kidney Dis*. 1987;9(3):206–210.

147. Allgren RL, et al. Anaritide in acute tubular necrosis. Auriculin Anaritide Acute Renal Failure Study Group. *N Engl J Med*. 1997;336(12):828–834.

148. Chatterjee PK, et al. Tempol, a membrane-permeable radical scavenger, reduces oxidant stress-mediated renal dysfunction and injury in the rat. *Kidney Int*. 2000;58(2):658–673.

149. Chiao H, et al. Alpha-melanocyte-stimulating hormone protects against renal injury after ischemia in mice and rats. *J Clin Invest*. 1997;99(6):1165–1172.

150. Hirschberg R, et al. Multicenter clinical trial of recombinant human insulin-like growth factor I in patients with acute renal failure. *Kidney Int*. 1999;55(6):2423–2432.

151. Jo SK, Rosner MH, Okusa MD. Pharmacologic treatment of acute kidney injury: why drugs haven't worked and what is on the horizon. *Clin J Am Soc Nephrol*. 2007;2(2):356–365.

152. Lange C, et al. Administered mesenchymal stem cells enhance recovery from ischemia/reperfusion-induced acute renal failure in rats. *Kidney Int*. 2005;68(4):1613–1617.

153. Molitoris BA. Transitioning to therapy in ischemic acute renal failure. *J Am Soc Nephrol*. 2003;14(1):265–267.

154. Weston CE, et al. Effect of oxidant stress on growth factor stimulation of proliferation in cultured human proximal tubule cells. *Kidney Int*. 1999;56(4):1274–1276.

155. Belsha CW, Kohaut EC, Warady BA. Dialytic management of childhood acute renal failure: a survey of North American pediatric nephrologists. *Pediatr Nephrol*. 1995;9(3):361–363.

156. Yu JE, Park MS, Pai KS. Acute peritoneal dialysis in very low birth weight neonates using a vascular catheter. *Pediatr Nephrol*. 2010;25(2):367–371.

157. Ellis EN, et al. Outcome of infants on chronic peritoneal dialysis. *Adv Perit Dial*. 1995;11:266–269.

158. Golej J, et al. Low-volume peritoneal dialysis in 116 neonatal and paediatric critical care patients. *Eur J Pediatr*. 2002;161(7):385–389.

159. Ledermann SE, et al. Long-term outcome of peritoneal dialysis in infants. *J Pediatr*. 2000;136(1):24–29.

160. McNiece KL, et al. Adequacy of peritoneal dialysis in children following cardiopulmonary bypass surgery. *Pediatr Nephrol*. 2005;20(7):972–976.

161. Rainey KE, DiGeronimo RJ, Pascual-Baralt J. Successful long-term peritoneal dialysis in a very low birth weight infant with renal failure secondary to feto-fetal transfusion syndrome. *Pediatrics*. 2000;106(4):849–851.

162. Sadowski RH, Harmon WE, Jabs K. Acute hemodialysis of infants weighing less than five kilograms. *Kidney Int*. 1994;45(3):903–906.

163. Wiegand C, et al. The management of life-threatening hyperammonemia: a comparison of several therapeutic modalities. *J Pediatr*. 1980;96(1):142–144.

18

164. Silver SM, Sterns RH, Halperin ML. Brain swelling after dialysis: old urea or new osmoles? *Am J Kidney Dis*. 1996;28(1):1–13.

165. Falk MC, et al. Continuous venovenous haemofiltration in the acute treatment of inborn errors of metabolism. *Pediatr Nephrol*. 1994;8(3):330–333.

166. Ronco C, et al. Treatment of acute renal failure in newborns by continuous arterio-venous hemofiltration. *Kidney Int*. 1986;29(4):908–915.

167. Symons JM, et al. Continuous renal replacement therapy in children up to 10 kg. *Am J Kidney Dis*. 2003;41(5):984–989.

168. Zobel G, et al. Continuous renal replacement therapy in critically ill patients. *Kidney Int Suppl*. 1998;66:S169–S173.

169. Santiago MJ, et al. The use of continuous renal replacement therapy in series with extracorporeal membrane oxygenation. *Kidney Int*. 2009;76(12):1289–1292.

170. Ronco C, et al. Continuous renal replacement therapy in neonates and small infants: development and first-in-human use of a miniaturised machine (CARPEDIEM). *Lancet*. 2014;383(9931):1807–1813.

171. Coulthard MG, et al. Haemodialysing babies weighing <8 kg with the Newcastle infant dialysis and ultrafiltration system (Nidus): comparison with peritoneal and conventional haemodialysis. *Pediatr Nephrol*. 2014;29(10):1873–1881.

172. Ronco C, Ricci Z, Goldstein SL. (R)evolution in the Management of Acute Kidney Injury in Newborns. *Am J Kidney Dis*. 2015;66(2):206–211.

173. Askenazi D, et al. Smaller circuits for smaller patients: improving renal support therapy with Aquadex. *Pediatr Nephrol*. 2016;31(5):853–860.

174. Sanchez-Pinto LN, et al. Association Between Progression and Improvement of Acute Kidney Injury and Mortality in Critically Ill Children. *Pediatr Crit Care Med*. 2015;16(8):703–710.

175. Askenazi DJ, et al. Acute kidney injury is independently associated with mortality in very low birthweight infants: a matched case-control analysis. *Pediatr Nephrol*. 2009;24(5):991–997.

176. Askenazi DJ, et al. 3-5 year longitudinal follow-up of pediatric patients after acute renal failure. *Kidney Int*. 2006;69(1):184–189.

177. Sutherland SM, et al. AKI in hospitalized children: epidemiology and clinical associations in a national cohort. *Clin J Am Soc Nephrol*. 2013;8(10):1661–1669.

178. Mammen C, et al. Long-term risk of CKD in children surviving episodes of acute kidney injury in the intensive care unit: a prospective cohort study. *Am J Kidney Dis*. 2012;59(4):523–530.

179. White SL, et al. Is low birth weight an antecedent of CKD in later life? A systematic review of observational studies. *Am J Kidney Dis*. 2009;54(2):248–261.

180. Bruel A, et al. Renal outcome in children born preterm with neonatal acute renal failure: IRENEO—a prospective controlled study. *Pediatr Nephrol*. 2016;31(12):2365–2373.

181. Rodriguez-Soriano J, et al. Long-term renal follow-up of extremely low birth weight infants. *Pediatr Nephrol*. 2005;20(5):579–584.

182. Jones C, Judd B. Long-term follow-up of extremely low birth weight infants. *Pediatr Nephrol*. 2006;21(2):299.

183. Jones CA, et al. Hypercalciuria in ex-preterm children, aged 7-8 years. *Pediatr Nephrol*. 2001;16(8):665–671.

184. Bacchetta J, et al. Both extrauterine and intrauterine growth restriction impair renal function in children born very preterm. *Kidney Int*. 2009;76(4):445–452.

185. Hsu CW, Symons JM. Acute kidney injury: can we improve prognosis? *Pediatr Nephrol*. 2010;25(12):2401–2412.

CHAPTER 19

Hereditary Tubulopathies

Israel Zelikovic, MD

Hereditary tubular transport disorders comprise a group of diseases that lead to profound derangements in the homeostasis of electrolytes, minerals, or organic solutes in the body and can be associated with significant morbidity.[1–5]

For decades, the study of inherited tubular transport disorders has focused on the physiologic and metabolic alterations leading to impaired solute handling by the tubular epithelial cell. Over the past two decades, the breakthrough in molecular biology and molecular genetics has provided the tools to investigate hereditary tubulopathies at the molecular level. As a result, exciting discoveries have been made, and the underlying molecular defects in many of these disorders have been defined.[1–4] The molecular study of hereditary tubulopathies has been important not only in clarifying the genetic basis of these disorders but also in providing new and important insight into the function of specific transport proteins and into the physiology of renal tubular reclamation of solutes.

Generally, tubular transport disorders are subdivided into two large groups: (1) *primary isolated tubulopathies,* which are mostly hereditary and involve an impairment in a single tubular function; and (2) *generalized tubulopathies,* which are hereditary or acquired and are caused by complex tubular derangements involving more than one transport system. A variety of primary inherited tubulopathies alter specific renal epithelial transport functions.[1,2] In most instances, the change in transport function leads to the loss of an essential substance in the urine and either impaired homeostasis of this substance in the body (as in renal tubular acidosis [RTA] or Bartter syndrome) or precipitation of the substance in the kidney (as in cystinuria or hypercalciuria). In some of these disorders, however, the defect in tubular function leads to accumulation of a substance in the body (as in pseudohypoaldosteronism type II).

Hereditary tubulopathies can affect children at all ages, but usually, children with these disorders present in the neonatal period or in the first year of life. Clinical manifestations of hereditary tubulopathies are commonly nonspecific and may include failure to thrive, stunted growth, poor feeding, recurrent vomiting, diarrhea, constipation, polyuria, polydipsia, or recurrent febrile episodes.[1] In some instances, however, more specific manifestations such as rickets, urolithiasis, or hypertension aid in the diagnosis of a specific tubulopathy. In most of these disorders, the principle of therapy is replacement of the substance lost in the urine or prevention of precipitation of the substance in the kidney. Some of the tubulopathies (e.g., isolated glycosuria) are benign and require no therapy. In addition to a detailed history and careful examination of the child, simultaneous and accurate assessment of the serum and urine concentration of the substance involved in the tubulopathy holds the key to the correct diagnosis.[1] Renal ultrasonography and bone radiography are helpful studies in most tubulopathies.

This chapter summarizes the general characteristics of hereditary tubular transport disorders, reviews the molecular pathophysiology and genetic aspects of the diseases, describes the clinical feature of the tubulopathies, and briefly summarizes their therapy. The focus of this chapter is on disorders resulting from primary gene defects in transporters or channels operating along the renal tubule. Some tubular transport disorders secondary to defects in receptors (e.g., as Ca^{2+}-sensing receptor or antidiuretic hormone receptor), enzymes (e.g., with no K [lysine] serine-threonine protein kinases, WNKs), or regulatory proteins (e.g., melanoma-associated antigen D2, MAGE-D2) resulting in isolated tubulopathies are also discussed. Generalized tubulopathies involving several transport systems (e.g., Fanconi syndrome) or resulting from mitochondrial cytopathies are not discussed or only briefly mentioned. Inherited tubular disorders of calcium, magnesium, and phosphorus are discussed in Chapter 20. In Tables 19.1 through 19.4, the disorders reviewed are summarized and grouped by the nephron segment affected.

Proximal Tubule

Proximal Renal Tubular Acidosis

General Characteristics

Proximal renal tubular acidosis (pRTA; RTA type 2) is characterized by normal anion gap, hyperchloremic metabolic acidosis caused by impaired capacity of the proximal tubule to reabsorb HCO_3^- (Fig. 19.1).[4,6,7] Thus, at normal plasma HCO_3^- concentration, large amounts of HCO_3^- (>15% of the filtered load) escape proximal reabsorption and reach the distal tubule. This load overwhelms the limited capacity of the distal tubule to reabsorb HCO_3^-, substantial bicarbonaturia occurs, urine pH increases, net acid secretion ceases, and metabolic acidosis develops.[7-9] This HCO_3^- wasting is a transient phenomenon, and when the serum HCO_3^- level stabilizes in the acidemia range, the smaller amounts of HCO_3^- lost in the proximal tubule are completely reabsorbed by the distal tubule, and urine pH decreases to less

Text continued on p. 321

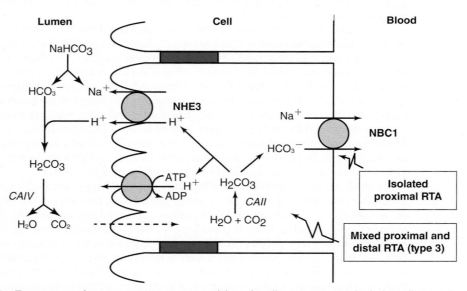

Fig. 19.1   Transport mechanisms participating in acid–base handling in a proximal tubular cell. H^+ and HCO_3^- are formed in the cell as a result of carbonic anhydrase II (CAII) action. H^+ exits the cell via the apical Na^+/H^+ exchanger (NHE3) and H^+-ATPase pump. HCO_3^- exit occurs via the basolateral Na^+/HCO_3^- cotransporter (NBC1). Hereditary renal tubular acidosis syndromes caused by defects in NBC1 and CAII, respectively, are depicted.

Table 19.1 HEREDITARY TUBULOPATHIES CAUSED BY TRANSPORT DEFECTS IN THE PROXIMAL TUBULE

Disorder	Defective Gene	Locus	Defective Protein	Mode of Inheritance	Localization of Defect	Clinical Features	OMIM Number[a]
Isolated proximal RTA (type 2)	*SLC4A4*	4q21	Na$^+$-HCO$_3^-$ cotransporter, NBC1	AR	Basolateral	Normal anion gap metabolic acidosis, failure to thrive, hypokalemia, polyuria, polydipsia, dehydration, muscle weakness, ocular abnormalities	604278
Classic cystinuria							
• Type I	*SLC3A1*	2p163	rBAT	AR	Luminal	Urinary stones, obstruction, infection	220100
• Non type I	*SLC7A9*	19q13.1	b$^{0,+}$AT	Incomplete AR	Luminal		
Lysinuric protein intolerance	*SLC7A7*	14q11	y$^+$LAT-1	AR	Basolateral	Failure to thrive, protein intolerance, vomiting, hypotonia, hyperammonemia, seizures, coma	222700
Hartnup disease	*SLC6A19*	5p15.33	AA transport system B^0	AR	Luminal	Skin rash, cerebellar ataxia, psychiatric illnesses	234500
Isolated hereditary glycosuria	*SLC5A2*	16p11.2	SGLT2	AR	Luminal	None	233100
Fanconi-Bickel syndrome	*SLC2A2*	3q26.1	GLUT2	AR	Basolateral	Failure to thrive, proximal tubulopathy, hepatomegaly, fasting hypoglycemia, postprandial hyperglycemia	227810

[a]Online Mendelian Inheritance in Man (database at http://www.ncbi.nlm.nih.gov/Omim).
AA, Amino acid; AR, autosomal recessive; b$^{0,+}$AT, light subunit of AA transport system b$^{0,+}$; GLUT2, facilitative glucose transporter; rBAT, heavy subunit of AA transport system b$^{0,+}$; SGLT2, Na$^+$-glucose cotransporter; y$^+$LAT-1, light subunit of AA transport system y$^+$L.

19

D

Table 19.2 TUBULOPATHIES CAUSED BY TRANSPORT DEFECTS IN THE LOOP OF HENLE

Disorder	Defective Gene	Locus	Defective Protein	Localization of Defect	Mode of Inheritance	Clinical Features	OMIM Number[a]
Antenatal Bartter syndrome (type I)	SLC12A1	15q21	Na$^+$-K$^+$-2Cl$^-$ cotransporter, NKCC2	Luminal	AR	Renal salt wasting, hypokalemia, hypochloremic metabolic alkalosis, failure to thrive, polyuria, dehydration, muscle weakness, hypercalciuria	601678
Antenatal Bartter syndrome (type II)	KCNJ1	11q24	K$^+$ channel, ROMK	Luminal	AR	Renal salt wasting, hypokalemia, hypochloremic metabolic alkalosis, failure to thrive, polyuria, dehydration, muscle weakness, hypercalciuria	241200
Classic Bartter syndrome (type III)	CLCNKB	1p36	Cl$^-$ channel, ClC-Kb	Basolateral	AR	Renal salt wasting, hypokalemia, hypochloremic metabolic alkalosis, failure to thrive, polyuria, dehydration, muscle weakness, ± hypercalciuria	602023
Bartter syndrome with deafness (type IV)	BSND	1p31	Barttin (β subunit of ClC-Ka/ClC-KB)	Basolateral	AR	Renal salt wasting, hypokalemia, hypochloremic metabolic alkalosis, failure to thrive, polyuria, dehydration, muscle weakness, ± hypercalciuria, chronic renal failure, sensorineural deafness	602522
Autosomal dominant hypocalcemia with Bartter syndrome (type V)	CASR	3q21	CaSR	Basolateral	AD	Renal salt wasting, hypokalemia, hypochloremic metabolic alkalosis, failure to thrive, polyuria, dehydration, muscle weakness, hypercalciuria	601198
Transient antenatal Bartter syndrome	MAGED2	Xp11	MAGE-D2	Luminal	X-linked	Severe polyhydramnios, transient renal salt wasting, hypokalemia, hypochloremic metabolic alkalosis, polyuria, dehydration, hypercalciuria	300971

[a]Online Mendelian Inheritance in Man (database at http://www.ncbi.nlm.nih.gov/Omim).
AD, Autosomal dominant; AR, autosomal recessive; CaSR, Ca^{2+}/Mg^{2+} sensing receptor; ClC-Ka, basolateral Cl$^-$ channel; ClC-Kb, basolateral Cl$^-$ channel; NKCC2, Na$^+$, K$^+$, 2Cl$^-$ cotransporter; MAGE-D2, melanoma-associated antigen D2; ROMK, renal outer medullary potassium channel.

Table 19.3 HEREDITARY TUBULOPATHIES CAUSED BY TRANSPORT DEFECTS IN THE DISTAL CONVOLUTED TUBULE

Disorder	Defective Gene	Locus	Defective Protein	Localization of Defect	Mode of Inheritance	Clinical Features	OMIM Number[a]
Gitelman syndrome	SLC12A3 CLCNKB	16q13 1p36	Na⁺-Cl⁻ cotransporter, TSC (NCCT) Cl⁻ channel, ClC-Kb	Luminal Basolateral	AR	Mild renal salt wasting, hypokalemia, hypochloremic, metabolic alkalosis, muscle weakness, tetany, hypomagnesemia, hypocalciuria	263800
EAST, SESAME syndrome	KCNJ10	1q23	K⁺ channel, Kir4.1	Basolateral	AR	Epilepsy, ataxia, sensorineural deafness, Gitelman-like tubulopathy	612780
Pseudohypoaldosteronism type 2 (Gordon syndrome)	WNK4 WNK1 KLHL3 CUL3	17q21 12p13 5q31 2q36	WNK4 WNK1 Kelch-like 3 Cullin 3	Cytoplasmic/luminal	AD	Thiazide-sensitive hypertension, hyperkalemia, hyperchloremic metabolic acidosis	601844 605232 605775 614496

[a]Online Mendelian Inheritance in Man (database at http://www.ncbi.nlm.nih.gov/Omim).
AD, Autosomal dominant; AR, autosomal recessive; ClC-Kb, basolateral Cl⁻ channel; EAST, epilepsy, ataxia, sensorineural deafness and tubulopathy; SESAME, seizures, sensorineural deafness, ataxia, mental retardation, and electrolyte imbalance; WNK, with no K [lysine] serine-threonine protein kinase.

Table 19.4 HEREDITARY TUBULOPATHIES CAUSED BY TRANSPORT DEFECTS IN THE CORTICAL COLLECTING DUCT

Disorder	Defective Gene	Locus	Defective Protein	Cell Type Involved	Localization of Defect	Clinical Features	OMIM Number[a]
Distal RTA (Type 1)							
AD distal RTA	$SLC4A1$	17q21-22	AE1	α intercalated	Basolateral	Mild metabolic acidosis, hypokalemia, hypercalciuria, hypocitraturia, nephrolithiasis, nephrocalcinosis, rickets/osteomalacia	179800
AR distal RTA	$SLC4A1$	17q21-22	AE1	α intercalated	Basolateral	Metabolic acidosis, hemolytic anemia (Southeast Asia only)	602722
AR distal RTA with deafness	$ATP6V1B1$	2p13	B_1 subunit of H^+-ATPase	α intercalated	Luminal	Early metabolic acidosis, nephrocalcinosis, vomiting, dehydration, growth retardation, rickets, bilateral sensorineural hearing loss	267300
AR distal RTA without or with late onset deafness	$ATP6VOA4$	7q33	a4 subunit of H^+-ATPase	α intercalated	Luminal	Early metabolic acidosis, nephrocalcinosis, vomiting, dehydration, growth retardation, rickets, late onset sensorineural hearing loss or normal hearing	602772
Mixed proximal and distal RTA (type 3)	$CA2$	8q22	Carbonic anhydrase II	Proximal tubule and α intercalated	Cytoplasm	Metabolic acidosis, hypokalemia, osteopetrosis, blindness, deafness, early nephrocalcinosis	259730
RTA Type 4							
AD pseudohypoaldosteronism type 1	$NR3C2$	4q31	Mineralocorticoid receptor	Principal	Cytoplasm	Mild hyponatremia, hyperkalemia, metabolic acidosis	177735
AR pseudohypoaldosteronism type 1	$SCNN1A$ $SCNN1B$ $SCNN1C$	12p13,1 16p13 16p12	Na^+ channel ENaC (α,β,γ subunits)	Principal	Luminal	Neonatal salt wasting, severe dehydration, hyperkalemic metabolic acidosis, hyponatremia, respiratory disease	264350
Nephrogenic Diabetes Insipidus							
X-linked NDI	$AVPR2$	Xq28	Vasopressin type-2 receptor, V2R	Principal	Basolateral	Polydipsia, polyuria, hyposthenuria, hypernatremic dehydration, failure to thrive, neurologic deficit	304800
AR or AD NDI	$AQP2$	12q13	H_2O channel, AQP2	Principal	Luminal	Polydipsia, polyuria, hyposthenuria, hypernatremic dehydration, failure to thrive, neurologic deficit	125800
Nephrogenic syndrome of inappropriate diuresis	$AVPR2$	Xq28	Vasopressin type-2 receptor, V2R	Principal	Basolateral	Hyponatremia, seizures, hypertonic urine	300539

[a]Online Mendelian Inheritance in Man (database at http://www.ncbi.nlm.nih.gov/Omim).
AD, Autosomal dominant; AE1, anion exchanger 1; AQP2, aquaporin 2; AR, autosomal recessive; ENaC, epithelial Na^+ channel; NDI, nephrogenic diabetes insipidus; RTA, renal tubular acidosis; V2R, vasopressin type 2 receptor.

than 5.5.[6,7] In pRTA, serum K^+ level is usually diminished. Hypokalemia develops because increased delivery of Na^+ to the distal nephron results in enhanced secretion of K^+ in the principal cell of the cortical collecting duct (CCD), and mild volume depletion secondary to Na^+ loss results in secondary hyperaldosteronism that increases K^+ secretion.[7-9]

pRTA occurs either as a manifestation of a generalized proximal tubular dysfunction (Fanconi syndrome) or as an isolated entity. Inheritance of isolated pRTA is autosomal recessive and occurs consistently in association with ocular abnormalities, including glaucoma, band keratopathy, and cataracts (see Table 19.1 and Fig. 19.1).[10-12] Additional manifestations include short stature, calcification of the basal ganglia, and mental retardation (see later discussion).[4,11]

Molecular Pathophysiology

Normally, most (80%–90%) of the filtered load of HCO_3^- is reabsorbed in the proximal tubule. Several membrane transport proteins participate in acid–base handling in the proximal tubule (see Fig. 19.1).[6-8,13] H^+ and HCO_3^- are formed in the proximal tubular cell as a result of the action of intracellular carbonic anhydrase II (CAII). H^+ efflux from cell to lumen occurs via the apical Na^+/H^+ exchanger (NHE3) and to a small extent via the apical H^+-ATPase pump. HCO_3^- exit to blood is mediated by the basolateral membrane Na^+-HCO_3^- cotransporter (NBC1).

The Na^+/HCO_3^- cotransporter NBC1 (see Fig. 19.1), encoded by the *SLC4A4* gene located on chromosome 4q21, has been implicated in autosomal recessive proximal RTA.[10,11] NBC1 belongs to the HCO_3^- transporter superfamily, to which the Cl^-/HCO_3^- exchanger also belongs.[6,14] Igarashi et al.[10] identified two homozygous missense mutations in kidney NBC1 in two individuals with autosomal recessive pRTA and ocular abnormalities (see Table 19.1). Both patients had cataracts, glaucoma, and band keratopathy. A number of other mutations have subsequently been described.[15,16] In addition to reduced functional activity, defects of intracellular trafficking have been demonstrated for some of these mutations.[15-17] Severe isolated proximal RTA was recently described in NBC1 W561X knock-in mouse.[18] It is possible that defective corneal NBC1 function in patients with isolated pRTA results in impaired HCO_3^- transport, which in turn leads to abnormal calcium carbonate deposition in the cornea and band keratopathy.[11,12]

Clinical Features

The most prominent clinical feature of pRTA is failure to thrive. Other manifestations, which are related to untreated hypokalemia, include polyuria, polydipsia, dehydration, vomiting, anorexia, constipation, and muscle weakness (see Table 19.1).[6,7] Hypercalciuria, nephrocalcinosis, and nephrolithiasis typically are not observed. Metabolic bone disease usually occurs in patients with Fanconi syndrome and is attributed to hypophosphatemia and impaired vitamin D metabolism, but may also be induced by the bone Ca^{2+}-depleting effect of chronic acidosis in isolated pRTA.[4,11]

The diagnosis of pRTA is usually straightforward and can be based on several simple laboratory data. These include (1) normal anion gap, hyperchloremic metabolic acidosis; (2) hypokalemia; (3) low urine pH during acidemia; and (4) a negative urinary anion gap (calculated as $[Na^+] + [K^+] - [Cl^-]$) indicating substantial urinary ammonium concentration, in the absence of extrarenal losses of HCO_3^- such as gastroenteritis[19,20] (as opposed to the positive urinary anion gap in distal RTA; see later discussion). Although usually not necessary, demonstration of increased (>15%) fractional excretion of HCO_3^- by the HCO_3^- titration curve can support the diagnosis. Children with pRTA require large doses of alkali (up to 20 mEq/kg per day). Hypokalemia should be treated by correcting hypovolemia and by using KCl supplements.[19,20]

Hereditary Aminoacidurias

Only negligible amounts of amino acids are normally present in the final urine, reflecting very efficient reabsorption mechanisms for these organic solutes in the proximal tubule. Aminoacidurias are a group of disorders in which a single amino acid or a group of amino acids are excreted in excess amounts in the urine.[21] The defective tubular reabsorption is assumed to result from a genetic defect in a specific transport system that directs the reabsorption of these amino acids under normal conditions. Some of these disorders also involve a similar transport abnormality in the intestine. As opposed to inborn errors of amino acid metabolism, in which plasma levels of amino acids are elevated resulting in overflow aminoaciduria, plasma levels of amino acids in hereditary aminoacidurias are largely normal. The aminoacidurias are generally categorized into five major groups according to the group-specific transport pathway presumed to be affected.[21] Discussed in this chapter are the cationic aminoacidurias, classic cystinuria, and lysinuric protein intolerance (LPI), as well as the neutral aminoaciduria, Hartnup disease (see Table 19.1 and Fig. 19.1). The genetic defects in these three membrane transport disorders, which are associated with significant morbidity, have been identified.

Classic Cystinuria

General Characteristics

Cystinuria is a disorder of amino acid transport characterized by excessive urinary excretion of cystine and the dibasic amino acids lysine, arginine, and ornithine.[21] The pathogenic mechanism of cystinuria is defective transepithelial transport of these amino acids in the proximal tubule and the small intestine.[21-23] The high-affinity, low-capacity amino acid transport system shared by cystine and the dibasic amino acids (i.e., $b^{0,+}$; Fig. 19.2) is defective in classic cystinuria.[21,24]

The very low solubility of cystine in the urine results in cystine stone formation in homozygous patients. Urinary cystine calculi may produce considerable morbidity, including urinary obstruction; colic; infection; and in severe cases, loss of kidney function. Cystinuria accounts for 1% to 2% of all urolithiasis and 6% to 8% of urolithiasis in children.[24,25]

Classic cystinuria is inherited in an autosomal recessive fashion. It is a common disorder with an overall prevalence of 1 in 7000 to 1 in 15,000 and an estimated gene frequency of 0.01.[22] A very high prevalence, 1 in 2500, is observed in Israeli Jews of Libyan origin.[21,24]

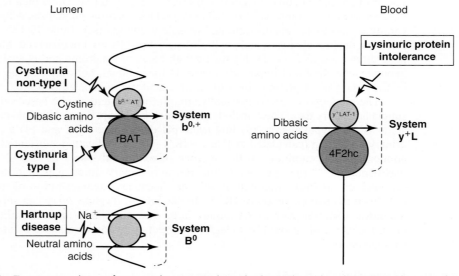

Fig. 19.2 Transport pathways for several amino acids at the luminal and basolateral membranes of a proximal tubular cell. *Large circles* represent the heavy subunits and *small circles* the light subunits of the heteromeric dibasic amino acid transporters $b^{0,+}$ and y^+L. Depicted are hereditary aminoacidurias caused by defects in these transporters.

Cystinuria has been classified into three phenotypes based on the degree of intestinal uptake of cystine by homozygotes and the level of urinary dibasic amino acids in heterozygotes.[24,25] Type I cystinuria is inherited as an autosomal recessive trait, and obligate heterozygotes have normal urinary amino acid profiles. In contrast, obligate heterozygotes for type II and type III cystinuria show various degrees of hyperexcretion of cystine and dibasic amino acids in the urine. In addition, genetic compounds of cystinuria, such as types I/III, can occur.[26]

Molecular Pathophysiology

Type I cystinuria is caused by mutations in the gene *SLCA3A1* localized to chromosome 2p21. The gene encodes a protein termed rBAT, which constitutes the heavy subunit of the proximal tubular, brush-border membrane-bound, heteromeric dibasic amino acid transporter $b^{0,+}$ (see Fig. 19.2).[21,27] To date, more than 130 different rBAT mutations have been reported in patients with type I cystinuria.[21,24] These mutations include nonsense, missense, splice site, frameshift mutations, and large deletions.[24,28] Cystinuria types II and III are caused by mutations in the gene *SLC7A9*, which is localized to chromosome 19q13.1 and encodes the $b^{0,+}$ AT protein that constitutes the light subunit of the heteromeric amino acid transporter $b^{0,+}$ (see Fig. 19.2).[6,29] To date, more than 95 different mutations have been identified in nontype I cystinuria patients.[21,24] Recently, the International Cystinuria Consortium (ICC) has introduced an additional classification of cystinuria subtypes based on genotype rather than phenotype.[21,24] This new classification includes: Type A—due to two mutations on *SLCA3A1* on chromosome 2; Type B—due to two mutations on *SLC7A9* on chromosome 19; and Type AB—due to one mutation on each *SLCA3A1* and *SLC7A9* (compound heterozygote).

Clinical Features

The simplest diagnostic test in cystinuria is the microscopic examination of the urinary sediment of a freshly voided morning urine.[22,25] The presence of typical flat hexagonal cystine crystals is diagnostic. The best screening procedure is the cyanide–nitroprusside test.[22] The definite test is a measurement of cystine and the dibasic amino acids concentrations by ion exchange chromatography.

Cystine stones are radiopaque because of the density of the sulfur molecule, and on radiography, they appear smooth. Cystine also may act as nidus for calcium oxalate, so mixed stones may be found.[21]

The disease usually presents with renal colic. Occasionally, infection, hypertension, or renal failure may be the first manifestation (see Table 19.1).[22,23,25] Most patients have recurrent stone formation. Cystinuric patients who receive a kidney transplant have normal urinary cystine and dibasic amino acid excretion after transplantation.[21]

Treatment

Cystine crystalluria occurs when the cystine content of the urine exceeds 300 mg/L at a pH of 4.5 to 7.0. Cystine solubility increases sharply at a urine pH above 7.0.[22] The major therapeutic approaches to cystinuria are designed to increase the solubility of cystine, reduce excretion cystine, and convert cystine to more soluble compounds.[22,24,30] Therapies used in the management of cystinuria include the following:

1. Increased oral fluid intake to increase urine volume and cystine solubility. Because patients with cystinuria excrete 0.5 to 1.0 g/day of cystine, intake of at least twice normal maintenance fluid volume for age could be required to keep the urinary cystine concentration below 300 mg/L.[21,22]
2. Oral alkali in addition to high fluid intake to further increase cystine solubility in the urine.[21] A urine pH of 7.5 to 8.0 can be maintained by the provision of 1 to 2 mEq/kg per day of bicarbonate or citrate in divided doses. Because high sodium intake increases cystine excretion, potassium citrate is preferred.[22,25] Because urine alkalinization may result in formation of mixed Ca^{2+}-containing stones, adherence to high fluid intake is crucial.

3. Na$^+$ restriction to reduce cystine excretion. Dietary Na$^+$ restriction is recommended in patients with cystinuria because urinary excretion of cystine and dibasic amino acids correlates with urinary Na$^+$ excretion.[31]

4. Pharmacologic therapy to increase cystine solubility and decrease cystine excretion. The sulfhydryl-binding compound D-penicillamine (β-dimethylcysteine) leads to the formation of the mixed disulfide penicillamine–cysteine after a disulfide exchange reaction. This mixed disulfide is far more water soluble than cystine. Unfortunately, penicillamine produces serious side effects, including rashes, fever, arthralgia, nephrotic syndrome, pancytopenia, and loss of taste.[22,32] Mercaptopropionyl glycine (MPG), another agent undergoing a disulfide exchange reaction, is as effective as D-penicillamine in the treatment of patients with cystinuria. Because of the lower toxicity of MPG, this compound is the pharmacologic agent of choice in the therapy of cystinuria.[24,33] It has been proposed that meso-1,3 dimercaptosuccinic acid (DMSA), an additional compound forming disulfide linkage with cysteine, might also be a useful therapeutic agent in those with cystinuria.[21] Recently, α-lipoic acid has been shown to increase urinary cystine solubility and to prevent cystine urolithiasis in a mouse model of cystinuria.[34] This widely used nutritional supplement with few adverse side effects is an attractive candidate for assessment in individuals with cystinuria.

5. Urologic procedures that have been used to treat cysteine stones include chemolysis of stones by irrigation through a percutaneous nephrostomy, extracorporeal shockwave lithotripsy, and lithotomy.[24,35]

Lysinuric Protein Intolerance

General Characteristics

LPI is a rare autosomal recessive disorder characterized by excessive urinary excretion of dibasic amino acids (especially lysine), normal cystine excretion, and poor intestinal absorption of dibasic amino acids.[21,36] Plasma values of dibasic amino acids are subnormal. The disease is relatively common in Finland, where the prevalence of the disease is 1 in 60,000, and in Italy.[36] Homozygous patients show massive dibasic aminoaciduria, as well as hyperammonemia, after a protein overload. The clinical manifestations in homozygotes for LPI are protein malnutrition and postprandial hyperammonemia. They include failure to thrive, marked protein intolerance, vomiting, diarrhea, hepatosplenomegaly, muscle hypotonia, interstitial lung disease, osteoporosis, seizures, and coma (see Table 19.1).[21,36–38]

Molecular Pathophysiology

The pathogenic mechanism of LPI appears to be defective, high-affinity, dibasic amino acid transport system y$^+$L (see Fig. 19.2) at the basolateral membrane of renal and intestinal epithelial cells, resulting in impaired efflux of these amino acids from cell to interstitium.[21,38,39] Nonepithelial cells such as hepatocytes, granulocytes, and cultures akin fibroblasts from patients with LPI also show impaired transport of dibasic amino acids. The defective hepatic transport of dibasic amino acids is associated with disturbances in the urea cycle and consequent hyperammonemia.[38]

LPI is caused by mutations in the gene *SLC7A7* encoding y$^+$LAT-1, a member of the family of light subunits that combine with 4F2hc (a heavy subunit) to form heteromeric amino acid transporters.[6,36] The 4F2hc/y$^+$LAT-1 transporter has been shown to have the activity of amino acid transport system y$^+$L that is responsible for the efflux of basic amino acids at the basolateral plasma membrane of epithelial cells (see Fig. 19.2).[40] The *SLC7A7* gene is localized to chromosome 14q11-13. To date, approximately 50 *SLC7A7* mutations, spread along the entire gene, have been found in LPI patients from different ethnic groups.[39,41]

Treatment

Therapy of patients with LPI consists of protein restriction to prevent hyperammonemia, as well as oral supplements of arginine, ornithine, and (most important) citrulline.[36,42] Administration of the latter amino acid, which corrects the hepatic deficiency in ornithine and arginine, results in clinical improvement and catch-up growth.

Hartnup Disease
General Characteristics

Hartnup disease, which may have afflicted Julius Caesar and his family,[43] was first recognized in two siblings in England in 1956.[44] This disease is characterized by intestinal malabsorption and massive aminoaciduria of the neutral monoamino monocarboxylic amino acids alanine, serine, threonine, valine, leucine, isoleucine, phenylalanine, tyrosine, tryptophan, histidine, glutamine, and asparagine (see Table 19.1).[45,46] Most patients also have increased excretion of indolic compounds that originate in the gut from bacterial degradation of tryptophan.[45] Transport of other neutral amino acids, including cystine, imino acids, glycine, and β-amino acids, is unaffected. The disease is inherited as an autosomal recessive trait and has an estimated incidence of 1 in 20,000 live births. Heterozygotes have normal urinary acid excretion under physiologic conditions. Clinical features in homozygotes may include photosensitive rash, cerebellar ataxia, and a variety of psychiatric manifestations resembling the features of pellagra (see Table 19.1).[45,46] These pellagra-like manifestations are primarily caused by intestinal malabsorption and urinary loss of tryptophan, an amino acid that is required for niacin synthesis. The diagnosis should be suspected in any patient with pellagra who has no history of niacin or nicotinamide deficiency and should be made by chromatographic analysis of the urine.[45]

Molecular Pathophysiology

A defect in the broad-specificity neutral, α-amino acid transport mechanism in the renal and intestinal brush-border membrane was presumed to be the pathogenic mechanism underlying this disorder.[21] The transport characteristics and the epithelial distribution of the Na^+-dependent neutral amino acid transport B° (see Fig. 19.2) have led to the conclusion that this transporter is the defective one in Hartnup disorder. In 2001, the gene responsible for Hartnup disease was localized to chromosome 5p15.[47] Subsequently, Bröer's group[48] cloned from the syntenic region in the mouse the B°AT1 (SLC6A19) gene. This SLC6 gene encodes a Na^+-dependent neutral amino acid transporter, which is expressed in the brush-border membrane of the early proximal tubule and the intestine and corresponds to the B° transport system.[49]

In 2004, two groups[50,51] cloned the human SLC6A19 gene from chromosome 5p15 and have found several mutations in this gene in British, Japanese, and Australian patients with Hartnup disease, thereby identifying SLC6A19 as the disease-causing gene. To date, a total of 21 mutations have been identified that cause Hartnup disorder.[21] Interestingly, it has been demonstrated[21] that most of the probands with Hartnup disease analyzed so far display allelic heterogeneity in that they are compound heterozygotes for the SLC6A19 mutation.

Treatment

Patients with Hartnup disease respond well to oral therapy with 40 to 100 mg/day of nicotinamide.[21] Oral administration of tryptophan ethyl ester, a lipid-soluble form of tryptophan, has been shown to increase serum tryptophan and reverse clinical symptoms in patients with Hartnup disease.[52]

Hereditary Glycosurias

Glycosurias are a group of disorders in which specific defects in glucose transporters in the renal tubule result in excretion of significant quantities of glucose in the urine.[21] This group includes hereditary isolated glycosuria and Fanconi-Bickel syndrome (see Table 19.1 and Fig. 19.3).

PROXIMAL CONVOLUTED TUBULE

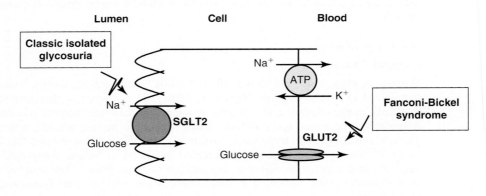

PROXIMAL STRAIGHT TUBULE

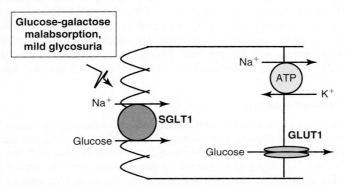

Fig. 19.3 Schematic model for the distribution of glucose transporters in renal tubular epithelium. Glucose transport from lumen to cell in the proximal convoluted tubule and the proximal straight tubule is mediated by the luminal Na+-dependent glucose transporters SGLT2 and SGLT1, respectively. Glucose exit from cells in these two nephron segments occurs via the basolateral, facilitative Na+-independent glucose transporters GLUT2 and GLUT1, respectively. Depicted are hereditary glycosurias caused by defects in these transporters. (Adapted with permission from Zelikovic I. Aminoaciduria and glycosuria in children. In: Avner ED, Harmon N, Niaudet P, et al., eds. *Pediatric Nephrology.* 7th ed. Berlin Heidelberg: Springer-Verlag; 2015:1155-1200.)

Hereditary Isolated Glycosuria

General Characteristics

Hereditary isolated glycosuria is an abnormality in which variable amounts of glucose are excreted in the urine at normal concentrations of blood glucose.[21,53] The renal defect is specific for glucose, and there is no increase in the urinary excretion of other sugars. Renal glycosuria is a benign condition without symptoms or physical consequences except during pregnancy or prolonged starvation—when dehydration and ketosis may develop.[53] The metabolism, storage, and use of carbohydrates as well as insulin secretion are normal. The condition exists from infancy throughout adult life, and diagnosis usually is done on routine urine analysis. The distinction between renal glycosuria and diabetes mellitus is made with a fasting blood glucose level and a glucose tolerance test. The genetic pattern in renal glycosuria is autosomal recessive.[21,53]

Molecular Pathophysiology

Transport of glucose at the brush-border membrane of the convoluted segment of the proximal tubule occurs by a low-affinity, high-capacity Na+-glucose cotransporter,

SGLT2 (see Fig. 19.3), which reabsorbs the bulk (90%) of the filtered glucose.[21,54,55] The residual glucose reabsorption occurs in the straight segment of the proximal tubule by the high-affinity, low-capacity Na^+-glucose cotransporter SGLT1.[54,55] Both SGLT2 and SGLT1 are members of the SLC5 Na^+/glucose cotransport family.[54,56] Glucose exit from proximal tubular cells is mediated by the facilitative, Na^+-independent glucose transporters GLUT2 and GLUT1, which belong to the SLC2 family of facilitative hexose transporters and are located in the basolateral membrane of the proximal convoluted and the proximal straight segments, respectively (see Fig. 19.3).[21,57,58]

Hereditary isolated glycosuria is caused by mutations in the gene *SLC5A2*, which is located on chromosome 16p11.2 and encodes SGLT2 (see Table 19.1 and Fig. 19.3). To date, more than 30 different *SLC5A2* mutations have been identified in patients with isolated glycosuria.[55,59,60] In some cases, the glycosuria in patients with *SLC5A2* mutations is accompanied by aminoaciduria, the pathophysiology of which is unknown.[61]

It is important to consider the relationships between renal glycosuria, a benign condition, and intestinal glucose–galactose malabsorption, a potentially lethal disease. Glucose–galactose malabsorption, an autosomal recessive disease, is characterized in homozygotes by a neonatal onset of severe watery diarrhea that results in death unless glucose and galactose are removed from the diet.[53] Glucose–galactose malabsorption is caused by mutations in the intestinal brush-border SGLT1 Na^+-glucose cotransporter.[56,62] Patients with glucose–galactose malabsorption who have been studied show a mild defect in renal tubular reabsorption of glucose.[21,56] In contrast, patients with isolated renal glycosuria show no defect in intestinal D-glucose absorption. This has indicated that the SGLT1 Na^+-glucose cotransporter affected in glucose–galactose malabsorption is shared between the intestine and the kidney (see Fig. 19.3).

Fanconi-Bickel Syndrome

Mutations in the gene for GLUT2 *(SLC2A2)*, the facilitative glucose transporter operating in all membranes of various tissues, including the hepatocyte and proximal convoluted tubule, are associated with glycosuria in the Fanconi-Bickel syndrome (see Table 19.1 and Fig. 19.3).[21,63] This autosomal recessive disorder is characterized by hepatorenal glycogen accumulation, Fanconi syndrome including proximal RTA, fasting hypoglycemia, postprandial hyperglycemia, impaired utilization of glucose and galactose, rickets, and markedly stunted growth.[63,64] The renal loss of glucose is attributable to the transport defect for monosaccharides across the renal basolateral membrane, which also leads to accumulation of glucose and secondarily glycogen within proximal tubular cells, resulting in toxic effects on these cells. To date, more than 30 different mutations in *SLC2A2* have been detected in patients with Fanconi-Bickel syndrome[21]; the clinical phenotype can be very heterogenous.[64,65] Therapy of patients with Fanconi-Bickel syndrome is symptomatic and includes stabilization of glucose homeostasis, treatment of rickets, replacement of renal solute losses, and promotion of growth.

Loop of Henle

Bartter Syndrome

General Characteristics

Bartter syndrome is a group of closely related hereditary tubulopathies. All variants of the syndrome share several clinical characteristics, including renal salt wasting, hypokalemic metabolic alkalosis, hyperreninemic hyperaldosteronism with normal blood pressure, and hyperplasia of the juxtaglomerular apparatus.[66–70] All forms of the syndrome are transmitted as autosomal recessive traits; the only exception is transient neonatal Bartter syndrome due to *MAGED2* mutation[71] (see later discussion) which is an x-linked entity.

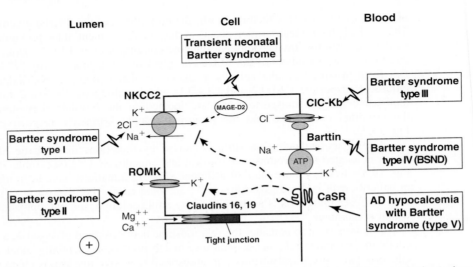

Fig. 19.4 Transcellular and paracellular transport pathways in the TAL. Cl⁻ reabsorption across the luminal membrane occurs via the Na⁺, K⁺, 2Cl⁻ cotransporter (NKCC2). This cotransporter is driven by the low intracellular Na⁺ and Cl⁻ concentrations generated by the basolateral Na⁺, K⁺-ATPase, and ClC-Kb, respectively. In addition, renal outer medullary potassium channel (ROMK) enables function of NKCC2 by recycling K⁺ back to the lumen. The lumen-positive electrical potential, which is generated by Cl entry into the cell and K⁺ exit from the cell, drives paracellular, claudin-16–, and claudin-19–mediated Ca²⁺ and Mg²⁺ transport from lumen to blood. Activation of the basolateral calcium/magnesium sensing receptor (CaSR) by high concentrations of extracellular Ca²⁺ or Mg²⁺ triggers a series of intracellular signaling events, resulting in an inhibition of the luminal ROMK channel and the luminal NKCC2 channel. This in turn results in decreased NaCl reabsorption and (secondary to the reduction in the intraluminal positive potential) increased urinary Ca²⁺ and Mg²⁺ excretion. Hereditary tubulopathies caused by defects in these transport mechanisms are depicted. *AD*, Autosomal dominant; *BSND*, Bartter syndrome with deafness; *MAGE-D2*, melanoma-associated antigen D2.

Molecular Pathophysiology

Generally, Bartter syndrome results from defective transepithelial transport of Cl⁻ in the thick ascending limb of the loop of Henle (TAL) or the distal convoluted tubule (DCT).[66,68,69] Transepithelial Cl⁻ transport in the TAL is a complex process that involves coordinated interplay among the luminal, bumetanide-sensitive Na⁺, K⁺, 2Cl⁻cotransporter (NKCC2); the luminal, K⁺ channel (renal outer medullary potassium channel [ROMK]); the basolateral Cl⁻ channel (ClC-Kb); as well as other cotransporters and channels (Fig. 19.4).[66,72–74] Chloride is reabsorbed across the luminal membrane of the TAL cell by the activity of NKCC2. This cotransporter is driven by the low intracellular Na⁺ and Cl⁻ concentration generated by Na⁺, K⁺-ATPase and ClC-Kb, respectively. In addition, ROMK enables functioning of NKCC2 by recycling K⁺ back to the renal tubular lumen. Normally, the lumen-to-cell flux of Cl⁻ via the NKCC2 cotransporter in the TAL and the exit of K⁺ from cell to lumen generate lumen-positive electrical potential, which in turn drives paracellular Ca²⁺ and Mg²⁺ transport from the lumen to the blood, mediated by the tight junction proteins claudin 16 and claudin 19 (see Fig. 19.4). The Ca²⁺/Mg²⁺-sensing receptor (CaSR), a G protein–coupled receptor expressed in the basolateral membrane of the TAL,[75,76] also appears to participate in electrolyte and mineral handling in this nephron segment. Activation of the CaSR by hypercalcemia or hypermagnesemia triggers a series of intracellular signaling events. This action inhibits NKCC2 and ROMK activity, decreases Cl⁻ reabsorption, reduces lumen positive voltage, and hence inhibits Mg²⁺ and Ca²⁺ reabsorption in the TAL, which results in urinary loss of these divalent cations (see later discussion; Fig. 19.4).[75,76] Chloride transport in the DCT occurs primarily via the luminal, thiazide-sensitive NaCl cotransporter (TSC; NCCT; see later discussion; Fig. 19.5).[72,73,77] Cl⁻ exit to blood in the DCT is mediated via basolateral Cl⁻ channels.

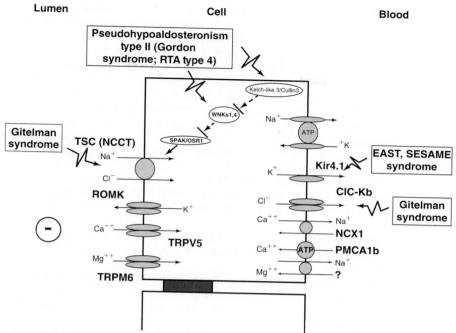

Fig. 19.5 Transport mechanisms in the distal convoluted tubule. Na$^+$ and Cl$^-$ reabsorption occurs via the luminal, thiazide-sensitive NaCl cotransporter (TSC; NCCT). The activity of NCCT is modulated, among other factors, by a complex multiprotein system that includes the intracellular serine/threonine protein kinases, WNK4 and WNK1, When stimulated by physiologic needs or mutation, WNK4/WNK1 will activate NCCT via phosphorylation of Ste20-like proline/alanine-rich kinase (SPAK) and oxidative stress-responsive kinase 1 (OSR1), or directly by increasing NCCT trafficking to the apical membrane. The Kelch-like 3 and Cullin 3 proteins form a RING-type E3-ubiquitin ligase complex that mediates WNK1 and WNK4 abundance by controlling their disposal. Na$^+$ exits the DCT cell via the basolateral Na$^+$, K$^+$-ATPase, and Cl$^-$ exit to blood is mediated by the basolateral Cl$^-$ channel ClC-Kb. K$^+$ is secreted from cell to lumen via apical ROMK, and exits the cell to interstitium via the basolateral K$^+$ channel Kir 4.1. The latter channel recycles K$^+$ entering the cell via the Na$^+$, K$^+$-ATPase back into the interstitium. Ca^{2+} enters the cell via the luminal Ca^{2+} channel TRPV5, is transported transcellularly by vitamin D–dependent calbindin-D28K (not shown), and exits the cell via the Ca^{2+}-ATPase, PMCA1B, and the Na$^+$/Ca^{2+} exchange, NCX1. Mg^{2+} enters the cell via the luminal Mg^{2+} channel, TRPM6, and exits the cell via a putative basolateral Na$^+$/Mg^{2+} exchanger. TRPM6-mediated Mg^{2+} entry into the cell is promoted by the negative intracellular membrane potential, which is maintained by the activity of the Na$^+$, K$^+$-ATPase, as well as by the action of the luminal K$^+$ channel ROMK and the basolateral K$^+$ channel Kir4.1. Hereditary tubulopathies caused by defects in these transport mechanisms are depicted.

The genetic variants of Bartter syndrome that have been identified include (see Table 19.2 and Figs. 19.4 and 19.5):[66,68,69,71,78–81]

1. Bartter syndrome type I is caused by mutations in the NKCC2 gene, *SLC12A1*. This gene belongs to the family of electroneutral chloride-coupled cotransporter genes[82,83] and resides on chromosome 15q15-21. This genetic variant leads to antenatal Bartter syndrome, which is the most severe form of the disease. It is characterized by polyhydramnios, premature birth, life-threatening episodes of salt and water loss in the neonatal period, hypokalemic alkalosis and failure to thrive, as well as osteopenia, hypercalciuria, and early-onset nephrocalcinosis.[66,69,78,84] This form of Bartter syndrome is mimicked by prolonged treatment with furosemide, a NKCC2 inhibitor.

2. Bartter syndrome type II is caused by mutations in the ROMK gene *(KCNJ1)*, which is located on chromosome 11q24-25.[66,68,85] ROMK mutations lead to the clinical phenotype of antenatal Bartter syndrome.[69,79]

3. Bartter syndrome type III is caused by mutations in the ClC-Kb gene, *CLCNKB*.[80] This gene, which is located on chromosome 1p36, belongs to the family of genes encoding voltage-gated Cl$^-$ channels.[66,86] Patients with *CLCNKB* mutation usually have classic Bartter syndrome, which occurs in infancy or early childhood. It is

characterized by marked salt wasting and hypokalemia, leading to polyuria, polydipsia, volume contraction, muscle weakness, and growth retardation. Hypercalciuria and nephrocalcinosis may occur.[66,69]

4. Bartter syndrome type IV is caused by mutations in the barttin gene, *BSND*. Barttin serves as a β subunit for ClC-Ka and ClC-Kb chloride channels (see Fig. 19.4).[87–89] A hereditary defect in barttin leads to antenatal Bartter syndrome associated with sensorineural deafness and renal failure. Barttin colocalizes with the subunit of the Cl⁻ channel in basolateral membranes of the renal tubule and inner ear epithelium[88] and has been shown to activate ClC-K function by modulating its gating.[90]

5. Bartter syndrome type V is caused by gain-of-function mutations in the gene *CASR*, encoding CaSR (see Fig. 19.4). This genetic defect leads to autosomal dominant hypocalcemia with Bartter syndrome.[91,92] As indicated earlier, activation of the basolateral CaSR inhibits the luminal NKCC2 cotransporter and the ROMK channel, resulting in decreased NaCl reabsorption and increased urinary Ca^{2+} and Mg^{2+} excretion.

6. Gitelman syndrome is caused by mutations in the gene *SLC12A3* encoding the thiazide-sensitive NaCl cotransporter (NCCT) operating in the DCT (see later discussion).

Recent data, however, have suggested that the genotype–phenotype correlation is not so clear-cut and that phenotypic overlap may occur. It has been shown that mutations in *CLCNKB* can also cause phenotypes that overlap with either antenatal or Gitelman syndrome.[93,94]

Recently, a new variant of neonatal Bartter syndrome has been reported.[71] This form of the syndrome is caused by loss-of-function mutations in the *MAGED2* gene which encodes myeloma–associated antigen D2 (MAGE-D2), maps to the x chromosome, and is expressed in the developing kidney. MAGE-D2 mutations cause x-linked polyhydramnios with prematurity and a severe but transient form of antenatal Bartter syndrome.[71] MAGE-D2 appears to affect the expression and function of the TAL-based NKCC2 and the DCT-based NCCT, and, hence, is essential for fetal renal salt reabsorption, amniotic fluid homeostasis, and the maintenance of pregnancy.[71,95]

The loss-of-function mutations in the genes of TAL cell transporters in Bartter syndrome lead to derangements in tubular handling of minerals observed in this syndrome.[66,72–74] Normally, the NKCC2-mediated entry of Cl⁻ from lumen to the TAL cell and the ROMK-mediated K⁺ exit from cell to lumen generate lumen-positive electrical potential, which in turn drives paracellular Ca^{2+} and Mg^{2+} transport from lumen to blood (see earlier; see Fig. 19.4). Impaired function of NKCC2 or ROMK in antenatal Bartter syndrome results in reduction of intraluminal positive charge, which leads to hypercalciuria and nephrocalcinosis. However, normal serum Ca^{2+} levels are maintained. Possible mechanisms responsible for the maintenance of normocalcemia include a 1.25(OH) vitamin D–induced increase in intestinal Ca^{2+} absorption and parathyroid hormone (PTH)–induced retrieval of Ca^{2+} from bone.[72,73] The transport defect in the TAL should have resulted in inhibition of Mg^{2+} reabsorption and hypomagnesemia. The absence of hypomagnesemia in patients with antenatal Bartter syndrome has been explained by compensatory stimulation of Mg^{2+} reabsorption in the DCT induced by the high level of aldosterone, which is a characteristic of the syndrome.[66]

Therapy

Treatment of patients with all variants of Bartter syndrome involves correction of hypovolemia as well as supplementation of lost electrolytes. This therapy includes increased oral fluid and salt intake and KCl supplements. Occasionally, Aldactone or amiloride (or both) can be added to correct the hypokalemia. Therapy with the nonsteroidal antiinflammatory drug, indomethacin, should be used only in neonatal Bartter syndrome or severe cases of Bartter syndrome unresponsive to other therapies. However, attention should be paid to potential gastrointestinal or renal toxicity of this drug. Patients with Gitelman syndrome should also receive $MgSO_4$ or $MgCl_2$ supplementation.

Distal Convoluted Tubule

Gitelman Syndrome

General Characteristics

Gitelman syndrome, which appears to be the most frequent hereditary tubulopathy,[96] is a variant of Bartter syndrome that is characterized by a mild clinical presentation in older children and adults.[66–68] Patients may be asymptomatic or present with transient muscle weakness, abdominal pain, symptoms of neuromuscular irritability, or unexplained hypokalemia.[68,96] Patients display mild renal salt wasting and hypochloremic metabolic alkalosis. Hypocalciuria and hypomagnesemia are typical (see Table 19.3).[66,67,96]

Molecular Pathophysiology

Gitelman syndrome is usually caused by mutations in the gene *SLC12A3* encoding the DCT apical membrane thiazide-sensitive NCCT (see Fig. 19.5).[81] Hence, the Gitelman phenotype is mimicked by prolonged treatment with thiazide, a potent NCCT blocker. However, mutations in the gene *CLCNKB* encoding the basolateral membrane Cl^- channel ClC-Kb have also been reported to result in Gitelman syndrome phenotype.[93,94]

The hypokalemia and alkalosis in Gitelman syndrome are the result of increased Na^+ delivery to the more distal CCD, leading to increased Na^+ reabsorption in this nephron segment, which in turn stimulates electrogenic secretion of K^+ and H^+. The exact mechanisms underlying the hypocalciuria and hypomagnesemia in Gitelman syndrome remain to be elucidated. It has been hypothesized that the loss-of-function mutation in NCCT causes hypocalciuria by the same mechanism as thiazides (see Fig. 19.5).[6,97] According to this hypothesis, impaired Na^+ reabsorption across the luminal membrane of the DCT cell causes the cell to hyperpolarize. This in turn stimulates entry of Ca^{2+} into the cell via the luminal voltage-activated Ca^{2+} channels, TRPV5.[97,98] In addition, the lowering of intracellular Na^+ concentration facilitates Ca^{2+} exit via the basolateral Na^+/Ca^{2+} exchanger, NCX1, and the Ca^{2+}-ATPase, PMCA1b.[98] Other studies have suggested that the hypocalciuria in Gitelman syndrome or in chronic thiazide administration is secondary to volume contraction, which increases proximal tubular Na^{2+} reabsorption and hence, facilitates hyperabsorption of Ca^{2+} in the proximal tubule.[99,100] The renal Mg^{2+} wasting and hypomagnesemia typical of Gitelman syndrome could be secondary to decreased abundance of the DCT luminal Mg^{2+} channel, TRPM6.[100]

Pseudohypoaldosteronism Type II

General Characteristics

Pseudohypoaldosteronism type II (PHAII), or Gordon syndrome, is an autosomal dominant disorder characterized by hypertension, hyperkalemia, hyperchloremic metabolic acidosis (RTA type 4; see later), and low plasma aldosterone levels.[101–103] PHAII phenotype is essentially the mirror image of Gitelman syndrome. The underlying pathogenic mechanism of PHAII is NaCl retention as well as K^+ retention, and the disease is highly responsive to low-dose thiazide treatment.[101,103]

Molecular Pathophysiology

Pseudohypoaldosteronism type II is caused by mutations in each of four genes which encode for a complex multiprotein system that regulates electrolyte transport in the distal nephron (see Fig. 19.5).[77,104–106] Two of these genes encode for with no K [lysine] serine-threonine protein kinases, WNK1 and WNK4. The other two genes encode for two proteins, Kelch-like 3 *(KLHL3)* and Cullin 3 *(CUL3)*, which form a RING-type E3-ubiquitin ligase complex that regulates WNK1 and WNK4 abundance by marking them for proteasomal degradation.[105,107] WNK1 and WNK4 modulate the activity of NCCT either via the phosphorylation of two other serine-threonine protein kinases, namely Ste20-like proline/alanine-rich kinase (SPAK) and oxidative stress-responsive kinase 1 (OSR1), or by controlling the trafficking of NCCT from cytoplasm to apical membrane (see Fig. 19.5).[77,104,105] In the baseline state, WNK4 (which is controlled, among other factors, by WNK1) is switched off and NCCT trafficking and activity are suppressed. Modulation of this complex multiprotein regulatory system plays a major role in the physiology of NaCl reabsorption/volume regulation and K[+] secretion in the distal nephron. However, disruption of this complex signaling pathway by any of the gene mutations in PHAII leads to increased surface expression and activity of the NCCT in the DCT.[77,101,103,104] Consequent decreased Na[+] delivery to the CCD results in reduced Na[+] reabsorption, which in turn results in decreased electrogenic secretion of H[+] and K[+].

It should be noted that WNKs also regulate the activity of NKCC2 in the TAL, the epithelial sodium channel (ENaC) in the CCD (see later discussion), and ROMK in the distal nephron.[105,106] Aberrant activation of WNK signaling in PHAII increases endocytosis of luminal, secretory ROMK channels further aggravating the hyperkalemia in this disease.[102,105,106]

EAST or SESAME Syndrome

Recently, two groups reported a new entity which involves the DCT.[108,109] EAST (epilepsy, ataxia, sensorineural deafness, and tubulopathy) or SESAME (seizures, sensorineural deafness, ataxia, mental retardation, and electrolyte imbalance) syndrome includes the indicated central nervous system and inner ear manifestations and a Gitelman syndrome–like tubulopathy with normotensive hypokalemic metabolic alkalosis and hypomagnesemia (see Table 19.3).[108,109] The syndrome is caused by a defect in the gene *KCNJ10* encoding the basolateral K[+] channel Kir4.1, which drives K[+] efflux from DCT cell (see Fig. 19.5). Kir4.1 malfunction leads to reduced basolateral K[+] cycling, which in turn impedes electrogenic Na[+], K[+]-ATPase transport.[106,110] This results in depolarization of the DCT apical membrane and inhibition of NCCT-driven NaCl reabsorption and TRPM6-driven Mg[2+] reabsorption, explaining the Gitelman syndrome–like phenotype. Kir4.1 disruption inhibits NaCl reabsorption in the DCT also by increasing intracellular Cl[−] concentration which, in turn, prevents WNK/SPAK/OSR1-mediated phosphorylation and activation of NCCT (see Fig. 19.5).[106,111,112]

Collecting Duct

Distal Renal Tubular Acidosis

General Characteristics

Distal renal tubular acidosis (dRTA; RTA type 1) is characterized by normal anion gap, hyperchloremic metabolic acidosis caused by failure of hydrogen ion secretion in the distal nephron (Fig. 19.6).[4,8,15,113] Patients fail to appropriately lower pH even in the presence of systemic acidosis.[4,8] Urine pH usually remains above 6. The defective H[+] secretion results in persistent bicarbonaturia (5%–15% of filtered load in infants and children), reduced net acid secretion (see later discussion), and metabolic acidosis.[8,15,113] Untreated dRTA is characterized by renal wasting of Na[+] and K[+]. As in proximal RTA, the urinary K[+] loss in dRTA is caused by extracellular fluid volume contraction and secondary hyperaldosteronism.[7,8]

Distal RTA in children is most commonly a primary entity. Primary dRTA is inherited as either an autosomal-dominant or autosomal-recessive trait (see Table 19.4).[6,15,113,114] Whereas patients with the autosomal-dominant form usually have a mild disease, those with autosomal-recessive dRTA may be severely affected in infancy with growth retardation and early nephrocalcinosis, leading to renal failure.[6,15,114] Autosomal recessive dRTA is subdivided into two variants with or without sensorineural hearing loss (see later discussion; see Table 19.4).[4,113,115,116]

Molecular Pathophysiology

Acid–base handling in the distal tubule occurs primarily in the CCD. There are two classes of cells in the CCD, which can be distinguished by morphologic and functional criteria: the principal cell and the intercalated cell (see Fig. 19.6).[117–119] The principal cells are involved in sodium, potassium, and water transport, and the intercalated

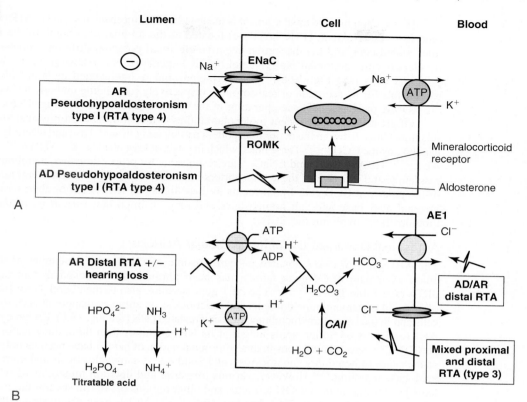

Fig. 19.6 Transport mechanisms involved in electrolyte and acid–base handling in principal cell (A) and α-intercalated cell (B) of the cortical collecting duct. (A) Aldosterone-mineralocorticoid receptor complex interacts with hormone-responsive elements of DNA in the nucleus of the principal cell. This results in production of specific proteins, which stimulate epithelial Na^+ channel (ENaC)–mediated Na^+ entry (and renal outer medullary potassium channel [ROMK]–mediated K^+ exit) at the luminal membrane and Na^+, K^+-ATPase at the basolateral membrane. (B) H^+ and HCO_3^- are formed in the α-intercalated cell as a result of intracellular carbonic anhydrase (CAII) action. H^+ is secreted into the lumen via H^+-ATPase and H^+-K^+–ATPase and binds to the major urinary buffers, HPO_4^{2-} and NH_3, to form titratable acid and ammonium ion, respectively. Depicted are hereditary renal tubular acidosis syndromes caused by defects in these transport mechanisms. *AD,* Autosomal dominant; *AR,* autosomal recessive.

cells, which make up one-third of the cells in the CCD, are responsible for acid–base transport (i.e., proton and bicarbonate secretion and reabsorption) in this nephron segment.[118,119]

H^+ and HCO_3^- are formed in the CCD cell as a result of the action of intracellular carbonic anhydrase (see Fig. 19.6). The CCD is capable of secreting H^+ or HCO_3^-, depending on the acid–base status of the body.[120,121] Two functionally distinct subtypes of intercalated cells have been identified in the CCD: α (or type A) and β (or type B). α (or type A) intercalated cells secrete protons to the lumen and reabsorb HCO_3^- to the blood (see Fig. 19.6).[119,120,122] These cells harbor the H^+-ATPase (proton pump) and the H^+/K^+-ATPase in the luminal membrane and the kidney splice variant of anion exchanger 1 (AE1), a Cl^-/HCO_3^- exchanger, in the basolateral membrane. β (or type B) intercalated cells (not depicted) operate in the reverse orientation: they reabsorb protons to the blood and secrete HCO_3^- (in exchange for Cl^-) across the apical membrane into the lumen.[119,120,121]

Secretion of H^+ in the α intercalated cells results in (1) reabsorption of 10% to 20% of the filtered HCO_3^- that escaped absorption in the proximal tubule, and (2) titration of the major urinary buffers HPO_4^{2-} and NH_3 to form $H_2PO_4^-$ (titratable acid) and ammonium ion (NH_4), respectively (see Fig. 19.6). NH_3 is synthesized primarily in the proximal tubule and reaches the distal tubular lumen by a series of specialized transport processes.[120,121]

H^+ secretion into the tubular lumen is mediated by two mechanisms: (1) H^+-ATPase (and to a lesser extent, H^+-K^+–ATPase) located at the luminal membrane of the α intercalated cells and (2) the lumen negative electrical potential difference created by electrogenic, epithelial Na^+ channel (ENaC)–mediated Na^+ reabsorption in the principal cells (see Fig. 19.6).[118,119,120] Principal and α intercalated cells are also responsible for K^+ secretion or reabsorption, respectively (depending on body needs), via ROMK or H^+-K^+–ATPase operating in the luminal membrane (see Fig. 19.6).

Of great interest are recent molecular studies demonstrating tight physical and functional links between the major transporters participating in acid–base and electrolyte handling by the CCD.[123–125] These links, which involve, at least, the Na^+-K^+–ATPase,[123,125] AE1,[123,124] H^+-ATPase,[124] and ENaC,[125] are responsible for proper targeting, membrane residency, and function of these transporters in the luminal or basolateral membrane of the polarized CCD cell. Impairments in these links can lead to major aberrations in renal acid–base and salt homeostasis and play an important role in hereditary tubulopathies involving the CCD.

Autosomal Dominant Distal Renal Tubular Acidosis

The AE1 gene, *SLC4A1*, located on chromosome 17q21-22 and a member of the anion exchanger *SLC4* gene family, has been implicated in autosomal dominant dRTA (see Table 19.4).[4,15,126,127] The AE1 gene product, also termed band 3, consists of 12 to 14 transmembrane domains and functions as an anion exchanger in erythroid cells and in the basolateral membrane of α-intercalated cells (see Fig. 19.6). Erythrocyte AE1 (eAE1) is 65 amino acids longer at its NH_2 terminus than the kidney isoform (kAE1).[126,127] Several mutations in this N-terminal region of band 3 have been identified as the cause of hereditary spherocytosis and Southeast Asian ovalocytosis and normal acid–base handling.[4,128] However, various missense and deletion mutations of AE1 have been found in the COOH terminus and other regions of AE1 in several families with autosomal dominant dRTA (see Fig. 19.6).[113,129,130] It has been demonstrated that AE1 mutations associated with autosomal dominant dRTA have normal function, but cause abnormalities in trafficking and targeting of AE1 to the renal basolateral membrane.[113,130–132] It is noteworthy that AE1 mutations causing autosomal recessive dRTA in association with hemolytic anemia have been demonstrated in Southeast Asian kindreds.[4,15]

Autosomal Recessive Distal Renal Tubular Acidosis

The *ATP6V1B1* gene, localized on chromosome 12q13 and encoding the B_1-subunit of the apical proton pump expressed in α-intercalated cells, has been implicated in autosomal recessive dRTA with early-onset sensorineural deafness (see Table 19.4 and Fig. 19.6).[133–135] The B_1-containing H^+-ATPase is a member of the vacuolar (V)-ATPase family that has a complex structure of at least 10 subunits.[135,136] An intracellular domain of H^+-ATPase, which, among other subunits, contains three B subunits, catalyzes ATP hydrolysis, providing energy for active H^+ transport across the membrane-spanning Vo domain.[4,136] Various mutations causing autosomal recessive dRTA with sensorineural deafness have been identified within the *ATP6V1B1* gene.[4,15,134,137,138] Consistent with the finding of hearing loss, expression of *ATP6V1B1* in the cochlea and endolymphatic sac has been demonstrated.[4,133] This suggests that mutations in inner ear H^+-ATPase likely affect auditory function by altering the normally acidic endolymphatic pH.[4,133]

Several homozygous mutations in the *ATP6V0A4* gene, located on chromosome 7q33-34 and encoding the a4 accessory subunit of H^+-ATPase, were found to cause dRTA without or with later onset deafness (see Table 19.4).[137–140] Recently, an *Atp6v0a4* knockout mouse was shown to recapitulate the loss of H^+-ATPase function seen in human dRTA.[141]

Clinical Features

Prominent clinical manifestations of dRTA include failure to thrive, polyuria, polydipsia, constipation, vomiting, dehydration, muscle weakness, nephrocalcinosis, and nephrolithiasis.[7,19,114] The factors promoting the nephrocalcinosis and stone formation in dRTA are hypercalciuria, hypocitraturia, and alkaline urine. The hypercalciuria is probably related to chronic accumulation of acid that is buffered by Ca^{2+} release from bone as well as inhibition of distal tubular Ca^{2+} reabsorption by chronic metabolic acidosis.[4] The hypocitraturia is secondary to intracellular acidosis that promotes citrate uptake from the tubular lumen.[142]

The diagnosis of primary, classical dRTA can be based on (1) normal anion gap, hyperchloremic metabolic acidosis; (2) hypokalemia (as opposed to the hyperkalemia observed in voltage-dependent defect); (3) urine pH greater than 5.5 during spontaneous acidosis; and (4) a positive urinary anion gap (see proximal RTA) indicating low urinary ammonium concentration.[7,19,20] Although usually not necessary, the diagnosis of dRTA can be substantiated by the demonstration of an inability to maximally acidify the urine after NH_4Cl loading or by the finding of urine–blood PCO_2 (U-BPCO_2 <20 mm Hg after alkali loading).[19,20] The evaluation of dRTA should include examination of urinary Ca^{2+} and citrate levels as well as renal ultrasonography to investigate for the presence of nephrocalcinosis.

Treatment

The goals of dRTA therapy are to improve growth, prevent nephrocalcinosis and nephrolithiasis, and prevent progressive renal insufficiency. Infants and young children with dRTA may require up to 5 mEq/kg per day of alkali to correct acidemia, depending on the magnitude of renal HCO_3^- wasting.[7,114] As renal HCO_3^- wasting decreases with age, alkali requirements decrease. Hypokalemia, which can be significant, should be corrected. Provision of HCO_3^- by using citrate salts provides the additional advantage of exogenous citrate to prevent nephrocalcinosis and nephrolithiasis.[19]

Mixed Proximal and Distal Renal Tubular Acidosis (Type 3)

This variant of RTA shares the features of both proximal (reduced HCO_3^- reabsorption) and distal (impaired urine acidification) RTA (see Table 19.4; Figs. 19.1 and 19.6). It is caused by autosomal recessive mutations of the *CAII* gene located on chromosome 8q22 and expressed in kidney, bone, and brain.[7,113,143,144] Because CAII is present in the cytosol of both proximal and distal tubules, these mutations lead to this mixed syndrome. Because the expression of *CAII* is affected also in bone and brain, additional manifestations include osteopetrosis, cerebral calcifications, and mental retardation.[143,144] The osteopetrosis, which is secondary to osteoclast dysfunction, is a condition of increased bone density but also increased bone fragility leading to increased fracture risk.[4] Excess bone growth leads to conductive deafness and can also cause blindness through compression of the optic nerve.

Hyperkalemic Renal Tubular Acidosis (Type 4)

Hyperkalemic RTA is characterized by a normal ability to acidify the urine during acidosis, but reduced urinary concentration of ammonium and hence of net acid.[4,7,8] The primary pathogenic mechanism in type 4 RTA is aldosterone deficiency or resistance that results in impairment of H^+ and K^+ secretion in the principal cells of the collecting tubule (see Fig. 19.6). The ensuing hyperkalemia leads to an impairment of ammonium production. Decreased ENaC-mediated Na^+ reabsorption by principal cells also contributes to impaired electrogenic secretion of H^+ by intercalated cells.

Two hereditary aldosterone resistance states, PHAI (discussed later) and PHAII (discussed earlier; see DCT), lead to type 4 RTA (see Table 19.4).

Pseudohypoaldosteronism Type I

General Characteristics and Clinical Features

Pseudohypoaldosteronism type I (PHAI) is a rare inherited disorder characterized by renal salt wasting and end-organ unresponsiveness to mineralocorticoids.[6,8,145] The manifestations of the disease include hyponatremia, hyperkalemia, hyperchloremic metabolic acidosis, and elevated plasma aldosterone and plasma renin activity. The disorder is divided into two forms of inheritance with distinct pathophysiologic and clinical features. The autosomal dominant form is a relatively mild disease that remits with age and is restricted to the kidney.[146] The autosomal recessive form presents with severe Na^+ transport defects in all aldosterone target tissues, including the kidney, colon, and salivary and sweat glands, as well as in the lungs.[6,147,148] Autosomal recessive PHAI is characterized by neonatal salt wasting with dehydration, hypotension, life-threatening hyperkalemia, type 4 RTA, and failure to thrive.[145,147,148] The sweat test result is usually positive. The manifestations of the disease do not respond to mineralocorticoids, but do improve with salt supplementation. Neonatal respiratory distress syndrome and respiratory tract infections in affected children are common.[149]

Molecular Pathophysiology

The amiloride-sensitive ENaC, located at the apical membrane of Na^+ transporting epithelia such as the kidney, colon, lung, and ducts of the exocrine glands, plays an essential role in Na^+ and fluid reabsorption. In the kidneys, ENaC, which is composed of a combination of three similar subunits, α, β, and γ, is found primarily in the principal cells of the collecting duct, where it mediates the entry of Na^+ across the luminal membrane, a process driven by the basolateral Na^+, K^+-ATPase (see Fig. 19.6).[118,147,148] Hence, ENaC has a central role in controlling extracellular fluid homeostasis and blood pressure. The activity of ENaC is under the tight control of hormones, such as aldosterone (see Fig. 19.6) and vasopressin.[118,150] Whereas the milder, autosomal dominant PHAI is caused by heterozygous loss-of-function mutations in the mineralocorticoid receptor gene, *NR3C2*,[146] autosomal recessive PHAI is caused by homozygous or compound heterozygous loss-of-function mutations, which have been described in each of the three genes, *SCNN1A*, *SCNN1B*, and *SCNN1C*, encoding for the subunits α, β, and γ, respectively, of ENaC (see Fig. 19.6).[6,147,151,152]

Nephrogenic Diabetes Insipidus

General Characteristics and Clinical Features

Congenital nephrogenic diabetes insipidus (NDI) is characterized by an inability of the kidney to concentrate urine in response to the ADH arginine vasopressin (AVP).[153,154] Polydipsia and polyuria, hyposthenuria, dehydration, constipation, and hypernatremia are the hallmarks of NDI in infants and children.[154,155] Failure to thrive is common, and recurrent episodes of dehydration may cause severe neurologic sequelae. Older children can present with poor growth, nocturia, and enuresis and learning and behavior difficulties.[153,155]

Clinical diagnosis of NDI can be established by a water deprivation test demonstrating inappropriate urinary concentration unresponsive to DDAVP (desmopressin) administration. The evaluation of an infant or a child with NDI should include renal ultrasonography to evaluate for NDI secondary to disorders that result in impaired ability to concentrate the urine. These include conditions such as dysplastic and polycystic kidneys, renal scars, and nephrocalcinosis.[153,155]

Molecular Pathophysiology

The movement of water across the renal tubular epithelial membrane is of central importance in maintaining water and electrolyte balance. Reabsorption of water in the renal tubule occurs mainly through aquaporin (AQP) water channels, the activity of which is controlled by the vasopressin type 2 receptor (V2R) (see below). AQPs are members of a large family of pore-forming intrinsic membrane proteins.[156,157] There are now 13 well-characterized mammalian AQPs, AQP 0 to 12, of which eight (AQPs 1, 2, 3, 4, 6, 7, 8, and 11) are expressed in the kidney.[154,157,158] Ultrastructural studies have shown that AQPs have a barrel-like structure and are assembled in tetramers.[157,159]

AQP2 is the vasopressin-responsive AQP in the principal cells of the renal collecting duct, where 10% of the filtered volume is reabsorbed (Fig. 19.7). AQP2 is localized to the apical side of the principal cell (whereas AQP3 and AQP4 are expressed at the basolateral membrane).[118] Binding of the antidiuretic hormone AVP to the V2R at the basolateral side of the principal cell activates G protein (G_s) and

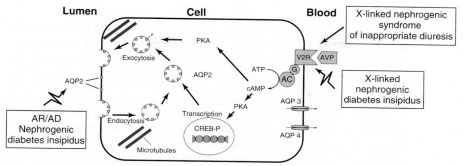

Fig. 19.7 Regulation of aquaporin 2 (AQP2) recycling in a principal cell of the collecting duct. Binding of arginine vasopressin (AVP) to the G protein-coupled vasopressin type 2 receptor (V2R) at the basolateral membrane triggers a signaling cascade, which results in protein kinase A (PKA)-induced phosphorylation of AQP2 in intracellular vesicles. After phosphorylation, AQP2-containing vesicles translocate to the apical membrane (a process that involves the microtubular machinery), thereby increasing the water permeability of the membrane. Also, PKA-mediated phosphorylation of the transcription factor, cAMP-responsive element binding protein (CREB), results in synthesis of new AQP2 channels. The entering water leaves the cell via the basolateral membrane-bound AQP3 and AQP4 channels. Upon dissociation of AVP from its receptor, AQP2 is retrieved endocytically from the apical membrane, and the cell returns to its water-impermeable state. Hereditary tubulopathies caused by defects in these pathways are depicted. *ATP,* Adenosine triphosphate.

increases intracellular cyclic adenosine monophosphate (cAMP) levels, resulting in phosphorylation of several residues in the C-terminus of AQP2 by cAMP-dependent protein kinase (see Fig. 19.7).[153,158] This in turn triggers intracellular clathrin-coated vesicles containing AQP2 to fuse with the apical membrane, rendering the cell water permeable. cAMP also enhances transcription of AQP2 via the activity of the nuclear factor, cAMP-responsive element binding protein (CREB), thereby generating new AQP2 channels. Reabsorbed water exits the cell to the interstitium via the basolateral, constitutively expressed, AQP3 and AQP4 channels. Upon dissociation of AVP from its receptor, AQP2 is internalized by ubiquitination-triggered endocytosis via the clathrin-coated vesicles, and the cell returns to its water-impermeable state.[153,154,156]

X-Linked Nephrogenic Diabetes Insipidus

X-linked NDI is caused by mutations in the V2 receptor gene, *AVPR2,* which resides on the long arm of chromosome X (Xq28).[160,161] Most (>90%) of the patients with congenital NDI have mutations in the *AVPR2* gene.[158] To date, over 200 different disease-causing mutations in the *AVPR2* gene have been reported in more than 300 families.[153,162] When studied in vitro, most *AVPR2* mutations are functional but lead to receptors that are trapped in the endoplasmic reticulum and are unable to reach the plasma membrane.[161]

Autosomal Recessive and Autosomal Dominant Nephrogenic Diabetes Insipidus

Congenital NDI can be transmitted as an autosomal recessive or autosomal dominant trait. In these cases, the disease is caused by mutations in the *AQP2* gene, located on chromosome 12q13.[163,164] Generally, there is no difference in clinical phenotype between the x-linked and autosomal recessive forms of NDI.[154] To date, more than 50 different disease-causing mutations in the *AQP2* gene have been reported in autosomal recessive NDI.[154,158] Most of these are missense mutations. Similar to AVPR2 mutants, mutations in the *AQP2* gene lead to an impaired routing of channel proteins to the plasma membrane caused by misfolding and retention in the endoplasmic reticulum.

At present, 10 NDI families with autosomal dominant inheritance have been identified.[154,158] This form of NDI is caused by various mutations in the *AQP2* gene that change the transport signal of the AQP2 protein with consequent misrouting to the Golgi compartment or to late endosomes.[154,158] Autosomal dominant NDI patients have a milder phenotype than those with autosomal recessive disease.[154]

Therapy

The hallmarks of long-term therapy of NDI include[153–155,158] (1) replacement of urinary water losses by adequate supply of fluid (if necessary, via nasogastric or gastric tube); (2) reduction of dietary solute load by restricting Na^+ intake and by providing protein intake not higher than the recommended daily allowance; and (3) pharmacologic therapy, including (a) thiazide and/or amiloride (which decrease urine volume most likely secondary to diuretic-induced reduction in extracellular fluid volume leading to enhanced proximal tubular reabsorption of the glomerular filtrate), and (b) (if indicated) indomethacin (which decreases water diuresis independent of AVP). (4) Finally, of great interest are recent studies investigating the yield of pharmacologic chaperones in rescuing misfolded V2R and AQP2 proteins trapped in the endoplasmic reticulum.[165,166] Similarly promising is a novel treatment approach for patients with AVPR2 mutations focusing on enhancing cAMP production in the principal cell independent of AVPR2 using compounds such as prostaglandin E[167] or secretin[168] receptor agonists. The findings of these studies may provide a basis for future design of therapeutic strategies for some forms of NDI.

Nephrogenic Syndrome of Inappropriate Diuresis

General Characteristics

The nephrogenic syndrome of inappropriate diuresis (NSIAD) is a rare, recently described genetic disorder of water balance affecting male infants.[169,170] The clinical and laboratory features of NSIAD resemble those of the syndrome of inappropriate secretion of antidiuretic hormone (SIADH) and include hyponatremia, seizures, and inappropriately hypertonic urine.[171,172] However, in contrast to the markedly elevated plasma AVP levels in SIADH, NSIAD is characterized by undetectable or very low AVP levels in plasma.[169,172]

Molecular Pathophysiology

NSIAD is caused by a gain of function mutation in the V2 receptor gene, *AVPR2*, which leads to constitutive activation of the receptor (see Table 19.4 and Fig. 19.7).[149] The two unrelated male infants included in the first report on this syndrome,[169] as well as few cases subsequently reported,[172] display missense mutations, resulting in the substitution of arginine to cysteine or leucine in codon 137 (R137C/L). Interestingly, whereas the R137C/L mutation causes NSIAD, a missense mutation converting arginine to histidine (R137H) leads to the opposite disease phenotype, NDI.[173] Several additional mutations, E229V,[174] I130N,[175] and L312S,[176] have been recently reported to cause NSIAD. All these mutations have differential effects on trafficking of the V2 receptor; however, the mechanism whereby these mutations cause constitutive activation of the receptor is unclear.

Interestingly, the manifestations of the disease mostly occur after the age of a few months. It has been suggested that limited concentrating capacity of the renal tubule in neonates combined with high insensible water loss might have a protective role and postpone the appearance of the disease.[172]

Therapy

The simplest therapy of NSIAD is fluid restriction, which, however, is not feasible during early life because of its consequence of caloric deficiency.[170,172] Administration of urea to induce osmotic diuresis or furosemide with salt supplementation, both therapies used in SIADH,[171,173] are potential therapies in NSIAD that have not been tested in this syndrome and can lead to serious side effects. Of great interest are recent functional studies in renal cells demonstrating AVP-induced internalization and silencing of constitutive activity of some of the mutant V2Rs by the inverse V2R agonists, tolvaptan and satavaptan.[174–176] The findings of these studies raise the possibility that administration of these compounds could have a therapeutic value for NSIAD by reducing steady-state surface receptor levels and/or constitutive signaling activity, thus lowering basal cAMP production and accumulation that most likely underlies NSIAD.

Conclusion

In the past decade, remarkable progress has been made in our understanding of the molecular pathogenesis of hereditary tubulopathies. Molecular genetics and molecular biology studies have led to the identification of numerous tubular disease-causing mutations, have provided important insight into the defective molecular mechanisms underlying various tubulopathies, and have greatly increased our understanding of the physiology of renal tubular transport. Nevertheless, numerous issues remain unsettled and warrant additional research. Future studies will shed more light on the molecular mechanisms and functional defects underlying the impaired transport in various tubulopathies. These studies may significantly improve our understanding of the mechanisms underlying renal salt homeostasis, urinary mineral excretion, and blood pressure regulation in health and disease. The identification of the molecular defects in inherited tubulopathies may provide a basis for future design of targeted therapeutic interventions and, possibly, strategies for gene therapy of these complex disorders.

Acknowledgment

I am indebted to Mrs. Ora Bider for her expert secretarial assistance, and to Mrs. Sarah Dichter for her assistance in creating the figures.

REFERENCES

1. Devuyst O, Belge H, Konard M, et al. Renal tubular disorders of electrolyte regulation in children. In: Avner ED, Harmon WE, Niaudet P, et al, eds. *Pediatric Nephrology*. 7th ed. Berlin-Heidelberg: Springer-Verlag; 2015:1201–1272.
2. Hildebrandt F. Genetic kidney diseases. *Lancet*. 2010;375:1287–1295.
3. Bonnardeaux A, Bichet DG. Inherited disorders of the renal tubule. In: Skorecki K, Chertow GM, Mardsen PA, et al, eds. *Brenner & Rector's The Kidney*. 10th ed. Philadelphia: Elsevier; 2016:1434–1474.
4. Fry AC, Karet FE. Inherited renal acidoses. *Physiology*. 2007;22:202–211.
5. Khosravi M, Walsh SB. The long-term complications of the inherited tubulopathies: an adult perspective. *Pediatr Nephrol*. 2015;30:385–395.
6. Zelikovic I. Molecular pathophysiology of tubular transport disorders. *Pediatr Nephrol*. 2001;16:919–935.
7. Soriano JR. Renal tubular acidosis: the clinical entity. *J Am Soc Nephrol*. 2002;13:2160–2170.
8. Krapf R, Seldin DW, Alpern RJ. Clinical syndromes of metabolic acidosis. In: Alpern RJ, Moe OW, Caplan M, eds. *Seldin and Giebisch's The Kidney, Physiology and Pathophysiology*. 5th ed. Philadelphia: Elsevier; 2013:2049–2111.
9. Gil-Pena H, Mejia N, Santos F. Renal tubular acidosis. *J Pediatr*. 2014;164:691–698.
10. Igarashi T, Inatomi J, Sekine T, et al. Mutations in SLC4A4 cause permanent isolated proximal renal tubular acidosis with ocular abnormalities. *Nat Genet*. 1999;23:264–266.
11. Igarashi T, Sekine T, Inatomi J, et al. Unraveling the molecular pathogenesis of isolated proximal renal tubular acidosis. *J Am Soc Nephrol*. 2002;13:2171–2177.
12. Usui T, Hara M, Satoh H, et al. Molecular basis of ocular abnormalities associated with proximal renal tubular acidosis. *J Clin Invest*. 2001;108:107–115.
13. Curthoys NP, Moe OW. Proximal tubule function and response to acidosis. *Clin J Am Soc Nephrol*. 2014;9:1627–1638.
14. Soleimani M, Burnham CE. Physiologic and molecular aspects of the Na^+/HCO_3^- cotransporter in health and disease processes. *Kidney Int*. 2000;57:371–384.
15. Alper SL. Familial renal tubular acidosis. *J Nephrol*. 2010;23:S57–S76.
16. Haque SK, Ariceta G, Batlle D. Proximal renal tubular acidosis: a not so rare disorder of multiple etiologies. *Nephrol Dial Transplant*. 2012;27:4273–4287.
17. Toye AM, Parker MD, Daly CM, et al. The human NBCe1-A mutant R881C, associated with proximal renal tubular acidosis, retains function but is mistargeted in polarized renal epithelia. *Am J Physiol Cell Physiol*. 2006;291:C788–C801.
18. Lo YF, Yang SS, Seki G, et al. Severe metabolic acidosis causes early lethality in NBC1 W516X knock-in mice as a model of human isolated proximal renal tubular acidosis. *Kidney Int*. 2011;79:730–741.
19. Zelikovic I. Renal tubular acidosis. *Pediatr Ann*. 1995;24:48–54.
20. Santos F, Ordonez FA, Taberner DC, et al. Clinical and laboratory approaches in the diagnosis of renal tubular acidosis. *Pediatr Nephrol*. 2015;30:2099–2107.
21. Zelikovic I. Aminoaciduria and glycosuria in children. In: Avner ED, Harmon N, Niaudet P, Yoshikawa N, eds. *Pediatric Nephrology*. 7th ed. Berlin Heidelberg: Springer-Verlag; 2015:1155–1200.
22. Palacin M, Goodyer P, Nunes V, et al. Cystinuria. In: Scriver CR, Beaudet AL, Sly WS, et al, eds. *The Metabolic and Molecular Bases of Inherited Disease*. New York: McGraw-Hill; 2001:4909–4932.
23. Mattoo A, Goldfarb DS. Cystinuria. *Semin Nephrol*. 2008;28:181–191.

19

24. Chillaron J, Font-Llitjos M, Fort J, et al. Pathophysiology and treatment of cystinuria. *Nat Rev Nephrol.* 2010;6:424–434.
25. Claes DJ, Jackson E. Cystinuria: mechanisms and management. *Pediatr Nephrol.* 2012;27:2031–2038.
26. Goodyer P, Saadi I, Ong P, et al. Cystinuria subtype and the risk of nephrolithiasis. *Kidney Int.* 1998;54:56–61.
27. Chillaron J, Roca R, Valencia A, et al. Heteromeric amino acid transporters: biochemistry, genetics, and physiology. *Am J Physiol.* 2001;281:F995–F1018.
28. Palacin M, Borsani G, Sebastio G. The molecular bases of cystinuria and lysinuric protein intolerance. *Curr Opin Genet Dev.* 2001;11:328–335.
29. Wagner CA, Lang F, Bröer S. Function and structure of heterodimeric amino acid transporters. *Am J Physiol.* 2001;281:C1077–C1093.
30. Sumorok N, Goldfarb DS. Update on cystinuria. *Curr Opin Nephrol Hypertens.* 2013;22:427–431.
31. Jaeger P, Portmann L, Saunders A, et al. Anticystinuric effects of glutamine and of dietary sodium restriction. *N Engl J Med.* 1986;315:1120–1123.
32. Jaffe IA. Adverse effects profile of sulfhydryl compounds in man. *Am J Med.* 1986;80:471–476.
33. Pak CYC, Fuller C, Sakhaee K, et al. Management of cystine nephrolithiasis with alpha-mercaptopropionylglycine. *J Urol.* 1986;136:1003–1008.
34. Zee T, Bose N, Zee J, et al. α-Lipoic acid treatment prevents cystine urolithiasis in a mouse model of cystinuria. *Nature Med.* 2017;23:288–290.
35. Saravakos P, Kokkinou V. Glannatos E. Cystinuria: current diagnosis and management. *J Urol.* 2014;83:693–699.
36. De Baulny HO, Schiff M, Dionisi-Vici C. Lysinuric protein intolerance (LPI): a multi organ disease by far more complex than a classic urea cycle disorder. *Mol Genet Metab.* 2012;106:12–17.
37. Mauhin W, Habarou F, Gobin S, et al. Update on lysinuric protein intolerance, a multi-faceted disease retrospective cohort analysis from birth to adulthood. *Orphanet J Rare Dis.* 2017;12:3.
38. Simell O. Lysinuric protein intolerance and other cationic aminoacidurias. In: Scriver CR, Beaudet AL, Sly WS, et al, eds. *The Metabolic and Molecular Bases of Inherited Disease.* New York: McGraw-Hill; 2001:4933–4956.
39. Sebastio G, Sperandeo MP, Andria G. Lysinuric protein intolerance: reviewing concepts on a multisystem disease. *Am J Med Genet Part C.* 2011;157:54–62.
40. Palacin M, Bertran J, Zorzano A. Heteromeric amino acid transporters explain aminoacidurias. *Curr Opin Nephrol Hypertens.* 2000;9:547–553.
41. Llitjos MF, Santiago BR, Espino M, et al. Novel SLC7A7 large rearrangements in lysinuric protein intolerance patients involving the same AluY repeat. *Eur J Hum Genet.* 2009;17:71–79.
42. Rajantie J, Simell O, Rapola J, et al. Lysinuric protein intolerance: a two year trial of dietary supplementation therapy with citrulline and lysine. *J Pediatr.* 1980;97:927–932.
43. Dirckx JH. Julius Caesar and the Julian emperors: a family cluster with Hartnup disease? *Am J Dermatopathol.* 1986;8:351–357.
44. Baron DN, Dent CE, Harris H, et al. Hereditary pellagra-like skin rash with temporary cerebellar ataxia, constant renal aminoaciduria and other bizarre biochemical features. *Lancet.* 1956;1:421–428.
45. Levy HL. Hartnup disorder. In: Scriver CR, Beaudet Al, Sly WS, et al, eds. *The Metabolic and Molecular Bases of Inherited Disease.* New York: McGraw-Hill; 2001:4957–4969.
46. Broer S. The role of the neutral amino acid transporter B^{0}AT1 (SLC6A19) in Hartnup disorder and protein nutrition. *IUBMB Life.* 2009;61:591–599.
47. Nozaki J, Dakeishi M, Ohura T, et al. Homozygosity mapping to chromosome 5p15 of a gene responsible for Hartnup disorder. *Biochem Biophys Res Comm.* 2001;284:255–260.
48. Bröer A, Klingel K, Kowalczuk S, et al. Molecular cloning of mouse amino acid transport system B^0, a neutral amino acid transporter related to Hartnup disorder. *J Biol Chem.* 2004;279:24467–24476.
49. Bröer S. Amino acid transport across mammalian intestinal and renal epithelia. *Physiol Rev.* 2008;88:249–280.
50. Kleta R, Romeo E, Ristic Z, et al. Mutations in SLC6A19, encoding B0AT1, cause Hartnup disorder. *Nature Genet.* 2004;36:999–1002.
51. Seow HF, Bröer S, Bröer A, et al. Hartnup disorder is caused by mutations in the gene encoding the neutral amino acid transporter SLC6A19. *Nature Genet.* 2004;36:1003–1007.
52. Jonas AJ, Butler IJ. Circumvention of defective neutral amino acid transport in Hartnup disease using tryptophan ethyl ester. *J Clin Invest.* 1989;84:200–204.
53. Wright E, Martin MG, Turk E. Familial glucose-galactose malabsorption and hereditary glycosuria. In: Scriver CR, Beaudet AL, Sly WS, et al, eds. *The Metabolic and Molecular Bases of Inherited Disease.* New York: McGraw-Hill; 2001:4891–4908.
54. Wright EM, Turk E. The sodium/glucose cotransport family SLC5. *Pflugers Arch.* 2004;447:510–518.
55. Wright EM, Loo DDF, Hirayama BA. Biology of human sodium glucose transporters. *Physiol Rev.* 2011;91:733–794.
56. Hummel CS, Wright EM. Glucose reabsorption in the kidney. In: Alpern RJ, Moe OW, eds. *Seldin and Giebisch's The Kidney, Physiology and Pathophysiology.* 5th ed. Philadelphia: Elsvier; 2013:2393–2404.
57. Uldry M, Thorens B. The SLC2 family of facilitated hexose and polyol transporters. *Pflugers Arch.* 2004;447:480–489.
58. Mueckler M, Thorens B. The SLC2 (GLUT) of membrane transporters. *Mol Aspects Med.* 2013;34:121–138.

59. Calado J, Sznajer Y, Metzger D, et al. Twenty-one additional cases of familial renal glucosuria: absence of genetic heterogeneity, high prevalence of private mutations and further evidence of volume depletion. *Nephrol Dial Transplant*. 2008;23:3874–3879.

60. Santer R, Calado J. Familial renal glucosuria and SGLT2: from a mendelian trait to a therapeutic target. *Clin J Am Soc Nephrol*. 2010;5:133–141.

61. Magen D, Sprecher E, Zelikovic I, et al. A novel missense mutation in SLC5A2 encoding SGLT2 underlies autosomal recessive renal glucosuria and aminoaciduria. *Kidney Int*. 2005;67:34–41.

62. Turk E, Zabel B, Mundlos S, et al. Glucose/galactose malabsorption caused by a defect in the Na$^+$/glucose cotransporter. *Nature*. 1991;350:354–356.

63. Santer R, Schneppenheim R, Dombrowski A, et al. Mutations in GLUT2, the gene for the liver-type glucose transporter, in patients with Fanconi-Bickel syndrome. *Nat Genet*. 1997;17:324–326.

64. Santer R, Groth S, Kinner M, et al. The mutation spectrum of the facilitative glucose transporter gene SLC2A2 (GLUT2) in patients with Fanconi-Bickel syndrome. *Hum Genet*. 2002;110:21–29.

65. Mannstadt M, Magen D, Segawa H, et al. Fanconi-Bickel syndrome and autosomal recessive proximal tubulopathy with hypercalciuria (ARPTH) are allelic variants caused by GLUT2 mutations. *J Clin Endocrinol Metab*. 2012;97:E1978–E1986.

66. Zelikovic I. Hypokalemic salt-losing tubulopathies: an evolving story. *Nephrol Dial Transpl*. 2003;18:1696–1700.

67. Knoers NVAM. Gitelman syndrome. *Adv Chronic Kidney Dis*. 2006;13:148–154.

68. Jain G, Ong S, Warnock DG. Genetic disorders of potassium homeostasis. *Semin Nephrol*. 2013;33:300–309.

69. Scholl UI, Lifton RP. Inherited disorders of renal salt homeostasis: insights from molecular genetics studies. In: Alpern RJ, Moe OW, eds. *Seldin and Giebisch's The Kidney, Physiology and Pathophysiology*. 5th ed. Philadelphia: Elsvier; 2013:1213–1240.

70. Seyberth HW. Pathophysiology and clinical presentations of salt-losing tubulopathies. *Pediatr Nephrol*. 2016;31:407–418.

71. Laghmani K, Beck BB, Yang SS, et al. Polyhdramnios, transient antenatal Bartter's syndrome, and MAGED2 mutations. *N Engl J Med*. 2016;374:1853–1863.

72. Mount DB. Transport of sodium, chloride and potassium. In: Skorecki K, Chertow GM, Mardsen PA, eds. *Brenner & Rector's The Kidney*. 10th ed. Philadelphia: Elsevier; 2016:144–184.

73. Bazua-Valenti SB, Castaneda-Bueno MC, Gamba G. Physiological role of SLC12 family members in the kidney. *Am J Physiol Renal Physiol*. 2016;311:F131–F144.

74. Mount DB. Thick ascending limb of the loop of Henle. *Clin J Am Soc Nephrol*. 2014;9:1974–1986.

75. Riccardi D, Valenti G. Localization and function of the renal calcium-sensing receptor. *Nat Rev Nephrol*. 2016;12:414–423.

76. Toka HR, Pollak MR, Houillier P. Calcium sensing in the renal tubule. *Physiology*. 2015;30:317–326.

77. Subramanya AR, Ellison DH. Distal convoluted tubule. *Clin J Am Soc Nephrol*. 2014;9:2147–2163.

78. Simon DB, Karet FE, Hamdan JM, et al. Bartter's syndrome, hypokalemic alkalosis with hypercalciuria, is caused by mutations in the Na-K-2Cl cotransporter NKCC2. *Nat Genet*. 1996;13:183–188.

79. Simon DB, Karet FE, Rodriguez-Soriano J, et al. Genetic heterogeneity of Bartter's syndrome revealed by mutations in the K+ channel, ROMK. *Nat Genet*. 1996;14:152–156.

80. Simon DB, Bindra RS, Mansfield TA, et al. Mutations in the chloride channel gene, CLCNKB, cause Bartter's syndrome type III. *Nat Genet*. 1997;17:171–178.

81. Simon DB, Nelson-Williams C, Bia MJ, et al. Gitelman's variant of Bartter's syndrome, inherited hypokalemic alkalosis, is caused by mutations in the thiazide-sensitive Na-Cl contransporter. *Nat Genet*. 1996;12:24–30.

82. Gamba G. Electroneutral chloride coupled cotransporters. *Curr Opin Nephrol Hypertens*. 2000;9:535–540.

83. Castrop H, Schiebl IM. Physiology and pathophysiology of the renal Na-K-2CI cotransporter (NKCC2). *Am J Physiol Renal Physiol*. 2014;307:F991–F1002.

84. Seyberth HW, Rascher W, Schweer H, et al. Congenital hypokalemia with hypercalciuria in pre-term infants: a hyperprostaglandinuric tubular syndrome different from Bartter syndrome. *J Pediatr*. 1985;107:694–701.

85. Welling PA, Ho K. A comprehensive guide to the ROMK potassium channel: form and function in health and disease. *Am J Physiol Renal Physiol*. 2009;297:F849–F863.

86. Andrini O, Keck M, Briones R, et al. CIC-K chloride channels: emerging pathophysiology of Bartter syndrome type 3. *Am J Physiol Renal Physiol*. 2015;308:F1324–F1334.

87. Birkenhager R, Otto E, Schurmann MJ, et al. Mutation of BSND causes Bartter syndrome with sensorineural deafness and kidney failure. *Nat Genet*. 2001;29:310–314.

88. Estevez R, Boettger T, Stein V, et al. Barttin is a Cl$^-$ channel beta-subunit crucial for renal Cl$^-$ reabsorption and inner ear K$^+$ secretion. *Nature*. 2001;414:558–561.

89. Janssen AGH, Scholl U, Domeyer C, et al. Disease-causing dysfunctions of barttin in Bartter syndrome type IV. *J Am Soc Nephrol*. 2009;20:145–153.

90. Fischer M, Janssen AGH, Fahlke C. Barttin activates CIC-K channel function by modulating gating. *J Am Soc Nephrol*. 2010;21:1281–1289.

91. Vargas-Poussou R, Huang C, Hulin P, et al. Functional characterization of a calcium-sensing receptor mutation in severe autosomal dominant hypocalcemia with a Bartter-like syndrome. *J Am Soc Nephron*. 2002;13:2259–2266.

92. Watanabe S, Fukumoto S, Chang H, et al. Association between activation mutations of calcium-sensing receptor and Bartter's syndrome. *Lancet*. 2002;360:692–694.

19

93. Jeck N, Konrad M, Peters M, et al. Mutations in the chloride channel gene, CLCNKB, leading to a mixed Bartter-Gitelman phenotype. *Pediatr Res*. 2000;48:754–758.
94. Zelikovic I, Szargel R, Hawash A, et al. A novel mutation in the chloride channel gene, CLCNKB, as a cause of Gitelman and Bartter syndromes. *Kidney Int*. 2003;63:24–32.
95. Quigley R, Saland J. Transient antenatal Bartter's syndrome and X-linked polyhydramnios: insights from the genetics of a rare condition. *Kidney Int*. 2016;90:719–723.
96. Blanchard A, Bockenhauer D, Bolignano D, et al. Gitelman syndrome: consensus and guidance from a kidney disease: improving global outcomes (KDIGO) controversies conference. *Kidney Int*. 2017;91:24–33.
97. Friedman PA. Codependence of renal calcium and sodium transport. *Annu Rev Physiol*. 1998;60:179–197.
98. Van de Graaf SFJ, Bindels RJM, Hoenderop JGJ. Physiology of epithelial Ca^{2+} and Mg^{2+} transport. *Rev Physiol Biochem Pharmacol*. 2007;158:77–160.
99. Nijenhuis T, Vallon V, Van der Kemp AW, et al. enhanced passive Ca^{2+} reabsorption and reduced Mg^{2+} channel abundance explains thiazide-induced hypocalciuria and hypomagnesemia. *J Clin Invest*. 2005;115:1651–1658.
100. Dimke H, Hoenderop JG, Bindels RJ. Hereditary tubular transport disorders: implications for renal handling of Ca^{2+} and Mg^{2+}. *Clin Science*. 2010;118:1–18.
101. Kahle KT, Wilson FH, Lifton RP. The syndrome of hypertension and hyperkalemia (pseudohypoaldosteronism type II): WNK kinases regulate the balance between renal salt reabsorption and potassium secretion. In: Lifton RP, Somlo S, Giebisch GH, et al, eds. *Genetic Diseases of the Kidney*. Philadelphia: Saunders Elsevier; 2009:313–329.
102. O'Shaughnessy KM. Gordon syndrome: a continuing story. *Pediatr Nephrol*. 2015;30:1903–1908.
103. Pathare G, Hoenderop JGJ, Bindels RJM, et al. A molecular update on pseudohypoaldosteronism type II. *Am J Physiol Renal Physiol*. 2013;305:F1513–F1520.
104. Bazua-Valenti SB, Gamba G. Revisiting the NaCl cotransporter regulation by with-no-lysine kinases. *Am J Physiol Renal Physiol*. 2015;308:C779–C791.
105. Hadchouel J, Ellison DH, Gamba G. Regulation of renal electrolyte transport by WNK and SPAK-OSRI Kinases. *Annu Rev Physiol*. 2016;78:367–389.
106. Welling PA. Roles and regulation of renal K channels. *Annu Rev Physiol*. 2016;78:415–435.
107. Uchida S. Regulation of blood pressure and renal electrolyte balance by Cullin-RING ligases. *Curr Opin Nephrol Hypertens*. 2014;23:487–493.
108. Bockenhauer D, Feather S, Stanescu HC, et al. Epilepsy, ataxia, sensorineural deafness, tubulopathy, and KCNJ10 mutations. *N Engl J Med*. 2009;360:1960–1970.
109. Scholl UI, Choi M, Liu T, et al. Seizures, sensorineural deafness, ataxia, mental retardation, and electrolyte imbalance (SeSAME syndrome) caused by mutations in KCNJ10. *PNAS*. 2009;106:5842–5847.
110. Palygin O, Pochynyuk O, Staruschenko A. Review: role and mechanisms of regulation of the basolateral $K_{ir}4.1/K_{ir}5.1$ K^+ channels in the distal tubules. *Acta Physiol*. 2017;219:260–273.
111. Zhang C, Wang L, Zhang J, et al. KCNJ10 determines the expression of the apical Na-Cl cotransporter (NCC) in the early distal convoluted tubule (DCT1). *PNAS*. 2014;111:11864–11869.
112. Bazua-Valenti SB, Chavez-Canales MC, Rojas-Vega LR, et al. The effect of WNK4 on the Na^+-Cl^- cotransporter is modulated by intracellular chloride. *J Am Soc Nephrol*. 2015;26:1781–1786.
113. Batlle D, Haque SK. Genetic causes and mechanisms of distal renal tubular acidosis. *Nephrol Dial Trnasplant*. 2012;27:3691–3704.
114. Quigley R, Wolf MTF. Renal tubular acidosis in children. In: Avner ED, Harmon WD, eds. *Pediatric Nephrology*. 7th ed. Berlin Heidelberg: Springer-Verlag; 2015:1273–1306.
115. Donckerwolcke RA, van Biervliet JP, Koorevaar G, et al. The syndrome of renal tubular acidosis with nerve deafness. *Acta Paediatr Scand*. 1976;65:100–104.
116. Brown MT, Cunningham MJ, Ingelfinger JR, et al. Progressive sensorineural hearing loss in association with distal renal tubular acidosis. *Arch Otolaryngol Head Neck Surg*. 1993;119:458–460.
117. Fenton RA, Praetorius J. Anatomy of the kidney. In: Skorecki K, Chertow GM, Mardsen PA, eds. *Brenner & Rector's The Kidney*. 10th ed. Philadelphia: Elsevier; 2016:42–82.
118. Pearce D, Soundararajan R, Trimpert C, et al. Collecting duct principal cell transport processes and their regulation. *Clin J Am Soc Nephrol*. 2015;10:135–146.
119. Roy A, Al-bataineh MM, Pastor-Soler NM. Collecting duct intercalated cell function and regulation. *Clin J Am Soc Nephrol*. 2015;10:305–324.
120. Hamm LL, Alpern RJ, Preisig PA. Cellular mechanisms of renal tubular acidification. In: Alpern RJ, Moe OW, Caplan M, eds. *Seldin and Giebisch's The Kidney, Physiology and Pathophysiology*. 5th ed. Philadelphia: Elsvier; 2013:1917–1978.
121. Hamm LL, Nakhoul N, Hering-Smith KS. Acid-base homeostasis. *Clin J Am Soc Nephrol*. 2015;10:2232–2242.
122. Wagner CA. Renal acid-base transport: old and new players. *Nephron Physiol*. 2006;103:1–6.
123. Su Y, Al-Lamki RS, Blake-Palmer KG, et al. Physical and functional links between anion exchanger-1 and sodium pump. *J Am Soc Nephrol*. 2015;26:400–409.
124. Mumtaz R, Trepiccione F, Hennings JC, et al. Intercalated cell depletion and vacuolar H^+-ATPase mistargeting in an AE1 R607H knockin model. *J Am Soc Nephrol*. 2017;28:1507–1520.
125. Feraille E, Dizin E. Coordinated control of ENaC and Na^+, K^+-ATPase in renal collecting duct. *J Am Soc Nephrol*. 2016;27:2554–2563.
126. Stewart AK, Alper SL. The SLC4 anion exchanger gene family. In: Alpern RJ, Moe OW, eds. *Seldin and Giebisch's The Kidney, Physiology and Pathophysiology*. 5th ed. Philadelphia: Elsevier; 2013:1861–1915.

127. Romero MF, Chen AP, Parker MD, et al. The SLC4 family of bicarbonate (HCO_3^-) transporters. *Mol Aspects Med.* 2013;34:159–182.
128. Gallagher PG. Red cell membrane disorders. *Hematology Am Soc Hematol Educ Program.* 2005;13–18.
129. Bruce LJ, Cope DL, Jones GK, et al. Familial distal renal tubular acidosis is associated with mutations in the red cell anion exchanger (Band 3 AE1) gene. *J Clin Invest.* 1997;100:1693–1707.
130. Shayakul C, Alper SL. Inherited renal tubular acidosis. *Curr Opin Nephrol Hypertens.* 2000;9:541–546.
131. Toye AM, Banting G, Tanner MJA. Regions of human kidney anion exchanger 1 (kAE1) required for basolateral targeting of kAE1 in polarised kidney cells: mis-targeting explains dominant renal tubular acidosis (dRTA). *J Cell Sci.* 2004;117:1399–1410.
132. Fry AC, Su Y, Viu V, et al. Mutation conferring apical-targeting motif on AE1 exchanger causes autosomal dominant distal RTA. *J Am Soc Nephrol.* 2012;23:1238–1249.
133. Karet FE, Finberg KE, Nelson RD, et al. Mutations in the gene encoding B1 subunit of H^+-ATPase cause renal tubular acidosis with sensorineural deafness. *Nat Genet.* 1999;21:84–90.
134. Blake-Palmer KG, Karet FE. Cellular physiology of the renal H^+ ATPase. *Curr Opin Nephrol Hypertens.* 2009;433–438.
135. Wagner CA, Finberg KE, Breton S, et al. Renal vacuolar-ATPase. *Physiol Rev.* 2004;84:1263–1314.
136. Jefferies KC, Cipriano DJ, Forgac M. Function, structure and regulation of the vacuolar (H^+)-ATPases. *Arch Biochem Biophys.* 2008;476:33–42.
137. Miura K, Sekine T, Takahashi K, et al. Mutational analyses of the *ATP6V1B1* and *ATP6V0A4* genes in patients with primary distal renal tubular acidosis. *Nephrol Dial Transplant.* 2013;28:2123–2130.
138. Gomez J, Gil-Pena H, Santos F, et al. Primary distal renal tubular acidosis: novel findings in patients studied by next-generation sequencing. *Pediatr Res.* 2016;79:496–501.
139. Smith AN, Skaug J, Choat KA, et al. Mutation in ATP6N1B, encoding a new kidney vacuolar proton pump 116-kD subunit, cause recessive distal renal tubular acidosis with preserved hearing. *Nat Genet.* 2000;26:71–75.
140. Stover EH, Borthwick KJ, Bavalia C, et al. Novel ATP6V1B1 and ATP6V0A4 mutations in autosomal recessive distal renal tubular acidosis with new evidence for hearing loss. *J Med Genet.* 2002;39:796–803.
141. Norgett EE, Golder ZJ, Canovas BL, et al. *Atp6vOa4* knockout mouse is a model of distal renal tubular acidosis with hearing loss, with additional external phenotype. *PNAS.* 2012;109:13775–13780.
142. Rothstein M, Obialo C, Hruska KA. Renal tubular acidosis. *Endocrinol Metab Clin North Am.* 1990;19:869–887.
143. Sly WS, Hewett-Emmett D, Whyte MP, et al. Carbonic anhydrase II deficiency identified as the primary defect in the autosomal recessive syndrome of osteopetrosis with renal tubular acidosis and cerebral calcification. *Proc Natl Acad Sci USA.* 1983;80:2752–2756.
144. Roth DE, Venta PJ, Tashian RE, et al. Molecular basis of human carbonic anhydrase H deficiency. *Proc Natl Acad Sci USA.* 1992;89:1804–1808.
145. Scheinman SJ, Guay-Woodford LM, Thakker RV, et al. Genetic disorders of renal electrolyte transport. *N Engl J Med.* 1999;340:1177–1187.
146. Geller DS, Rodriguez-Soriano J, Vallo A, et al. Mutations in the mineralocorticoid receptor gene cause autosomal dominant pseudohypoaldosteronism type I. *Nat Genet.* 1998;19:279–281.
147. Rossier BC. Cum grano salis: the epithelial sodium channel and the control of blood pressure. *J Am Soc Nephrol.* 1997;8:980–992.
148. Bonny O, Hummler E. Dysfunction of epithelial sodium transport: from human to mouse. *Kidney Int.* 2000;57:1313–1318.
149. Kerem E, Bistritzer T, Hanukoglu A, et al. Pulmonary epithelial sodium channel dysfunction and excess airway liquid in pseudohypoaldosteronism. *N Engl J Med.* 1999;341:156–162.
150. Staub O, Loffing J. Mineralocorticoid action in the aldosterone sensitive distal nephron. In: Alpern RJ, Moe OW, Caplan M, eds. *Seldin and Giebisch's the Kidney, Physiology and Pathophysiology.* 5th ed. Philadelphia: Elsevier; 2013:1181–1211.
151. Bonny O, Rossier BC. Disturbances of Na/K balance: pseudohypoaldosteronism revisited. *J Am Soc Nephrol.* 2002;13:2399–2414.
152. Chang SS, Grunder S, Hanukoglu A, et al. Mutations in subunits of the epithelial sodium channel cause salt wasting with hyperkalaemic acidosis, pseudohypoaldosteronism type 1. *Nat Genet.* 1996;12:248–253.
153. Bockenhauer D, Bichet DG. Pathophysiology, diagnosis and management of nephrogenic diabetes insipidus. *Nat Rev Nephrol.* 2015;11:576–588.
154. Knoers NVAM, Levtchenko EN. Nephrogenic diabetes insipidus in children. In: Avner ED, Harmon WE, Niaudet P, et al, eds. *Pediatric Nephrology.* 7th ed. Berlin Heidelberg: Springer Verlag; 2015:1307–1328.
155. Linshaw MA. Congenital nephrogenic diabetes insipidus. *Pediatr Rev.* 2007;28:372–380.
156. Loonen AJM, Knoers NVAM, Van Os CH, et al. Aquaporin 2 mutations in nephrogenic diabetes insipidus. *Semin Nephrol.* 2008;28:252–265.
157. Verkman AS. Aquaporins in clinical medicine. *Annu Rev Med.* 2012;63:303–316.
158. Kortenoeven MLA, Fenton RA. Renal aquaporins and water balance disorders. *Biochim Biophys Acta.* 2014;1840:1533–1549.
159. Kozono D, Yasui M, King LS, et al. Aquaporin water channels: atomic structure molecular dynamics meet clinical medicine. *J Clin Invest.* 2002;109:1395–1399.
160. Rosenthal W, Seibold A, Antaramian A, et al. Molecular identification of the gene responsible for congenital nephrogenic diabetes insipidus. *Nature.* 1992;359:233–235.
161. Bichet DG. Vasopressin receptor mutations in nephrogenic diabetes insipidus. *Semin Nephrol.* 2008;28:245–251.

19

162. Spainakis E, Milord E, Gragnoli C. AVPR2 variants and mutations in nephrogenic diabetes insipidus: review and missense mutation significance. *J Cell Physiol*. 2008;217:605–617.

163. Deen PMT, Verdijk MA, Knoers NVAM, et al. Requirement of human renal water channel aquaporin-2 for vasopressin-dependent concentration of urine. *Science*. 1994;264:92–95.

164. Mulders SM, Knoers AVAM, van Leiburg AF, et al. New mutations in the AQP2 gene in nephrogenic diabetes insipidus resulting in functional but misrouted water channels. *J Am Soc Nephrol*. 1997;8:242–248.

165. Cohen FE, Kelly JW. Therapeutic approaches to protein-misfolding diseases. *Nature*. 2003;426:905–909.

166. Bernier V, Morello J, Zarruk A, et al. Pharmacologic chaperones as a potential treatment for x-linked nephrogenic diabetes insipidus. *J Am Soc Nephrol*. 2006;17:232–243.

167. Olesen ETB, Rutzler MR, Moeller HB, et al. Vasopressin-independent targeting of aquaporin-2 by selective E-prostanoid receptor agonists alleviates nephrogenic diabetes insipidus. *PNAS*. 2011;108:12949–12954.

168. Procino G, Milano S, Carmosino M, et al. Combination of secretin and fluvastatin ameliorates the polyuria associated with x-linked nephrogenic diabetes insipidus in mice. *Kidney Int*. 2014;86:127–138.

169. Feldman BJ, Rosenthal SM, Vargas GA, et al. Nephrogenic syndrome of inappropriate antidiuresis. *N Engl J Med*. 2005;352:1884–1890.

170. Gitelman SE, Feldman BJ, Rosenthal SM. Nephrogenic syndrome of inappropriate antidiuresis: a novel disorder in water balance in pediatric patients. *Am J Med*. 2006;119:S54–S58.

171. Ellison DH, Berl T. The syndrome of inappropriate antidiuresis. *N Engl J Med*. 2007;356:2064–2072.

172. Levtchenko EN, Monnens LAH. Nephrogenic syndrome of inappropriate antidiuresis. *Nephrol Dial Transplant*. 2010;25:2839–2843.

173. Rochdi MD, Vargas GA, Carpentier E, et al. Functional characterization of vasopressin type 2 receptor substitutions (R137H/C/L) leading to nephrogenic diabetes insipidus and nephrogenic syndrome of inappropriate antidiuresis: implications for treatments. *Mol Pharmacol*. 2010;77:836–845.

174. Carpentier E, Greenbaum LA, Rochdi D, et al. Identification and characterization of an activating F229V substitution in the V2 vasopressin receptor in an infant with NSAID. *J Am Soc Nephrol*. 2012;23:1635–1640.

175. Erdelyi LS, Mann WA, Morris-Rosendahl DJ, et al. Mutation in the V2 vasopressin receptor gene, *AVPR2*, causes nephrogenic syndrome of inappropriate diuresis. *Kidney Int*. 2015;88:1070–1078.

176. Tiulpakov A, White CW, Abhayawardana RS, et al. Mutations of vasopressin receptor 2 including novel L3125 have differential effects on trafficking. *Mol Endocrinol*. 2016;30:889–904.

CHAPTER 20

Inherited Disorders of Calcium, Phosphate, and Magnesium

Jyothsna Gattineni, MD, Matthias Tilmann Wolf, MD

- Regulation of Calcium, Magnesium, and Phosphate Involves Multiple Hormones. Genetic Disorders Affecting Any of These Regulators Result in Dysregulation of These Minerals' Ions and Subsequently Cause Clinical Symptoms.
- All Three Mineral Ions Are Absorbed in a Transcellular and Paracellular Fashion (Absorption Through the Cell Versus Absorption in Between the Cells, Respectively).
- The Vast Majority of Calcium and Phosphorus Is Absorbed in the Proximal Tubule, Whereas Most of the Magnesium Is Absorbed in the Thick Ascending Limb.
- Fine-Tuning of Tubular Calcium and Magnesium Absorption Occurs in the Distal Convoluted Tubule. However, Fine-Tuning of Phosphorus in the Distal Tubule Has Not Been Described.
- A Major Driving Force for Calcium and Magnesium Absorption in the Thick Ascending Limb Is the Lumen-Positive Potential.
- A Requirement for Magnesium Absorption in the Distal Convoluted Tubule Is the Negative Membrane Potential.
- Patients With Magnesium Disturbances May Not Present With Renal but With Neurologic Symptoms.

Inherited Disorders of Calcium

Introduction

Calcium (Ca^{2+}) is critical for many biologic functions in the body, and the vast majority of Ca^{2+} is stored in the bone. Ca^{2+} is vital for bone formation in the form of calcium phosphate hydroxyapatite and plays crucial roles in enzymatic reactions, in signaling pathways, and electric membrane potentials.[1] The Ca^{2+} content of a term newborn is approximately 30 g compared with approximately 1000 g in an adult.[2,3] Serum Ca^{2+} represents approximately 1% of the total body Ca^{2+}. Ca^{2+} regulation is tightly controlled and involves a complex interplay between the bone, intestine, and kidneys (Fig. 20.1).

Intestinal Ca^{2+} absorption occurs in the small intestine in a saturable, transcellular fashion and in the ileum and colon in a nonsaturable, paracellular fashion.[4] Intestinal Ca^{2+} absorption depends highly on the systemic Ca^{2+} concentration. In the newborn, approximately 60% of the oral intake of Ca^{2+} is absorbed in the gastrointestinal tract.

The kidneys are a major regulator of Ca^{2+} homeostasis by modifying tubular Ca^{2+} reabsorption versus urinary loss.[5] Complexed and free Ca^{2+} is filtered by the renal glomerulus. Along the nephron, approximately 95% of the filtered Ca^{2+} is reabsorbed.[6] The vast majority of Ca^{2+} is absorbed in the proximal tubule (60%–70%) and the thick ascending limb of Henle (TAL) (20%) across the paracellular pathway

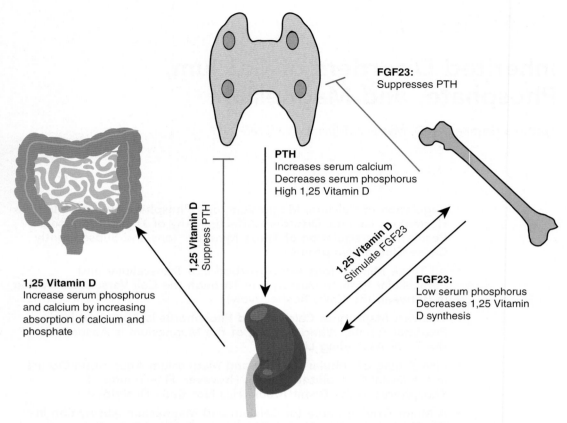

FGF23:
Suppresses PTH

PTH
Increases serum calcium
Decreases serum phosphorus
High 1,25 Vitamin D

1,25 Vitamin D
Suppress PTH

1,25 Vitamin D
Stimulate FGF23

FGF23:
Low serum phosphorus
Decreases 1,25 Vitamin
D synthesis

1,25 Vitamin D
Increase serum phosphorus
and calcium by increasing
absorption of calcium and
phosphate

Fig. 20.1   Summary of PTH, vitamin D, and FGF23 effects on calcium and phosphate homeostasis.

(between epithelial cells), in parallel with sodium (Na^+) and water.[4] In the TAL the major driving force for Ca^{2+} absorption is the lumen-positive potential difference.[7] Fine-tuning of renal Ca^{2+} reabsorption occurs in the distal convoluted tubule, where most of the remaining 10% of Ca^{2+} is reabsorbed in a transcellular fashion via the renal Ca^{2+} channel TRPV5 at the apical membrane (Fig. 20.2).[8] Inside the renal epithelial cell Ca^{2+} is bound to calbindin-D_{28K} to avoid the risk of calcium-induced cell death. Notably, the intracellular free Ca^{2+} concentration is approximately 100 nM (0.1 μmol/L), whereas the extracellular free Ca^{2+} concentration is approximately 1 mM (2.5 mmol/L). On the basolateral side, Ca^{2+} is extruded by the plasma membrane Ca^{2+} ATPase (PMCA) and the sodium/calcium exchanger (NCX) (see Fig. 20.2).[9] Parathyroid hormone (PTH) and 1,25-dihydroxy vitamin D3 (1,25 Vitamin D) both increase serum Ca^{2+}, whereas calcitonin decreases Ca^{2+} concentration (Fig. 20.1).

Regulators of Calcium Homeostasis

A complicated system consisting of hormones (PTH, FGF23, calcitonin), receptors (PTH receptor, CaSR), and vitamins (vitamin D) regulate Ca^{2+} homeostasis involving different organs, such as the parathyroid gland, intestine, bone, and kidneys. Dysfunction of these organs, hormones, vitamins, or their receptors results in disturbed Ca^{2+} homeostasis and causes either hypercalcemia or hypocalcemia. For a review of these different components of Ca^{2+}, PO_4^-, and Mg^{2+} regulation, please refer to the chapter "Perinatal Calcium and Phosphorus Metabolism."

Hypercalcemia

Neonatal hypercalcemia is defined as total serum Ca^{2+} concentrations greater than 10.5 mg/dL (>2.6 mmol/L).

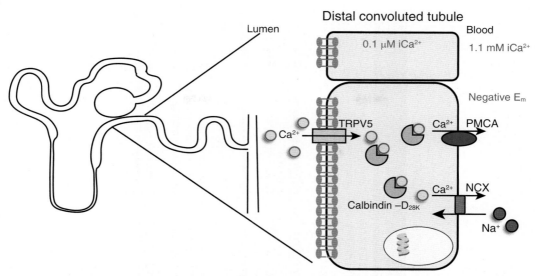

Fig. 20.2 Transcellular calcium (Ca^{2+}) absorption in the distal convoluted tubule occurs via the apical Ca^{2+} channel TRPV5. Ca^{2+} is bound inside the cell by calbindin-D_{28K} and exported at the basolateral side by the Ca^{2+} ATPase (PMCA) and the sodium/Ca^{2+} exchanger NCX.

Symptoms of Hypercalcemia

Hypercalcemia may remain asymptomatic or may cause polyuria, nephrocalcinosis, dehydration, renal failure, abdominal pain, constipation, nausea, pancreatitis, poor feeding, muscular hypotonia, bradycardia, shortened QTc interval, and lethargy.

A list of inherited causes of hypercalcemia is provided in Tables 20.1 and 20.2.

PTH-Dependent Hypercalcemia

Hypercalcemia Due to Hyperparathyroidism

Congenital Hyperparathyroidism/Primary Hyperparathyroidism. Primary hyperparathyroidism is a rare condition caused by parathyroid hyperplasia and occurs by sporadic or autosomal recessive inheritance. Clinical presentation includes symptoms listed previously but also hypophosphatemia, hypercalciuria, and hyperphosphaturia. Bone demineralization and even osteitis fibrosa and fractures can occur. A renal ultrasound may reveal nephrocalcinosis.

Parathyroid tumors are a rare event in neonates, with adenomas being the most common.[10] Parathyroid tumors occur either isolated or as part of a tumor syndrome (e.g., the multiple endocrine neoplasias [MENs] or hyperparathyroidism with jaw tumors).[11] Parathyroid tumors can be due to heterozygous somatic mutations (gain-of-function mutation) resulting in overexpression of oncogenes, such as *RET* (causing MEN2) or *PRAD1* (parathyroid adenoma 1) or recessive mutations in tumor-suppressor genes (loss-of-function mutation).[12,13] MEN type 1 is caused by autosomal dominant mutations in the *MEN1* gene (a tumor suppressor gene which encodes Menin) and is characterized by parathyroid, pancreatic, or pituitary tumors.[14,15] MEN type 2 (MEN2) is due to activating, heterozygous mutations in the proto-oncogene *RET1*.[16] These mutations typically result in hyperparathryroidism due to a parathyroid adenoma, medullary carcinoma of the thyroid, and pheochromocytoma. Parathyroid carcinoma and tumors of the mandible occur in a rare genetic syndrome called hyperparathyroidism–jaw tumor syndrome, which is caused by mutations in the gene *HRPT2* (which encodes the tumor suppressor parafibromin).[17,18]

The diagnosis of primary hyperparathyroidism is made by the detection of elevated PTH or inappropriately normal PTH levels given higher circulating Ca^{2+}

Table 20.1 LIST OF INHERITED FORMS OF HYPERCALCEMIA DUE TO HYPERPARATHYROIDISM OR ENHANCED PTH SIGNALING

Disorder	OMIM	Inheritance	Gene Locus	1,25 (OH)$_2$ Vitamin D	PTH	Serum Ca^{2+}	Urine Ca^{2+}	Gene (Protein)	Function	References
Congenital hyperparathyroidism	*168461	Sporadic	11q13.3	$n/\uparrow$	$\uparrow$	$\uparrow$	$\uparrow$	*CCND1/PRAD1* (Cyclin D1)	Phosphorylase which inactivates *RB* oncogene	12,13
Multiple endocrine neoplasias type 1	#131100	AD	11q13.1	$n/\uparrow$	$\uparrow$	$\uparrow$	$\uparrow$	*MEN1* (Menin)	Tumor suppressor	14,15
Multiple endocrine neoplasias type 2	#171400	AD	10q11.2	$n/\uparrow$	$\uparrow$	$\uparrow$	$\uparrow$	*RET* (RET)	RET protooncogene is overexpressed	16
Hyperparathyroidism–jaw tumor syndrome	#145001	AD	1q31.2	$n/\uparrow$	$\uparrow$	$\uparrow$	$\uparrow$	*HRPT2/CDC73* (Parafibromin)	Tumor suppressor	17,18
Familial hypocalciuric hypercalcemia type 1 (FHH1)	#145980	AD	3q13.3	$n/\uparrow$	$n/\uparrow$	$\uparrow$	$\downarrow$	*CASR* (CaSR)	Ca^{2+}-sensing receptor	22,33
FHH2	#145981	AD	19p13.3	$n/\uparrow$	$n/\uparrow$	$\uparrow$	$\downarrow$	*GNA11* (Gα$_{11}$)	G protein signaling	35
FHH3	#600740	AD	19q13.32	$n/\uparrow$	$n/\uparrow$	$\uparrow$	$\downarrow$	*AP2S1* (AP2σ1)	Clathrin adaptor protein	32
Neonatal severe hyperparathyroidism	#239200	AR	3q13.3	$n/\uparrow$	$\uparrow$	$\uparrow$	$\uparrow$	*CASR* (CaSR)	Ca^{2+}-sensing receptor	38,41–43
Jansen metaphyseal chondrodysplasia	#156400	AD	3p21	$n/\uparrow$	$n/\downarrow$	$\uparrow$	$\uparrow$	*PTHR1* (PTHR1)	Constitutive active PTH receptor	44–47

AD, Autosomal dominant; *n*, normal.

Table 20.2 LIST OF INHERITED FORMS OF PTH-INDEPENDENT HYPERCALCEMIAS

Disorder	OMIM	Inheritance	Gene Locus	1,25 (OH)$_2$ Vitamin D	PTH	Serum Ca^{2+}	Urine Ca^{2+}	Gene (Protein)	Function	References
Severe infantile hypophosphatasia	#241500	AR	1p36.12	n/↓	↓	↑	↑	ALPL (alkaline phosphatase)	Pyrophosphatase	51,53
Idiopathic infantile hypercalcemia	#143880	AR	20q13.2	n/↑	↓	↑	↑	CYP24A1 (25-hydroxyvitamin D 24-hydroxylase)	Vitamin D metabolism	56–58
Williams-Beuren syndrome	#194050	AD	7q11.23	n/↑	n/↑	n/↑	n/↑	ELN (elastin)	Connective tissue protein	63,64
Bartter syndrome type 1	#601678	AR	15q15-q21.1	n	n/↑	n/↑	↑	SLC12A1 (NKCC2)	Na$^+$-K$^+$-Cl$^-$ cotransporter	69
Bartter syndrome type 2	#241200	AR	11q24	n	n/↑	n	↑	KCNJ1 (ROMK)	K$^+$ channel	70
Bartter syndrome type 3	#607364	AR	1p36	n	n	n	n/↑	CLCNKB (CLC-Kb)	Chloride channel	76
Bartter syndrome type 4	#602522	AR	1p31	n	n	n	↑	BSND (Barttin)	Subunit of CLC-Kb channel	75
Bartter syndrome type 5	#300971	XLR	Xp11.21	n.d.	n.d.	n	↑	MAGED2 (melanoma associated antigen D2)	Modifies NCC and NKCC2	73

AD, Autosomal dominant; AR, autosomal recessive; n, normal; n.d., no data; XLR, x-linked recessive.

20

levels, 1,25 Vitamin D concentrations are elevated or normal, serum phosphate levels are low-normal or low, and alkaline phosphatase can be elevated due to bone disease. A spot urine Ca^{2+} to creatinine ratio (normally <1 in infants) and a 24-hour urine collection enable the diagnosis of hypercalciuria. A renal ultrasound may detect nephrocalcinosis, and an x-ray of the wrist may demonstrate bone involvement. The treatment of choice is total parathyroidectomy with partial autotransplantation. Preoperatively, hyperparathyroid adenomas are detected by technetium 99m sestamibi scan. Following parathyroidectomy the influx of Ca^{2+} into the healing bone may aggravate the duration of hypocalcemia, a phenomenon called "hungry bone syndrome."[19] In very low birth weight infants and newborns the removal of the parathyroid glands may be complicated by the small size of the parathyroid glands. Adjunct medical treatment in such cases is possible with the Ca^{2+}-sensing receptor (CaSR) mimetic Cinacalcet, which may provide intermittent relief until surgery is an option.[20]

Familial Hypocalciuric Hypercalcemia/Neonatal Severe Hyperparathyroidism. Characteristics of familial hypocalciuric hypercalcemia (FHH) are mild hypercalcemia, inappropriately normal or mildly elevated PTH, and hypocalciuria. Genetically, three different forms of FHH (FHH1-3) were identified by genetic linkage. For FHH1 and FHH2, there are usually no signs of hypercalcemia and no nephrocalcinosis, and PTH levels remain normal; there may be mild hypermagnesemia, but overall patients remain asymptomatic. Rarely, pancreatitis and chondrocalcinosis may occur.[21] For FHH1, inactivating mutations in the *CaSR* gene have been described that are inherited in an autosomal dominant fashion.[22] To maintain Ca^{2+} homeostasis within the body, a sensing mechanism for Ca^{2+} is required. This function is provided by CaSR, which is a seven transmembrane–spanning G protein–coupled receptor (GPCR).[23–25] The gene encoding the CaSR is most highly expressed in organs involved in Ca^{2+} homeostasis, such as the parathyroid glands, C cells of the thyroid gland, bone, and kidneys. CaSR recognizes surprisingly minor perturbations in extracellular Ca^{2+} concentration and reacts by adjusting PTH secretion. Stimulation of CaSR by Ca^{2+} binding reduces PTH secretion via G protein–coupled signaling via $G\alpha_{q/11}$, $G\alpha_i$, $G\alpha_{12/13}$, and $G\alpha_{qs}$ and other pathways such as MAPK.[24,26–28] In FHH1 the altered CaSR on the parathyroid gland does not respond appropriately to increasing serum Ca^{2+} concentrations so that higher serum Ca^{2+} concentrations are required to suppress PTH. This results in a shift of the set point for PTH release to the right. The CaSR mutation can also impair renal Ca^{2+} excretion, thereby contributing to the hypocalciuria. In the kidney, activation of CaSR increases Ca^{2+} excretion, acidifies urinary pH, and impairs urinary concentration in an attempt to reduce the risk of nephrocalcinosis and nephrolithiasis. In addition, in an attempt to maintain solubility of urinary Ca^{2+} salts and to prevent tubular Ca^{2+} precipitation, CaSR activation at the apical membrane of the collecting duct enhances acid secretion by stimulation of H^+-ATPase and inhibits water absorption by interference with vasopressin-induced aquaporin-2 (AQP2) insertion in the apical membrane.[29–31] Chronic hypercalcemia results in diabetes insipidus by AQP2 downregulation via the CaSR.

In the context of hypophosphatemia, hypocalciuria helps to distinguish FHH versus hyperparathyroidsim (which causes hypercalciuria). Approximately 65% of FHH patients have *CaSR* mutations.[32] The opposite pathophysiology can be seen with autosomal dominant hypocalcemia (see later). Gain-of-function mutations of the CaSR, which induce a higher sensitivity to extracellular Ca^{2+}, can also result in Bartter syndrome.[33,34] As these mutations imitate elevated extracellular Ca^{2+} concentrations, PTH secretion is suppressed and impairs renal Ca^{2+} and Mg^{2+} absorption.

Over the following years, FHH was found to be a genetically heterogeneous condition. Loss-of-function mutations in $G\alpha_{11}$, which encodes a protein involved in the signaling cascade of the CaSR, were found in FHH2 patients.[35] Because $G\alpha_{11}$ is part of the CaSR signaling cascade, it was a candidate gene for FHH2. *In vitro* experiments confirmed that loss-of-function mutations in the encoding gene *GNA11* decreased the sensitivity of the CaSR to extracellular Ca^{2+} and resulted in a rightward shift in the concentration-response curve, with significantly higher half-maximal effective concentration (EC50) values. Interestingly, gain-of-function mutations in the genes encoding $G\alpha_{11}$ result in the opposite phenotype of autosomal dominant hypocalcemia (see later).[35]

In FHH3, clinical characteristics can be different with elevated PTH levels, hypophosphatemia, and osteomalacia.[36,37] FHH3 is caused by dominant mutations in the adaptor protein-2 sigma subunit (AP2σ1, encoded by the *AP2S1* gene), which results in loss of function of the encoded protein, which is important as a component of clathrin-coated vesicles.[32] *AP2S1* mutations decrease the sensitivity of CaSR-expressing cells to extracellular Ca^{2+} and impair CaSR endocytosis by reducing the affinity for the dileucine motif.[22,32] Mutations were identified in 20% of FHH patients without *CASR* mutations.[32] Overall the disease severity in FHH is relatively mild, and some patients remain asymptomatic. Sporadic *CaSR* mutations are also possible.[38] FHH patients are usually treated with thiazides or calcimimetics. Parathyroidectomy is contraindicated.[39,40]

A more pronounced phenotype than FHH is associated with neonatal severe hyperparathyroidism (NSHPT), which is due to homozygous or compound heterozygous, inactivating mutations in the *CaSR* gene.[22,38,41–43] Symptoms include severe hypercalcemia, markedly elevated PTH levels, failure to thrive, polyuria, hypotonia, and hypophosphatemia. Infants with NSHPT often have pronounced bone disease. NSHPT patients are treated with rehydration, bisphosphonates, and calcimimetics. Patients who are not responding to medical treatment may benefit from parathyroidectomy.

Jansen Metaphyseal Chondrodysplasia

This rare, autosomal dominant condition is characterized by severe hypercalcemia, hypophosphatemia, abnormal chondrocyte proliferation, and normal or undetectable PTH or PTH-related peptide levels.[44] Affected patients display short stature and short extremities.[45] This condition is caused by heterozygous mutations of the PTH receptor result in constitutive activation of the receptor.[45,46] These PTH receptor mutations resulted in agonist-independent accumulation of cyclic adenosine monophosphate (cAMP), a secondary messenger of the PTH receptor. Some of the identified PTH receptor mutations yielded milder skeletal phenotypes and overall normal stature but hypercalcemia and a higher risk for hypercalciuria resulting in a higher risk of nephrolithiasis.[47] Bisphosphonates may be able to improve this condition.[48]

PTH-Independent Hypercalcemia

Severe Infantile Hypophosphatasia

Hypercalcemia, hypercalciuria, paradoxically low alkaline phosphatase levels, failure to thrive, poor feeding, increased intracranial pressure, papilledema, and nephrocalcinosis are found in a rare autosomal recessive condition named infantile hypophosphatasia.[49] In addition, loss of deciduous teeth is described in affected children. Symptoms can present perinatally, in infancy, in childhood, or in adolescence, spanning a surprisingly large clinical variability ranging from intrauterine death to unmineralized bone and dental complications. The variability is due to autosomal dominant versus recessive transmission of the gene defect with two affected alleles causing the more severe and earlier phenotypes.[50] This disorder is due to mutations in the gene *ALPL* encoding tissue-nonspecific isoenzyme alkaline phosphatase.[51] As a result, alkaline phosphatase activity is impaired in the liver, kidney, teeth, and bone. The encoded protein is a cell surface phosphohydrolase. When deficient, there is accumulation of the substrates for alkaline phosphatase, including inorganic pyrophosphate (alkaline phosphatase is a pyrophosphatase), a very potent inhibitor of mineralization, thereby explaining the dental and osseous phenotype. In the infantile form of hypophosphatasia, symptoms present prior to 6 months of age. Hypercalcemia and hyperphosphatemia with severe rickets are seen due to the inability of the patient's blocked entry of minerals into the skeleton with appropriately reduced PTH concentrations.[52] Infants may also present with pyridoxine-dependent seizures due to incomplete extracellular hydrolysis of pyridoxal 5′-phosphate, the major circulating form of vitamin B6. More than 300 *ALPL* mutations have been published. In the infantile form, approximately 50% of affected infants die.[53] A lethal outcome is likely in the context of pyridoxine-dependent seizures.[54] Diagnosis is made by elevated levels of phosphoethanolamine (serum and urine), inorganic pyrophosphate (serum and urine), and pyridoxal 5′-phosphate (serum). Radiographic signs for the infantile form include lack of mineralization, gracile ribs, poorly calcified metaphysis, fractures, progressive demineralization, and premature bony fusion. Treatment for these patients has improved with asfotase alfa, a bone-targeted recombinant enzyme replacement therapy.

Idiopathic Infantile Hypercalcemia (Lightwood Syndrome)

Idiopathic infantile hypercalcemia (IIH) occurs typically in the first year of life, with a peak between 5 and 8 months. Patients may develop failure to thrive, vomiting, hypercalciuria, and dehydration.[55] Overall the prognosis is good even though many patients may develop nephrocalcinosis. No syndromic features were discovered. In some instances, IIH resolves spontaneously. Typically, PTH levels are suppressed, and there are upper limits of normal to elevated 25(OH)$_2$D and 1,25 Vitamin D levels.[56] In the past, excessive vitamin D intake, increased sensitivity to vitamin D, and increased PTHrP secretion were thought to be involved in the pathogenesis. In 2011 Schlingmann and coworkers published recessive mutations in the CYP24A1 gene, which encodes the 25-hydroxyvitamin D 24-hydroxylase as the main cause for IIH.[57] Mutations were found in IIH patients and a second cohort of patients who displayed symptoms of vitamin D intoxication soon after receiving high-dose vitamin D prophylaxis. The encoded enzyme converts 1,25 Vitamin D to an inactive metabolite. The identified mutations were found to abolish 1,25 Vitamin D catabolism almost completely in vitro, resulting in higher levels of 1,25 Vitamin D and subsequently hypercalcemia.[57] Patients with CYP24A1 mutations developed severe hypercalcemia when they received vitamin D prophylaxis. Given the routine use of cholecalciferol supplementation in children, medical professionals should be aware of this condition causing this rare side effect of vitamin D supplementation. Interestingly, adult patients with nephrolithiasis and hypercalcemia were also found to have CYP24A1 mutations.[58]

A subgroup of IIH patients did not have CYP24A1 mutations but was characterized by pronounced hypophosphatemia and renal phosphate wasting, in addition to hypercalcemia, suppressed PTH, and nephrocalcinosis.[59] Interestingly, all patients also received vitamin D prophylaxis. Genome-wide linkage analysis pointed to SLC34A1, which encodes the renal sodium–phosphate cotransporter 2a (NaPi2a), and recessive mutations in 16 patients with IIH were identified. This cotransporter is responsible for combined sodium and phosphate absorption from the proximal tubule, and affected patients demonstrated urinary phosphate wasting in addition to symptomatic hypercalcemia in infancy. Functional studies of mutant NaPi2a showed impaired trafficking of the cotransporter to the plasma membrane and thereby resulted in less phosphate transport activity.

One may wonder how renal phosphate wasting results in hypercalcemia and nephrocalcinosis. The biologic activity of 1,25 Vitamin D is regulated by its activating enzyme 1α-hydroxylase (CYP27B1) and its deactivating enzyme 24-hydroxylase (CYP24A1). Both enzymes are regulated by 1,25 Vitamin D itself, phosphate, Ca^{2+}, PTH, and the fibroblast factor 23 (FGF23), a phosphatonin. FGF23 inhibits 1α-hydroxylase and promotes 1,25 Vitamin D degradation by enhancing 24-hydroxylase. A key role in the pathomechanism of this specific subgroup is the downregulation of FGF23 in the context of hypophosphatemia and hyperphosphaturia. The hypophosphatemia results in more active 1,25 Vitamin D synthesis and less 1,25 Vitamin D catabolism, thereby increasing the 1,25 Vitamin D level, serum Ca^{2+} concentration, and hypercalciuria.[59] As a proof of concept, treatment with furosemide, rehydration, corticosteroids, or ketoconazole or a low calcium diet does not improve the patient's hypercalcemia. Phosphate supplementation improves the hypercalcemia in affected patients.

Williams-Beuren Syndrome

Williams-Beuren syndrome (WBS) is characterized by elfin facies, supravalvular aortic stenosis, peripheral pulmonary stenosis, motor disabilities, dental abnormalities, developmental delay, and a friendly personality.[60] Hypercalcemia and hypercalciuria can occur with WBS and can result in severe nephrocalcinosis.[61] Additional endocrine disorders can include diabetes mellitus (DM), mild hypothyroidism, hyperparathyroidism, and impaired bone metabolism, and approximately 20% of patients may have congenital anomalies of the kidney and urogenital tract (CAKUT).[60,62] Approximately 90% of WBS patients carry a microdeletion of chromosome 7, which includes the *elastin* gene, causing a hemizygous continuous gene deletion syndrome of 25 to 30 genes.[63,64]

Bartter Syndrome

Bartter syndrome is characterized by salt wasting, polyuria, hypokalemia, metabolic alkalosis, massive polyuria, which can result in life-threatening dehydration, hyper-reninemic hyperaldosteronism, polyhydramnios, failure to thrive, hypercalciuria, nephrocalcinosis, osteopenia, and almost always prematurity.[65-68] The development of these features can take weeks to months. The causes for antenatal Bartter syndrome include recessive mutations of the Na^+-K^+-$2Cl^-$-cotransporter NKCC2 and the renal outer medullary potassium channel ROMK.[69,70] Mutations of the gene encoding ROMK frequently result in postnatal hyperkalemia in contrast to all other genes contributing to Bartter syndrome.[71,72] In the TAL CaSR is expressed at the basolateral membrane and impairs paracellular and transcellular NaCl and divalent cation reabsorption by inhibiting ROMK and NKCC2 (Fig. 20.3).[26] This results in a decrease of the lumen-positive potential and reduces the driving force for paracellular Na^+, Ca^{2+}, and Mg^{2+} reabsorption and causes urinary wasting of these electrolytes.[73,74]

A less common cause for antenatal Bartter syndrome are mutations of *Barttin*, which is a subunit of the basolateral chloride channel *CLCNKB*.[75] In addition to the symptoms described previously, these patients also have sensorineural deafness. Recessive mutations in *CLCNKB* cause classical Bartter syndrome.[76] Hypercalciuria, hyperparathyroidism, and nephrocalcinosis are detected with *NKCC2* mutations. In rare instances, hypercalcemia is described.[77,78] Transient hypercalciuria and nephrolcalcinosis were also noticed with *MAGED2* mutations, a novel cause for antenatal Bartter syndrome.[79] Bartter syndrome is discussed more in detail in a different chapter.

Hypocalcemia

Neonatal hypocalcemia is defined as total serum Ca^{2+} concentrations less than 7 mg/dL (<1.75 mmol/L) and for ionized Ca^{2+} less than 4.4 mg/dL (1.1 mmol/L) compared with adult hypocalcemia with Ca^{2+} concentrations less than 8.4 mg/dL (2.1 mmol/L). After delivery the maternal Ca^{2+} supply is interrupted and the main source of Ca^{2+} is the bone. Due to the low dietary Ca^{2+} intake on the first day of life, the nadir (4.4–5.4 mg/dL, 1.1–1.36 mmol/L) in full-term neonates is reached within 24 hours postdelivery and gradually increases thereafter.[80] Approximately 30% of preterm infants will encounter hypocalcemia within the first 48 hours. Serum Ca^{2+} concentrations correlate with gestational age. Therefore premature infants have a higher likelihood of developing hypocalcemia.[81] Low serum albumin levels are a common contributing factor for hypocalcemia, but ionized Ca^{2+} concentrations should remain normal.

Symptoms of Hypocalcemia

Symptoms of hypocalcemia may be mild but can manifest as neonatal jitteriness and convulsions (generalized and focal). Because hypocalcemia and hypomagnesemia may present in a similar fashion, both electrolytes should be measured. A chest x-ray may help to determine the thymic silhouette in case of suspicion for DiGeorge syndrome. An ECG may reveal increased corrected QT interval longer than 0.4 seconds.

A list of inherited causes of hypocalcemia is provided in Tables 20.3–20.5.

Hypocalcemia Due to PTH Abnormalities/Hypoparathyroidism

Congenital Hypoparathyroidism. Familial isolated hypoparathyroidism can be inherited as an autosomal recessive, dominant, or X-linked trait or it may occur

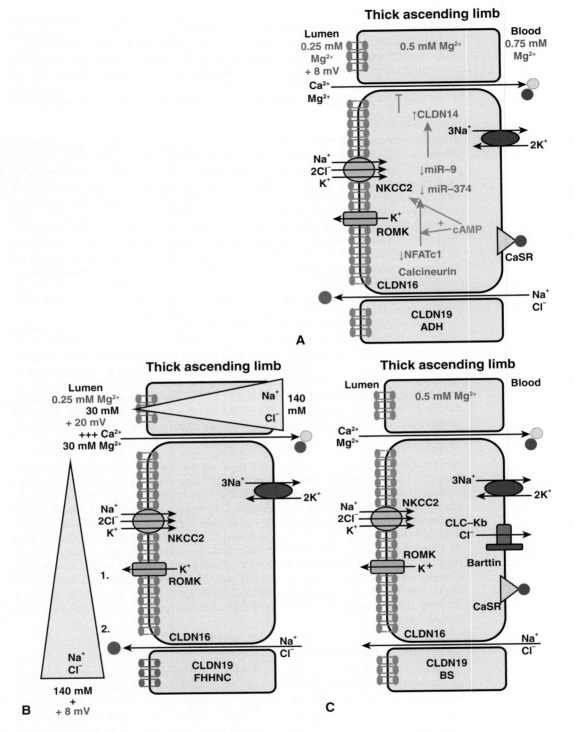

Fig. 20.3 Autosomal dominant hypocalcemia, FHHNC, and Bartter syndrome affect the TAL by disturbing the lumen-positive potential and are grouped together as hypercalciuric hypomagnesemias. (A) In the case of autosomal dominant hypocalcemia, CaSR activation results in hypomagnesemia by a number of different mechanisms. For example the lumen-positive potential difference is affected by downregulation of NKCC2 and ROMK via an inhibitable adenylcyclase and activation of inhibitory G proteins. This results in decreased intracellular cAMP levels, which usually stimulate NKCC2 and ROMK channels. A new intriguing pathway involving calcineurin signaling and downregulation of NFAT signaling has been published recently. This novel pathway includes regulation of miR9 and miR374. As CaSR is stimulated, miR9 and 374 are downregulated, which in turn enhances Claudin-14 expression. Claudin-14 inhibits activity of the Claudin-16/Claudin-19 complex and thereby interferes with the creation of the lumen-positive potential. (B) The lumen-positive potential in the TAL is due to the secretion of potassium via ROMK channels and the dilution potential. The dilution potential is created by the decreasing luminal Na+ concentration from the proximal to the distal part of the TAL, which decreases from 140 mM to 30 mM. Subsequently the interstitium surrounding the distal TAL contains much more Na+ and Cl− than the tissue around the proximal TAL. Overall, this forms a concentration gradient with a higher interstitial Na+ and Cl− concentration than in the lumen and a driving force for Na+ and Cl− to leak back into the lumen. Claudin-16 and -19 are responsible for the permeability of Na+ and Cl− from the interstitium to lumen. As mostly Na+ leaks back into the lumen this contributes to the lumen-positive potential. This mechanism increases the lumen potential from +8 to +20 mV. (C) Intracellular Cl− regulation is disturbed by mutations in CLCNKB and BSND causing Bartter syndrome. Intracellular Cl− is important for NCC and NKCC2 activity. The lumen-positive potential is reduced with decreased NKCC2 function, which may interfere with tubular Mg^{2+} absorption. Adapted from 157.

sporadically. Mutations occur in genes regulating parathyroid gland development or in the *PTH* gene (in the PTH precursor preproPTH).[82–85] Patients present with hypocalcemia, hyperphosphatemia, inappropriately low PTH, and low 1,25 Vitamin D concentrations. Due to the lack of renal PTH action, tubular absorption of Ca^{2+} is diminished, resulting in hypercalciuria and a higher risk for nephrocalcinosis and chronic kidney disease (CKD). Interestingly, *CASR* gene mutations have also been found to result in hypoparathyroidism in addition to causing autosomal dominant hypocalcemia (see later).[86,87]

Hypoparathyroidism, Deafness, and Renal Anomalies Syndrome. Hypoparathyroidism, deafness, and renal anomalies (HDR) syndrome is characterized by congenital hypoparathyroidism, bilateral sensorineural deafness, and renal dysplasia/cysts. HDR patients present with hypocalcemia and low to undetectable PTH concentrations. HDR syndrome is caused by heterozygous mutations in the transcription factor GATA3 on chromosome 10p14.[88–91] GATA3 expression during human and murine development (e.g., in otic vesicle, parathyroid glands, kidneys) is consistent with the HDR phenotype.[92–94]

DiGeorge Syndrome. Hypoparathyroidism can be part of DiGeorge syndrome, which is characterized by branchial cleft abnormalities including hypoplasia of pharyngeal arches, parathyroid glands, thymus, cardiac and craniofacial defects. This syndrome is due to chromosomal deletions of 22q11.2, which includes approximately 30 genes.[95–97] One of these genes is the *TBX1* gene, and mice lacking *Tbx1* and humans with *TBX1* point mutations develop DiGeorge syndrome.[98,99] *TBX1* encodes a transcription factor of the T-box family and is crucial in organogenesis. Another form of DiGeorge syndrome is due to a deletion of 10p.[100] Approximately 17% of DiGeorge patients have no detectable chromosomal abnormality.[101] In approximately 50% to 60% of DiGeorge patients, hypocalcemia is diagnosed.[102,103] Transient hypocalcemia at birth can be seen due to abrupt discontinuation of maternal Ca^{2+} supply and the delivery stress. Patients are treated with vitamin D and Ca^{2+} to keep serum Ca^{2+} concentrations in the low normal to avoid nephrocalcinosis and nephrolithiasis.

GCMB Mutations. Isolated parathyroid gland agenesis was published due to heterozygous (dominant negative) or recessive (loss-of-function) mutations in the glial cell missing B (*GCMB* or *GCM2*) gene, which encodes for a parathyroid specific transcription factor and contributes to regulation of PTH gene expression.[104–107]

Table 20.3 LIST OF INHERITED FORMS OF HYPOCALCEMIAS DUE TO HYPOPARATHYROIDISM

Disorder	OMIM	Inheritance	Gene Locus	1,25 (OH)$_2$ Vitamin D	PTH	Serum Ca^{2+}	Urine Ca^{2+}	Gene (Protein)	Function	References
Congenital hypoparathyroidism	#146200	AD	11p15.3	↓	↓	↓	↓	PTH (PreproPTH)	PTH hormone	82–85
Hypoparathyroidism, deafness, and renal anomalies (HDR)	#146255	AD	10p14	↓	↓	↓	↓	GATA3 (GATA3)	Transcription factor	88–91
DiGeorge syndrome	#188400	AD	22q11.2	↓-n	↓	↓	↓	Heterogenous gene deletion syndrome/TBX1	TBX1 encodes transcription factor	98,99,101
Parathyroid gland agenesis	#146200	AD/AR	6p24.2	↓	↓	↓	↓	GCMB/GCM2 (GCMB/GCM2)	Transcription factor	107
Autoimmune polyendocrine syndrome	#240300	AR	21q22.3	↓	↓	↓	↓	AIRE (AIRE)	Nuclear transcription factor	108
Kearns-Sayre syndrome	#530000	mito.	mito.	↓	↓	↓	↓	MTTL1 (MTTL1)	tRNA for leucine	110,111
MELAS syndrome	#540000	mito.	mito.	↓	↓	↓	↓	MTTL1, MTTQ, … (MTTL1, MTTQ)	tRNA for leucine, glutamine, …	110,111
Kenney-Caffey syndrome	#244460	AR	1q42.3	↓	↓	↓	↓	TBCE (TBCE)	Tubulin-specific chaperone	112,113
Blomstrand disease	#215045	AR	3p21.31	↓	n-↑	↓	↓	PTHR1 (PTH receptor)	PTH receptor	114,115

AD, Autosomal dominant; AR, autosomal recessive; mito., mitochondrial; n, normal.

Table 20.4 LIST OF INHERITED FORMS OF HYPOCALCEMIAS DUE TO CALCIUM SENSING RECEPTOR OR SIGNALING ABNORMALITIES

Disorder	OMIM	Inheritance	Gene Locus	1,25 (OH)$_2$ Vitamin D	PTH	Serum Ca^{2+}	Urine Ca^{2+}	Gene (Protein)	Function	References
Autosomal dominant hypocalcemia	#601198	AD	3q13.3-q21.1	↓	n-↓	↓	↑	*CASR* (CaSR) (gain-of-function)	Ca^{2+}-sensing receptor	121–124
Autosomal dominant hypocalcemia	#615361	AD	19p13.3	↓	n-↓	↓	↑	*GNA11* (Gα$_{11}$) (gain-of-function)	G protein signaling	35,126
Pseudohypoparathyroidism—type Ia	#103580	AD	20q13.32	↓	↑	↓	n.d.	*GNAS1* (Gα$_s$)	G protein signaling	128
Pseudohypoparathyroidism—type Ib	#603233	AD	20q13.32	↓	↑	↓	n.d.	*STX16* (Syntaxin 16)	Endosome-trans-Golgi-network	136
Pseudohypoparathyroidism—type II	%203330	AD	n.d.	↓	↑	↓	n.d.	n.d.		
Pseudopseudohypoparathyroidism	#612463	AD	20q13.32	↓	↑	↓	n.d.	*GNAS1* (Gα$_s$)	G protein signaling	133

AD, Autosomal dominant; *n*, normal; *n.d.*, no data.

20

Table 20.5 LIST OF INHERITED FORMS OF HYPOCALCEMIAS DUE TO VITAMIN D DISTURBANCES

Disorder	OMIM	Inheritance	Gene Locus	1,25 (OH)₂ Vitamin D	PTH	Serum Ca²⁺	Urine Ca²⁺	Gene (Protein)	Function	References
Vitamin D-dependent rickets type 1	#264700	AR	12q14.1	↓	↑	↓	n-↓	*CYP27B1* (25-(OH) vitamin D3-1-α-hydroxylase)	Enzyme	140
Vitamin D-dependent rickets type 2	#277440	AR	12q13.11	↑	↑	↓	n-↓	*VDR* (vitamin D receptor)	Receptor	141–143

AR, Autosomal recessive; *n*, normal.

Autoimmune Polyendocrine Syndrome. Another syndrome that includes hypoparathyroidism is autoimmune polyendocrine syndrome type 1 (APS1), which is caused by autosomal recessive mutations in the autoimmune regulator gene *(AIRE)*.[108] APS1 is characterized by multiple endocrine gland insufficiencies (e.g., hypoparathyroidism, adrenal insufficiency, hypogonadism, DM, hypothyroidism) and chronic mucocutaneous candidiasis in childhood. This gene encodes a nuclear transcription factor which eliminates self-reactive T cells in the thymus.[109] As a consequence the immune system fails to establish immunologic tolerance.

Mitochondrial Disorders Associated With Hypoparathyrodism. Three mitochondrial disorders are associated with hypoparathyroidism, including Kearns-Sayre syndrome (KSS), mitochondrial encephalopathy, lactic acidosis, and stroke-like episodes syndrome (MELAS), and mitochondrial trifunctional protein deficiency syndrome.[110,111]

Other Syndromes (e.g., Kenney-Caffey and Blomstrand Disease). In approximately 50% of patients with Kenney-Caffey syndrome (KCS), hypoparathyroidism has been described. Genetic heterogeneity with mutations in the genes encoding tubulin-specific chaperone *(TBCE)* and family with sequence similarity 111A *(FAM111A)* were described.[112,113]

Another rare, autosomal recessive cause for hypocalcemia is Blomstrand chondrodysplasia. This condition is characterized by accelerated bone maturation, advanced chondrocyte differentiation, hyperdensity of the skeleton, accelerated ossification, and early lethality.[114] The causes for this disease are mutations of the PTH receptor impairing its binding of PTH, function, or expression.[115]

Treatment for these conditions include Ca^{2+} and 1,25 Vitamin D supplements, which may be complicated by developing hypercalciuria and nephrocalcinosis. Thiazide diuretics may be able to improve hypercalciuria.[116] Recombinant PTH (1–84) and (1–34) have been successfully used to improve successfully Ca^{2+} homeostasis.[117–119] An orally active small molecule PTHR1 agonist called PCO371 was discovered as potential therapeutic option.[120]

Hypocalcemia Due to CaSR Abnormalities or Downstream Signaling

Autosomal Dominant (Hypercalciuric) Hypocalcemia. In autosomal dominant hypocalcemia type 1, approximately 50% of patients remain asymptomatic or have mild hypocalcemia. Hypocalcemia may be present in the neonatal period. The other 50% can develop seizures, paresthesia, and carpopedal spasms. Although overall rare, this condition may be responsible for up to a third of patients with idiopathic hypoparathyroidism.[121] Approximately 10% have hypercalciuria with nephrocalcinosis and kidney stones.[33,122] Patients with autosomal dominant hypocalcemia often present with hypomagnesemia and hypermagnesuria. Approximately one-third of patients have ectopic and basal ganglia calcifications.[33,122] PTH concentration may be normal or inappropriately low. As a cause for autosomal dominant hypocalcemia type 1, gain-of-function mutations in the CaSR were identified resulting in higher serum Ca^{2+} threshold for PTH release (see Fig. 20.3A).[123] This imitates higher extracellular calcium concentrations, and as a result PTH secretion is suppressed and renal Ca^{2+} and Mg^{2+} absorption is impaired. Some patients may present with hypokalemia and alkalosis, symptoms consistent with Bartter syndrome, which is thought to be due to the CaSR effect on sodium absorption in the TAL.[124] The Bartter syndrome phenotype is thought to be due to impaired NKCC2 and ROMK function induced by an inhibitable adenyl cyclase, thus reducing Na^+, K^+, and Cl^- reabsorption in the TAL (see Fig. 20.3A).[34,124,125]

In a cohort of autosomal dominant hypocalcemia patients without hypercalciuria, heterozygous gain-of-function mutations of *GNA11* were identified, also resulting in an increased sensitivity of CaSR-expressing cells to extracellular Ca^{2+}, thereby causing a leftward shift in the concentration-response curves.[35] *GNA11* encodes a G protein that connects CaSR sensing with the Ca^{2+}/IP3/PKC signaling pathway in the parathyroid gland.[126] Differentiation between autosomal dominant hypocalcemia and hypoparathyroidism is important because treatment of autosomal dominant hypocalcemia patients with calcium and vitamin D may aggravate hypercalciuria and may worsen nephrocalcinosis.[33,123]

D

Pseudohypoparathyroidism

Pseudohypoparathyroidism (PHP) is due to a partial or complete peripheral resistance of the biologic actions of PTH. PHP is a heterogeneous syndrome characterized by increased PTH concentrations but functional hypoparathyroidism.[127] Biochemical features of PHP are similar to hypoparathyroidism with hypocalcemia, hyperphosphatemia, and low 1,25 Vitamin D concentrations, but PHP patients have an elevated PTH level. PHP type 1a (PHP-Ia) is also called Albright hereditary osteodystrophy and is characterized by short stature, round facies, barrel chest, obesity and brachydactyly, shortening of the fourth and fifth metacarpals, and mild developmental delay.[128] This disorder is due to autosomal dominant inheritance of mutations in the *GNAS1* gene, which encodes the alpha subunit of the stimulatory G protein (Gα_s). Other forms of PHP include PHP-Ib and pseudo-PHP.[129]

Heterozygous loss-of-function mutations in the *GNAS1* gene, leading to a 50% reduction of Gα_s activity, cause PHP-Ia. However, the *GNAS1* gene is an imprinted gene and the clinical presentation depends on whether the mutant allele is inherited from the mother or the father.[130,131] In case the mutation is inherited from the mother the patient will present with PHP, whereas the patient will present with pseudo-PHP when the mutation is inherited from the father. Pseudo-PHP is characterized by the same physical characteristics as patients with PHP-Ia but lacks the endocrine abnormalities and also frequently does not show obesity.[132,133] In case of a maternally inherited mutation, only the paternal GNAS allele is available. Due to silencing/imprinting of the paternal GNAS allele in multiple tissues, including the proximal tubule, this results effectively in a complete *GNAS* knockout. These patients present with PHP-Ia or Albright hereditary osteodystrophy and do not respond appropriately with an increase of urinary cAMP and PO$_4^-$ excretion after PTH exposure due to resistance of the proximal tubule to PTH. Because Gα_s and cAMP are crucial in the downstream signaling of other peptide hormones, patients may develop resistance to hormones such as luteinizing hormone, follicle stimulating hormone, and thyroid-stimulating hormone (TSH).[134] In pseudo-PHP the patient inherits the *GNAS* mutation from the paternal allele. Because the paternal mutant *GNAS* gene will be silenced due to imprinting, many adult tissues will be left with one functional copy of *GNAS*. Therefore these patients do not develop PTH or other hormone resistance and are characterized by normal serum Ca^{2+} and phosphate concentrations.[128]

Patients with PHP-Ib do not develop the phenotype of Albright hereditary osteodystrophy but still exhibit PTH resistance limited to the kidney. PHP-Ib patients have a higher risk of TSH resistance and shortening of the fourth and fifth metacarpals.[135] These patients have mutations in regulatory elements of the *GNAS* gene which alter the control of paternal DNA methylation and its imprinting in the kidney.[136,137] Despite the limitation of PTH resistance to the kidney and laboratory tests indicating hypoparathyroidism, these patients' bones still respond to PTH and are therefore exposed to the skeletal complications of chronic PTH exposure, such as osteoporosis or osteitis fibrosa cystica.[138]

Another cohort of patients with hypoparathyroidism and inappropriate renal phosphaturic response to PTH but normal renal cAMP and Gα_s activity after PTH exposure is defined as pseudo-PHP type II. This condition is thought to be due to intracellular resistance to cAMP, possibly a defective cAMP-dependent kinase.[139] The different forms of PHP can be classified according to the renal and systemic response to PTH exposure (e.g., Ellsworth-Howard test).

Hypocalcemia Due to Disturbed Vitamin D Metabolism

Inherited forms of low vitamin D include vitamin D synthesis and the vitamin D receptor. Impaired 1α hydroxylation of 25(OH) vitamin D is due to recessive loss-of-function mutations in the *CYP27B1* gene, resulting in vitamin D–dependent rickets type 1.[140] These patients are characterized by hypocalcemia, hypophosphatemia, normal or elevated 25(OH)D, and very low 1,25 Vitamin D concentrations and elevated PTH levels. Infants present with rickets, osteomalacia, and seizures and respond well to treatment with 1,25 Vitamin D. A more common cause for impaired 1α hydroxylation of 25(OH) vitamin D is CKD.

Vitamin D–dependent rickets type 2 is characterized by resistance of the tissues to the biologic effects of calcitriol caused by recessive, inactivating mutations in the *VDR* gene.[141,142] The biochemical profile is very similar to patients with vitamin D–dependent rickets type 1 (e.g., hypocalcemia, hypophosphatemia, hyperparathyroidism), but in type 2 patients, elevated concentrations of 1,25 Vitamin D are detected. Infants present with rickets and seizures. Some patients also develop alopecia.[143] Patients are treated with large doses of 1,25 Vitamin D to overcome the vitamin D receptor resistance and may also need Ca^{2+} infusions.

Inherited Disorders of Magnesium

20

Introduction

Magnesium (Mg^{2+}) is the second most abundant intracellular cation but is frequently overlooked. Mg^{2+} plays important roles in human physiology by acting as a cofactor for more than 600 enzymes, participating in cardiac contractility and nerve conduction, providing stability against DNA and RNA damage via oxidative stress, controlling cell cycle and cell proliferation, and finally ATP has to bind Mg^{2+} to be biologically active.[144] An adult body contains a total of 27 g Mg^{2+}, whereas a term newborn has approximately 0.8 g. Similar to Ca^{2+} the vast majority (80%) of Mg^{2+} is accrued in the third trimester. Mg^{2+} is stored in three compartments: (1) the bone (65% of total body Mg^{2+}), (2) intracellular (34%), and (3) in the extracellular fluid (ECF) (1%). The role of Mg^{2+} in bone is not well understood, and the significance of Mg^{2+} for bone is frequently underestimated. Infants with extended fetal Mg^{2+} exposure from maternal treatment for tocolysis can develop congenital rickets.[145] Fetal Mg^{2+} toxicity leads to impaired bone mineralization and may cause fractures.[146] On the other hand, Mg^{2+} seems to be involved in bone metabolism by inducing osteoblast proliferation.

Due to the small Mg^{2+} content in ECF, plasma Mg^{2+} concentration may not provide the most reliable assessment of total body Mg^{2+} content.[147] Mg^{2+} is present as the free ion (55%), bound to protein (35%), and complexed by different anions (e.g., oxalate, phosphate) (15%).[147] Serum Mg^{2+} is controlled within tight limits (1.5–2.8 mg/dL or 0.62–1.16 mmol/L) and is the same for neonates, infants, children, and adults.[148] Preterm and term neonates have similar cord serum Mg^{2+} concentrations. After delivery, both display an initial decrease in serum Mg^{2+} which reaches a nadir at 48 hours with 1.87 mg/dL (0.77 mmol/L), after which serum Mg^{2+} increases in the first week of life.[149] Dependent on the accompanying disease process, serum Mg^{2+} may vary: increased Mg^{2+} concentrations are found with hyperbilirubinemia, acidosis, and preterm respiratory distress syndrome.[150–152]

Postdelivery, blood Mg^{2+} concentration reflects the balance between intestinal and renal Mg^{2+} excretion. Intestinal Mg^{2+} absorption occurs in the small intestine, cecum, and colon and ranges between 25% to 80%, depending on the total body Mg^{2+} content.[153,154] Intestinal Mg^{2+} absorption is higher in low Mg^{2+} states. In the small intestine, Mg^{2+} is absorbed in a paracellular fashion (in between epithelial cells), which is nonsaturable. In the cecum and colon, Mg^{2+} is absorbed in a transcellular, saturable fashion via apical Mg^{2+} channels transient receptor potential melastatin 6 (TRPM6) and TRPM7 in epithelial cells. Very little is known about Mg^{2+} handling in epithelial cells. A basolateral Mg^{2+} ATPase and/or Mg^{2+}-Na^+ exchanger has been hypothesized to facilitate basolateral Mg^{2+} extrusion.[154] *SLC41A3* encodes a basolateral Mg^{2+}-Na^+ exchanger in the distal convoluted tubule (DCT) and was published as a component for Mg^{2+} extrusion (Fig. 20.4A).[155]

In the kidney, approximately 80% of the total body Mg^{2+} is filtered by the glomerulus and 95% to 99% of the filtered Mg^{2+} is absorbed along the nephron. Finally, only approximately 100 mg of Mg^{2+} is excreted in urine per day.[156,157] Although the proximal tubule plays a key role for tubular absorption of most electrolytes such as potassium, sodium, and phosphorus, it is responsible for only 10% to 25% of renal Mg^{2+} absorption. In contrast, the vast majority of Mg^{2+} is absorbed in the TAL (65%–75%).[144,156] Mg^{2+} transport in the TAL occurs in a paracellular fashion, and

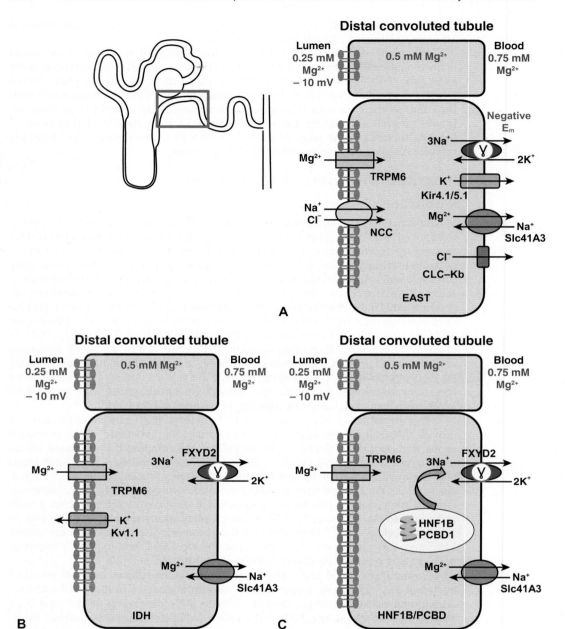

Fig. 20.4   EAST, IDH, and HNF1B/PCBD disturb the negative membrane potential of the DCT and cause Gitelman-like phenotype. (A) In EAST syndrome, recessive *Kir4.1* mutations affect the extrusion of K+ via the heteromeric Kir4.1/5.1 complex and interferes with the function of the basolateral Na+/K+-ATPase, which both result in forming a less negative membrane potential. This affects negatively the basolateral Cl− export and subsequently inhibits apical Na+ and Cl− absorption via NCC and Mg2+ by TRPM6. (B) IDH is caused by mutations in *FXYD2* and *KCNA1*, but the mechanisms are not well understood. *FXYD2* mutations may result in a dysfunctional γ subunit of the Na+/K+ ATPase and a lower intracellular K+ concentration. A different ratio of extracellular versus intracellular K+ affects the formation of the negative membrane potential. Alternatively, altered Na+/K+ ATPase function could alter the activity of the Mg2+-Na+ exchanger by altering intracellular Na+. *KCNA1* mutations affect the extrusion of K+ via Kv1.1, which contributes to the negative membrane potential. The latter is required for Mg2+ absorption via TRPM6. (C) In the nucleus HNF1B and PCBD1 form a complex regulate transcription of *FXYD2*, which modifies the activity of the Na+/K+-ATPase as the γ subunit. Adapted from 157.

the lumen-positive transepithelial potential difference is the main driving force.[158] Fine-tuning of renal Mg^{2+} absorption takes place in the DCT, where 10% of Mg^{2+} is reabsorbed. Here, Mg^{2+} is transported in a transcellular fashion via the epithelial, apical Mg^{2+} channels TRPM6 and TRPM7 (see Fig. 20.4A).[5,9,159]

Regulators of Magnesium Homeostasis

Similar to Ca^{2+}, Mg^{2+} regulation is dependent on bone, intestine, and kidneys.[9] The kidneys have the most intricate hormonal regulation for Mg^{2+} homeostasis. In particular, transcellular Mg^{2+} absorption in the DCT via TRPM6 is influenced by a number of hormones, including epidermal growth factor (EGF), insulin, and estrogen.

Epidermal Growth Factor

EGF was identified as the first magnesiotropic hormone in Dutch sisters with isolated recessive hypomagnesemia (IRH) (see later under "Isolated Recessive Hypomagnesemia").[160]

Insulin

Hypomagnesemia has been associated with type 2 DM (T2DM) and gestational DM.[161–164] Insulin phosphorylates at least two specific sites in the Mg^{2+} channel TRPM6 which are also known to associate with a higher risk of DM. Insulin increases TRPM6 activity by phosphoinositide 3-kinase and Rac1 signaling, thereby enhancing TRPM6 cell surface abundance.[164]

Estrogen

Because estrogen therapy in postmenopausal women improved hypermagnesuria, estrogen has also been discussed as a magnesiotropic hormone.[165,166] Renal Trpm6 mRNA level was decreased in ovariectomized rats. This effect was reversed by 17β-estradiol. This is consistent with estrogen enhancing Trpm6 transcription or mRNA stabilization.[167]

Other Hormone Interactions Involving Mg^{2+} Homeostasis

Overall, many of the same hormones regulating Ca^{2+} homeostasis are also involved in maintenance of Mg^{2+} concentration. For example, changes in Mg^{2+} affect PTH secretion similar to Ca^{2+}, with Mg^{2+} being less potent compared with Ca^{2+}.[168] Although short-term decrease in Mg^{2+} increases PTH secretion, chronic hypomagnesemia abolishes PTH secretion significantly, subsequently causing hypocalcemia. The latter effect is caused by alterations of the Ca^{2+}-sensitive, Mg^{2+}-dependent adenylate cyclase system, which is crucial for the secretion of PTH.[169,170] Thus Mg^{2+} deficiency may cause or aggravate hypocalcemia by blunting the PTH response to lower serum Ca^{2+} concentrations. The effect of calcitonin is thought to be minimal, but there are some indications that calcitonin is involved in fetal Mg^{2+} homeostasis because knockout mice lacking calcitonin displayed total body Mg^{2+} depletion and lower serum Mg^{2+} concentrations.[171,172] Moreover, calcitonin has been shown to enhance Mg^{2+} absorption in the DCT.[173] The effect of vitamin D seems minor and appears to be indirect, but pharmacologic dosages of vitamin D enhance intestinal Mg^{2+} absorption.[174] However, there is no correlation between serum Mg^{2+} concentration and plasma 1,25 Vitamin D.[175] Interestingly, Mg^{2+} is an essential cofactor of the 1,25-hydroxylation reaction in the renal tubular cells to form 1,25 Vitamin D, presumably due to its role as a cofactor for 1α-hydroxylase in the renal tubular cells.[176] Mg^{2+} deficiency increases FGF23 concentration and enhances renal 24,25-hydroxylase.[176,177] Other hormones known to have a mild to modest influence on Mg^{2+} homeostasis are thyroxine, aldosterone (both reduce Mg^{2+} absorption), epinephrine, glucocorticosteroids, and progesterone.[173,178–182]

Hypermagnesemia

Symptoms of Hypermagnesemia

Symptoms include muscle weakness, fatigue, and somnolence. Hypermagnesemia usually occurs in preeclamptic women and their offspring after Mg^{2+} therapy and in patients with end-stage renal disease (ESRD).

Hypomagnesemia

Symptoms of Hypomagnesemia

Although mild to moderate hypomagnesemia does not cause acute symptoms, more pronounced hypomagnesemia results in muscle spasms, arrhythmia, and seizures.

Hypomagnesemia is more common and can result as a side effect of medications, insufficient Mg^{2+} intake, or rare inherited renal defects. Here we will focus on inherited renal disorders causing Mg^{2+} abnormalities. These genetic conditions are divided into hypercalciuric, Gitelman-like, and other hypomagnesemias (Tables 20.6–20.8).

Hypercalciuric Hypomagnesemias

The disorders in this group are characterized by disruption of the lumen-positive transepithelial potential difference, which subsequently impairs paracellular Mg^{2+} and Ca^{2+} absorption in the TAL and causes hypermagnesuria and hypercalciuria.

Familial Hypomagnesemia With Hypercalciuria and Nephrocalcinosis

Familial hypomagnesemia with hypercalciuria and nephrocalcinosis (FHHNC) patients present with a wide spectrum of symptoms, including hypomagnesemia, hypocalcemia, nephrocalcinosis, and in some patients ocular involvement.[183,184] Hypomagnesemia is not sufficiently severe to cause neurologic symptoms. Affected individuals can develop CKD in their teens to twenties. Recessive mutations in *Claudin-16 (CLDN16)* were identified in FHHNC patients with earlier onset of ESRD with two loss-of-function mutations.[185,186] In patients with FHHNC and eye involvement, recessive mutations in the related *Claudin-19 (CLDN19)* gene were found.[187] Both Claudin-16 and -19 are expressed in the kidney, specifically in the TAL (see Fig. 20.3B).[185,187,188] Claudin-19 is also detected in the eye. Claudin-16 and -19 both colocalize to tight junctions in the TAL and DCT. Tight junctions represent protein complexes in between epithelial cells which are crucial for the permeability of the epithelial barrier.[188] Both proteins physically interact with each other and form heterodimers.[189,190] When *CLDN16* mutations were first identified the hypothesis was that aberrant Claudin-16 impairs tubular Mg^{2+} and Ca^{2+} by disturbing an Mg^{2+} or Ca^{2+} selective channel.[185] Over the years our understanding of the pathophysiology in FHHNC has advanced. The major driving force for paracellular Mg^{2+} and Ca^{2+} is the lumen-positive potential difference which is created by two mechanisms: (1) secretion of K^+ via ROMK and (2) the dilution potential (see Fig. 20.3B).[189] Apical ROMK and NKCC2 channels work as a unit, with electroneutral absorption of Na^+, K^+, and Cl^- via NKCC2. Due to the elevated intracellular K^+ concentration, K^+ is instantly secreted in the lumen via ROMK. The dilution potential is formed by the decrease of tubular Na^+ concentration from the beginning of the TAL (140 mM) to the further downstream TAL with a much lower tubular Na^+ concentration (30 mM). When the luminal Na^+ decreases from 140 to 30 mM, and the peritubular Na^+ increases to 140 mM in the further distal TAL, a major gradient is created for Na^+ and Cl^- between tubular lumen and the interstitium. This mechanism generates a driving force for both ions to leak back into the tubular lumen (see Fig. 20.3B). Claudin-16 and -19 in tight junctions determine the permeability for interstitial Na^+ and Cl^- to move back into the lumen. Claudin-16 enhances Na^+ permeability, whereas Claudin-19 decreases Cl^- permeability. Combined they result in a high permeability ratio for Na^+ to Cl^- with a strong cation selectivity for Na^+ which subsequently contributes to the lumen-positive potential. Why FHHNC patients develop ESRD remains unclear. Possibly, hypercalciuria and nephrocalcinosis contribute to ESRD. Thiazide treatment improves hypercalciuria but does not decrease the risk for ESRD.[191]

Autosomal Dominant Hypocalcemia

Autosomal dominant hypocalcemia has already been discussed previously in the calcium section. However, autosomal dominant hypocalcemia can also result in hypomagnesemia. In contrast to FHHNC, approximately half of patients develop neurologic symptoms with carpopedal spasms and seizures. Gain-of-function mutations enhance the sensitivity of CaSR, contributing to a higher receptor response despite

Table 20.6 LIST OF INHERITED FORMS OF HYPERCALCIURIC HYPOMAGNESEMIAS

Disorder	OMIM	Inheritance	Gene Locus	Serum Mg^{2+}	PTH	Serum Ca^{2+}	Urine Ca^{2+}	Gene (Protein)	Function	References
Familial hypomagnesemia with hypercalciuria and nephrocalcinosis	#248250	AR	3q28	↓	n-↑	↓	↑	CLDN16 (Claudin-16)	Tight junction proteins	185,186
Familial hypomagnesemia with hypercalciuria and nephrocalcinosis plus ocular involvement	#248190	AR	1p34	↓	n-↑	↓	↑	CLDN19 (Claudin-19)	Tight junction proteins	187
Classical Bartter syndrome (type 3)	#607364	AR	1p36	n-↓	↑	↓	↑	CLCNKB (ClC subunit B)	Basolateral chloride channel	195
Autosomal dominant hypocalcemia/Bartter syndrome (type 5)	#601198	AD	3q13	n-↓	↓	↓	↑	CASR (CaSR)	Calcium sensing receptor	123,192

AD, Autosomal dominant; *AR,* autosomal recessive; *n,* normal.

Table 20.7 LIST OF INHERITED FORMS OF GITELMAN-LIKE HYPOMAGNESEMIAS

Disorder	OMIM	Inheritance	Gene Locus	Serum Mg^{2+}	PTH	Serum Ca^{2+}	Urine Ca^{2+}	Gene (Protein)	Function	References
Gitelman syndrome	#263800	AR	16q13	↓	n	n-↓	↓	SLC12A3 (NCC)	Na^+-Cl^- cotransporter	199
Antenatal Bartter syndrome with sensorineural deafness (type 4)	#602522	AR	1p31	↓	n	n	n-↑	BSND (Barttin)	Subunit of ClC-Ka/b	75
EAST/SeSAME syndrome	#612780	AR	1q23	↓	n	n	↓	KCNJ10 (Kir4.1)	Apical potassium channel	206,209
Isolated dominant hypomagnesemia	#154020	AD	11q23	↓	n	n	↓	FXYD2 (FXYD2)	Na^+/K^+-ATPase (γ subunit)	212
	*176260	AD	12p13	↓	n	n	↓	KCNA1 (Kv1.1)	Apical potassium channel	213
HNF1B nephropathy	#137920	AD	17q12	↓	n	n	n	HNF1B (HNF1beta)	Transcription factor	222
Hypomagnesemia after transient neonatal hyperphenyl-alaninemia	#264070	AR	10q22	↓	n.d.	n.d.	n.d.	PCBD1 (PCBD1)	Tetrahydrobiopterin metabolism	225

AD, Autosomal dominant; AR, autosomal recessive; n, normal; n.d., no data.

Table 20.8 LIST OF INHERITED FORMS OF OTHER HYPOMAGNESEMIAS

Disorder	OMIM	Inheritance	Gene Locus	Serum Mg^{2+}	PTH	Serum Ca^{2+}	Urine Ca^{2+}	Gene (Protein)	Function	References
Isolated recessive hypomagnesemia	#611718	AR	4q25	$\downarrow$	n	n	n	*EGF* (Pro-EGF)	Epidermal growth factor	160
Hypomagnesemia with secondary hypocalcemia	#602014	AR	9q22	$\downarrow$	$\downarrow$	$\downarrow$	n-$\uparrow$	*TRPM6* (TRPM6)	Apical Mg^{2+} channel	229,230
Hypomagnesemia with impaired brain development	#616418	AD/AR	10q24	$\downarrow$	n.d.	n.d.	n.d.	*CNNM2* (CNNM2)	Cyclin M2	238,239
Hypomagnesemia with metabolic syndrome	#500005	Maternal	mtDNA	$\downarrow$	n	n	$\downarrow$	*MTTI* (MTTI)	Mitochondrial tRNA for isoleucine	241

AD, Autosomal dominant; *AR*, autosomal recessive; *n*, normal; *n.d.*, no data.

physiologic extracellular Ca^{2+} concentrations, imitating hypercalcemia (see Fig. 20.3A).[24] As a consequence, PTH is suppressed and renal Mg^{2+} and Ca^{2+} absorption is decreased.[24,192] A very recent study implicated CaSR activation with calcineurin signaling, NFAT pathway, miRNAs, and Claudin-14.[193,194] Specifically, CaSR stimulation enhanced Claudin-14 expression, which is a negative regulator of Claudins-16 and -19 (see Fig. 20.3A). This reduces the strength of the dilution potential and the lumen-positive potential, thus causing urinary Mg^{2+} and Ca^{2+} wasting.

Bartter Syndrome

Patients with classical Bartter syndrome (type III) are characterized by polyuria, renal salt wasting, concentration defect, hypokalemic metabolic alkalosis, and hypercalciuria.[67] With advanced age, patients can develop a Gitelman-like phenotype with hypomagnesemia and hypocalciuria.[195] The genes causing Bartter syndrome have been discussed previously (see Fig. 20.3C). *CLCNBK* and *BSND* mutations disturb intracellular Cl^- regulation which interferes with NCC and NKCC2 function, thereby disturbing the lumen-positive potential and paracellular Mg^{2+} absorption (see Fig. 20.3C).[65,66]

Gitelman-Like Hypomagnesemias

In the DCT, Mg^{2+} absorption requires the negative membrane potential. Published mutations in this group affect proteins regulating Na^+, K^+, or Cl^- transport in the DCT (see Fig. 20.4). This disturbs the negative membrane potential. All disorders in this group are characterized by hypocalciuria, volume contraction, hypotension, and renin-angiotensin system (RAS) activation (see Table 20.7). This enhances K^+ and H^+ secretion and contributes to hypokalemia and metabolic alkalosis.

Gitelman Syndrome (GS)

With a prevalence of $1:40,000$, this is one of the most common tubulopathies in humankind.[196] The characteristics of GS are hypokalemic alkalosis, hypocalciuria, and hypomagnesemia.[197] Patients display muscle weakness, salt craving, fatigue, thirst, nocturia, and carpopedal spasms.[198] GS is caused by recessive mutations in the *SLC12A3* gene, which encodes the Na-Cl-cotransporter NCC.[199] However, in a significant number of patients (up to 40%) the second mutation may not be identified because they may be located deep into the intron or may be caused by genomic rearrangements.[200–202] A *Ncc* knockout mouse displayed a phenotype similar to human GS with hypomagnesemia and hypocalciuria, but no metabolic alkalosis or volume contraction was described.[203,204] Due to the volume contraction in GS, compensatory enhanced paracellular absorption of water, Na^+, and Ca^{2+} occur, leading to hypocalciuria.[204,205] Regarding the hypomagnesemia, a variety of hypotheses have been suggested, including dysfunctional Mg^{2+} absorption, atrophy of the DCT, renal Mg^{2+} wasting, and K^+ depletion. Less apical Trpm6 expression was found in $Ncc^{-/-}$ mice and wild-type mice after thiazide treatment, explaining the urinary Mg^{2+} wasting.[205] Patients with GS require Mg^{2+} and K^+ supplementation. Spironolactone, amiloride, or eplerenone may be used as additional options to maintain normal K^+ concentrations.

EAST Syndrome (Epilepsy, Ataxia, Sensorineural Deafness, Tubulopathy)

This is a rare syndrome characterized by epilepsy, ataxia, sensorineural deafness, and salt loosing tubulopathy.[206] In early infancy, these patients develop speech and motor delay, seizures, hearing impairment, ataxia, tremor, dysdiadochokinesia.[207] As EAST patients get older, they develop hypocalciuria, hypokalemic metabolic alkalosis, and hypomagnesemia.[208] Recessive mutations in the *KCJN10* gene were described as the cause, encoding for the basolateral, inwardly rectifying K^+ channel Kir4.1.[206,209] The encoded protein was found in the stria vascularis of the inner ear, the brain, and then DCT.[206] The encoded Kir4.1 channel associated with another K^+ channel Kir 5.1 and forms heteromeric complexes (see Fig. 20.4A).[210] The basolateral Kir4.1/5.1 complex works together with the basolateral Na^+/K^+-ATPase by recycling K^+ ions that entered the cell in exchange for extruding Na^+.[209,211] The correct distribution of extracellular versus intracellular K^+ is crucial for the generation of the negative membrane potential (see Fig. 20.4A). The seizures may be caused by the depolarization of neurons which lower the threshold for convulsions.[209]

Isolated Dominant Hypomagnesemias (IDHs)

Patients with IDH present with onset of seizures in childhood, hypocalciuria, severe hypomagnesemia, developmental delay (possibly due to frequent seizures), and urinary Mg^{2+} wasting but do not have hypokalemic metabolic alkalosis, salt wasting, or RAS stimulation. Heterozygous mutations in two genes, *FXYD2* and *KCNA1*, result in IDH (see Fig. 20.4B).[212,213] FXYD2 encodes the γ subunit of the Na^+/K^+-ATPase. FXYD2 decreases Na^+ and enhances ATP affinity in a tissue-specific manner.[214,215] The *FXYD2* mutation is thought to have a dominant negative effect which impairs trafficking and causes perinuclear accumulation of the mutant protein. The exact mechanism how *FXYD2* mutations contribute to hypomagnesemia remains unclear.

The second IDH gene *KCNA1* encodes the apical voltage-gated channel Kv1.1 (see Fig. 20.4B).[213] Although urinary Mg^{2+} wasting was found, no Ca^{2+} abnormalities were detected. Patients are characterized by muscle cramps, tetany, tremors, and muscle weakness. In all affected patients, ataxia and myokymia, an involuntary form of localized muscle trembling, were described. It is remarkable that in addition to IDH, *KCNA1* mutations were previously described in patients with ataxia and myokymia.[216] However, only the N255D mutation results in hypomagnesemia.[213] Although the potassium channel Kv1.1 colocalizes with TRPM6 in the DCT, Kv1.1 does not regulate the Mg^{2+} channel TRPM6. Coexpression of wild-type and mutant Kv1.1 channel results in a dominant negative effect of the potassium channel complex as Kv1.1 forms tetramers. Gating of the channel pore is probably affected, which diminishes the negative membrane potential.

HNF1B Nephropathy

HNF1B encodes the transcription factor hepatocyte nuclear transcription factor 1β, which is crucial for pancreatic and renal development. Patients with heterozygous *HNF1B* mutations are characterized by a wide spectrum of different symptoms, including maturity-onset diabetes of the young type 5 (MODY5), hyperechogenic kidneys, multicystic and glomerulocystic kidney disease, renal hypoplasia, renal agenesis, hyperuricemic nephropathy, and renal cysts and diabetes syndrome.[217–221] Hypomagnesemia is identified in approximately half of all *HNF1B* patients and is due to urinary Mg^{2+} losses.[222] In addition, hypocalciuria can be seen. *HNF1B* mutations are inherited in an autosomal dominant fashion and frequently also occur *de novo*. The encoded HNF1B protein regulates other regulators of renal Mg^{2+} homeostasis such as FXYD2 by binding to the *FXYD2* gene promoter (see Fig. 20.4C).[222] Mutations in *HNF1B* impair transcription of the Na^+/K^+-ATPase subunit FXYD2.[223]

Transient Neonatal Hyperphenylalaninemia and Primapterinuria

This rare condition is usually a benign, neonatal self-limiting syndrome without long-term sequela.[224] Nevertheless, in three adult patients with recessive mutations in the gene *PCBD1*, which causes transient neonatal hyperphenylalaninemia and primapterinuria, hypomagnesemia, renal Mg^{2+} losses, and MODY were diagnosed.[225] *PCBD1* encodes the protein Pterin-4α carbinolamine dehydratase, which forms a heterotetrameric complex and physically interacts with HNF1B.[225] PCBD1 is a crucial factor for dimerization, and, in case of mutant *PCBD1,* dimerization with HNF1B is impaired, resulting in proteolytic instability of the PCBD1-HNF1B complex (see Fig. 20.4C). Subsequently, this results in impaired HNF1B-mediated activation of the *FXYD2* promoter.

Other Hypomagnesemias

The conditions in this group do not fit in one of the previously outlined groups and are summarized in Table 20.8.

Isolated Recessive Hypomagnesemia

This condition is caused by recessive mutations in the *pro-EGF* gene, and affected patients develop seizures in infancy, developmental delay, and hypomagnesemia because of urinary Mg^{2+} wasting but lack other electrolyte abnormalities.[160,226] The *pro-EGF* gene encodes for the precursor of the EGF, which undergoes further maturation. Although pro-EGF is a large transmembrane protein with 1207 amino acids (aa), which is eventually cleaved from the membrane, the final EGF protein is part of the extracellular protein domain and is surprisingly small with 53 aa. The identified mutation was found in the cytosolic C-terminus of the large pro-EGF protein affecting a sorting motif, which subsequently impairs EGF secretion. Wild-type EGF is secreted at the basolateral side of the DCT where it binds to the EGF receptor, thereby activating a tyrosine kinase which stimulates TRPM6 (Fig. 20.5).[160] A novel chemotherapeutic treatment with a chimeric human/mouse anti-EGF antibody called cetuximab confirmed the significance of EGF as an autocrine magnesiotropic hormone because patients treated with cetuximab become hypomagnesemic.[227]

Hypomagnesemia With Secondary Hypocalcemia (HSH)

This disorder manifests in early infancy with generalized seizures, profound hypomagnesemia, and hypocalcemia.[228] Affected patients have renal and intestinal Mg^{2+} losses. Recessive mutations in the *TRPM6* gene, which encodes the TRPM6 channel, were identified in these patients (see Fig. 20.5).[229,230] TRPM6 is a member of the extensive TRP channel family and contains in addition to the Mg^{2+} channel a C-terminal kinase domain. TRPM6 is the only true Mg^{2+} channel involved in hypomagnesemic disorders outlined in this chapter. The TRPM6 channels are located in the gut and the kidney, thereby enhancing intestinal and renal Mg^{2+} absorption.[231,232] TRPM6 is highly homologous to TRPM7, another channel permeable to Ca^{2+} and Mg^{2+}, and both channels form heteromers, interact, and modify each other.[233] Upregulation of TRPM6 has been shown for hypomagnesemia, insulin, and estrogen, whereas calcineurin inhibitors decrease TRPM6 activity.[164,167,234,235] It is not well understood why HSH patients develop hypocalcemia.[236] Most likely, hypomagnesemia impairs PTH secretion as HSH patients have inappropriately low PTH concentrations. HSH patients usually do not respond to Ca^{2+} or vitamin D supplementation; however, hypocalcemia improves with Mg^{2+} therapy.[237]

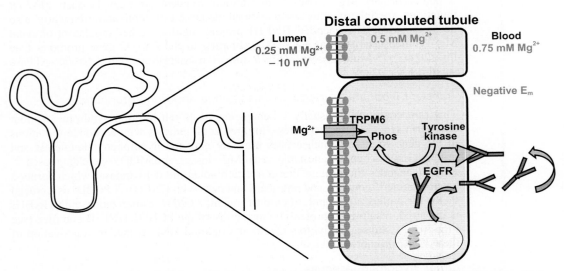

Fig. 20.5 IRH and HSH affect Mg^{2+} absorption in the DCT. IRH affects proper secretion of EGF, which activates the basolateral EGFR in an autocrine/paracrine fashion. EGFR activation stimulates TRPM6 via a tyrosine kinase. Adapted from 157.

Hypomagnesemia With Impaired Brain Development

The patients are characterized by hypomagnesemia, seizures, muscle weakness, vertigo, and headaches. Both heterozygous and homozygous *CNNM2* mutations were found in affected individuals.[238] However, other mutation carriers remained asymptomatic. *CNNM2* encodes the protein transmembrane cyclin M2, which is localized at the basolateral membrane of the TAL and DCT. Nonsense and missense mutations were identified and reduced Mg^{2+} sensitive current.[238,239] The CNNM2 function in physiology remains unclear; a role as an Mg^{2+} transporter or Mg^{2+} sensor is discussed.[238,240]

Mitochondrial Hypomagnesemia

Several mitochondrial conditions have been linked to hypomagnesemia. For example, hypomagnesemia was found in a large kindred with hypercholesterolemia and hypertension.[241] Only females were affected, which raised concern for mitochondrial inheritance. Because affected individuals also displayed hypocalciuria, it was suspected that the DCT was affected. The mitochondrially encoded isoleucine tRNA gene was found to be altered by a mutation altering a thymidine residue next to the anticodon triplet, a highly conserved site which is crucial for codon-anticodon recognition.

Inherited Disorders of Phosphate

Introduction

Phosphate plays a critical role in numerous biologic processes in humans and other vertebrates. Phosphate is the oxidized form of phosphorus and is found in the body in both inorganic and organic forms. The organic form of phosphate is mostly found in phospholipids and plasma lipoproteins. The inorganic form of phosphate is the primary circulating form of phosphate in the ECF. In an adult, 85% of phosphate is present in bones and teeth. The remaining 15% of phosphate is distributed in the soft tissues (14%) and ECF (1%). At a physiologic pH, inorganic phosphate exists in the ratio of HPO_4^{-2} to $H_2PO_4^{-1}$ as $4:1$. In addition to being an important component of bone, cell membrane, and nucleic acids, phosphate plays an important role in energy metabolism and phosphorylation of proteins responsible for intracellular signaling and is an important component of 2,3-diphosphoglycerate (2,3-DPG) for oxygen carriage in the blood. Other functions of phosphate include maintenance of pH in the human body as phosphate is an important urinary and blood buffer.[242]

Measurable serum phosphate is the extracellular inorganic phosphate and, as it represents 1% of the total body phosphate stores, does not accurately represent the total body phosphate levels. However, maintenance of measurable serum phosphate levels within the normal range is critical for many functions of the human body. Although phosphate homeostasis in a neonate is in a positive balance due to growth, adults are in a neutral phosphate balance. Phosphate balance involves complex interaction between gastrointestinal absorption, urinary excretion, and bone remodeling which results in exchange of phosphate between bone, the ECF, and recycling of phosphate in the body.

Transport of phosphate in the gastrointestinal tract occurs via transcellular and paracellular pathways. Transcellular phosphate transport is a saturable, active sodium-dependent transport via sodium phosphate cotransporter 2b (NaPi-2b, Slc34a2). NaPi-2b is regulated by 1,25 vitamin D, pH, and dietary phosphate content.[243–245] Dietary phosphate comes in both inorganic and organic forms; phosphatases in the gastrointestinal tract metabolize the organic form to inorganic form, and thus inorganic phosphate is the phosphate that is primarily absorbed from the gastrointestinal tract.[246] On the other hand, paracellular phosphate transport is not saturable and diffusion based, and thus, with increasing content of phosphate in the diet, there is a linear increase in phosphate absorption. Of the circulating serum phosphate, approximately 10% to 20% is protein bound, and 5% is complexed with other circulating cations, making 85% of the circulating phosphorus filterable across the glomerulus. Of the filtered phosphorus, approximately 80% to 90% is reabsorbed by the proximal tubule in the kidney. The principal renal transporters for phosphate reabsorption include sodium phosphate cotransporter 2a and 2c, NaPi-2a (Slc34a1), and NaPi-2c (Slc34a3). Another family of phosphate transporters, Slc20 are type 3 sodium-dependent phosphate transporters, PiT-1 and PiT-2.[247] Originally identified as retroviral receptors, they have now been shown to mediate phosphate transport. PiT-1 and PiT-2 are ubiquitously present in the body and have been shown to be present in the kidney. PiT-2 has been shown to be present in the proximal tubule and regulated by FGF23, phosphate intake, and metabolic acidosis. However, they play a minor role in regulating renal phosphate reabsorption under basal conditions.[248,249] Until recently, the basolateral phosphate transporter has been elusive; recent data indicate that a retroviral receptor, xenotropic and polytropic retrovirus receptor 1 (XPR1), potentially could be a basolateral phosphate transporter. Further studies are needed to confirm the role of XPR1 as a basolateral phosphate transporter.[250–252]

Regulators of Phosphate Homeostasis

Regulation of phosphate homeostasis involves an intricate interplay involving many organ systems, hormones, and receptors. Complex interaction between the gastrointestinal tract, parathyroid gland, bone, and the kidney keeps the serum phosphorus within the physiologic range for normal functioning of the human body. This will be discussed in detail in a different chapter; however, will provide a brief overview here.

Fibroblast Growth Factor 23

FGF23 is a phosphaturic hormone that is primarily produced by the osteocytes in the bone. FGF23 causes urinary phosphate wasting by decreasing the expression of sodium phosphate cotransporters (NaPi-2a and NaPi-2c) on the brush border membrane of the proximal tubule.[253] In addition, FGF23 also inhibits the expression of 1α-hydroxylase and increases the expression of 24-hydroxylase,[254] resulting in a decrease in circulating levels of 1,25 vitamin D. Klotho is an important coreceptor for FGF23. In children and adults, elevated levels of FGF23 cause hypophosphatemic rickets. On the contrary, deficiency of FGF23 results in hyperphosphatemia and tumoral calcinosis. These will be discussed in detail later in this chapter. Intact FGF23 is biologically active, and FGF23 is degraded by proteases such as furin to N-terminal and C-terminal fragments.

The role of FGF23 in fetal and neonatal phosphate homeostasis has recently been explored. Using mouse models of FGF23 null mice or FGF23 excess seen in *Hyp* mice (mouse model of X-linked hypophosphatemic rickets), there was no difference in fetal serum phosphorus, calcium, or PTH levels. In addition, there were no changes in the total body phosphorus or skeletal mineralization.[255,256] Furthermore, fetal serum phosphorus levels were normal in *Klotho*$^{-/-}$ fetuses, whereas these mice have significantly elevated FGF23 levels. On the other hand, *Pth*$^{-/-}$ fetuses have elevated serum phosphorus levels, reiterating the importance of PTH in fetal phosphate homeostasis. The same group of authors also studied double mutant mice with deletion of PTH and FGF23 *(Fgf23*$^{-/-}$*/Pth*$^{-/-}$*)* and the serum phosphorus levels in these double mutants were comparable to the *Pth*$^{-/-}$ mice, indicating once again that FGF23 does not play an important role in fetal phosphate homeostasis. The authors also studied postnatal phosphate homeostasis in *Klotho*$^{-/-}$, *Fgf23*$^{-/-}$, and *Hyp* mice. Although *Fgf23*$^{-/-}$ mice and *Klotho*$^{-/-}$ mice had normal phosphate homeostasis at birth, they did develop hyperphosphatemia at approximately 1 week of age. In contrast, *Hyp* mice became hypophosphatemic approximately 12 hours after birth.[257]

In humans, Takaiwat and coworkers studied healthy term infants and compared FGF23 levels in the cord blood with day 5 of life and in healthy adults. It is interesting to note that the intact FGF23 was quite low in the cord blood compared with healthy adults. Intact FGF23 was comparable in 5-day-old infants and healthy adults; however, the C-terminal FGF23 was significantly higher in the cord blood and 5-day-old infants compared with adults. These data suggest that there is increased degradation of FGF23 in the cord blood and during early postpartum period leading to lower intact (functioning) FGF23 levels. This is important as within the first 24 hours neonates develop hypocalcemia with a compensatory increase in PTH and 1,25 vitamin D levels in response to transient hypocalcemia. As FGF23 decreases 1,25 vitamin D levels, it is important that intact FGF23 levels remain low in the early postpartum period to prevent a decrease in 1,25 vitamin D levels. In addition, it is possible that low FGF23 levels also contribute to the higher serum phosphate levels in neonates, which is critical for skeletal mineralization.[258]

Parathyroid Hormone

PTH is discussed in detail earlier in this chapter and is critical for calcium homeostasis. PTH decreases serum phosphate by increasing urinary phosphate wasting with downregulation of NaPi-2a and NaPi-2c. However, PTH increases the circulating levels of 1,25 vitamin D by increasing the expression of 1α-hydroxylase and decreasing the expression of 24-hydroxylase. Increased 1,25 vitamin D increases gastrointestinal absorption of calcium and phosphate. In addition, PTH increases bone resorption, which releases calcium and phosphate into the circulation. PTH prevents hyperphosphatemia by increasing urinary excretion of phosphate.

Animal models have shown that fetal PTH is important for calcium, phosphate, and magnesium homeostasis. In the absence of PTH, fetuses exhibit hypocalcemia, hyperphosphatemia, and hypomagnesemia.[259–261] PTH is low in humans at birth and increases rapidly within 24 hours of age.[262,263]

1,25 Vitamin D

1,25 Vitamin D is discussed earlier in the chapter in the calcium section because it also regulates calcium homeostasis. 1,25 Vitamin D is the biologically active form of vitamin D and is also important for phosphate homeostasis. 1α-hydroxylase (CYP27B1) converts 25 vitamin D to 1,25 vitamin D primarily in the kidney, where it is tightly regulated.[264,265] Under physiologic conditions, the kidney is the main source of circulating levels of 1,25 vitamin D, although 1,25 vitamin D is synthesized in many organs, where it acts in a paracrine/autocrine fashion.[266] Although hypophosphatemia and PTH induce 1α-hydroxylase, FGF23 and hyperphosphatemia decrease the expression of 1α-hydroxylase.[267–270] 1,25 Vitamin D is metabolized by 24-hydroxylase (CYP24) to 24,25 vitamin D, which is biologically inactive. Expression of 24-hydroxylase is increased by FGF23 and 1,25 vitamin D. FGF23 decreases circulating levels of 1,25 vitamin D, and 1,25 vitamin D upregulates FGF23 expression, completing a feedback loop as shown in Fig. 20.1.[269]

Fetuses of animal models where vitamin D receptor was deleted demonstrated no abnormalities in their serum mineral marker concentrations and no changes in skeletal mineralization. In addition, there appears to be no transplacental transport of 1,25 vitamin D.[271,272] However, in the neonate, 1,25 vitamin D plays an important role in mineral ion homeostasis. Various mouse models of vitamin D receptor deletion and Cyp27b1 deletion have been studied, and until weaning, there appears to be no major disturbances in their mineral concentration, but after weaning, they are hypocalcemic and hypophosphatemic and have elevated PTH levels, along with signs of rickets. Rescue diet with calcium and phosphate restores their serum calcium, phosphate, and PTH levels and normalizes their bone mineralization.[273–278] These data support that calcium and phosphate are critical for bone mineralization in the growing skeleton.

In humans, the effects of vitamin D deficiency (nutritional rickets) are not evident at birth in the majority of cases, with a few exceptions when the mother's stores of vitamin D are almost negligible.[279,280] Even in infants born with 1α-hydroxylase deficiency (vitamin D–dependent rickets type I) or a vitamin D receptor or postreceptor defect (vitamin D–dependent rickets type II and III), the infants do not present at birth but at approximately 3 to 12 months of age with low serum calcium and phosphate along with signs of rickets.

Klotho

Klotho is a coreceptor for FGF23 which is necessary for binding of FGF23 to its receptor.[281] Klotho can cause phosphaturia independent of FGF23.[282] Although the precise role of Klotho in phosphate homeostasis in the fetus and the neonate is not well studied at this time, Klotho plays an important role in the complex interdependent regulatory pathways involving FGF23 and 1,25 vitamin D, as demonstrated in murine models and in humans. Klotho mRNA is decreased in transgenic mice overexpressing FGF23, and administration of recombinant FGF23 to wild-type mice decreases Klotho mRNA levels.[283,284] However, serum Klotho levels measured in patients with X-linked hypophosphatemic rickets, a condition of FGF23 excess, were noted to be comparable to healthy subjects.[285] FGF23 decreases serum levels of 1,25 vitamin D, and in turn 1,25 vitamin D upregulates Klotho expression.[286,287] Moreover, deletion of Klotho in mouse models results in elevated 1,25 vitamin D levels, and thus Klotho also appears to participate in a negative feedback regulatory loop of 1,25 vitamin D homeostasis.[288] Klotho deletion in mice results in elevated FGF23 levels, along with hyperphosphatemia and hypercalcemia, and these biochemical abnormalities can be improved by placing the mice either on a low phosphate or low vitamin D diet, indicating that the regulation of FGF23 by Klotho is dependent on serum phosphate and 1,25 vitamin D levels.[287,288]

Hypophosphatemia

Normal serum phosphorus in a term neonate is higher than the adults, and the acceptable range is 5.6 to 8.4 mg/dL.[246] In a premature infant the acceptable range for serum phosphorus levels is 4 to 8 mg/dL.[289]

Symptoms of Hypophosphatemia

Mild to moderate hypophosphatemia can remain asymptomatic in the acute period, but prolonged hypophosphatemia can cause impaired bone mineralization in the neonate. Because phosphate is an important component of ATP, many organ systems can be affected with intracellular depletion of ATP. These organ systems include muscle, central nervous system, cardiopulmonary system, hematologic system, and the gastrointestinal tract. The red blood cells in hypophosphatemia can have a decrease in 2,3-diphosphoglycerate levels which will prevent efficient delivery of oxygen to tissues.[290] The signs and symptoms of moderate to severe hypophosphatemia include decreased cardiac output, respiratory insufficiency/failure, myopathy, jitteriness, irritability, seizures, ileus, platelet and leucocyte dysfunction, rhabdomyolysis, and hemolysis.[291–296] Chronic hypophosphatemia causes bone pain and affects bone structure and strength, resulting in rickets in children.[254] In addition, chronic hypophosphatemia can lead to proximal and distal renal tubular defect, causing glycosuria, bicarbonaturia, hypercalciuria, and hypermagnesuria.[297] Moreover, hypophosphatemia can induce insulin resistance, impaired gluconeogenesis, and metabolic acidosis with decreased ammonia generation and hydrogen ion excretion. The next section will discuss the inherited disorders of hypophosphatemia.

Disorders of Hypophosphatemia
Disorders of FGF23 Excess

Autosomal Dominant Hypophosphatemic Rickets (ADHR). ADHR is due to activating mutations of the *FGF23* gene.[298,299] The resultant mutant FGF23 protein is resistant to cleavage by subtilisin-like proprotein converstase (furin-like protease), which results in increased circulating levels of FGF23.[300] Elevated levels of FGF23 result in urinary phosphate wasting, low serum phosphorus levels, and low or inappropriately normal 1,25 vitamin D levels. Econs and coworkers studied a large kindred of patients with ADHR and demonstrated that there was incomplete penetrance and dichotomous presentation in patients with ADHR.[301] One group of patients with ADHR presented in childhood with complaints of delayed walking, short stature, bone pain, leg deformities, poor growth, and dental anomalies. The biochemical phenotype includes abnormalities as described previously. Although the presentation is not in the neonatal period, the clinician should be on the lookout for these biochemical abnormalities if the family history is positive for ADHR. A second group of patients present as adults who were primarily females where pregnancy was noted to be an important triggering factor. When patients present in adulthood, their primary complaint is bone pain, fractures, and muscle weakness but lack the lower extremity deformities. Iron deficiency has been associated with development of the biochemical phenotype in patients with ADHR, which could explain the presentation in females during pregnancy.[302]

Treatment options include phosphate supplementation, along with 1,25 vitamin D, which would increase gastrointestinal phosphate absorption.

X-Linked Hypophosphatemic Rickets (XLH). XLH is inherited in an X-linked dominant fashion and is the most common inherited form of rickets, with an incidence of 1 : 20,000. This disease was first described by Winters and coworkers.[303] There is no male-to-male transmission, and all daughters of an affected male will have XLH. This disease is due to inactivating mutations in the *PHEX* gene (*ph*osphate regulating gene with *h*omologies to *e*ndopeptidases on the *X* chromosome).[304] PHEX is highly expressed in bones and teeth.[305] Initially the disease was thought to be an inherent defect in the kidney, but when a patient with XLH underwent renal transplantation, the patient's biochemical phenotype did not improve after transplantation, suggesting that the primary defect was due to a circulating factor.[306] Because ADHR and XLH shared similar biochemical phenotype and because FGF23 was established as the causative factor in ADHR, it was logical to measure FGF23 levels in patients with XLH and the murine models of XLH. FGF23 was elevated in mouse models of XLH and in the vast majority of patients with XLH.[307,308] Until recently it was unknown as to how mutations in the *PHEX* gene resulted in elevated FGF23 levels because FGF23 is not a substrate for PHEX.[309] Using a mouse model of XLH, the Hyp mouse, Yuan and coworkers elegantly demonstrated that a decrease in a chaperone protein 7B2 results in decreased 7B2:PC2 enzyme activity, which directly effects FGF23 degradation and indirectly enhances FGF23 transcript in the bone, resulting in increased circulating FGF23.[310]

Children with XLH usually present before the age of 2 years. Due to excess FGF23, the serum biochemical abnormalities including hypophosphatemia, phosphaturia, and inappropriately normal or low levels of 1,25 vitamin D are similar to those seen in ADHR. Serum calcium and PTH are usually normal, but these patients do have elevated alkaline phosphatase. Due to the biochemical abnormalities and age at presentation, patients usually present with delayed walking, leg deformities, short stature, and dental abscesses. A genotype-phenotype correlation has been described in XLH patients, with a severe phenotype seen in patients with deletions, nonsense mutations, and spliced mutations leading to premature stop codon, whereas patients with missense mutations appear to have a milder phenotype.[311] Moreover, gene dosage effect was also examined by studying female *Hyp* mice. Even with comparable FGF23 levels, the skeletal phenotype was worse in homozygous female *Hyp* mice compared with the heterozygous female *Hyp* mice.[312] Although patients with XLH do not present in the neonatal period, physicians need to monitor children of patients with XLH. An interesting observation was made by studying 4 infants of parents with XLH. Serum phosphate was low in all of them between 2 and 6 weeks of age, with increased fractional excretion of phosphate noted at 6 months of age except in one infant. Rickets was noted on x-rays at approximately 3 to 6 months of age.[313]

Treatment is symptomatic with phosphate supplements and 1,25 vitamin D. Hyperparathyroidism is a well-described complication in XLH patients on treatment, and Cinacalcet has been used as an additive agent. Patients on therapy have increased risk of nephrocalcinosis, which can lead to CKD. The use of monoclonal FGF23 antibody KRN23 in children (unpublished) and adults has shown promising results, with sustained improvement in serum phosphate and 1,25 vitamin D levels.[313a,313b] This KRN23 antibody might revolutionize the treatment of patients with XLH because it can be started at the time of diagnosis and prevent the iatrogenic complications such as secondary hyperparathyroidism and nephrocalcinosis.

Autosomal Recessive Hypophosphatemic Rickets. Autosomal recessive hypophosphatemic rickets (ARHR) is an extremely rare disease associated with inactivating homozygous mutations in the genes encoding for dentin matrix protein-1 (DMP-1), ectonucleotide pyrophosphate/phosphodiesterase-1 (ENPP1), and families with

20

sequence similarity 20-member C (FAM20c).[314–320] The biochemical phenotype is similar to patients with XLH and ADHR which includes urinary phosphate wasting, hypophosphatemia, and low or inappropriately normal 1,25 vitamin D. Serum calcium and PTH levels are usually normal in these patients. Mouse models for these genes have been studied, and all have elevated FGF23 levels. DMP-1 is present in teeth and bone and regulates the mineralization process.[321,322] ENPP1 is a mineralization inhibitor, and FAM20c is responsible for phosphorylation of the cleavage site of FGF23.[317,323] Lack of FAM20c promotes O-glycosylation of the cleavage site, stabilizing FGF23 protein and resulting in elevated FGF23 levels. Like patients with XLH and ADHR, these patients also present at 6 to 24 months of age. Treatment of these patients includes standard of care with phosphate and 1,25 vitamin D supplementation.

Fibrous Dysplasia. Fibrous dysplasia is a disorder in which normal bone is replaced by fibrous dysplastic tissue and is due to an activating mutation of GNAS1 that encodes for the alpha subunit of G protein, $G_s\alpha$. FGF23 has been shown to be produced by this dysplastic tissue in a cyclic AMP-dependent manner, and the disease severity varies with the burden of the bone lesions. Elevated FGF23 results in urinary phosphate wasting, hypophosphatemia, and low or inappropriately normal 1,25 vitamin D levels. Fibrous dysplasia can occur in isolation or can be associated with McCune-Albright syndrome. Patients with McCune-Albright syndrome are characterized by precocious puberty, thyrotoxicosis, café au lait spots, and polyostotic bone lesions.[324–328]

Klotho Overexpression

Hypophosphatemic Rickets and Hyperparathyroidism. One patient with hypophosphatemic rickets and hyperparathyroidism has been described to have overexpression of Klotho due to a translocation within a breakpoint adjacent to the *Klotho* gene; this patient presented at the age of 13 months with poor growth and macrocephaly. She was noted to have hypophosphatemia, increased fractional excretion of phosphate, elevated PTH levels, inappropriately low 1,25 vitamin D levels, and radiologic evidence of rickets. She was initially treated for hypophosphatemic rickets with 1,25 vitamin D and phosphate supplements, to which she had some response but a few years later continued to have hypercalcemia and hyperparathyroidism. Despite ¾ parathyroidectomy, she developed hypercalcemia and hyperplasia of the remaining parathyroid gland. Serum Klotho levels were elevated, and this is the first human care report of elevated Klotho levels associated with hypophosphatemia. There are many unanswered questions as to why FGF23 and PTH were elevated despite hypophosphatemia, and the data from this one patient might suggest that PTH, FGF23, and Klotho play an important role in phosphate homeostasis, although it remains unclear how they regulate/interact with each other.[329]

PTH Disorders

Hyperparathyroidism and Disorders of 1,25 Vitamin D Homeostasis

Conditions of hyperparathyroidism and vitamin D homeostasis are discussed in detail; they can affect serum phosphate and are discussed previously.

Proximal Tubulopathies

Patients with proximal tubular disorders, including but not limited to Fanconi syndrome, Lowes syndrome, and Dent disease, should be considered in the differential diagnosis of hypophosphatemia. These conditions are associated with urinary phosphate wasting and hypophosphatemia, in addition to metabolic acidosis, glycosuria, and failure to thrive. Detailed discussion of these conditions is beyond the scope of this chapter.

Disorders of Sodium Phosphate Cotransporters

The principal renal transporters for phosphate reabsorption include sodium phosphate cotransporter 2a and 2c, NaPi-2a (Slc34a1), and NaPi-2c (Slc34a3).

Hereditary Hypophosphatemic Rickets With Hypercalciuria. Hereditary hypophosphatemic rickets with hypercalciuria (HHRH) is inherited in an autosomal recessive fashion and is due to inactivating mutations of NaPi-2c.[330,331] Tieder and coworkers first described the clinical phenotype of HHRH in a consanguineous Bedouin family.[332] NaPi-2c appears to be an essential renal phosphate transporter in humans. Patients usually present in the first couple of years of life with rickets, bone pain, muscle weakness, short stature, and lower extremity deformities. Biochemical phenotype includes hypophosphatemia, phosphaturia, elevated 1,25 vitamin D levels, hypercalciuria, and suppressed PTH levels. Elevated 1,25 vitamin D levels in these patients result in increased calcium absorption from the gastrointestinal tract which results in transient hypercalcemia, suppressed PTH levels, and hypercalciuria. Patients with this condition also develop nephrolithiasis. An important differentiating feature between HHRH and conditions of FGF23 excess is high elevated 1,25 vitamin D levels in HHRH, whereas they are low or inappropriately normal in conditions of FGF23 excess. Treatment for HHRH is phosphate supplementation. These patients should not receive 1,25 vitamin D because this will worsen hypercalciuria and nephrolithiasis.

Autosomal Recessive Fanconi's Syndrome With Hypophosphatemic Rickets. Two adult siblings who were initially thought to have HHRH with proximal tubulopathy later developed renal insufficiency along with low 1,25 vitamin D levels and normocalciuria. Genetic studies on these two patients revealed homozygous mutations in *NaPi-2a* gene. Expression of the mutant NaPi2a in *Xenopus laevis* oocytes demonstrated that the mutant NaPi-2a protein does not reach the brush border membrane and accumulates intracellularly. FGF23 levels were in the low-normal range.[333]

Idiopathic Infantile Hypercalcemia With Hypophosphatemia. As described in the hypercalcemia section of this chapter, a group of investigators identified mutations in the *NaPi-2a* gene in a subset of patients with IIH who did not have *CYP24A1* mutations. The mutant protein demonstrated defective trafficking to the brush border membrane, where NaPi-2a is responsible for phosphate reabsorption. In humans the importance of NaPi-2a relative to NaPi-2c remains to be studied.[59]

A list of inherited causes of hypophosphatemia is provided in Table 20.9.

Hyperphosphatemia

Symptoms of Hyperphosphatemia

Symptoms of acute hyperphosphatemia are primarily due to hypocalcemia that have been described in the "Hypocalcemia" section. Use of high-dose phosphate enemas can cause acute kidney injury and phosphate nephropathy, as seen in renal biopsy. Chronic symptoms of hyperphosphatemia are commonly seen in CKD and ESRD and have been associated with vascular calcification. Inherited conditions of hyperphosphatemia are discussed later.

Disorders of FGF23 Deficiency

Hyperphosphatemic Familial Tumoral Calcinosis (HFTC). HFTC is inherited in an autosomal dominant or in an autosomal recessive fashion. This is due to deficiency of FGF23. FGF23 undergoes proteolytic cleavage at the "RXXR" site. O-glycosylation of the threonine residue in the RXXR site is important for the secretion of intact FGF23 protein. This O-glycosylation is performed by GALNT3, which encodes for UDP-N-acetyl-alpha-D-galactosamine:polypeptide N-acetylgalactosaminyl transferase 3. Thus patients with inactivating mutations of GALNT3 have decreased circulating levels of FGF23.[334,335] Inactivating mutations of the conserved region of the *FGF23* gene itself have been demonstrated to cause familial tumoral calcinosis. The resultant mutant FGF23 protein is either prone to degradation by proteases or is not secreted in its intact form and thereby results in decreased circulating levels of FGF23.[336] The biochemical phenotype of this disease includes hyperphosphatemia, elevated 1,25 vitamin D levels, sometimes hypercalcemia, and painful deposition of calcium and phosphate in the soft tissue skin and joints. This is a highly debilitating and painful disorder, and treatment options include phosphate binders. Surgical

Table 20.9   LIST OF INHERITED HYPOPHOSPHATEMIC AND HYPERPHOSPHATEMIC DISORDERS DUE TO HORMONE DYSREGULATION

Disorder	OMIM	Inheritance	Gene Locus	Serum Phosphate	1,25 Vitamin D	FePhos	PTH	Gene (Protein)	Function	References
Hypophosphatemic Disorders										
Conditions of FGF23 Excess										
ADHR	193100	AD	12p.13.32	↓	n-↓	↑	n	*FGF23* (FGF23)	Phosphaturic hormone, activating mutation of FGF23	298,299
XLH	307800	XLD	Xp22.11	↓	n-↓	↑	n	*PHEX* (PHEX)	Endopeptidase, increased FGF23 from bone	304,307,308
ARHR1	241520	AR	4q22.1	↓	n-↓	↑	n	*DMP1* (DMP1)	Bone mineralization, SIBLING protein family.	314,315
ARHR2	613312	AR	6q23.2	↓	n-↓	↑	n	*ENPP1* (ENPP1)	Enzyme, nucleotide pyrophosphatase	316,318
ARHR3	259775	AR	7p22.3	↓	n-↓	↑	n	*FAM20c* (FAM20c)	Kinase	319,320
MAS	174800	Sporadic	20q13.32	↓	n-↓	↑	n	*GNAS1*	Signaling protein	325,326
Condition of Klotho Excess										
HRHPT	612089	Translocation	9q21.1/13q13.1	↓	↓	↑	↑	*KLOTHO* (KLOTHO)	Coreceptor	329
Hyperphosphatemic Disorders										
Conditions of FGF23 Deficiency										
HFTC	211900	AD/AR	2q24.3 12p13.32	↑	↑	↓	n	*FGF23* (FGF23) *GALNT3* (GALNT3)	Phosphaturic hormone Enzyme	336 334,335
Condition of Klotho Deficiency										
HFTC	211900	AR	13q13.1	↑	↑	↓	↑	*KLOTHO* (KLOTHO)	Coreceptor	337

AD, Autosomal dominant; *ADHR*, autosomal dominant hypophosphatemic rickets; *AR*, autosomal recessive; *ARHR*, autosomal recessive hypophosphatemic rickets; *HFTC*, hyperphosphatemic familial tumoral calcinosis; *HRHPT*, hypophosphatemic rickets and hyperparathyroidism; *MAS*, McCune-Albright syndrome; *n*, normal; *XLD*, X-linked dominant; *XLH*, X-linked hypophosphatemic rickets.

removal of the lesions provides only temporary relief because in many cases the lesions recur.

Loss of Klotho Function

Loss of function of Klotho was first described in a 13-year-old girl who presented with tumoral calcinosis, hyperphosphatemia, hypercalcemia, and elevated 1,25 vitamin D and FGF23 levels. The absence of Klotho causes resistance to the phosphaturic actions of FGF23.[337]

PTH Disorders

Hypoparathyroidism is associated with hyperphosphatemia along with hypocalcemia which is described previously.

A list of inherited causes of hyperphosphatemia is provided in Table 20.9.

REFERENCES

1. Ramasamy I. Recent advances in physiological calcium homeostasis. *Clin Chem Lab Med.* 2006;44:237–273.
2. Ziegler EE, O'Donnell AM, Nelson SE, Fomon SJ. Body composition of the reference fetus. *Growth.* 1976;40:329–341.
3. Matkovic V, Heaney RP. Calcium balance during human growth: evidence for threshold behavior. *Am J Clin Nutr.* 1992;55:992–996.
4. Hoenderop JG, Nilius B, Bindels RJ. Calcium absorption across epithelia. *Physiol Rev.* 2005;85:373–422.
5. Hoenderop JG, Bindels RJ. Epithelial Ca2+ and Mg2+ channels in health and disease. *J Am Soc Nephrol.* 2005;16:15–26.
6. Frick KK, Bushinsky DA. Molecular mechanisms of primary hypercalciuria. *J Am Soc Nephrol.* 2003;14:1082–1095.
7. Dimke H, Hoenderop JG, Bindels RJ. Hereditary tubular transport disorders: implications for renal handling of Ca2+ and Mg2+. *Clin Sci.* 2010;118:1–18.
8. Dimke H, Hoenderop JG, Bindels RJ. Molecular basis of epithelial Ca2+ and Mg2+ transport: insights from the TRP channel family. *J Physiol.* 2011;589:1535–1542.
9. Hoenderop JG, Bindels RJ. Calciotropic and magnesiotropic TRP channels. *Physiology (Bethesda).* 2008;23:32–40.
10. Marx SJ. Hyperparathyroid and hypoparathyroid disorders. *N Engl J Med.* 2000;343:1863–1875.
11. Trump D, Farren B, Wooding C, et al. Clinical studies of multiple endocrine neoplasia type 1 (MEN1). *QJM.* 1996;89:653–669.
12. Cryns VL, Thor A, Xu HJ, et al. Loss of the retinoblastoma tumor-suppressor gene in parathyroid carcinoma. *N Engl J Med.* 1994;330:757–761.
13. Motokura T, Bloom T, Kim HG, et al. A novel cyclin encoded by a bcl1-linked candidate oncogene. *Nature.* 1991;350:512–515.
14. Chandrasekharappa SC, Guru SC, Manickam P, et al. Positional cloning of the gene for multiple endocrine neoplasia-type 1. *Science.* 1997;276:404–407.
15. Thakker RV. Genetics of endocrine and metabolic disorders: parathyroid. *Rev Endocr Metab Disord.* 2004;5:37–51.
16. Guru SC, Goldsmith PK, Burns AL, et al. Menin, the product of the MEN1 gene, is a nuclear protein. *Proc Natl Acad Sci USA.* 1998;95:1630–1634.
17. Pepe J, Cipriani C, Pilotto R, et al. Sporadic and hereditary primary hyperparathyroidism. *J Endocrinol Invest.* 2011;34:40–44.
18. Shane E, Bilezikian JP. Parathyroid carcinoma: a review of 62 patients. *Endocr Rev.* 1982;3:218–226.
19. Brasier AR, Nussbaum SR. Hungry bone syndrome: clinical and biochemical predictors of its occurrence after parathyroid surgery. *Am J Med.* 1988;84:654–660.
20. Peacock M, Bilezikian JP, Klassen PS, et al. Cinacalcet hydrochloride maintains long-term normocalcemia in patients with primary hyperparathyroidism. *J Clin Endocrinol Metab.* 2005;90:135–141.
21. Thakker RV. Diseases associated with the extracellular calcium-sensing receptor. *Cell Calcium.* 2004;35:275–282.
22. Pollak MR, Brown EM, Chou YH, et al. Mutations in the human Ca(2+)-sensing receptor gene cause familial hypocalciuric hypercalcemia and neonatal severe hyperparathyroidism. *Cell.* 1993;75:1297–1303.
23. Brown EM, Gamba G, Riccardi D, et al. Cloning and characterization of an extracellular Ca(2+)-sensing receptor from bovine parathyroid. *Nature.* 1993;366:575–580.
24. Brown EM, MacLeod RJ. Extracellular calcium sensing and extracellular calcium signaling. *Physiol Rev.* 2001;81:239–297.
25. Riccardi D, Kemp PJ. The calcium-sensing receptor beyond extracellular calcium homeostasis: conception, development, adult physiology, and disease. *Annu Rev Physiol.* 2012;74:271–297.
26. Riccardi D, Brown EM. Physiology and pathophysiology of the calcium-sensing receptor in the kidney. *Am J Physiol Renal Physiol.* 2010;298:F485–F499.

27. Mamillapalli R, VanHouten J, Zawalich W, Wysolmerski J. Switching of G-protein usage by the calcium-sensing receptor reverses its effect on parathyroid hormone-related protein secretion in normal versus malignant breast cells. *J Biol Chem*. 2008;283:24435–24447.

28. Mamillapalli R, Wysolmerski J. The calcium-sensing receptor couples to Galpha(s) and regulates PTHrP and ACTH secretion in pituitary cells. *J Endocrinol*. 2010;204:287–297.

29. Renkema KY, Velic A, Dijkman HB, et al. The calcium-sensing receptor promotes urinary acidification to prevent nephrolithiasis. *J Am Soc Nephrol*. 2009;20:1705–1713.

30. Sands JM, Naruse M, Baum M, et al. Apical extracellular calcium/polyvalent cation-sensing receptor regulates vasopressin-elicited water permeability in rat kidney inner medullary collecting duct. *J Clin Invest*. 1997;99:1399–1405.

31. Hebert SC. Extracellular calcium-sensing receptor: implications for calcium and magnesium handling in the kidney. *Kidney Int*. 1996;50:2129–2139.

32. Nesbit MA, Hannan FM, Howles SA, et al. Mutations in AP2S1 cause familial hypocalciuric hypercalcemia type 3. *Nat Genet*. 2013;45:93–97.

33. Pearce SH, Williamson C, Kifor O, et al. A familial syndrome of hypocalcemia with hypercalciuria due to mutations in the calcium-sensing receptor. *N Engl J Med*. 1996;335:1115–1122.

34. Watanabe S, Fukumoto S, Chang H, et al. Association between activating mutations of calcium-sensing receptor and Bartter's syndrome. *Lancet*. 2002;360:692–694.

35. Nesbit MA, Hannan FM, Howles SA, et al. Mutations affecting G-protein subunit alpha11 in hypercalcemia and hypocalcemia. *N Engl J Med*. 2013;368:2476–2486.

36. McMurtry CT, Schranck FW, Walkenhorst DA, et al. Significant developmental elevation in serum parathyroid hormone levels in a large kindred with familial benign (hypocalciuric) hypercalcemia. *Am J Med*. 1992;93:247–258.

37. Nesbit MA, Hannan FM, Graham U, et al. Identification of a second kindred with familial hypocalciuric hypercalcemia type 3 (FHH3) narrows localization to a <3.5 megabase pair region on chromosome 19q13.3. *J Clin Endocrinol Metab*. 2010;95:1947–1954.

38. Pearce SH, Trump D, Wooding C, et al. Calcium-sensing receptor mutations in familial benign hypercalcemia and neonatal hyperparathyroidism. *J Clin Invest*. 1995;96:2683–2692.

39. Egbuna OI, Brown EM. Hypercalcaemic and hypocalcaemic conditions due to calcium-sensing receptor mutations. *Best Pract Res Clin Rheumatol*. 2008;22:129–148.

40. Lietman SA, Germain-Lee EL, Levine MA. Hypercalcemia in children and adolescents. *Curr Opin Pediatr*. 2010;22:508–515.

41. Pollak MR, Chou YH, Marx SJ, et al. Familial hypocalciuric hypercalcemia and neonatal severe hyperparathyroidism. Effects of mutant gene dosage on phenotype. *J Clin Invest*. 1994;93:1108–1112.

42. Bai M, Pearce SH, Kifor O, et al. In vivo and in vitro characterization of neonatal hyperparathyroidism resulting from a de novo, heterozygous mutation in the Ca2+-sensing receptor gene: normal maternal calcium homeostasis as a cause of secondary hyperparathyroidism in familial benign hypocalciuric hypercalcemia. *J Clin Invest*. 1997;99:88–96.

43. Ward BK, Cameron FJ, Magno AL, et al. A novel homozygous deletion in the calcium-sensing receptor ligand-binding domain associated with neonatal severe hyperparathyroidism. *J Pediatr Endocrinol Metab*. 2006;19:93–100.

44. Juppner H. Functional properties of the PTH/PTHrP receptor. *Bone*. 1995;17:39s–42s.

45. Schipani E, Kruse K, Juppner H. A constitutively active mutant PTH-PTHrP receptor in Jansen-type metaphyseal chondrodysplasia. *Science*. 1995;268:98–100.

46. Schipani E, Langman CB, Parfitt AM, et al. Constitutively activated receptors for parathyroid hormone and parathyroid hormone-related peptide in Jansen's metaphyseal chondrodysplasia. *N Engl J Med*. 1996;335:708–714.

47. Bastepe M, Raas-Rothschild A, Silver J, et al. A form of Jansen's metaphyseal chondrodysplasia with limited metabolic and skeletal abnormalities is caused by a novel activating parathyroid hormone (PTH)/PTH-related peptide receptor mutation. *J Clin Endocrinol Metab*. 2004;89:3595–3600.

48. Onuchic L, Ferraz-de-Souza B, Mendonca BB, et al. Potential effects of alendronate on fibroblast growth factor 23 levels and effective control of hypercalciuria in an adult with Jansen's metaphyseal chondrodysplasia. *J Clin Endocrinol Metab*. 2012;97:1098–1103.

49. Fraser D. Hypophosphatasia. *Am J Med*. 1957;22:730–746.

50. Whyte MP, Zhang F, Wenkert D, et al. Hypophosphatasia: validation and expansion of the clinical nosology for children from 25 years experience with 173 pediatric patients. *Bone*. 2015;75:229–239.

51. Weiss MJ, Cole DE, Ray K, et al. A missense mutation in the human liver/bone/kidney alkaline phosphatase gene causing a lethal form of hypophosphatasia. *Proc Natl Acad Sci USA*. 1988;85: 7666–7669.

52. Whyte MP, Greenberg CR, Salman NJ, et al. Enzyme-replacement therapy in life-threatening hypophosphatasia. *N Engl J Med*. 2012;366:904–913.

53. Whyte MP. Hypophosphatasia—aetiology, nosology, pathogenesis, diagnosis and treatment. *Nat Rev Endocrinol*. 2016;12:233–246.

54. Baumgartner-Sigl S, Haberlandt E, Mumm S, et al. Pyridoxine-responsive seizures as the first symptom of infantile hypophosphatasia caused by two novel missense mutations (c.677T>C, p.M226T; c.1112C>T, p.T371I) of the tissue-nonspecific alkaline phosphatase gene. *Bone*. 2007;40:1655–1661.

55. Lightwood R, Stapleton T. Idiopathic hypercalcaemia in infants. *Lancet*. 1953;265:255–256.

56. Castanet M, Mallet E, Kottler ML. Lightwood syndrome revisited with a novel mutation in CYP24 and vitamin D supplement recommendations. *J Pediatr*. 2013;163:1208–1210.

57. Schlingmann KP, Kaufmann M, Weber S, et al. Mutations in CYP24A1 and idiopathic infantile hypercalcemia. *N Engl J Med*. 2011;365:410–421.

58. Nesterova G, Malicdan MC, Yasuda K, et al. 1,25-(OH)2D-24 Hydroxylase (CYP24A1) Deficiency as a Cause of Nephrolithiasis. *Clin J Am Soc Nephrol*. 2013;8:649–657.
59. Schlingmann KP, Ruminska J, Kaufmann M, et al. Autosomal-Recessive Mutations in SLC34A1 Encoding Sodium-Phosphate Cotransporter 2A Cause Idiopathic Infantile Hypercalcemia. *J Am Soc Nephrol*. 2016;27:604–614.
60. Pober BR. Williams-Beuren syndrome. *N Engl J Med*. 2010;362:239–252.
61. Sindhar S, Lugo M, Levin MD, et al. Hypercalcemia in Patients with Williams-Beuren Syndrome. *J Pediatr*. 2016;178:254–260.e4.
62. Stagi S, Manoni C, Scalini P, et al. Bone mineral status and metabolism in patients with Williams-Beuren syndrome. *Hormones (Athens)*. 2016;15:404–412.
63. Ewart AK, Morris CA, Atkinson D, et al. Hemizygosity at the elastin locus in a developmental disorder, Williams syndrome. *Nat Genet*. 1993;5:11–16.
64. Lowery MC, Morris CA, Ewart A, et al. Strong correlation of elastin deletions, detected by FISH, with Williams syndrome: evaluation of 235 patients. *Am J Hum Genet*. 1995;57:49–53.
65. Hebert SC. Bartter syndrome. *Curr Opin Nephrol Hypertens*. 2003;12:527–532.
66. Kleta R, Bockenhauer D. Bartter syndromes and other salt-losing tubulopathies. *Nephron Physiol*. 2006;104:p73–p80.
67. Bartter FC, Pronove P, Gill JR Jr, Maccardle RC. Hyperplasia of the juxtaglomerular complex with hyperaldosteronism and hypokalemic alkalosis. A new syndrome. *Am J Med*. 1962;33:811–828.
68. Seys E, Andrini O, Keck M, et al. Clinical and Genetic Spectrum of Bartter Syndrome Type 3. *J Am Soc Nephrol*. 2017;28(8):2540–2552.
69. Simon DB, Karet FE, Hamdan JM, et al. Bartter's syndrome, hypokalaemic alkalosis with hypercalciuria, is caused by mutations in the Na-K-2Cl cotransporter NKCC2. *Nat Genet*. 1996;13:183–188.
70. Simon DB, Karet FE, Rodriguez-Soriano J, et al. Genetic heterogeneity of Bartter's syndrome revealed by mutations in the K+ channel, ROMK. *Nat Genet*. 1996;14:152–156.
71. Finer G, Shalev H, Birk OS, et al. Transient neonatal hyperkalemia in the antenatal (ROMK defective) Bartter syndrome. *J Pediatr*. 2003;142:318–323.
72. Peters M, Jeck N, Reinalter S, et al. Clinical presentation of genetically defined patients with hypokalemic salt-losing tubulopathies. *Am J Med*. 2002;112:183–190.
73. Gamba G, Friedman PA. Thick ascending limb: the Na(+) : K(+) : 2Cl(−) co-transporter, NKCC2, and the calcium-sensing receptor, CaSR. *Pflugers Arch*. 2009;458:61–76.
74. Wang W, Lu M, Balazy M, Hebert SC. Phospholipase A2 is involved in mediating the effect of extracellular Ca2+ on apical K+ channels in rat TAL. *Am J Physiol*. 1997;273:F421–F429.
75. Birkenhager R, Otto E, Schurmann MJ, et al. Mutation of BSND causes Bartter syndrome with sensorineural deafness and kidney failure. *Nat Genet*. 2001;29:310–314.
76. Simon DB, Bindra RS, Mansfield TA, et al. Mutations in the chloride channel gene, CLCNKB, cause Bartter's syndrome type III. *Nat Genet*. 1997;17:171–178.
77. Gross I, Siedner-Weintraub Y, Simckes A, Gillis D. Antenatal Bartter syndrome presenting as hyperparathyroidism with hypercalcemia and hypercalciuria: a case report and review. *J Pediatr Endocrinol Metab*. 2015;28:943–946.
78. Wongsaengsak S, Vidmar AP, Addala A, et al. A novel SLC12A1 gene mutation associated with hyperparathyroidism, hypercalcemia, nephrogenic diabetes insipidus, and nephrocalcinosis in four patients. *Bone*. 2017;97:121–125.
79. Laghmani K, Beck BB, Yang SS, et al. Polyhydramnios, Transient Antenatal Bartter's Syndrome, and MAGED2 Mutations. *N Engl J Med*. 2016;374:1853–1863.
80. Kovacs CS. Bone development and mineral homeostasis in the fetus and neonate: roles of the calciotropic and phosphotropic hormones. *Physiol Rev*. 2014;94:1143–1218.
81. Venkataraman PS, Tsang RC, Steichen JJ, et al. Early neonatal hypocalcemia in extremely preterm infants. High incidence, early onset, and refractoriness to supraphysiologic doses of calcitriol. *Am J Dis Child*. 1986;140:1004–1008.
82. Arnold A, Horst SA, Gardella TJ, et al. Mutation of the signal peptide-encoding region of the preproparathyroid hormone gene in familial isolated hypoparathyroidism. *J Clin Invest*. 1990;86:1084–1087.
83. Karaplis AC, Lim SK, Baba H, et al. Inefficient membrane targeting, translocation, and proteolytic processing by signal peptidase of a mutant preproparathyroid hormone protein. *J Biol Chem*. 1995;270:1629–1635.
84. Datta R, Waheed A, Shah GN, Sly WS. Signal sequence mutation in autosomal dominant form of hypoparathyroidism induces apoptosis that is corrected by a chemical chaperone. *Proc Natl Acad Sci USA*. 2007;104:19989–19994.
85. Parkinson DB, Thakker RV. A donor splice site mutation in the parathyroid hormone gene is associated with autosomal recessive hypoparathyroidism. *Nat Genet*. 1992;1:149–152.
86. De Luca F, Ray K, Mancilla EE, et al. Sporadic hypoparathyroidism caused by de Novo gain-of-function mutations of the Ca(2+)-sensing receptor. *J Clin Endocrinol Metab*. 1997;82:2710–2715.
87. Baron J, Winer KK, Yanovski JA, et al. Mutations in the Ca(2+)-sensing receptor gene cause autosomal dominant and sporadic hypoparathyroidism. *Hum Mol Genet*. 1996;5:601–606.
88. Nesbit MA, Bowl MR, Harding B, et al. Characterization of GATA3 mutations in the hypoparathyroidism, deafness, and renal dysplasia (HDR) syndrome. *J Biol Chem*. 2004;279:22624–22634.
89. Ali A, Christie PT, Grigorieva IV, et al. Functional characterization of GATA3 mutations causing the hypoparathyroidism-deafness-renal (HDR) dysplasia syndrome: insight into mechanisms of DNA binding by the GATA3 transcription factor. *Hum Mol Genet*. 2007;16:265–275.

20

90. Pandolfi PP, Roth ME, Karis A, et al. Targeted disruption of the GATA3 gene causes severe abnormalities in the nervous system and in fetal liver haematopoiesis. *Nat Genet*. 1995;11:40–44.

91. Van Esch H, Groenen P, Nesbit MA, et al. GATA3 haplo-insufficiency causes human HDR syndrome. *Nature*. 2000;406:419–422.

92. van der Wees J, van Looij MA, de Ruiter MM, et al. Hearing loss following Gata3 haploinsufficiency is caused by cochlear disorder. *Neurobiol Dis*. 2004;16:169–178.

93. van Looij MA, van der Burg H, van der Giessen RS, et al. GATA3 haploinsufficiency causes a rapid deterioration of distortion product otoacoustic emissions (DPOAEs) in mice. *Neurobiol Dis*. 2005;20:890–897.

94. Grigorieva IV, Mirczuk S, Gaynor KU, et al. Gata3-deficient mice develop parathyroid abnormalities due to dysregulation of the parathyroid-specific transcription factor Gcm2. *J Clin Invest*. 2010;120:2144–2155.

95. Greenberg F. Hypoparathyroidism and the DiGeorge syndrome. *N Engl J Med*. 1989;320:1146–1147.

96. Lichtner P, Konig R, Hasegawa T, et al. An HDR (hypoparathyroidism, deafness, renal dysplasia) syndrome locus maps distal to the DiGeorge syndrome region on 10p13/14. *J Med Genet*. 2000;37:33–37.

97. Scambler PJ. The 22q11 deletion syndromes. *Hum Mol Genet*. 2000;9:2421–2426.

98. Jerome LA, Papaioannou VE. DiGeorge syndrome phenotype in mice mutant for the T-box gene, Tbx1. *Nat Genet*. 2001;27:286–291.

99. Yagi H, Furutani Y, Hamada H, et al. Role of TBX1 in human del22q11.2 syndrome. *Lancet*. 2003;362:1366–1373.

100. Monaco G, Pignata C, Rossi E, et al. DiGeorge anomaly associated with 10p deletion. *Am J Med Genet*. 1991;39:215–216.

101. Stoller JZ, Epstein JA. Identification of a novel nuclear localization signal in Tbx1 that is deleted in DiGeorge syndrome patients harboring the 1223delC mutation. *Hum Mol Genet*. 2005;14:885–892.

102. Ryan AK, Goodship JA, Wilson DI, et al. Spectrum of clinical features associated with interstitial chromosome 22q11 deletions: a European collaborative study. *J Med Genet*. 1997;34:798–804.

103. Novelli A, Sabani M, Caiola A, et al. Diagnosis of DiGeorge and Williams syndromes using FISH analysis of peripheral blood smears. *Mol Cell Probes*. 1999;13:303–307.

104. Kawahara M, Iwasaki Y, Sakaguchi K, et al. Involvement of GCMB in the transcriptional regulation of the human parathyroid hormone gene in a parathyroid-derived cell line PT-r: effects of calcium and 1,25(OH)2D3. *Bone*. 2010;47:534–541.

105. Sticht H, Hashemolhosseini S. A common structural mechanism underlying GCMB mutations that cause hypoparathyroidism. *Med Hypotheses*. 2006;67:482–487.

106. Bowl MR, Mirczuk SM, Grigorieva IV, et al. Identification and characterization of novel parathyroid-specific transcription factor Glial Cells Missing Homolog B (GCMB) mutations in eight families with autosomal recessive hypoparathyroidism. *Hum Mol Genet*. 2010;19:2028–2038.

107. Ding C, Buckingham B, Levine MA. Familial isolated hypoparathyroidism caused by a mutation in the gene for the transcription factor GCMB. *J Clin Invest*. 2001;108:1215–1220.

108. Alimohammadi M, Bjorklund P, Hallgren A, et al. Autoimmune polyendocrine syndrome type 1 and NALP5, a parathyroid autoantigen. *N Engl J Med*. 2008;358:1018–1028.

109. Gardner JM, Fletcher AL, Anderson MS, Turley SJ. AIRE in the thymus and beyond. *Curr Opin Immunol*. 2009;21:582–589.

110. Dionisi-Vici C, Garavaglia B, Burlina AB, et al. Hypoparathyroidism in mitochondrial trifunctional protein deficiency. *J Pediatr*. 1996;129:159–162.

111. Labarthe F, Benoist JF, Brivet M, et al. Partial hypoparathyroidism associated with mitochondrial trifunctional protein deficiency. *Eur J Pediatr*. 2006;165:389–391.

112. Unger S, Gorna MW, Le Bechec A, et al. FAM111A mutations result in hypoparathyroidism and impaired skeletal development. *Am J Hum Genet*. 2013;92:990–995.

113. Diaz GA, Khan KT, Gelb BD. The autosomal recessive Kenny-Caffey syndrome locus maps to chromosome 1q42-q43. *Genomics*. 1998;54:13–18.

114. Blomstrand S, Claesson I, Save-Soderbergh J. A case of lethal congenital dwarfism with accelerated skeletal maturation. *Pediatr Radiol*. 1985;15:141–143.

115. Jobert AS, Zhang P, Couvineau A, et al. Absence of functional receptors for parathyroid hormone and parathyroid hormone-related peptide in Blomstrand chondrodysplasia. *J Clin Invest*. 1998;102:34–40.

116. Porter RH, Cox BG, Heaney D, et al. Treatment of hypoparathyroid patients with chlorthalidone. *N Engl J Med*. 1978;298:577–581.

117. Winer KK, Fulton KA, Albert PS, Cutler GB Jr. Effects of pump versus twice-daily injection delivery of synthetic parathyroid hormone 1-34 in children with severe congenital hypoparathyroidism. *J Pediatr*. 2014;165:556–563.e1.

118. Linglart A, Rothenbuhler A, Gueorgieva I, et al. Long-term results of continuous subcutaneous recombinant PTH (1-34) infusion in children with refractory hypoparathyroidism. *J Clin Endocrinol Metab*. 2011;96:3308–3312.

119. Clarke BL, Vokes TJ, Bilezikian JP, et al. Effects of parathyroid hormone rhPTH(1-84) on phosphate homeostasis and vitamin D metabolism in hypoparathyroidism: REPLACE phase 3 study. *Endocrine*. 2017;55:273–282.

120. Tamura T, Noda H, Joyashiki E, et al. Identification of an orally active small-molecule PTHR1 agonist for the treatment of hypoparathyroidism. *Nat Commun*. 2016;7:13384.

121. Lienhardt A, Bai M, Lagarde JP, et al. Activating mutations of the calcium-sensing receptor: management of hypocalcemia. *J Clin Endocrinol Metab*. 2001;86:5313–5323.

122. Yamamoto M, Akatsu T, Nagase T, Ogata E. Comparison of hypocalcemic hypercalciuria between patients with idiopathic hypoparathyroidism and those with gain-of-function mutations in the calcium-sensing receptor: is it possible to differentiate the two disorders? *J Clin Endocrinol Metab*. 2000;85:4583–4591.

123. Pollak MR, Brown EM, Estep HL, et al. Autosomal dominant hypocalcaemia caused by a Ca(2+)-sensing receptor gene mutation. *Nat Genet*. 1994;8:303–307.

124. Vargas-Poussou R, Huang C, Hulin P, et al. Functional characterization of a calcium-sensing receptor mutation in severe autosomal dominant hypocalcemia with a Bartter-like syndrome. *J Am Soc Nephrol*. 2002;13:2259–2266.

125. Vezzoli G, Arcidiacono T, Paloschi V, et al. Autosomal dominant hypocalcemia with mild type 5 Bartter syndrome. *J Nephrol*. 2006;19:525–528.

126. Li D, Opas EE, Tuluc F, et al. Autosomal dominant hypoparathyroidism caused by germline mutation in GNA11: phenotypic and molecular characterization. *J Clin Endocrinol Metab*. 2014;99:E1774–E1783.

127. Tafaj O, Juppner H. Pseudohypoparathyroidism: one gene, several syndromes. *J Endocrinol Invest*. 2016;40(4):347–356.

128. Levine MA, Ahn TG, Klupt SF, et al. Genetic deficiency of the alpha subunit of the guanine nucleotide-binding protein Gs as the molecular basis for Albright hereditary osteodystrophy. *Proc Natl Acad Sci USA*. 1988;85:617–621.

129. Bastepe M. The GNAS locus and pseudohypoparathyroidism. *Adv Exp Med Biol*. 2008;626:27–40.

130. Wilson LC, Oude Luttikhuis ME, Clayton PT, et al. Parental origin of Gs alpha gene mutations in Albright's hereditary osteodystrophy. *J Med Genet*. 1994;31:835–839.

131. Yu S, Yu D, Lee E, et al. Variable and tissue-specific hormone resistance in heterotrimeric Gs protein alpha-subunit (Gsalpha) knockout mice is due to tissue-specific imprinting of the gsalpha gene. *Proc Natl Acad Sci USA*. 1998;95:8715–8720.

132. Schuster V, Eschenhagen T, Kruse K, et al. Endocrine and molecular biological studies in a German family with Albright hereditary osteodystrophy. *Eur J Pediatr*. 1993;152:185–189.

133. Long DN, McGuire S, Levine MA, et al. Body mass index differences in pseudohypoparathyroidism type 1a versus pseudopseudohypoparathyroidism may implicate paternal imprinting of Galpha(s) in the development of human obesity. *J Clin Endocrinol Metab*. 2007;92:1073–1079.

134. Levine MA, Downs RW Jr, Moses AM, et al. Resistance to multiple hormones in patients with pseudohypoparathyroidism. Association with deficient activity of guanine nucleotide regulatory protein. *Am J Med*. 1983;74:545–556.

135. Weber TJ, Liu S, Indridason OS, Quarles LD. Serum FGF23 levels in normal and disordered phosphorus homeostasis. *J Bone Miner Res*. 2003;18:1227–1234.

136. Juppner H, Schipani E, Bastepe M, et al. The gene responsible for pseudohypoparathyroidism type Ib is paternally imprinted and maps in four unrelated kindreds to chromosome 20q13.3. *Proc Natl Acad Sci USA*. 1998;95:11798–11803.

137. Yu S, Gavrilova O, Chen H, et al. Paternal versus maternal transmission of a stimulatory G-protein alpha subunit knockout produces opposite effects on energy metabolism. *J Clin Invest*. 2000;105:615–623.

138. Murray TM, Rao LG, Wong MM, et al. Pseudohypoparathyroidism with osteitis fibrosa cystica: direct demonstration of skeletal responsiveness to parathyroid hormone in cells cultured from bone. *J Bone Miner Res*. 1993;8:83–91.

139. Drezner M, Neelon FA, Lebovitz HE. Pseudohypoparathyroidism type II: a possible defect in the reception of the cyclic AMP signal. *N Engl J Med*. 1973;289:1056–1060.

140. Kitanaka S, Takeyama K, Murayama A, et al. Inactivating mutations in the 25-hydroxyvitamin D3 1alpha-hydroxylase gene in patients with pseudovitamin D-deficiency rickets. *N Engl J Med*. 1998;338:653–661.

141. Yagi H, Ozono K, Miyake H, et al. A new point mutation in the deoxyribonucleic acid-binding domain of the vitamin D receptor in a kindred with hereditary 1,25-dihydroxyvitamin D-resistant rickets. *J Clin Endocrinol Metab*. 1993;76:509–512.

142. Malloy PJ, Weisman Y, Feldman D. Hereditary 1 alpha,25-dihydroxyvitamin D-resistant rickets resulting from a mutation in the vitamin D receptor deoxyribonucleic acid-binding domain. *J Clin Endocrinol Metab*. 1994;78:313–316.

143. Fraher LJ, Karmali R, Hinde FR, et al. Vitamin D-dependent rickets type II: extreme end organ resistance to 1,25-dihydroxy vitamin D3 in a patient without alopecia. *Eur J Pediatr*. 1986;145:389–395.

144. de Baaij JH, Hoenderop JG, Bindels RJ. Magnesium in man: implications for health and disease. *Physiol Rev*. 2015;95:1–46.

145. Lamm CI, Norton KI, Murphy RJ, et al. Congenital rickets associated with magnesium sulfate infusion for tocolysis. *J Pediatr*. 1988;113:1078–1082.

146. Wedig KE, Kogan J, Schorry EK, Whitsett JA. Skeletal demineralization and fractures caused by fetal magnesium toxicity. *J Perinatol*. 2006;26:371–374.

147. Ryan MF. The role of magnesium in clinical biochemistry: an overview. *Ann Clin Biochem*. 1991;28 (Pt 1):19–26.

148. Tsang RC. Neonatal magnesium disturbances. *Am J Dis Child*. 1972;124:282–293.

149. Atkinson SA, Radde IC, Anderson GH. Macromineral balances in premature infants fed their own mothers' milk or formula. *J Pediatr*. 1983;102:99–106.

150. Sarici SU, Serdar MA, Erdem G, Alpay F. Evaluation of plasma ionized magnesium levels in neonatal hyperbilirubinemia. *Pediatr Res*. 2004;55:243–247.

151. Sarici SU, Serdar MA, Erdem G, et al. Plasma ionized magnesium levels in neonatal respiratory distress syndrome. *Biol Neonate*. 2004;86:110–115.

152. Olofsson K, Matthiesen G, Rudnicki M. Whole blood ionized magnesium in neonatal acidosis and preterm infants: a prospective consecutive study. *Acta Paediatr*. 2001;90:1398–1401.
153. Fine KD, Santa Ana CA, Porter JL, Fordtran JS. Intestinal absorption of magnesium from food and supplements. *J Clin Invest*. 1991;88:396–402.
154. Quamme GA. Recent developments in intestinal magnesium absorption. *Curr Opin Gastroenterol*. 2008;24:230–235.
155. de Baaij JH, Arjona FJ, van den Brand M, et al. Identification of SLC41A3 as a novel player in magnesium homeostasis. *Sci Rep*. 2016;6:28565.
156. Chubanov V, Gudermann T, Schlingmann KP. Essential role for TRPM6 in epithelial magnesium transport and body magnesium homeostasis. *Pflugers Arch*. 2005;451:228–234.
157. Wolf MT. Inherited and acquired disorders of magnesium homeostasis. *Curr Opin Pediatr*. 2017;29:187–198.
158. Shareghi GR, Agus ZS. Magnesium transport in the cortical thick ascending limb of Henle's loop of the rabbit. *J Clin Invest*. 1982;69:759–769.
159. Brunette MG, Vigneault N, Carriere S. Micropuncture study of magnesium transport along the nephron in the young rat. *Am J Physiol*. 1974;227:891–896.
160. Groenestege WM, Thebault S, van der Wijst J, et al. Impaired basolateral sorting of pro-EGF causes isolated recessive renal hypomagnesemia. *J Clin Invest*. 2007;117:2260–2267.
161. Kao WH, Folsom AR, Nieto FJ, et al. Serum and dietary magnesium and the risk for type 2 diabetes mellitus: the Atherosclerosis Risk in Communities Study. *Arch Intern Med*. 1999;159:2151–2159.
162. Lopez-Ridaura R, Willett WC, Rimm EB, et al. Magnesium intake and risk of type 2 diabetes in men and women. *Diabetes Care*. 2004;27:134–140.
163. Pham PC, Pham PM, Pham SV, et al. Hypomagnesemia in patients with type 2 diabetes. *Clin J Am Soc Nephrol*. 2007;2:366–373.
164. Nair AV, Hocher B, Verkaart S, et al. Loss of insulin-induced activation of TRPM6 magnesium channels results in impaired glucose tolerance during pregnancy. *Proc Natl Acad Sci USA*. 2012;109:11324–11329.
165. McNair P, Christiansen C, Transbol I. Effect of menopause and estrogen substitutional therapy on magnesium metabolism. *Miner Electrolyte Metab*. 1984;10:84–87.
166. Muneyyirci-Delale O, Nacharaju VL, Dalloul M, et al. Serum ionized magnesium and calcium in women after menopause: inverse relation of estrogen with ionized magnesium. *Fertil Steril*. 1999;71:869–872.
167. Groenestege WM, Hoenderop JG, van den Heuvel L, et al. The epithelial Mg2+ channel transient receptor potential melastatin 6 is regulated by dietary Mg2+ content and estrogens. *J Am Soc Nephrol*. 2006;17:1035–1043.
168. Suh SM, Tashjian AH Jr, Matsuo N, et al. Pathogenesis of hypocalcemia in primary hypomagnesemia: normal end-organ responsiveness to parathyroid hormone, impaired parathyroid gland function. *J Clin Invest*. 1973;52:153–160.
169. Beck N, Kim KS, Wolak M, Davis BB. Inhibition of carbonic anhydrase by parathyroid hormone and cyclic AMP in rat renal cortex in vitro. *J Clin Invest*. 1975;55:149–156.
170. Bellorin-Font E, Martin KJ. Regulation of the PTH-receptor-cyclase system of canine kidney: effects of calcium, magnesium, and guanine nucleotides. *Am J Physiol*. 1981;241:F364–F373.
171. Shaul PW, Mimouni F, Tsang RC, Specker BL. The role of magnesium in neonatal calcium homeostasis: effects of magnesium infusion on calciotropic hormones and calcium. *Pediatr Res*. 1987;22:319–323.
172. McDonald KR, Fudge NJ, Woodrow JP, et al. Ablation of calcitonin/calcitonin gene-related peptide-alpha impairs fetal magnesium but not calcium homeostasis. *Am J Physiol Endocrinol Metab*. 2004;287:E218–E226.
173. Dai LJ, Ritchie G, Kerstan D, et al. Magnesium transport in the renal distal convoluted tubule. *Physiol Rev*. 2001;81:51–84.
174. Krejs GJ, Nicar MJ, Zerwekh JE, et al. Effect of 1,25-dihydroxyvitamin D3 on calcium and magnesium absorption in the healthy human jejunum and ileum. *Am J Med*. 1983;75:973–976.
175. Wilz DR, Gray RW, Dominguez JH, Lemann J Jr. Plasma 1,25-(OH)2-vitamin D concentrations and net intestinal calcium, phosphate, and magnesium absorption in humans. *Am J Clin Nutr*. 1979;32:2052–2060.
176. Matsuzaki H, Katsumata S, Kajita Y, Miwa M. Magnesium deficiency regulates vitamin D metabolizing enzymes and type II sodium-phosphate cotransporter mRNA expression in rats. *Magnes Res*. 2013;26:83–86.
177. Matsuzaki H, Katsumata S, Maeda Y, Kajita Y. Changes in circulating levels of fibroblast growth factor 23 induced by short-term dietary magnesium deficiency in rats. *Magnes Res*. 2016;29:48–54.
178. Simsek G, Andican G, Unal E, et al. Calcium, magnesium, and zinc status in experimental hyperthyroidism. *Biol Trace Elem Res*. 1997;57:131–137.
179. Delva P, Pastori C, Degan M, et al. Intralymphocyte free magnesium in patients with primary aldosteronism: aldosterone and lymphocyte magnesium homeostasis. *Hypertension*. 2000;35:113–117.
180. He Y, Yao G, Savoia C, Touyz RM. Transient receptor potential melastatin 7 ion channels regulate magnesium homeostasis in vascular smooth muscle cells: role of angiotensin II. *Circ Res*. 2005;96:207–215.
181. Djurhuus MS, Henriksen JE, Klitgaard NA. Magnesium, sodium, and potassium content and [3H] ouabain binding capacity of skeletal muscle in relatives of patients with type 2 diabetes: effect of dexamethasone. *Metabolism*. 2002;51:1331–1339.
182. Joborn H, Akerstrom G, Ljunghall S. Effects of exogenous catecholamines and exercise on plasma magnesium concentrations. *Clin Endocrinol (Oxf)*. 1985;23:219–226.

183. Weber S, Schneider L, Peters M, et al. Novel paracellin-1 mutations in 25 families with familial hypomagnesemia with hypercalciuria and nephrocalcinosis. *J Am Soc Nephrol*. 2001;12: 1872–1881.
184. Michelis MF, Drash AL, Linarelli LG, et al. Decreased bicarbonate threshold and renal magnesium wasting in a sibship with distal renal tubular acidosis. (Evaluation of the pathophysiological role of parathyroid hormone). *Metabolism*. 1972;21:905–920.
185. Simon DB, Lu Y, Choate KA, et al. Paracellin-1, a renal tight junction protein required for paracellular Mg2+ resorption. *Science*. 1999;285:103–106.
186. Konrad M, Hou J, Weber S, et al. CLDN16 genotype predicts renal decline in familial hypomagnesemia with hypercalciuria and nephrocalcinosis. *J Am Soc Nephrol*. 2008;19:171–181.
187. Konrad M, Schaller A, Seelow D, et al. Mutations in the tight-junction gene claudin 19 (CLDN19) are associated with renal magnesium wasting, renal failure, and severe ocular involvement. *Am J Hum Genet*. 2006;79:949–957.
188. Yu AS. Claudins and the kidney. *J Am Soc Nephrol*. 2015;26:11–19.
189. Hou J, Renigunta A, Konrad M, et al. Claudin-16 and claudin-19 interact and form a cation-selective tight junction complex. *J Clin Invest*. 2008;118:619–628.
190. Hou J, Renigunta A, Gomes AS, et al. Claudin-16 and claudin-19 interaction is required for their assembly into tight junctions and for renal reabsorption of magnesium. *Proc Natl Acad Sci USA*. 2009;106:15350–15355.
191. Zimmermann B, Plank C, Konrad M, et al. Hydrochlorothiazide in CLDN16 mutation. *Nephrol Dial Transplant*. 2006;21:2127–2132.
192. Bapty BW, Dai LJ, Ritchie G, et al. Mg2+/Ca2+ sensing inhibits hormone-stimulated Mg2+ uptake in mouse distal convoluted tubule cells. *Am J Physiol*. 1998;275:F353–F360.
193. Gong Y, Renigunta V, Himmerkus N, et al. Claudin-14 regulates renal Ca(+)(+) transport in response to CaSR signalling via a novel microRNA pathway. *EMBO J*. 2012;31:1999–2012.
194. Gong Y, Himmerkus N, Plain A, et al. Epigenetic regulation of microRNAs controlling CLDN14 expression as a mechanism for renal calcium handling. *J Am Soc Nephrol*. 2015;26:663–676.
195. Zelikovic I, Szargel R, Hawash A, et al. A novel mutation in the chloride channel gene, CLCNKB, as a cause of Gitelman and Bartter syndromes. *Kidney Int*. 2003;63:24–32.
196. Rudin A. Bartter's syndrome. A review of 28 patients followed for 10 years. *Acta Med Scand*. 1988; 224:165–171.
197. Gitelman HJ, Graham JB, Welt LG. A new familial disorder characterized by hypokalemia and hypomagnesemia. *Trans Assoc Am Physicians*. 1966;79:221–235.
198. Cruz DN, Shaer AJ, Bia MJ, et al. Gitelman's syndrome revisited: an evaluation of symptoms and health-related quality of life. *Kidney Int*. 2001;59:710–717.
199. Simon DB, Nelson-Williams C, Bia MJ, et al. Gitelman's variant of Bartter's syndrome, inherited hypokalaemic alkalosis, is caused by mutations in the thiazide-sensitive Na-Cl cotransporter. *Nat Genet*. 1996;12:24–30.
200. Nozu K, Iijima K, Nozu Y, et al. A deep intronic mutation in the SLC12A3 gene leads to Gitelman syndrome. *Pediatr Res*. 2009;66:590–593.
201. Lo YF, Nozu K, Iijima K, et al. Recurrent deep intronic mutations in the SLC12A3 gene responsible for Gitelman's syndrome. *Clin J Am Soc Nephrol*. 2011;6:630–639.
202. Vargas-Poussou R, Dahan K, Kahila D, et al. Spectrum of mutations in Gitelman syndrome. *J Am Soc Nephrol*. 2011;22:693–703.
203. Schultheis PJ, Lorenz JN, Meneton P, et al. Phenotype resembling Gitelman's syndrome in mice lacking the apical Na+-Cl– cotransporter of the distal convoluted tubule. *J Biol Chem*. 1998;273:29150–29155.
204. Loffing J, Vallon V, Loffing-Cueni D, et al. Altered renal distal tubule structure and renal Na(+) and Ca(2+) handling in a mouse model for Gitelman's syndrome. *J Am Soc Nephrol*. 2004;15:2276–2288.
205. Nijenhuis T, Vallon V, van der Kemp AW, et al. Enhanced passive Ca2+ reabsorption and reduced Mg2+ channel abundance explains thiazide-induced hypocalciuria and hypomagnesemia. *J Clin Invest*. 2005;115:1651–1658.
206. Bockenhauer D, Feather S, Stanescu HC, et al. Epilepsy, ataxia, sensorineural deafness, tubulopathy, and KCNJ10 mutations. *N Engl J Med*. 2009;360:1960–1970.
207. Cross JH, Arora R, Heckemann RA, et al. Neurological features of epilepsy, ataxia, sensorineural deafness, tubulopathy syndrome. *Dev Med Child Neurol*. 2013;55:846–856.
208. Bandulik S, Schmidt K, Bockenhauer D, et al. The salt-wasting phenotype of EAST syndrome, a disease with multifaceted symptoms linked to the KCNJ10 K+ channel. *Pflugers Arch*. 2011;461: 423–435.
209. Scholl UI, Choi M, Liu T, et al. Seizures, sensorineural deafness, ataxia, mental retardation, and electrolyte imbalance (SeSAME syndrome) caused by mutations in KCNJ10. *Proc Natl Acad Sci USA*. 2009;106:5842–5847.
210. Parrock S, Hussain S, Issler N, et al. KCNJ10 mutations display differential sensitivity to heteromerisation with KCNJ16. *Nephron Physiol*. 2013;123:7–14.
211. Zhang C, Wang L, Su XT, et al. KCNJ10 (Kir4.1) is expressed in the basolateral membrane of the cortical thick ascending limb. *Am J Physiol Renal Physiol*. 2015;308:F1288–F1296.
212. Meij IC, Koenderink JB, van Bokhoven H, et al. Dominant isolated renal magnesium loss is caused by misrouting of the Na(+),K(+)-ATPase gamma-subunit. *Nat Genet*. 2000;26:265–266.
213. Glaudemans B, van der Wijst J, Scola RH, et al. A missense mutation in the Kv1.1 voltage-gated potassium channel-encoding gene KCNA1 is linked to human autosomal dominant hypomagnesemia. *J Clin Invest*. 2009;119:936–942.

20

214. Jones DH, Li TY, Arystarkhova E, et al. Na,K-ATPase from mice lacking the gamma subunit (FXYD2) exhibits altered Na+ affinity and decreased thermal stability. *J Biol Chem*. 2005;280: 19003–19011.

215. Sweadner KJ, Arystarkhova E, Donnet C, Wetzel RK. FXYD proteins as regulators of the Na,K-ATPase in the kidney. *Ann N Y Acad Sci*. 2003;986:382–387.

216. Browne DL, Gancher ST, Nutt JG, et al. Episodic ataxia/myokymia syndrome is associated with point mutations in the human potassium channel gene, KCNA1. *Nat Genet*. 1994;8:136–140.

217. Horikawa Y, Iwasaki N, Hara M, et al. Mutation in hepatocyte nuclear factor-1 beta gene (TCF2) associated with MODY. *Nat Genet*. 1997;17:384–385.

218. Clissold RL, Hamilton AJ, Hattersley AT, et al. HNF1B-associated renal and extra-renal disease-an expanding clinical spectrum. *Nat Rev Nephrol*. 2015;11:102–112.

219. Gondra L, Decramer S, Chalouhi GE, et al. Hyperechogenic kidneys and polyhydramnios associated with HNF1B gene mutation. *Pediatr Nephrol*. 2016;31:1705–1708.

220. Verhave JC, Bech AP, Wetzels JF, Nijenhuis T. Hepatocyte Nuclear Factor 1beta-Associated Kidney Disease: More than Renal Cysts and Diabetes. *J Am Soc Nephrol*. 2016;27:345–353.

221. Bockenhauer D, Jaureguiberry G. HNF1B-associated clinical phenotypes: the kidney and beyond. *Pediatr Nephrol*. 2016;31:707–714.

222. Adalat S, Woolf AS, Johnstone KA, et al. HNF1B mutations associate with hypomagnesemia and renal magnesium wasting. *J Am Soc Nephrol*. 2009;20:1123–1131.

223. Ferre S, Veenstra GJ, Bouwmeester R, et al. HNF-1B specifically regulates the transcription of the gammaa-subunit of the Na+/K+-ATPase. *Biochem Biophys Res Commun*. 2011;404:284–290.

224. Thony B, Neuheiser F, Kierat L, et al. Mutations in the pterin-4alpha-carbinolamine dehydratase (PCBD) gene cause a benign form of hyperphenylalaninemia. *Hum Genet*. 1998;103:162–167.

225. Ferre S, de Baaij JH, Ferreira P, et al. Mutations in PCBD1 cause hypomagnesemia and renal magnesium wasting. *J Am Soc Nephrol*. 2014;25:574–586.

226. Geven WB, Monnens LA, Willems JL, et al. Isolated autosomal recessive renal magnesium loss in two sisters. *Clin Genet*. 1987;32:398–402.

227. Tejpar S, Piessevaux H, Claes K, et al. Magnesium wasting associated with epidermal-growth-factor receptor-targeting antibodies in colorectal cancer: a prospective study. *Lancet Oncol*. 2007;8:387–394.

228. Paunier L, Radde IC, Kooh SW, et al. Primary hypomagnesemia with secondary hypocalcemia in an infant. *Pediatrics*. 1968;41:385–402.

229. Schlingmann KP, Weber S, Peters M, et al. Hypomagnesemia with secondary hypocalcemia is caused by mutations in TRPM6, a new member of the TRPM gene family. *Nat Genet*. 2002;31:166–170.

230. Walder RY, Landau D, Meyer P, et al. Mutation of TRPM6 causes familial hypomagnesemia with secondary hypocalcemia. *Nat Genet*. 2002;31:171–174.

231. Milla PJ, Aggett PJ, Wolff OH, Harries JT. Studies in primary hypomagnesaemia: evidence for defective carrier-mediated small intestinal transport of magnesium. *Gut*. 1979;20:1028–1033.

232. Voets T, Nilius B, Hoefs S, et al. TRPM6 forms the Mg2+ influx channel involved in intestinal and renal Mg2+ absorption. *J Biol Chem*. 2004;279:19–25.

233. Chubanov V, Waldegger S, Mederos y Schnitzler M, et al. Disruption of TRPM6/TRPM7 complex formation by a mutation in the TRPM6 gene causes hypomagnesemia with secondary hypocalcemia. *Proc Natl Acad Sci USA*. 2004;101:2894–2899.

234. Cao G, van der Wijst J, van der Kemp A, et al. Regulation of the epithelial Mg2+ channel TRPM6 by estrogen and the associated repressor protein of estrogen receptor activity (REA). *J Biol Chem*. 2009;284:14788–14795.

235. Nijenhuis T, Hoenderop JG, Bindels RJ. Downregulation of Ca(2+) and Mg(2+) transport proteins in the kidney explains tacrolimus (FK506)-induced hypercalciuria and hypomagnesemia. *J Am Soc Nephrol*. 2004;15:549–557.

236. Anast CS, Mohs JM, Kaplan SL, Burns TW. Evidence for parathyroid failure in magnesium deficiency. *Science*. 1972;177:606–608.

237. Shalev H, Phillip M, Galil A, et al. Clinical presentation and outcome in primary familial hypomagnesaemia. *Arch Dis Child*. 1998;78:127–130.

238. Stuiver M, Lainez S, Will C, et al. CNNM2, encoding a basolateral protein required for renal Mg2+ handling, is mutated in dominant hypomagnesemia. *Am J Hum Genet*. 2011;88:333–343.

239. Arjona FJ, de Baaij JH, Schlingmann KP, et al. CNNM2 mutations cause impaired brain development and seizures in patients with hypomagnesemia. *PLoS Genet*. 2014;10:e1004267.

240. Sponder G, Mastrototaro L, Kurth K, et al. Human CNNM2 is not a Mg(2+) transporter per se. *Pflugers Arch*. 2016;468:1223–1240.

241. Wilson FH, Hariri A, Farhi A, et al. A cluster of metabolic defects caused by mutation in a mitochondrial tRNA. *Science*. 2004;306:1190–1194.

242. Amanzadeh J, Reilly RF Jr. Hypophosphatemia: an evidence-based approach to its clinical consequences and management. *Nat Clin Pract Nephrol*. 2006;2:136–148.

243. Danisi G, Bonjour JP, Straub RW. Regulation of Na-dependent phosphate influx across the mucosal border of duodenum by 1,25-dihydroxycholecalciferol. *Pflugers Arch*. 1980;388:227–232.

244. Hattenhauer O, Traebert M, Murer H, Biber J. Regulation of small intestinal Na-P(i) type IIb cotransporter by dietary phosphate intake. *Am J Physiol*. 1999;277:G756–G762.

245. Hilfiker H, Hattenhauer O, Traebert M, et al. Characterization of a murine type II sodium-phosphate cotransporter expressed in mammalian small intestine. *Proc Natl Acad Sci USA*. 1998;95: 14564–14569.

246. Medicine Io, ed. *Dietary Reference Intakes for Calcium, Phosphorus, Magnesium, Vitamin D, and Fluoride*. National Academy of Sciences; 1997.

247. Virkki LV, Biber J, Murer H, Forster IC. Phosphate transporters: a tale of two solute carrier families. *Am J Physiol Renal Physiol.* 2007;293:F643–F654.

248. Villa-Bellosta R, Ravera S, Sorribas V, et al. The Na+-Pi cotransporter PiT-2 (SLC20A2) is expressed in the apical membrane of rat renal proximal tubules and regulated by dietary Pi. *Am J Physiol Renal Physiol.* 2009;296:F691–F699.

249. Villa-Bellosta R, Sorribas V. Compensatory regulation of the sodium/phosphate cotransporters NaPi-IIc (SCL34A3) and Pit-2 (SLC20A2) during Pi deprivation and acidosis. *Pflugers Arch.* 2010;459: 499–508.

250. Ansermet C, Moor MB, Centeno G, et al. Renal Fanconi Syndrome and Hypophosphatemic Rickets in the Absence of Xenotropic and Polytropic Retroviral Receptor in the Nephron. *J Am Soc Nephrol.* 2017;28:1073–1078.

251. Giovannini D, Touhami J, Charnet P, et al. Inorganic phosphate export by the retrovirus receptor XPR1 in metazoans. *Cell Rep.* 2013;3:1866–1873.

252. Legati A, Giovannini D, Nicolas G, et al. Mutations in XPR1 cause primary familial brain calcification associated with altered phosphate export. *Nat Genet.* 2015;47:579–581.

253. Gattineni J, Bates C, Twombley K, et al. FGF23 decreases renal NaPi-2a and NaPi-2c expression and induces hypophosphatemia in vivo predominantly via FGF receptor 1. *Am J Physiol Renal Physiol.* 2009;297:F282–F291.

254. Gattineni J, Baum M. Genetic disorders of phosphate regulation. *Pediatr Nephrol.* 2012;27:1477–1487.

255. Ma Y, Samaraweera M, Cooke-Hubley S, et al. Neither absence nor excess of FGF23 disturbs murine fetal-placental phosphorus homeostasis or prenatal skeletal development and mineralization. *Endocrinology.* 2014;155:1596–1605.

256. Ohata Y, Yamazaki M, Kawai M, et al. Elevated fibroblast growth factor 23 exerts its effects on placenta and regulates vitamin D metabolism in pregnancy of Hyp mice. *J Bone Miner Res.* 2014;29:1627–1638.

257. Ma Y, Kirby BJ, Fairbridge NA, et al. FGF23 Is Not Required to Regulate Fetal Phosphorus Metabolism but Exerts Effects Within 12 Hours After Birth. *Endocrinology.* 2017;158:252–263.

258. Takaiwa M, Aya K, Miyai T, et al. Fibroblast growth factor 23 concentrations in healthy term infants during the early postpartum period. *Bone.* 2010;47:256–262.

259. Kovacs CS, Manley NR, Moseley JM, et al. Fetal parathyroids are not required to maintain placental calcium transport. *J Clin Invest.* 2001;107:1007–1015.

260. Kovacs CS, Chafe LL, Fudge NJ, et al. PTH regulates fetal blood calcium and skeletal mineralization independently of PTHrP. *Endocrinology.* 2001;142:4983–4993.

261. Simmonds CS, Karsenty G, Karaplis AC, Kovacs CS. Parathyroid hormone regulates fetal-placental mineral homeostasis. *J Bone Miner Res.* 2010;25:594–605.

262. Saggese G, Baroncelli GI, Bertelloni S, Cipolloni C. Intact parathyroid hormone levels during pregnancy, in healthy term neonates and in hypocalcemic preterm infants. *Acta Paediatr Scand.* 1991;80:36–41.

263. Loughead JL, Mimouni F, Ross R, Tsang RC. Postnatal changes in serum osteocalcin and parathyroid hormone concentrations. *J Am Coll Nutr.* 1990;9:358–362.

264. Fraser DR, Kodicek E. Unique biosynthesis by kidney of a biological active vitamin D metabolite. *Nature.* 1970;228:764–766.

265. Fraser DR. Regulation of the metabolism of vitamin D. *Physiol Rev.* 1980;60:551–613.

266. Dusso AS, Brown AJ, Slatopolsky E. Vitamin D. *Am J Physiol Renal Physiol.* 2005;289:F8–F28.

267. Fraser DR, Kodicek E. Regulation of 25-hydroxycholecalciferol-1-hydroxylase activity in kidney by parathyroid hormone. *Nat New Biol.* 1973;241:163–166.

268. Gattineni J, Twombley K, Goetz R, et al. Regulation of serum 1,25(OH)2 vitamin D3 levels by fibroblast growth factor 23 is mediated by FGF receptors 3 and 4. *Am J Physiol Renal Physiol.* 2011;301:F371–F377.

269. Liu S, Tang W, Zhou J, et al. Fibroblast growth factor 23 is a counter-regulatory phosphaturic hormone for vitamin D. *J Am Soc Nephrol.* 2006;17:1305–1315.

270. Shimada T, Hasegawa H, Yamazaki Y, et al. FGF-23 is a potent regulator of vitamin D metabolism and phosphate homeostasis. *J Bone Miner Res.* 2004;19:429–435.

271. Kovacs CS, Woodland ML, Fudge NJ, Friel JK. The vitamin D receptor is not required for fetal mineral homeostasis or for the regulation of placental calcium transfer in mice. *Am J Physiol Endocrinol Metab.* 2005;289:E133–E144.

272. Noff D, Edelstein S. Vitamin D and its hydroxylated metabolites in the rat. Placental and lacteal transport, subsequent metabolic pathways and tissue distribution. *Horm Res.* 1978;9:292–300.

273. Dardenne O, Prudhomme J, Hacking SA, et al. Rescue of the pseudo-vitamin D deficiency rickets phenotype of CYP27B1-deficient mice by treatment with 1,25-dihydroxyvitamin D3: biochemical, histomorphometric, and biomechanical analyses. *J Bone Miner Res.* 2003;18:637–643.

274. Dardenne O, Prud'homme J, Hacking SA, et al. Correction of the abnormal mineral ion homeostasis with a high-calcium, high-phosphorus, high-lactose diet rescues the PDDR phenotype of mice deficient for the 25-hydroxyvitamin D-1alpha-hydroxylase (CYP27B1). *Bone.* 2003;32:332–340.

275. Dardenne O, Prud'homme J, Arabian A, et al. Targeted inactivation of the 25-hydroxyvitamin D(3)-1(alpha)-hydroxylase gene (CYP27B1) creates an animal model of pseudovitamin D-deficiency rickets. *Endocrinology.* 2001;142:3135–3141.

276. Li YC, Amling M, Pirro AE, et al. Normalization of mineral ion homeostasis by dietary means prevents hyperparathyroidism, rickets, and osteomalacia, but not alopecia in vitamin D receptor-ablated mice* * This work was supported by NIH Grants DK-46974 (to M.B.D.) and DE-04724 (to R.B.) and a NIH National Research Service Award (to Y.C.L.). *Endocrinology.* 1998;139:4391–4396.

20

277. Li YC, Pirro AE, Amling M, et al. Targeted ablation of the vitamin D receptor: an animal model of vitamin D-dependent rickets type II with alopecia. *Proc Natl Acad Sci USA*. 1997;94:9831–9835.
278. Panda DK, Miao D, Tremblay ML, et al. Targeted ablation of the 25-hydroxyvitamin D 1alpha-hydroxylase enzyme: evidence for skeletal, reproductive, and immune dysfunction. *Proc Natl Acad Sci USA*. 2001;98:7498–7503.
279. Teotia M, Teotia SP, Nath M. Metabolic studies in congenital vitamin D deficiency rickets. *Indian J Pediatr*. 1995;62:55–61.
280. Teotia M, Teotia SP. Nutritional and metabolic rickets. *Indian J Pediatr*. 1997;64:153–157.
281. Kurosu H, Ogawa Y, Miyoshi M, et al. Regulation of fibroblast growth factor-23 signaling by klotho. *J Biol Chem*. 2006;281:6120–6123.
282. Hu MC, Shi M, Zhang J, et al. Klotho: a novel phosphaturic substance acting as an autocrine enzyme in the renal proximal tubule. *FASEB J*. 2010;24:3438–3450.
283. Marsell R, Krajisnik T, Goransson H, et al. Gene expression analysis of kidneys from transgenic mice expressing fibroblast growth factor-23. *Nephrol Dial Transplant*. 2008;23:827–833.
284. Dai B, David V, Martin A, et al. A comparative transcriptome analysis identifying FGF23 regulated genes in the kidney of a mouse CKD model. *PLoS ONE*. 2012;7:e44161.
285. Carpenter TO, Insogna KL, Zhang JH, et al. Circulating levels of soluble klotho and FGF23 in X-linked hypophosphatemia: circadian variance, effects of treatment, and relationship to parathyroid status. *J Clin Endocrinol Metab*. 2010;95:E352–E357.
286. Haussler MR, Haussler CA, Whitfield GK, et al. The nuclear vitamin D receptor controls the expression of genes encoding factors which feed the "Fountain of Youth" to mediate healthful aging. *J Steroid Biochem Mol Biol*. 2010;121:88–97.
287. Tsujikawa H, Kurotaki Y, Fujimori T, et al. Klotho, a gene related to a syndrome resembling human premature aging, functions in a negative regulatory circuit of vitamin D endocrine system. *Mol Endocrinol*. 2003;17:2393–2403.
288. Segawa H, Yamanaka S, Ohno Y, et al. Correlation between hyperphosphatemia and type II Na-Pi cotransporter activity in klotho mice. *Am J Physiol Renal Physiol*. 2007;292:F769–F779.
289. Williford AL, Pare LM, Carlson GT. Bone mineral metabolism in the neonate: calcium, phosphorus, magnesium, and alkaline phosphatase. *Neonatal Netw*. 2008;27:57–63.
290. Lichtman MA, Miller DR, Cohen J, Waterhouse C. Reduced red cell glycolysis, 2, 3-diphosphoglycerate and adenosine triphosphate concentration, and increased hemoglobin-oxygen affinity caused by hypophosphatemia. *Ann Intern Med*. 1971;74:562–568.
291. Jacob HS, Amsden T. Acute hemolytic anemia with rigid red cells in hypophosphatemia. *N Engl J Med*. 1971;285:1446–1450.
292. Schubert L, DeLuca HF. Hypophosphatemia is responsible for skeletal muscle weakness of vitamin D deficiency. *Arch Biochem Biophys*. 2010;500:157–161.
293. Knochel JP. The pathophysiology and clinical characteristics of severe hypophosphatemia. *Arch Intern Med*. 1977;137:203–220.
294. Knochel JP. Hypophosphatemia and rhabdomyolysis. *Am J Med*. 1992;92:455–457.
295. Newman JH, Neff TA, Ziporin P. Acute respiratory failure associated with hypophosphatemia. *N Engl J Med*. 1977;296:1101–1103.
296. O'Connor LR, Wheeler WS, Bethune JE. Effect of hypophosphatemia on myocardial performance in man. *N Engl J Med*. 1977;297:901–903.
297. Goldfarb S, Westby GR, Goldberg M, Agus ZS. Renal tubular effects of chronic phosphate depletion. *J Clin Invest*. 1977;59:770–779.
298. ADHR Consortium. Autosomal dominant hypophosphataemic rickets is associated with mutations in FGF23. *Nat Genet*. 2000;26:345–348.
299. Econs MJ, McEnery PT, Lennon F, Speer MC. Autosomal dominant hypophosphatemic rickets is linked to chromosome 12p13. *J Clin Invest*. 1997;100:2653–2657.
300. White KE, Carn G, Lorenz-Depiereux B, et al. Autosomal-dominant hypophosphatemic rickets (ADHR) mutations stabilize FGF-23. *Kidney Int*. 2001;60:2079–2086.
301. Econs MJ, McEnery PT. Autosomal dominant hypophosphatemic rickets/osteomalacia: clinical characterization of a novel renal phosphate-wasting disorder. *J Clin Endocrinol Metab*. 1997;82:674–681.
302. Imel EA, Peacock M, Gray AK, et al. Iron modifies plasma FGF23 differently in autosomal dominant hypophosphatemic rickets and healthy humans. *J Clin Endocrinol Metab*. 2011;96:3541–3549.
303. Winters RW, Graham JB, Williams TF, et al. A genetic study of familial hypophosphatemia and vitamin D resistant rickets with a review of the literature. 1958. *Medicine (Baltimore)*. 1991;70:215–217.
304. Consortium HYP. A gene (PEX) with homologies to endopeptidases is mutated in patients with X-linked hypophosphatemic rickets. The HYP Consortium. *Nat Genet*. 1995;11:130–136.
305. Du L, Desbarats M, Viel J, et al. cDNA cloning of the murine Pex gene implicated in X-linked hypophosphatemia and evidence for expression in bone. *Genomics*. 1996;36:22–28.
306. Morgan JM, Hawley WL, Chenoweth AI, et al. Renal transplantation in hypophosphatemia with vitamin D-resistant rickets. *Arch Intern Med*. 1974;134:549–552.
307. Yamazaki Y, Okazaki R, Shibata M, et al. Increased circulatory level of biologically active full-length FGF-23 in patients with hypophosphatemic rickets/osteomalacia. *J Clin Endocrinol Metab*. 2002;87:4957–4960.
308. Liu S, Zhou J, Tang W, et al. Pathogenic role of Fgf23 in Hyp mice. *Am J Physiol Endocrinol Metab*. 2006;291:E38–E49.
309. Liu S, Guo R, Simpson LG, et al. Regulation of fibroblastic growth factor 23 expression but not degradation by PHEX. *J Biol Chem*. 2003;278:37419–37426.

310. Yuan B, Feng JQ, Bowman S, et al. Hexa-D-arginine treatment increases 7B2*PC2 activity in hyp-mouse osteoblasts and rescues the HYP phenotype. *J Bone Miner Res.* 2013;28:56–72.
311. Morey M, Castro-Feijoo L, Barreiro J, et al. Genetic diagnosis of X-linked dominant Hypophosphatemic Rickets in a cohort study: tubular reabsorption of phosphate and 1,25(OH)2D serum levels are associated with PHEX mutation type. *BMC Med Genet.* 2011;12:116.
312. Ichikawa S, Gray AK, Bikorimana E, Econs MJ. Dosage effect of a Phex mutation in a murine model of X-linked hypophosphatemia. *Calcif Tissue Int.* 2013;93:155–162.
313. Moncrieff MW. Early biochemical findings in familial hypophosphataemic, hyperphosphaturic rickets and response to treatment. *Arch Dis Child.* 1982;57:70–72.
313a. Imel EA, Zhang X, Ruppe MD, et al. Prolonged Correction of Serum Phosphorus in Adults With X-Linked Hypophosphatemia Using Monthly Doses of KRN23. *J Clin Endocrinol Metab.* 2015;100(7):2565–2573.
313b. Carpenter TO, Imel EA, Ruppe MD, et al. Randomized trial of the anti-FGF23 antibody KRN23 in X-linked hypophosphatemia. *J Clin Invest.* 2014;124(4):1587–1597.
314. Feng JQ, Ward LM, Liu S, et al. Loss of DMP1 causes rickets and osteomalacia and identifies a role for osteocytes in mineral metabolism. *Nat Genet.* 2006;38:1310–1315.
315. Lorenz-Depiereux B, Bastepe M, Benet-Pages A, et al. DMP1 mutations in autosomal recessive hypophosphatemia implicate a bone matrix protein in the regulation of phosphate homeostasis. *Nat Genet.* 2006;38:1248–1250.
316. Lorenz-Depiereux B, Schnabel D, Tiosano D, et al. Loss-of-function ENPP1 mutations cause both generalized arterial calcification of infancy and autosomal-recessive hypophosphatemic rickets. *Am J Hum Genet.* 2010;86:267–272.
317. Rutsch F, Ruf N, Vaingankar S, et al. Mutations in ENPP1 are associated with 'idiopathic' infantile arterial calcification. *Nat Genet.* 2003;34:379–381.
318. Levy-Litan V, Hershkovitz E, Avizov L, et al. Autosomal-recessive hypophosphatemic rickets is associated with an inactivation mutation in the ENPP1 gene. *Am J Hum Genet.* 2010;86:273–278.
319. Rafaelsen SH, Raeder H, Fagerheim AK, et al. Exome sequencing reveals FAM20c mutations associated with fibroblast growth factor 23-related hypophosphatemia, dental anomalies, and ectopic calcification. *J Bone Miner Res.* 2013;28:1378–1385.
320. Wang X, Wang S, Li C, et al. Inactivation of a novel FGF23 regulator, FAM20C, leads to hypophosphatemic rickets in mice. *PLoS Genet.* 2012;8:e1002708.
321. Liu S, Zhou J, Tang W, et al. Pathogenic role of Fgf23 in Dmp1-null mice. *Am J Physiol Endocrinol Metab.* 2008;295:E254–E261.
322. Lu Y, Yuan B, Qin C, et al. The biological function of DMP-1 in osteocyte maturation is mediated by its 57-kDa C-terminal fragment. *J Bone Miner Res.* 2011;26:331–340.
323. Tagliabracci VS, Engel JL, Wiley SE, et al. Dynamic regulation of FGF23 by Fam20C phosphorylation, GalNAc-T3 glycosylation, and furin proteolysis. *Proc Natl Acad Sci USA.* 2014;111:5520–5525.
324. Imel EA, Econs MJ. Fibrous dysplasia, phosphate wasting and fibroblast growth factor 23. *Pediatr Endocrinol Rev.* 2007;4(suppl 4):434–439.
325. Weinstein LS, Yu S, Warner DR, Liu J. Endocrine manifestations of stimulatory G protein alpha-subunit mutations and the role of genomic imprinting. *Endocr Rev.* 2001;22:675–705.
326. Yamamoto T, Imanishi Y, Kinoshita E, et al. The role of fibroblast growth factor 23 for hypophosphatemia and abnormal regulation of vitamin D metabolism in patients with McCune-Albright syndrome. *J Bone Miner Metab.* 2005;23:231–237.
327. Boyce AM, Bhattacharyya N, Collins MT. Fibrous dysplasia and fibroblast growth factor-23 regulation. *Curr Osteoporos Rep.* 2013;11:65–71.
328. Bhattacharyya N, Wiench M, Dumitrescu C, et al. Mechanism of FGF23 processing in fibrous dysplasia. *J Bone Miner Res.* 2012;27:1132–1141.
329. Brownstein CA, Adler F, Nelson-Williams C, et al. A translocation causing increased alpha-klotho level results in hypophosphatemic rickets and hyperparathyroidism. *Proc Natl Acad Sci USA.* 2008;105:3455–3460.
330. Lorenz-Depiereux B, et Pages A, Eckstein G, et al. Hereditary hypophosphatemic rickets with hypercalciuria is caused by mutations in the sodium-phosphate cotransporter gene SLC34A3. *Am J Hum Genet.* 2006;78:193–201.
331. Bergwitz C, Roslin NM, Tieder M, et al. SLC34A3 mutations in patients with hereditary hypophosphatemic rickets with hypercalciuria predict a key role for the sodium-phosphate cotransporter NaPi-IIc in maintaining phosphate homeostasis. *Am J Hum Genet.* 2006;78:179–192.
332. Tieder M, Modai D, Samuel R, et al. Hereditary hypophosphatemic rickets with hypercalciuria. *N Engl J Med.* 1985;312:611–617.
333. Magen D, Berger L, Coady MJ, et al. A loss-of-function mutation in NaPi-IIa and renal Fanconi's syndrome. *N Engl J Med.* 2010;362:1102–1109.
334. Topaz O, Shurman DL, Bergman R, et al. Mutations in GALNT3, encoding a protein involved in O-linked glycosylation, cause familial tumoral calcinosis. *Nat Genet.* 2004;36:579–581.
335. Frishberg Y, Ito N, Rinat C, et al. Hyperostosis-hyperphosphatemia syndrome: a congenital disorder of O-glycosylation associated with augmented processing of fibroblast growth factor 23. *J Bone Miner Res.* 2007;22:235–242.
336. Benet-Pages A, Orlik P, Strom TM, Lorenz-Depiereux B. An FGF23 missense mutation causes familial tumoral calcinosis with hyperphosphatemia. *Hum Mol Genet.* 2005;14:385–390.
337. Ichikawa S, Imel EA, Kreiter ML, et al. A homozygous missense mutation in human KLOTHO causes severe tumoral calcinosis. *J Clin Invest.* 2007;117:2684–2691.

20

CHAPTER 21

Congenital Urinary Tract Obstruction—Diagnosis and Management in the Fetus

Douglas G. Matsell, MDCM

- Fetal Kidney Development Continues Through the Late Third Trimester of Pregnancy in Humans
- A Number of In Utero Insults, Including Urinary Tract Obstruction, Can Significantly Alter Normal Nephrogenesis, Resulting in a Reduction in Nephron Number, a Disruption in Normal Glomerular and Tubular Function, and an Alteration in the Normal Structure of the Kidney
- The Timing, Location, and Severity of Obstruction Will Dictate the Likelihood of Problems in the Postnatal Period
- Severe Bladder Outlet Obstruction May Result in Severe Kidney Dysplasia, a Lack of Kidney Function, and Consequent Oligohydramnios and Pulmonary Hypoplasia
- Present Predictors of Postnatal Outcome Including Antenatal Imaging and Fetal Urine Analysis Continue to Lack Optimal Sensitivity and Specificity
- Biased and Unbiased Approaches for Identifying Fetal Biomarkers Using Small Amounts of Urine Hold Out Promise for Predicting Those Fetuses With a Poor Outcome
- While In Utero Intervention Has Been Disappointing, the Results Have Been Affected by a Lack of Standardized and Stratified Patient Selection, Due in Part to the Low Prevalence of the Problem and the Inherent Bias of Referring Physicians and Families
- As Our Diagnostic Tools Improve, So Will Our Ability to Appropriately Select Fetuses That Would Benefit From Relief of Urinary Tract Obstruction During Early Fetal Life

Introduction

Congenital kidney anomalies including those that cause urinary tract obstruction are the most common abnormalities discovered on screening antenatal ultrasounds and are the most common causes of long-term postnatal kidney problems in children. Perinatologists, neonatologists, and health care professionals caring for women with high-risk pregnancies and for preterm infants should therefore arm themselves with a working knowledge of kidney development, the effects of prenatal injury on the developing kidney, and the accuracy of antenatal assessments in predicting postnatal outcomes.

In this chapter we will review normal human kidney development with a focus on the events that occur around and after 20 weeks' gestation. This midpoint in fetal life and in fetal kidney development is the time at which most screening antenatal ultrasounds are performed and at which decisions around continuation of the pregnancy are made. We will highlight the controversies and difficulties in accurately diagnosing urinary tract obstruction in the fetus, in determining the extent and clinical relevance, if any, of this obstruction, and the limited array of valid markers in the affected fetus that accurately predict postnatal outcome.

Definitions and Scope of Congenital Urinary Tract Obstruction

Congenital urinary tract obstruction (CUTO) refers to anomalies of the developing urinary tract resulting in obstruction to urinary flow. Obstruction can occur anywhere along the urinary tract from the urethra to the developing kidney calyces (Box 21.1). Most commonly encountered and clinically significant are anomalies causing bladder outlet obstruction, which are predominant in male fetuses, and either due to a posterior urethral valve (PUV) or urethral atresia. Bladder outlet or lower urinary tract obstruction in females tends to be due to more complex anomalies such as developmental anomalies of the cloaca and in syndromes such as megacystis microcolon. CUTO due to PUV is the most common anomaly, occurring in approximately 1:3000 live male births, and is found exclusively in male fetuses.[1] It is the most common cause of chronic kidney disease in young boys and the single most common cause for needing a kidney transplant.[2,3]

The severity of kidney injury in cases with PUV is related to both the timing and the severity of the urethral obstruction. In some cases, bladder outlet obstruction is evident as early as 18 to 20 weeks' gestation, at the time of the first screening antenatal ultrasound. In other cases, the obstruction is apparent only later in gestation in the third trimester and after 32 weeks' gestation. Additionally, the severity of obstruction can vary from mild, going undetected until later in life, to severe, resulting in significant bilateral developmental kidney injury, oligohydramnios, and fetal death. The explanation for this variation in clinical phenotype is unknown. It may be related to a spectrum of alterations in the pattern of development of the urethra, including anterior fusion of the developing plicae of the prostatic and membranous urethra, lack of normal canalization of the urethra, or an anomaly in the insertion of the Wolffian duct.[1] Other anomalies include urethral atresia, which is much less common, with a prevalence of 1:30,000 births.[4] It may be seen in association with other urogenital anomalies and as part of a more extensive cloacal anomaly of development. Uretero-pelvic junction (UPJ) obstruction is the most common anatomical cause of hydronephrosis in the fetus and newborn, occurring in 1:500 to 1:2000 live births.[5] The causes of UPJ obstruction are varied, including extrinsic compression of the ureter at the level of the junction of the kidney pelvis; however, most cases are intrinsic and result from abnormal ureteric development and in the surrounding muscular layers. As with PUV and urethral obstruction, most cases of ureteric obstruction are incomplete or partial, rendering predictions of postnatal outcome and decisions around the need for surgical correction difficult. Severe UPJ obstruction also results in significant developmental kidney injury, and in cases with bilateral involvement (20%–25%), results in significant fetal morbidity and mortality. Uretero-vesico junction (UVJ) obstruction also causes hydronephrosis that may be detectable in the developing fetus. It is less common than UPJ obstruction but, like UPJ obstruction, if severe and early, it can result in significant developmental kidney injury.

Box 21.1   CAUSES OF CONGENITAL URINARY TRACT OBSTRUCTION

Bladder outlet obstruction
  Posterior urethral valve
  Urethral atresia
Megacystis microcolon
Cloacal dysgenesis
Ureteric obstruction
  Uretero-pelvic junction obstruction
  Uretero-vesico junction obstruction

Megaureter
Extrinsic compression
Ureterocoele
Syringocoele
Abdominal tumor (teratoma)
Hydrocolpos

An important consideration in the antenatal assessment of a fetus with CUTO is the potential association with other anomalies either within or outside the urinary tract, due either to a genetic syndrome where the gene mutation affects multiple sites along the urinary tract[6,7] or other organ systems,[8] or to a field defect where multiple systems are affected during development. Collectively these are referred to as CAKUT (congenital anomalies of the kidney and urinary tract). The precise number of CAKUT cases that are due to genetic mutations is unknown; however new generation sequencing approaches have identified new gene mutations in up to 23% of cases with multiple malformations and in 15% of individuals with isolated urinary tract anomalies.[9]

Antenatal Diagnosis of Congenital Urinary Tract Obstruction

The hallmark diagnostic test for urinary tract obstruction in the fetus is the identification of hydronephrosis by imaging studies. Most cases of CUTO are identified by second trimester screening ultrasound. Fetal hydronephrosis is found in approximately 1% to 5% of all pregnancies screened routinely by antenatal ultrasound.[10–13] However, not all antenatal hydronephrosis (ANH) is due to urinary tract obstruction. In fact, the majority of cases with antenatally diagnosed hydronephrosis (50%–70% of cases) have transient or functional hydronephrosis that resolves spontaneously over time with no intervention. In a meta-analysis of a large number of pregnancies screened with antenatal ultrasounds (104,572), only 1.6% had documented postnatal urinary tract pathology.[14] Importantly, in cases of documented ANH, increasing severity of hydronephrosis, as defined by an increase in antero-posterior diameter (APD) of the renal pelvis, increased the likelihood of finding postnatal pathology, and in particular, an obstructive urinary tract condition. Of the obstructive conditions, UPJ obstruction was the most common, occurring in 54.3% of cases with severe ANH (as defined as an APD > 15 mm in the third trimester), PUV occurred in 5.3%, while other causes of ureteric obstruction were seen in 5.3% of the cases. The severity of ANH, therefore, is an important determinant of the likelihood of postnatal pathology. It can be used in a standardized care plan to help direct antenatal consultation and immediate postnatal investigation and follow-up (Fig. 21.1). In particular, in cases of an isolated unilateral ANH, even in severe cases, a postnatal ultrasound before 1 month of age would be indicated to confirm the antenatal findings. In moderate to severe cases, further staged testing would be performed to evaluate the severity of obstruction, associated urinary tract anomalies, and the need for surgical consultation

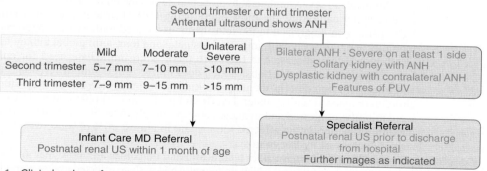

Fig. 21.1   Clinical pathway for postnatal imaging of antenatally detected hydronephrosis (ANH). In mild, moderate, and unilateral severe ANH detected in the second or third trimester, follow-up ultrasound (US) imaging should be performed in the first month after birth. Subsequent specialist referrals will depend on the severity of hydronephrosis at that point. In situations where the hydronephrosis is severe and bilateral, where the contralateral kidney is abnormal, or where there are features of posterior urethral valves (PUV), specialist referral is recommended prior to delivery and also immediately after birth. Postnatal imaging should be performed prior to discharge from hospital. (Adapted from van den Brekel A. Postnatal investigation of antenatally detected hydronephrosis. UBC Faculty of Medicine series: This Changed My Practice, 2015. http://thischangedmypractice.com/postnatal-investigation -hydronephrosis/.)

and intervention. While there is experimental evidence in animal models that supports the benefit of relieving obstruction on longer-term kidney function,[15] the indications and timing for this surgery in human fetuses are unclear and controversial. Clinical indications for surgical intervention in the postnatal period include progression of hydronephrosis on ultrasound, differential kidney function less than 40% on nuclear renogram, a drop in differential function of more than 10% on consecutive scans, or clinical complications such as febrile urinary tract infection or pain.[16] Both the severity of hydronephrosis and the loss of function in the hydronephrotic kidney are predictive of the likelihood of requiring surgery.

Fetuses in which the hydronephrosis on screening antenatal ultrasound is bilateral and severe on at least one side, where there is a solitary kidney with hydronephrosis, where there is unilateral hydronephrosis and an abnormal contralateral kidney, or where there are features of bladder outlet obstruction are at risk for the complications of kidney failure. These situations therefore require antenatal consultation with a maternal fetal specialist, pediatric nephrologist, and/or pediatric urologist (see Fig. 21.1).

Detailed ultrasound examination of the fetal urinary tract detects the majority of obstructive kidney anomalies, particularly when performed by an experienced operator.[17] Fetal magnetic resonance imaging (MRI) can complement ultrasound studies by providing a more comprehensive assessment of the fetal urinary tract,[18] which may be indicated in complex syndromes, associated CAKUT, or pregnancies with severe oligohydramnios and pulmonary hypoplasia.[19] However, predictive values of MRI for CUTO are lacking and further prospective, comparative studies in larger patient populations are needed to justify the inherent cost, and in the newborn infant, the need for sedation with MRI studies.[20]

Postnatal Outcomes of Antenatally Diagnosed Congenital Urinary Tract Obstruction

An understanding of the postnatal outcomes of the various conditions associated with fetal urinary tract obstruction is required to direct further antenatal counseling, investigation, consultation, and intervention. As discussed in the previous sections, the postnatal outcome of mild hydronephrosis is excellent and in most cases there is complete resolution of the antenatal findings, as seen in up to 97% of cases in a large prospective observational cohort.[21] Therefore, in the face of an otherwise normal fetus, the hydronephrosis can be further evaluated with postnatal ultrasound imaging within the first month after birth.

Moderate to severe unilateral hydronephrosis, on the other hand, is often indicative of underlying pathology, the most likely being UPJ obstruction. Isolated unilateral UPJ obstruction diagnosed in the fetus is not associated with increased morbidity or mortality and ultimately with impaired postnatal and long-term global kidney function or chronic kidney disease and therefore there is no immediate need for antenatal intervention. However, UPJ obstruction does impact single-unit differential function and long-term outcome in the affected kidney. In prospective follow-up studies of children diagnosed with unilateral ANH and postnatal UPJ obstruction, in cases that were initially monitored and managed conservatively, over 50% required surgery for declining function in the affected kidney and in almost 90% of those who had more severe degrees of hydronephrosis.[22]

Conditions that may affect fetal health and outcomes are those that involve both kidneys, including bilateral ANH, unilateral ANH with an affected contralateral kidney, or bladder outlet obstruction. The likelihood that the condition will be life-threatening to the fetus and will significantly impact postnatal outcome is directly related to the severity of the obstruction and the extent of injury caused to the developing kidney, that is, the degree of developmental kidney injury. The challenge is to accurately estimate the extent of this injury. These estimates will inform decisions around the continuation of the pregnancy and, potentially, decisions about intervention within the antenatal or immediate postnatal period.

The Effects of Urinary Tract Obstruction on the Developing Kidney

Urinary tract obstruction during fetal life disrupts normal kidney development. This consists of the acquisition and development of new nephrons, the functional units of the kidney, of morphogenesis, the enlargement and growth of the existing kidney structures, and of segment-specific differentiation or the development of the specific and unique functions of the kidney. Active nephrogenesis begins at about 6 to 8 weeks' gestation and continues through to 36 weeks.[23] New nephron formation results from a reciprocal induction of the ureteric duct and the pluripotent cells of the metanephric mesenchyme, derived from the embryonic mesoderm layer.[24] During that time the human fetus acquires the full complement of approximately 600,000 to 1 million nephrons. The initiation of glomerular filtration begins with vascularization of the developing glomeruli at about 8 to 10 weeks' gestation, resulting in the production of fetal urine.[25] Over the course of gestation, the full complement of glomeruli are acquired, the nephron undergoes segmental differentiation, and the nephrons grow and extend to eventually form a well-demarcated cortex and medulla region.

The acquisition of renal function also occurs during fetal gestation and mirrors the morphologic changes. Glomerular filtration begins with vascularization of the kidney and glomeruli, with the development and regulation of renal blood and plasma flow, and with the de novo expression of protein and ion transporters through the length of the nephron. The fetal kidney develops the capacity to dilute urine through the regulated reabsorption of minerals such as Na^+, K^+, Cl^-, and the capacity to concentrate the urine through the reabsorption of water through the development of water channels under the influence of the circulating hormone vasopressin.

The induction of nephrogenesis, the transition of progenitor mesenchymal cells to differentiated epithelia, and the differentiated maturation of tubular segments are all events initiated and orchestrated by a precise temporal and spatial expression of a hierarchy of genes and the proteins they encode. The fundamental importance of this expression occurs early in the development of the mammalian kidney, as early as the mesonephros stage of development where genes responsible for axial orientation and kidney cell determination are expressed.[26] The process of induction of directed gene expression occurs throughout fetal life and into the postnatal period, where genetically directed kidney tubule cell growth and differentiation continue to occur.

While the specifics of gene expression are beyond the scope of this discussion, in principle, a disruption in the normal pattern of kidney development gene expression can result in abnormally formed kidneys that function abnormally. A number of in utero events may be responsible for this disruption, including in utero exposure to toxins, gene mutations, hypoxia, protein restriction, preterm birth, and intrauterine growth restriction, among others (Fig. 21.2).[27–31] In the case of monogenic mutations, the severity of the phenotype depends on the hierarchical importance of the gene, as downstream genes controlling a multitude of essential developmental processes are also likely to be affected. More often, the developmental kidney defect is part of a polygenic disorder and is associated with a number of other phenotypic malformations.

Fetal urinary tract obstruction, like gene mutations or in utero exposure to toxins, also affects normal kidney development when it occurs during the critical stages of nephrogenesis. In addition to hydronephrosis, significant obstruction results in renal hypodysplasia (RHD), characterized by a reduction in the normal parenchyma; disrupted architecture, often with reduced formation of the medulla; a reduction in the number of glomeruli; cystic transformation of the glomeruli and tubules along the full length of the nephron; remodeling of the developing collecting ducts; and marked expansion and fibrosis of the kidney interstitium.[32–34] Mechanistically, obstruction to urinary flow disrupts the normal induction of nephrons, leading to a glomerular deficit and abnormally formed glomeruli, a proximal tubular deficit and alteration in segment-determining genes, and a remodeling of the collecting duct with alteration in the normal cell populations.[35] In addition, obstruction of urinary flow in both the proximal tubule and the collecting duct causes a phenotypic change in the epithelia,

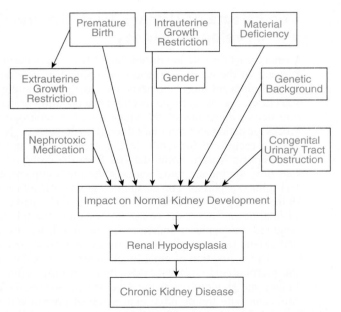

Fig. 21.2 Antenatal factors that influence fetal kidney outcomes. Urinary tract obstruction, in addition to a number of other antenatal insults, can affect long-term kidney outcome in the fetus. Severe obstruction disrupts normal nephrogenesis, resulting in a decrease in nephron endowment and consequent predisposition to chronic kidney disease.

with the formation of peritubular smooth muscle collars, remodeling of the pericyte and peritubular capillary network, and recruitment and expansion of the interstitial fibroblast population.

The Effects of Urinary Tract Obstruction on Fetal Kidney Function

Given its effects on the normal development of kidney architecture, urinary tract obstruction in the fetus impacts both fetal and postnatal kidney function. However, kidney function in the fetus is difficult to determine, given developmental changes over gestation, the complexity and array of functional changes, the interposition of the placenta, and the technical and ethical limitations of studying and sampling fetal blood and urine. Our knowledge of normal human fetal kidney function has been extrapolated from experimental animal models, postnatal observations in preterm human infants, and from histopathologic analyses of human fetal kidneys. Unlike in the newborn infant, the effects of obstruction on kidney function at specific times of fetal evaluation have not been well described. Most routine antenatal screening ultrasounds occur at 18 to 20 weeks' gestation; significant urinary tract obstruction at that time manifests as hydronephrosis, hydroureters, and bladder and urethral anomalies. While these effects on kidney anatomy are easily appreciated, their effects on actual "real-time" kidney function may be difficult to measure.

The development of normal fetal kidney function involves the acquisition of normal glomerular numbers that determine normal fetal glomerular filtration rate (GFR), of mechanisms that regulate this fetal GFR, and of fetal kidney tubular function, that are responsible for the establishment and maintenance of Na^+, H_2O, and acid-base balance.

Development of glomeruli, the glomerular vasculature, and the glomerular filtration barrier occurs between 8 and 36 weeks' gestation in humans.[36] Fetal GFR increases steadily over this time, reflecting new nephron development, an increase in the number of glomeruli, and, most importantly, an increase in glomerular surface area.[37–39]

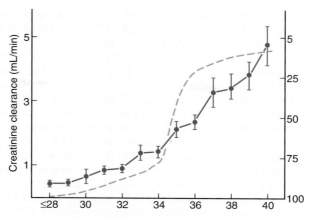

Fig. 21.3 Relationship between fetal glomerular filtration rate (GFR) and fetal kidney weight and gestational age. Pattern of change in GFR and persistence of the nephrogenic zone of the human fetal kidney cortex. As the gestational age increases, the nephrogenic zone decreases and disappears by 36 weeks' gestation. This is associated with a corresponding increase in GFR as reflected by creatinine clearance. Data from 205 neonates, N ranging from 7 to 26 in each group at different gestational ages. (Reproduced with permission from Trnka P, Hiatt MJ, Tarantal AF, Matsell DG. Congenital urinary tract obstruction: defining markers of developmental kidney injury. *Pediatr Res.* 2012;72:446-454.)

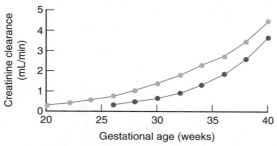

Gestational age (weeks)

Fig. 21.4 Increase in fetal glomerular filtration rate (GFR) during gestation. Creatinine clearance was calculated from fetal urine and blood sample values during fetal life and in preterm infants, and used as a surrogate measure of fetal GFR. In both the fetus *(lighter dots, upper line)* and in the preterm infant *(darker dots, lower line)*, creatinine clearance increased with increasing gestational age. (Reproduced with permission from Haycock GB. Development of glomerular filtration and tubular sodium reabsorption in the human fetus and newborn. *Br J Urol.* 1998;81 Suppl 2:33-38.)

After the completion of nephrogenesis, GFR rapidly increases during the later stages of gestation,[40] due in part to the enlargement of the glomeruli and filtration area with increase in body mass of the fetus,[41,42] and to renal blood redistribution and recruitment of the outer cortical nephrons (Fig. 21.3).[43] While the absolute creatinine clearance (a standard measure of kidney function) for a 20 weeks' gestation fetus is estimated to be less than 1 mL/min, over the subsequent period of nephrogenesis, and at term, the GFR increases approximately fivefold to 4 to 5 mL/min (Fig. 21.4).[36]

In addition to being due to an increase in the number of functional glomeruli, the increase in fetal GFR also results from developmental changes in the variables that determine single nephron function: an increase in mean arterial pressure, which increases glomerular capillary hydrostatic pressure[44,45]; an increase in renal blood flow[46-49]; and a decrease in renal vascular resistance.[50,51] In turn, regulators of normal fetal GFR physiology also undergo maturational changes during fetal life, including an upregulation of the components of the renin-angiotensin system, which controls systemic blood pressure by maintaining systemic and renal vascular resistance[52,53]; the sympathetic nervous system, which increases renal vascular resistance, preferentially increasing the afferent arteriolar tone of the fetal glomerulus and decreasing GFR[54]; and endothelin, prostaglandins (PGE2, PGD2, and PGI2), and nitric oxide, which are important fetal kidney vasoregulators.[55-59]

As the fetal kidney develops glomerular function it also acquires complex, differentiated, segment-specific tubular function. Fetal kidneys are unable to fully dilute and concentrate urine.[60,61] Urine concentrating ability increases with increasing gestational age, reflecting the fetal kidney's increased responsiveness to antidiuretic hormone,[62,63] water channel development,[64-66] and renal medullary maturation.[67-70] Important changes also occur in sodium transport. Urinary sodium losses, as reflected by the fractional excretion of sodium (FENa), decrease with increasing gestational age and fetal kidney maturity. The FENa in term infants is less than 1%, while in preterm and small-for-gestational-age infants it approaches 2.4%, being higher in more preterm infants (Fig. 21.5).[71,72] Likewise, a number of maturational changes occur in sodium handling in the developing fetal kidney,[73] including an increase in the abundance of sodium transporters (Na-K-ATPase, NHE3 exchanger, Na-K-2Cl cotransporter, and the ENaC channel),[74-79] enhanced paracellular transport,[80] increased responsiveness to circulating hormones,[81-83] and a postnatal decrease in circulating atrial natriuretic peptide.[84] The capacity of the fetal kidney to regulate acid-base balance is less than in the adult kidney, but increases with gestational age.[85-87] In the proximal tubule, the expression of the sodium transporters NHE3, Na-K-ATPase, and type IV carbonic anhydrase increase with kidney maturation.[88-90] Similarly, the fetal kidney has a reduced ability to secrete both organic and inorganic acids.[91] In the fetal cortical collecting duct, the intercalated cell population, in particular the alpha-intercalated cells responsible for acid excretion, is significantly reduced compared to the postnatal kidney.[92,93]

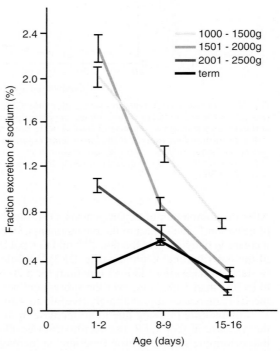

Fig. 21.5 Changes in sodium excretion in the developing kidney. At birth, urinary sodium losses, measured by the fractional excretion of sodium (FENa), decrease with increasing gestational age. For example, the FENa is significantly higher in the infant born between 1000 and 1500 g (*lightest red line*) than in the term infant (*black line*). In the preterm and low-birth-weight infant, the fractional excretion of sodium decreases after birth and by 2 to 3 weeks approaches that of the term infant. (Modified from Bueva A, Guignard JP. Renal function in preterm neonates. *Pediatr Res.* 1994;36:572-577.)

The precise effects of obstruction on these various elements of normal kidney function in the human fetus have not been described, but can be extrapolated from observations in infants born with urinary tract obstruction, particularly those born preterm, from autopsy specimens of fetuses with severe bladder outlet obstruction, and from experimental animal models. In a large cohort of children with RHD and small kidneys, PUV was responsible for approximately 30% of the cases, while other forms of CAKUT, including cases of hydronephrosis, were responsible for another 25%.[8] Similarly in children with PUV, approximately 75% have been shown to have at least one small kidney when evaluated postnatally.[94] These observations support the experimental evidence that urinary tract obstruction results in a nephron deficit, which translates into a decrease in fetal GFR and predisposes to postnatal progression of chronic kidney disease. While in experimental animals the expression of regulatory factors of GFR is altered, with persistent fetal expression of renin in the microvasculature,[95] activation of the RAS,[96] and downregulation of eNOS[97] in the obstructed developing kidney, similar studies in human fetuses are lacking.

In human and nonhuman primate fetuses, urinary tract obstruction causes substantial collecting duct tubular injury and has a particular effect on collecting duct development and postnatal function. This is reflected in collecting duct epithelial remodeling noted in early fetal life, with a dropout of normal intercalated cell populations evident by late gestation.[35,98] Similarly, proximal tubule epithelial cell injury has been reported with abundant cell death in obstructed developing rat kidneys. The functional consequences of these injuries on tubular function are difficult to quantify in the fetus. However in newborn infants, affected by severe PUV, particularly those born preterm, alterations in kidney function are commonly seen, including a decrease in GFR, and tubular abnormalities including polyuria (due to a defect in concentrating ability), urinary salt wasting (due to a decrease in tubular Na^+ reabsorption), and metabolic acidosis (due to an altered expression in collecting duct intercalated cell expression).

The Measurement of Fetal Kidney Function

The evaluation of fetal kidney function is complex, imperfect, and controversial. Precise evaluation of fetal kidney function, however, would enable an estimate of the severity of injury at the time of evaluation and help with further discussions around immediate and postnatal prognosis. Estimates of fetal kidney health and function include imaging studies, fetal blood and urine sample estimates of fetal GFR, and amniotic fluid (AF) sampling, including the concentrations of analytes, fluid volumes, and fetal urine flow rates.

Screening ultrasound during the second trimester of pregnancy identifies most cases of severe CUTO. Occasionally, the obstruction becomes clinically significant in later stages of pregnancy. Most cases of significant upper and lower urinary tract obstruction affecting one or both kidneys are associated with hydronephrosis. Lower tract obstruction, and in particular bladder outlet obstruction, can also result in posterior urethral dilatation (keyhole sign) and bladder involvement with a distended thick-walled bladder. The ultrasound findings of significant obstruction are correlated with the underlying histopathologic changes. Increased echogenicity of the affected kidneys reflects parenchymal disruption, a poorly defined cortico-medullary border reflects abnormal kidney architecture and underdevelopment or hypoplasia of the renal medulla, and cystic changes reflect tubular dilatation and cystic transformation of the injured developing tubules. All of these ultrasound findings are indicative of abnormal kidney development resulting from the effects of obstruction to urinary flow in the developing kidney.[99]

While radiologic imaging of the fetal kidney is an imperfect measure of kidney function, direct measurement of fetal GFR would be an ideal determinant. However, estimating fetal GFR is technically challenging given the need for fetal blood sampling. Consequently, there are limited normative data in uncomplicated pregnancies. In humans, fetal GFR has been estimated as early as 20 weeks' gestation.[36,100–102] Fetal blood levels of β_2-microglobulin, the light chain of the class I major histocompatibility antigens, have been used to estimate fetal GFR.[103–107] Fetuses with urinary tract obstruction have been shown to have higher serum levels than those without obstruction, reflecting a decrease in urinary clearance as a result of kidney injury, and β_2-microglobulin is a better predictor of postnatal kidney function than either α_1-microglobulin or cystatin C.[107] In a cohort of fetuses with urinary tract malformations including urinary tract obstruction, a fetal serum β_2-microglobulin above the cutoff of 5.6 mg/L had a sensitivity of 80%, a specificity of 98.6%, a positive predictive value of 88.9%, and a negative predictive value of 97.1% for postnatal renal failure.[103] The usefulness of β_2-microglobulin is hampered by the lack of robust normative data, resulting from sampling of a small number of patients, by measurements at different stages of gestation, and by variable measures of outcome.

More commonly, the concentrations of fetal urine electrolytes have been used in the antenatal evaluation of fetal kidney function in fetuses identified with significant lower urinary tract obstruction. In the developing fetal kidney, the ability to reabsorb electrolytes such as Na^+, Cl^-, Ca^{2+}, and water increases with increasing gestational age. In the cases of kidney injury that occurs during kidney development, this tubular reabsorption is presumably impaired, resulting in higher than normal urinary concentrations. Fetal urinary values have been correlated with clinical outcomes, kidney histology, and postnatal kidney function.[106,108–116] Significant kidney injury resulting in impaired postnatal function is associated with high fetal concentrations of electrolytes (high specificity, low false positive rate), but these electrolyte findings have low sensitivity to predict outcome (high false-negative rate).[117] A recent comprehensive systematic review of the published studies of fetal urine analysis revealed that there is currently no individual analyte or threshold which, as a diagnostic test, can accurately predict postnatal renal function.[118] The studies reviewed were hampered by selection bias, by small numbers, by variation in the thresholds of the most widely investigated analytes, and by lack of correlation with gestational age. The value of fetal urine, fetal blood, or AF cystatin C levels in assessing fetal kidney function is unknown. During normal pregnancy, AF cystatin C levels decrease with increasing gestational age, but are increased in pregnancies associated with fetal uropathy.[119]

Fetal urinary flow rates and AF volume have also been used as indirect measures of fetal GFR during the second half of pregnancy and can be calculated from changes in fetal bladder volumes on repeat ultrasound examinations over time.[120,121] In the early fetal period, most of the AF is produced by the amnion, placenta, and umbilical cord. AF volume increases from approximately 25 mL at 10 weeks' gestation to approximately 400 mL at 20 weeks' gestation when fetal kidneys become the main source, although the total volume of AF can vary substantially. By 28 weeks' gestation, AF volume reaches a plateau of approximately 800 mL until term, with a slight decline postterm.[122] Any impairment of fetal kidney function, including urinary tract obstruction, will manifest as oligohydramnios from mid-trimester onwards; however, this is a coarse estimation of absolute fetal GFR with poor correlation with actual GFR.

The Prediction of Postnatal Outcome

Antenatal ultrasound evaluation of the developing fetus has become routine care in the management of healthy pregnancies. Consequently, urinary tract abnormalities, including those that result in urinary tract obstruction, are being diagnosed in utero. Before the advent of antenatal screening, the clinical presentation of these conditions was variable, from in utero death, death in the immediate postnatal period from respiratory or kidney failure, presentation later in life with various stages of chronic kidney disease (CKD) or with recurrent urinary tract infections, pyelonephritis, urosepsis, or voiding abnormalities, to being entirely asymptomatic and having the kidney anomaly diagnosed serendipitously. The value therefore of an antenatal diagnosis of urinary tract obstruction in a fetus is the potential to predict the postnatal prognosis and risk for death, CKD, or the need for dialysis and transplantation; the usefulness of helping plan postnatal management including support, consultation, and further investigation around the time of delivery; and planning and counseling around the decision to continue the pregnancy.

In order to predict postnatal outcomes in fetuses with urinary tract obstruction, the antenatal assessment needs to be stratified according to the type of kidney anomaly. Unilateral obstructive anomalies, such as UPJ or UVJ obstruction, a duplicate ureter with ureterocoele, or a multicystic dysplastic kidney, rarely need intervention in the antenatal period and are rarely associated with mortality in the fetal or immediate neonatal period. As previously discussed, these anomalies sometimes involve other organ systems, as seen in a number of genetic syndromes; this should be considered in the antenatal evaluation.

Unilateral ureteric obstruction can affect normal development, function, and outcome of the affected kidney. Like lower tract obstruction, not all obstructions affect outcome, so therefore, not all obstructions need intervention. In severe cases of unilateral kidney obstruction, there is no immediate indication for fetal surgical intervention, given the technical challenges and the risk of surgery to the fetus and the mother, which outweighs the potential for improvement in long-term postnatal outcome. Even in the postnatal period, the selection of cases ultimately "needing" surgery is not well defined, but those who do proceed to surgery do so after an extended period of investigation and observation, during which time the severity of hydronephrosis and change in differential kidney function are monitored. Surgery in the first year is uncommon and often related to developing complications such as infection and pyelonephritis rather than preserving of kidney function.[16,22]

Long-term observational studies in children with isolated solitary kidneys, due to nongenetic forms of renal agenesis, unilateral nephrectomy, or multicystic dysplastic kidney, have demonstrated an increased risk for long-term kidney complications, including loss of kidney function over time.[123–126] Factors that predict a poorer outcome in these children include the association of other anatomical anomalies and the lack of compensatory growth in the solitary kidney. Similarly in the fetus, a lack of compensatory growth of the kidney contralateral to the obstruction would signal significant compromised development, which would put the fetus at long-term risk of progressive kidney injury in the postnatal period. While not affecting the immediate management of the fetus in utero, it would indicate the need for closer long-term follow-up after birth.

More concerning is the fetus with both kidneys affected by the urinary tract obstruction, as seen in bladder outlet obstruction due to PUV, in bilateral ureteric obstruction, as seen in bilateral UPJ obstructions, megaureters, large bladder ureterocoeles obstructing both kidneys, or in a solitary kidney with any degree of urinary tract obstruction. CUTO due to PUV is the single most important cause of CKD and end-stage renal disease (ESRD) in young boys.[3,123,127–133] A number of clinical characteristics in the postnatal period have been associated with a poor outcome in these boys, including delayed diagnosis and surgical intervention,[134,135] the presence of high-grade vesicoureteral reflux,[128,132] impaired kidney function when evaluated postnatally at various times,[130,136] an elevated nadir serum creatinine,[137] and upper-tract surgical diversion.[94] A lower than normal estimated GFR 1 year after birth[133,138] or a best postnatal estimated GFR less than 60 mL/min per 1.73 m^2 is associated with developing end-stage renal disease.[94] While these findings emphasize important postnatal factors that predict outcome in CUTO, they also highlight the importance of prenatal kidney injury in the pathogenesis of progressive renal failure.[139–143]

Prediction of outcome based on fetal characteristics is more difficult and less accurate. The typical antenatal ultrasound findings of PUV include a male fetus, oligohydramnios, a thickened bladder wall with a dilated posterior urethra, hydroureteronephrosis, and renal parenchymal changes, which may be apparent as early as the first screening ultrasound at 18 to 20 weeks' gestation. These features in various combinations and with varying severity have been used to predict outcome, to select cases for in utero intervention, and to decide about pregnancy termination. Their value in predicting postnatal and long-term kidney outcome, however, is still unclear given that published reports are heterogeneous, retrospective in nature, have small sample sizes, and lack standardized measures of long-term outcome.[108,130,139,144–156] The antenatal ultrasound parameter with the best predictive accuracy for postnatal kidney function is the presence of oligohydramnios. Despite its qualitative nature, a history of oligohydramnios during pregnancy in studies without a specified threshold has a high predictive accuracy (sensitivity 0.75–1.0, specificity 0.67–0.75) for impaired kidney function in the postnatal period[157] and for ESRD in boys with PUV.[94] Renal cortical parenchymal appearance, including renal cystic changes and increased kidney echogenicity, has the best predictive value for postnatal renal function in survivors.[157] In a large contemporaneous single-center cohort with a well-defined outcome, measures of end-stage renal disease and CKD, oligohydramnios, and renal parenchymal injury (renal cortical cysts and increased renal echogenicity) had a high positive likelihood ratio to predict postnatal ESRD, with a high test specificity and significantly increased odds and hazard ratios.[94] While these features may not help to inform the selection of cases for in utero vesico-amniotic shunting,[158] they have value in predicting poor long-term kidney outcome. This information is vital in discussions around pregnancy counseling for the parents of a fetus with PUV, as the decision to terminate their pregnancy is often based on a prediction of the long-term kidney prognosis.

Strategies to identify biomarkers other than ultrasound findings and urine electrolytes in the fetus affected by urinary tract obstruction include both biased and unbiased approaches. Biased approaches attempt to measure the changes in the production or expression of a particular biologic product shown, through other experimental systems or models, to be involved in the pathogenesis of the disease. The characteristics of ideal biomarkers of developmental kidney injury have recently been reviewed.[41] In CUTO, the histopathologic characteristics of kidney injury depend on multiple factors, such as the anatomical site, severity, completeness, and duration of the obstruction. A number of animal models have helped define the histopathologic changes which occur with severe, early, and often complete ureteric obstruction,[159] including marked alteration in normal kidney development, with small kidneys, cyst formation from all segments of the nephron, abnormal glomerular development and final glomerular number, and underdevelopment of the renal medulla, while obstruction later in gestation causes hydronephrosis without these changes.[32,160–162] In particular, the nonhuman primate model of obstructive nephropathy[34] highlights the significant decrease in glomerular number[30] and tubulointerstitial changes associated with fetal urinary tract obstruction.[98] These experimental findings mirror the changes seen in the obstructed human fetal kidney.[163]

The pathogenesis of developmental kidney injury in the obstructed fetal kidney therefore involves a reduction in glomerular number, marked tubular epithelial injury and reorganization, and extensive interstitial remodeling and fibrosis. These characteristics can be used to inform a biased approach to developing fetal biomarkers to predict postnatal outcome. It is currently not possible to accurately approximate the number of glomeruli in the kidney at any stage of gestation or the extent of tubulointerstitial damage caused by obstruction. A number of key proteins in these events, however, are altered or differentially expressed in obstructed fetal kidneys[98,163] and can be measured in whole urine and exosomes in children with obstructive nephropathy.[41,164] The change in urinary excretion of select proteins can reflect the severity of epithelial injury, as seen, for example, with scaffolding transmembrane epithelial proteins involved in cell-cell adhesion, with a decrease in normal E-cadherin and N-cadherin excretion, and in an increase in L1 cell adhesion molecule (L1CAM) excretion. Similarly, flow-sensing epithelial proteins such as the transient receptor potential cation channel subfamily V member 4 (TRPV4) are also increased in the urine of cases with urinary obstruction.[164] Other potential candidate biomarker proteins include changes in the excretion of mesenchymal proteins such as vimentin and α-smooth muscle actin, proteins expressed specifically by differentiated principal and intercalated cells of the collecting duct including aquaporin-2 and vacuolar-type H^+-ATPase,[164] components of the renin-angiotensin system,[165] inflammatory markers including monocyte chemotactic peptide-1,[166,167] or adhesion molecules such as intercellular adhesion molecule-1.[168] Several studies have confirmed the utility of elevated urinary transforming growth factor-β excretion as a marker of the severity of renal dysplasia in both upper and lower urinary tract obstruction in the postnatal period[169–172] and as a biomarker of prenatal developmental kidney injury.[164]

For various reasons, including the difficulty and safety of obtaining antenatal fetal kidney tissue samples and the limited quantity of fetal urine available for study, studies of the correlations of fetal candidate biomarkers and postnatal outcome are lacking. In boys with PUV, the urinary excretion of transforming growth factor-β and L1CAM measured postnatally was shown to correlate with the progression of CKD and the development of ESRD.[164]

Similarly, there are limited data on unbiased approaches to studying potential fetal kidney proteins that predict outcome. Recently, Klein et al. employed capillary electrophoresis coupled with mass spectrometry (which required only 150 μl of fetal urine) to analyze the urinary peptidome of fetuses with PUV, in an attempt to discriminate those fetuses at risk of early end-stage renal disease.[173] Twenty-six peptides were identified from a total of over 4000 candidates. The peptide biomarker profile had high predictive value for mortality and for postnatal end-stage renal disease in the PUV group. Interestingly, of the 26 peptides identified, 25 were collagen peptides, and all increased in abundance in the urine of obstructed fetuses.

In a different approach to defining the fetal urinary proteome, candidate proteins were identified by antibody array and quantified with enzyme-linked immunosorbent assay from the urine of preterm infants immediately after birth and compared after 12 months of postnatal maturation. Preterm infants at birth were found to have elevated levels of insulin-like growth factor binding protein-1, -2, and -6, monocyte chemotactic protein-1, CD14, and sialic acid-binding Ig-like lectin 5, which declined to levels similar to those of full-term infants by 2 to 6 months of life. While cases of fetal urinary tract obstruction were not included, the results highlighted that normal urinary protein patterns change over time with nephrogenesis and renal maturation.[174]

In Utero Intervention

The aim of antenatal intervention in lower urinary tract obstruction is to relieve obstruction in fetuses that would benefit from such shunting.[41] In most cases, the decision to proceed with surgery, as well as the decision to terminate the pregnancy, has been based in part on the results of fetal imaging and of fetal urine and AF analysis. Given the limited sensitivity and specificity of the studies used to predict long-term kidney outcomes, there has been difficulty in predicting and selecting cases that would benefit from intervention. Over the past 30 years, a number of centers have reported their experience with in utero surgery for lower urinary tract obstruction. A large systematic review of 16 observational and 7 controlled studies involving 342 cases demonstrated that vesico-amniotic shunting improved perinatal survival when compared to no intervention (OR 2.53, 95% CI 1.08–5.93).[175] However, many of the studies suffered from site-specific selection bias, small sample size, and none of the studies identified in the systematic review were randomized trials. A large single-center retrospective review studied the outcomes of pregnancies complicated by urinary tract obstruction and oligohydramnios in which vesico-amniotic shunting was performed. Not surprisingly, given the inherent drawbacks of the selection criteria, they report a 47% perinatal survival after successful shunting; however, 40% of survivors developed end-stage renal disease on follow-up.[176] Similarly, long-term outcome studies show a high prevalence of bladder dysfunction requiring regular catheterization or placement of a vesicostomy, urinary tract infections, and the development of asthma and recurrent respiratory infections due to pulmonary hypoplasia.[177] Thus, fetal urinary diversion has not resulted in the anticipated improvement in outcomes in pregnancies complicated by severe CUTO.

Recently, the PLUTO (Percutaneous vesico-amniotic shunting versus conservative management for fetal lower urinary tract obstruction) study analyzed the survival benefit of in utero intervention in fetuses with bladder outlet obstruction.[158] This was a multicenter, international, nonrandomized cohort of pregnancies with a planned sample size of 150, which was stopped after 31 women were enrolled because of poor recruitment. There were no differences in the severity of oligohydramnios, hydronephrosis, cortical cysts, or kidney echogenicity in fetuses between the treatment and nontreatment groups. Although the treated group may have had a slight survival advantage, there were no differences in the longer-term kidney outcomes in both groups, suggesting that these antenatal features may not be useful in identifying those fetuses that may benefit from in utero bladder decompression. As highlighted by Morris et al., given the logistic problems with recruitment, as well as physician and patient biases and preferences, as well as the low incidence of lower urinary tract obstruction (LUTO), future prospective randomized intervention trials for this condition will be challenging.[178] The ideal study would be able to stratify the patients according to an antenatal assessment of severity of obstruction to analyze the effects of intervention. The previous studies have been challenged by their retrospective nature, their small numbers, by center-specific selection bias, and a lack of standardized inclusion and exclusion criteria. To demonstrate the benefit of in utero surgery, a precise estimate of kidney injury at the time of intervention is required. Not all fetuses with obstruction need intervention, as their obstruction is mild and not associated with long-term ESRD. Some fetuses are severely affected by the obstruction with severe kidney dysplasia and oligohydramnios (which may be related to the gestational age when the obstruction is detected) and would not benefit from intervention, as the injury is irreversible and not salvageable. The challenge is to identify those fetuses with significant obstruction that is detected early, which can be assessed to be impacting further development and long-term outcome, but in whom the existing kidney structure and function at the time of evaluation appear salvageable.

REFERENCES

1. Farrugia MK. Fetal bladder outlet obstruction: embryopathology, in utero intervention and outcome. *J Pediatr Urol.* 2016;12(5):296–303.
2. Wong CS, Pierce CB, Cole SR, et al. Association of proteinuria with race, cause of chronic kidney disease, and glomerular filtration rate in the chronic kidney disease in children study. *Clin J Am Soc Nephrol.* 2009;4(4):812–819.
3. Ardissino G, Dacco V, Testa S, et al. Epidemiology of chronic renal failure in children: data from the ItalKid project. *Pediatrics.* 2003;111(4 Pt 1):e382–e387.
4. Malin G, Tonks AM, Morris RK, et al. Congenital lower urinary tract obstruction: a population-based epidemiological study. *BJOG.* 2012;119(12):1455–1464.
5. Becker A, Baum M. Obstructive uropathy. *Early Hum Dev.* 2006;82(1):15–22.
6. Sanyanusin P, Schimmenti LA, McNoe LA, et al. Mutation of the PAX2 gene in a family with optic nerve colobomas, renal anomalies and vesicoureteral reflux. *Nat Genet.* 1995;9(4):358–364.
7. Abdelhak S, Kalatzis V, Heilig R, et al. A human homologue of the Drosophila eyes absent gene underlies branchio-oto-renal (BOR) syndrome and identifies a novel gene family. *Nat Genet.* 1997;15(2):157–164.
8. Matsell DG, Cojocaru D, Matsell EW, Eddy AA. The impact of small kidneys. *Pediatr Nephrol.* 2015;30(9):1501–1509.
9. Sanna-Cherchi S, Kiryluk K, Burgess KE, et al. Copy-number disorders are a common cause of congenital kidney malformations. *Am J Hum Genet.* 2012;91(6):987–997.
10. Blyth B, Snyder HM, Duckett JW. Antenatal diagnosis and subsequent management of hydronephrosis. *J Urol.* 1993;149(4):693–698.
11. Gunn TR, Mora JD, Pease P. Antenatal diagnosis of urinary tract abnormalities by ultrasonography after 28 weeks' gestation: incidence and outcome. *Am J Obstet Gynecol.* 1995;172(2 Pt 1):479–486.
12. Livera LN, Brookfield DS, Egginton JA, Hawnaur JM. Antenatal ultrasonography to detect fetal renal abnormalities: a prospective screening programme. *BMJ.* 1989;298(6685):1421–1423.
13. Sairam S, Al-Habib A, Sasson S, Thilaganathan B. Natural history of fetal hydronephrosis diagnosed on mid-trimester ultrasound. *Ultrasound Obstet Gynecol.* 2001;17(3):191–196.
14. Lee RS, Cendron M, Kinnamon DD, Nguyen HT. Antenatal hydronephrosis as a predictor of postnatal outcome: a meta-analysis. *Pediatrics.* 2006;118(2):586–593.
15. Chevalier RL, Thornhill BA, Chang AY, et al. Recovery from release of ureteral obstruction in the rat: relationship to nephrogenesis. *Kidney Int.* 2002;61(6):2033–2043.
16. Longpre M, Nguan A, Macneily AE, Afshar K. Prediction of the outcome of antenatally diagnosed hydronephrosis: a multivariable analysis. *J Pediatr Urol.* 2012;8(2):135–139.
17. Robyr R, Benachi A, Daikha-Dahmane F, et al. Correlation between ultrasound and anatomical findings in fetuses with lower urinary tract obstruction in the first half of pregnancy. *Ultrasound Obstet Gynecol.* 2005;25(5):478–482.
18. Martin C, Darnell A, Duran C, et al. Magnetic resonance imaging of the intrauterine fetal genitourinary tract: normal anatomy and pathology. *Abdom Imaging.* 2004;29(3):286–302.
19. Kajbafzadeh AM, Payabvash S, Sadeghi Z, et al. Comparison of magnetic resonance urography with ultrasound studies in detection of fetal urogenital anomalies. *J Pediatr Urol.* 2008;4(1):32–39.

20. McMann LP, Kirsch AJ, Scherz HC, et al. Magnetic resonance urography in the evaluation of prenatally diagnosed hydronephrosis and renal dysgenesis. *J Urol.* 2006;176(4 Pt 2):1786–1792.
21. Madden-Fuentes RJ, McNamara ER, Nseyo U, et al. Resolution rate of isolated low-grade hydronephrosis diagnosed within the first year of life. *J Pediatr Urol.* 2014;10(4):639–644.
22. Chertin B, Pollack A, Koulikov D, et al. Conservative treatment of ureteropelvic junction obstruction in children with antenatal diagnosis of hydronephrosis: lessons learned after 16 years of follow-up. *Eur Urol.* 2006;49(4):734–738.
23. Quaggin SE, J K. Embryology of the kidney. In: Brenner BM, ed. *Brenner and Rector's The Kidney.* Vol. 1. 8th ed. Philadelphia: Saunders Elsevier; 2008:1–24.
24. Dressler GR. The cellular basis of kidney development. *Annu Rev Cell Dev Biol.* 2006;22:509–529.
25. Dressler GR. Advances in early kidney specification, development and patterning. *Development.* 2009;136(23):3863–3874.
26. Narlis M, Grote D, Gaitan Y, et al. Pax2 and pax8 regulate branching morphogenesis and nephron differentiation in the developing kidney. *J Am Soc Nephrol.* 2007;18(4):1121–1129.
27. Chaturvedi S, Ng KH, Mammen C. The path to chronic kidney disease following acute kidney injury: a neonatal perspective. *Pediatr Nephrol.* 2017;32(2):227–241.
28. Carmody JB, Charlton JR. Short-term gestation, long-term risk: prematurity and chronic kidney disease. *Pediatrics.* 2013;131(6):1168–1179.
29. Schreuder MF, Nauta J. Prenatal programming of nephron number and blood pressure. *Kidney Int.* 2007;72(3):265–268.
30. Matsell DG, Mok A, Tarantal AF. Altered primate glomerular development due to in utero urinary tract obstruction. *Kidney Int.* 2002;61(4):1263–1269.
31. Saint-Faust M, Boubred F, Simeoni U. Renal development and neonatal adaptation. *Am J Perinatol.* 2014;31(9):773–780.
32. Peters CA, Carr MC, Lais A, et al. The response of the fetal kidney to obstruction. *J Urol.* 1992;148(2 Pt 2):503–509.
33. Chevalier RL. Growth factors and apoptosis in neonatal ureteral obstruction. *J Am Soc Nephrol.* 1996;7(8):1098–1105.
34. Tarantal AF, Han VK, Cochrum KC, et al. Fetal rhesus monkey model of obstructive renal dysplasia. *Kidney Int.* 2001;59(2):446–456.
35. Hiatt MJ, Ivanova L, Toran N, et al. Remodeling of the fetal collecting duct epithelium. *Am J Pathol.* 2010;176(2):630–637.
36. Haycock GB. Development of glomerular filtration and tubular sodium reabsorption in the human fetus and newborn. *Br J Urol.* 1998;81(suppl 2):33–38.
37. Robillard JE, Kulvinskas C, Sessions C, et al. Maturational changes in the fetal glomerular filtration rate. *Am J Obstet Gynecol.* 1975;122(5):601–606.
38. Manalich R, Reyes L, Herrera M, et al. Relationship between weight at birth and the number and size of renal glomeruli in humans: a histomorphometric study. *Kidney Int.* 2000;58(2):770–773.
39. Hughson M, Farris AB 3rd, Douglas-Denton R, et al. Glomerular number and size in autopsy kidneys: the relationship to birth weight. *Kidney Int.* 2003;63(6):2113–2122.
40. Arant BS Jr. Developmental patterns of renal functional maturation compared in the human neonate. *J Pediatr.* 1978;92(5):705–712.
41. Trnka P, Hiatt MJ, Tarantal AF, Matsell DG. Congenital urinary tract obstruction: defining markers of developmental kidney injury. *Pediatr Res.* 2012;72(5):446–454.
42. Hill KJ, Lumbers ER. Renal function in adult and fetal sheep. *J Dev Physiol.* 1988;10(2):149–159.
43. Seikaly MG, Arant BS Jr. Development of renal hemodynamics: glomerular filtration and renal blood flow. *Clin Perinatol.* 1992;19(1):1–13.
44. Spitzer A, Edelmann CM Jr. Maturational changes in pressure gradients for glomerular filtration. *Am J Physiol.* 1971;221(5):1431–1435.
45. Ichikawa I, Maddox DA, Brenner BM. Maturational development of glomerular ultrafiltration in the rat. *Am J Physiol.* 1979;236(5):F465–F471.
46. Aperia A, Herin P. Development of glomerular perfusion rate and nephron filtration rate in rats 17-60 days old. *Am J Physiol.* 1975;228(5):1319–1325.
47. Allison ME, Lipham EM, Gottschalk CW. Hydrostatic pressure in the rat kidney. *Am J Physiol.* 1972;223(4):975–983.
48. Rudolph AM, Heymann MA. The fetal circulation. *Annu Rev Med.* 1968;19:195–206.
49. Veille JC, Hanson RA, Tatum K, Kelley K. Quantitative assessment of human fetal renal blood flow. *Am J Obstet Gynecol.* 1993;169(6):1399–1402.
50. Gruskin AB, Edelmann CM Jr, Yuan S. Maturational changes in renal blood flow in piglets. *Pediatr Res.* 1970;4(1):7–13.
51. Aperia A, Broberger O, Herin P, Joelsson I. Renal hemodynamics in the perinatal period. A study in lambs. *Acta Physiol Scand.* 1977;99(3):261–269.
52. Wolf G. Angiotensin II and tubular development. *Nephrol Dial Transplant.* 2002;17(suppl 9):48–51.
53. Robillard JE, Weismann DN, Gomez RA, et al. Renal and adrenal responses to converting-enzyme inhibition in fetal and newborn life. *Am J Physiol.* 1983;244(2):R249–R256.
54. DiBona GF, Kopp UC. Neural control of renal function. *Physiol Rev.* 1997;77(1):75–197.
55. Abadie L, Blazy I, Roubert P, et al. Decrease in endothelin-1 renal receptors during the 1st month of life in the rat. *Pediatr Nephrol.* 1996;10(2):185–189.
56. Guignard J, Gouyon JB. Glomerular filtration in neonates. In: Polin R, ed. *Nephrology and Fluid/Electrolyte Physiology: Neonatology Questions and Controversies.* 2nd ed. Philadelphia: Elsevier; 2012:117–135.

57. Solhaug MJ, Ballevre LD, Guignard JP, et al. Nitric oxide in the developing kidney. *Pediatr Nephrol.* 1996;10(4):529–539.
58. Solhaug MJ, Wallace MR, Granger JP. Nitric oxide and angiotensin II regulation of renal hemodynamics in the developing piglet. *Pediatr Res.* 1996;39(3):527–533.
59. Han KH, Lim JM, Kim WY, et al. Expression of endothelial nitric oxide synthase in developing rat kidney. *Am J Physiol Renal Physiol.* 2005;288(4):F694–F702.
60. Rodriguez-Soriano J, Vallo A, Castillo G, Oliveros R. Renal handling of water and sodium in infancy and childhood: a study using clearance methods during hypotonic saline diuresis. *Kidney Int.* 1981; 20(6):700–704.
61. Sujov P, Kellerman L, Zeltzer M, Hochberg Z. Plasma and urine osmolality in full-term and pre-term infants. *Acta Paediatr Scand.* 1984;73(6):722–726.
62. Horster MF, Zink H. Functional differentiation of the medullary collecting tubule: influence of vasopressin. *Kidney Int.* 1982;22(4):360–365.
63. Hadeed AJ, Leake RD, Weitzman RE, Fisher DA. Possible mechanisms of high blood levels of vasopressin during the neonatal period. *J Pediatr.* 1979;94(5):805–808.
64. Yasui M, Marples D, Belusa R, et al. Development of urinary concentrating capacity: role of aquaporin-2. *Am J Physiol.* 1996;271(2 Pt 2):F461–F468.
65. Baum M, Quigley R, Satlin L. Maturational changes in renal tubular transport. *Curr Opin Nephrol Hypertens.* 2003;12(5):521–526.
66. Bonilla-Felix M, Jiang W. Aquaporin-2 in the immature rat: expression, regulation, and trafficking. *J Am Soc Nephrol.* 1997;8(10):1502–1509.
67. Waters A. Functional development of the nephron. In: Geary D, Schaefer F, eds. *Comprehensive Pediatric Nephrology.* Philadelphia: Elsevier; 2008:111–129.
68. Madsen K, Tinning AR, Marcussen N, Jensen BL. Postnatal development of the renal medulla; role of the renin-angiotensin system. *Acta Physiol (Oxf).* 2013;208(1):41–49.
69. Cha JH, Kim YH, Jung JY, et al. Cell proliferation in the loop of henle in the developing rat kidney. *J Am Soc Nephrol.* 2001;12(7):1410–1421.
70. Song R, Yosypiv IV. Development of the kidney medulla. *Organogenesis.* 2012;8(1):10–17.
71. Siegel SR, Oh W. Renal function as a marker of human fetal maturation. *Acta Paediatr Scand.* 1976;65(4):481–485.
72. Bueva A, Guignard JP. Renal function in preterm neonates. *Pediatr Res.* 1994;36(5):572–577.
73. Baum M, Quigley R. Ontogeny of renal sodium transport. *Semin Perinatol.* 2004;28(2):91–96.
74. Schmidt U, Horster M. Na-K-activated ATPase: activity maturation in rabbit nephron segments dissected in vitro. *Am J Physiol.* 1977;233(1):F55–F60.
75. Guillery EN, Karniski LP, Mathews MS, Robillard JE. Maturation of proximal tubule Na+/H+ antiporter activity in sheep during transition from fetus to newborn. *Am J Physiol.* 1994;267(4 Pt 2):F537–F545.
76. Igarashi P, Vanden Heuvel GB, Payne JA, Forbush B 3rd. Cloning, embryonic expression, and alternative splicing of a murine kidney-specific Na-K-Cl cotransporter. *Am J Physiol.* 1995;269(3 Pt 2):F405–F418.
77. Schmitt R, Ellison DH, Farman N, et al. Developmental expression of sodium entry pathways in rat nephron. *Am J Physiol.* 1999;276(3 Pt 2):F367–F381.
78. Vehaskari VM, Hempe JM, Manning J, et al. Developmental regulation of ENaC subunit mRNA levels in rat kidney. *Am J Physiol.* 1998;274(6 Pt 1):C1661–C1666.
79. Watanabe S, Matsushita K, McCray PB Jr, Stokes JB. Developmental expression of the epithelial Na+ channel in kidney and uroepithelia. *Am J Physiol.* 1999;276(2 Pt 2):F304–F314.
80. Quigley R, Baum M. Developmental changes in rabbit proximal straight tubule paracellular permeability. *Am J Physiol Renal Physiol.* 2002;283(3):F525–F531.
81. Chevalier RL, Thornhill BA, Belmonte DC, Baertschi AJ. Endogenous angiotensin II inhibits natriuresis after acute volume expansion in the neonatal rat. *Am J Physiol.* 1996;270(2 Pt 2):R393–R397.
82. Sulyok E. Dopaminergic control of neonatal salt and water metabolism. *Pediatr Nephrol.* 1988; 2(1):163–165.
83. Beck JC, Lipkowitz MS, Abramson RG. Ontogeny of Na/H antiporter activity in rabbit renal brush border membrane vesicles. *J Clin Invest.* 1991;87(6):2067–2076.
84. Bierd TM, Kattwinkel J, Chevalier RL, et al. Interrelationship of atrial natriuretic peptide, atrial volume, and renal function in premature infants. *J Pediatr.* 1990;116(5):753–759.
85. Gibson KJ, McMullen JR, Lumbers ER. Renal acid-base and sodium handling in hypoxia and subsequent mild metabolic acidosis in foetal sheep. *Clin Exp Pharmacol Physiol.* 2000;27(1–2):67–73.
86. Schwartz GJ, Haycock GB, Edelmann CM Jr, Spitzer A. Late metabolic acidosis: a reassessment of the definition. *J Pediatr.* 1979;95(1):102–107.
87. Edelmann CM, Soriano JR, Boichis H, et al. Renal bicarbonate reabsorption and hydrogen ion excretion in normal infants. *J Clin Invest.* 1967;46(8):1309–1317.
88. Schwartz GJ, Evan AP. Development of solute transport in rabbit proximal tubule. I. HCO-3 and glucose absorption. *Am J Physiol.* 1983;245(3):F382–F390.
89. Schwartz GJ, Brown D, Mankus R, et al. Low pH enhances expression of carbonic anhydrase II by cultured rat inner medullary collecting duct cells. *Am J Physiol.* 1994;266(2 Pt 1):C508–C514.
90. Winkler CA, Kittelberger AM, Watkins RH, et al. Maturation of carbonic anhydrase IV expression in rabbit kidney. *Am J Physiol Renal Physiol.* 2001;280(5):F895–F903.
91. Mehrgut FM, Satlin LM, Schwartz GJ. Maturation of HCO3– transport in rabbit collecting duct. *Am J Physiol.* 1990;259(5 Pt 2):F801–F808.

92. Kim J, Tisher CC, Madsen KM. Differentiation of intercalated cells in developing rat kidney: an immunohistochemical study. *Am J Physiol*. 1994;266(6 Pt 2):F977–F990.
93. Satlin LM, Matsumoto T, Schwartz GJ. Postnatal maturation of rabbit renal collecting duct. III. Peanut lectin-binding intercalated cells. *Am J Physiol*. 1992;262(2 Pt 2):F199–F208.
94. Matsell DG, Yu S, Morrison SJ. Antenatal Determinants of Long-Term Kidney Outcome in Boys with Posterior Urethral Valves. *Fetal Diagn Ther*. 2016;39(3):214–221.
95. Chevalier RL, Kim A, Thornhill BA, Wolstenholme JT. Recovery following relief of unilateral ureteral obstruction in the neonatal rat. *Kidney Int*. 1999;55(3):793–807.
96. Chevalier RL, Thornhill BA, Forbes MS, Kiley SC. Mechanisms of renal injury and progression of renal disease in congenital obstructive nephropathy. *Pediatr Nephrol*. 2010;25(4):687–697.
97. Silverstein DM, Travis BR, Thornhill BA, et al. Altered expression of immune modulator and structural genes in neonatal unilateral ureteral obstruction. *Kidney Int*. 2003;64(1):25–35.
98. Butt MJ, Tarantal AF, Jimenez DF, Matsell DG. Collecting duct epithelial-mesenchymal transition in fetal urinary tract obstruction. *Kidney Int*. 2007;72(8):936–944.
99. Winyard P, Chitty L. Dysplastic and polycystic kidneys: diagnosis, associations and management. *Prenat Diagn*. 2001;21(11):924–935.
100. Moniz CF, Nicolaides KH, Bamforth FJ, Rodeck CH. Normal reference ranges for biochemical substances relating to renal, hepatic, and bone function in fetal and maternal plasma throughout pregnancy. *J Clin Pathol*. 1985;38(4):468–472.
101. Nicolaides KH, Cheng HH, Snijders RJ, Moniz CF. Fetal urine biochemistry in the assessment of obstructive uropathy. *Am J Obstet Gynecol*. 1992;166(3):932–937.
102. Nava S, Bocconi L, Zuliani G, et al. Aspects of fetal physiology from 18 to 37 weeks' gestation as assessed by blood sampling. *Obstet Gynecol*. 1996;87(6):975–980.
103. Berry SM, Lecolier B, Smith RS, et al. Predictive value of fetal serum beta 2-microglobulin for neonatal renal function. *Lancet*. 1995;345(8960):1277–1278.
104. Cobet G, Gummelt T, Bollmann R, et al. Assessment of serum levels of alpha-1-microglobulin, beta-2-microglobulin, and retinol binding protein in the fetal blood. A method for prenatal evaluation of renal function. *Prenat Diagn*. 1996;16(4):299–305.
105. Dommergues M, Muller F, Ngo S, et al. Fetal serum beta2-microglobulin predicts postnatal renal function in bilateral uropathies. *Kidney Int*. 2000;58(1):312–316.
106. Muller F, Dreux S, Audibert F, et al. Fetal serum ss2-microglobulin and cystatin C in the prediction of post-natal renal function in bilateral hypoplasia and hyperechogenic enlarged kidneys. *Prenat Diagn*. 2004;24(5):327–332.
107. Nguyen C, Dreux S, Heidet L, et al. Fetal serum alpha-1 microglobulin for renal function assessment: comparison with beta2-microglobulin and cystatin C. *Prenat Diagn*. 2013;33(8):775–781.
108. Glick PL, Harrison MR, Golbus MS, et al. Management of the fetus with congenital hydronephrosis II: prognostic criteria and selection for treatment. *J Pediatr Surg*. 1985;20(4):376–387.
109. Crombleholme TM, Harrison MR, Golbus MS, et al. Fetal intervention in obstructive uropathy: prognostic indicators and efficacy of intervention. *Am J Obstet Gynecol*. 1990;162(5):1239–1244.
110. Mandelbrot L, Dumez Y, Muller F, Dommergues M. Prenatal prediction of renal function in fetal obstructive uropathies. *J Perinat Med*. 1991;19(suppl 1):283–287.
111. Eugene M, Muller F, Dommergues M, et al. Evaluation of postnatal renal function in fetuses with bilateral obstructive uropathies by proton nuclear magnetic resonance spectroscopy. *Am J Obstet Gynecol*. 1994;170(2):595–602.
112. Freedman AL, Bukowski TP, Smith CA, et al. Fetal therapy for obstructive uropathy: diagnosis specific outcomes [corrected]. *J Urol*. 1996;156(2 Pt 2):720–723, discussion 723–724.
113. Guez S, Assael BM, Melzi ML, et al. Shortcomings in predicting postnatal renal function using prenatal urine biochemistry in fetuses with congenital hydronephrosis. *J Pediatr Surg*. 1996;31(10):1401–1404.
114. Bunduki V, Saldanha LB, Sadek L, et al. Fetal renal biopsies in obstructive uropathy: feasibility and clinical correlations—preliminary results. *Prenat Diagn*. 1998;18(2):101–109.
115. Muller F, Bernard MA, Benkirane A, et al. Fetal urine cystatin C as a predictor of postnatal renal function in bilateral uropathies. *Clin Chem*. 1999;45(12):2292–2293.
116. Miguelez J, Bunduki V, Yoshizaki CT, et al. Fetal obstructive uropathy: is urine sampling useful for prenatal counselling? *Prenat Diagn*. 2006;26(1):81–84.
117. Abdennadher W, Chalouhi G, Dreux S, et al. Fetal urine biochemistry at 13-23 weeks of gestation in lower urinary tract obstruction: criteria for in-utero treatment. *Ultrasound Obstet Gynecol*. 2015;46(3):306–311.
118. Morris RK, Quinlan-Jones E, Kilby MD, Khan KS. Systematic review of accuracy of fetal urine analysis to predict poor postnatal renal function in cases of congenital urinary tract obstruction. *Prenat Diagn*. 2007;27(10):900–911.
119. Mussap M, Fanos V, Pizzini C, et al. Predictive value of amniotic fluid cystatin C levels for the early identification of fetuses with obstructive uropathies. *BJOG*. 2002;109(7):778–783.
120. Rabinowitz R, Peters MT, Vyas S, et al. Measurement of fetal urine production in normal pregnancy by real-time ultrasonography. *Am J Obstet Gynecol*. 1989;161(5):1264–1266.
121. Hedriana HL. Ultrasound measurement of fetal urine flow. *Clin Obstet Gynecol*. 1997;40(2):337–351.
122. Underwood MA, Gilbert WM, Sherman MP. Amniotic fluid: not just fetal urine anymore. *J Perinatol*. 2005;25(5):341–348.
123. Sanna-Cherchi S, Ravani P, Corbani V, et al. Renal outcome in patients with congenital anomalies of the kidney and urinary tract. *Kidney Int*. 2009;76(5):528–533.

21

124. Westland R, Kurvers RA, van Wijk JA, Schreuder MF. Risk factors for renal injury in children with a solitary functioning kidney. *Pediatrics*. 2013;131(2):e478–e485.

125. Westland R, Schreuder MF, Bokenkamp A, et al. Renal injury in children with a solitary functioning kidney—the KIMONO study. *Nephrol Dial Transplant*. 2011;26(5):1533–1541.

126. Mansoor O, Chandar J, Rodriguez MM, et al. Long-term risk of chronic kidney disease in unilateral multicystic dysplastic kidney. *Pediatr Nephrol*. 2011;26(4):597–603.

127. Seikaly MG, Ho PL, Emmett L, et al. Chronic renal insufficiency in children: the 2001 Annual Report of the NAPRTCS. *Pediatr Nephrol*. 2003;18(8):796–804.

128. Ansari MS, Gulia A, Srivastava A, Kapoor R. Risk factors for progression to end-stage renal disease in children with posterior urethral valves. *J Pediatr Urol*. 2010;6(3):261–264.

129. Heikkila J, Holmberg C, Kyllonen L, et al. Long-term risk of end stage renal disease in patients with posterior urethral valves. *J Urol*. 2011;186(6):2392–2396.

130. Sarhan OM, El-Ghoneimi AA, Helmy TE, et al. Posterior urethral valves: multivariate analysis of factors affecting the final renal outcome. *J Urol*. 2011;185(6 suppl):2491–2495.

131. Holmdahl G, Sillen U. Boys with posterior urethral valves: outcome concerning renal function, bladder function and paternity at ages 31 to 44 years. *J Urol*. 2005;174(3):1031–1034, discussion 1034.

132. DeFoor W, Clark C, Jackson E, et al. Risk factors for end stage renal disease in children with posterior urethral valves. *J Urol*. 2008;180(4 suppl):1705–1708, discussion 1708.

133. Pohl M, Mentzel HJ, Vogt S, et al. Risk factors for renal insufficiency in children with urethral valves. *Pediatr Nephrol*. 2012;27(3):443–450.

134. Lal R, Bhatnagar V, Mitra DK. Long-term prognosis of renal function in boys treated for posterior urethral valves. *Eur J Pediatr Surg*. 1999;9(5):307–311.

135. Ziylan O, Oktar T, Ander H, et al. The impact of late presentation of posterior urethral valves on bladder and renal function. *J Urol*. 2006;175(5):1894–1897, discussion 1897.

136. Denes ED, Barthold JS, Gonzalez R. Early prognostic value of serum creatinine levels in children with posterior urethral valves. *J Urol*. 1997;157(4):1441–1443.

137. Drozdz D, Drozdz M, Gretz N, et al. Progression to end-stage renal disease in children with posterior urethral valves. *Pediatr Nephrol*. 1998;12(8):630–636.

138. Lopez Pereira P, Espinosa L, Martinez Urrutina MJ, et al. Posterior urethral valves: prognostic factors. *BJU Int*. 2003;91(7):687–690.

139. Harvie S, McLeod L, Acott P, et al. Abnormal antenatal sonogram: an indicator of disease severity in children with posterior urethral valves. *Can Assoc Radiol J*. 2009;60(4):185–189.

140. Reinberg Y, de Castano I, Gonzalez R. Prognosis for patients with prenatally diagnosed posterior urethral valves. *J Urol*. 1992;148(1):125–126.

141. Hutton KA, Thomas DF, Arthur RJ, et al. Prenatally detected posterior urethral valves: is gestational age at detection a predictor of outcome? *J Urol*. 1994;152(2 Pt 2):698–701.

142. Roth KS, Carter WH Jr, Chan JC. Obstructive nephropathy in children: long-term progression after relief of posterior urethral valve. *Pediatrics*. 2001;107(5):1004–1010.

143. Kousidis G, Thomas DF, Morgan H, et al. The long-term outcome of prenatally detected posterior urethral valves: a 10 to 23-year follow-up study. *BJU Int*. 2008;102(8):1020–1024.

144. Morris RK, Kilby MD. An overview of the literature on congenital lower urinary tract obstruction and introduction to the PLUTO trial: percutaneous shunting in lower urinary tract obstruction. *Aust N Z J Obstet Gynaecol*. 2009;49(1):6–10.

145. Hutton KA, Thomas DF, Davies BW. Prenatally detected posterior urethral valves: qualitative assessment of second trimester scans and prediction of outcome. *J Urol*. 1997;158(3 Pt 2):1022–1025.

146. Bernardes LS, Salomon R, Aksnes G, et al. Ultrasound evaluation of prognosis in fetuses with posterior urethral valves. *J Pediatr Surg*. 2011;46(7):1412–1418.

147. Kibar Y, Ashley RA, Roth CC, et al. Timing of posterior urethral valve diagnosis and its impact on clinical outcome. *J Pediatr Urol*. 2011;7(5):538–542.

148. Daikha-Dahmane F, Dommergues M, Muller F, et al. Development of human fetal kidney in obstructive uropathy: correlations with ultrasonography and urine biochemistry. *Kidney Int*. 1997;52(1):21–32.

149. Jee LD, Rickwood AM, Turnock RR. Posterior urethral valves. Does prenatal diagnosis influence prognosis? *Br J Urol*. 1993;72(5 Pt 2):830–833.

150. Zaccara A, Giorlandino C, Mobili L, et al. Amniotic fluid index and fetal bladder outlet obstruction. Do we really need more? *J Urol*. 2005;174(4 Pt 2):1657–1660.

151. Sarhan O, Zaccaria I, Macher MA, et al. Long-term outcome of prenatally detected posterior urethral valves: single center study of 65 cases managed by primary valve ablation. *J Urol*. 2008;179(1):307–312, discussion 312–313.

152. Kaefer M, Peters CA, Retik AB, Benacerraf BB. Increased renal echogenicity: a sonographic sign for differentiating between obstructive and nonobstructive etiologies of in utero bladder distension. *J Urol*. 1997;158(3 Pt 2):1026–1029.

153. Anumba DO, Scott JE, Plant ND, Robson SC. Diagnosis and outcome of fetal lower urinary tract obstruction in the northern region of England. *Prenat Diagn*. 2005;25(1):7–13.

154. El-Ghoneimi A, Desgrippes A, Luton D, et al. Outcome of posterior urethral valves: to what extent is it improved by prenatal diagnosis? *J Urol*. 1999;162(3 Pt 1):849–853.

155. Coplen DE, Hare JY, Zderic SA, et al. 10-year experience with prenatal intervention for hydronephrosis. *J Urol*. 1996;156(3):1142–1145.

156. Oliveira EA, Rabelo EA, Pereira AK, et al. Prognostic factors in prenatally-detected posterior urethral valves: a multivariate analysis. *Pediatr Surg Int*. 2002;18(8):662–667.

157. Morris RK, Malin GL, Khan KS, Kilby MD. Antenatal ultrasound to predict postnatal renal function in congenital lower urinary tract obstruction: systematic review of test accuracy. *BJOG.* 2009; 116(10):1290–1299.
158. Morris RK, Malin GL, Quinlan-Jones E, et al. Percutaneous vesicoamniotic shunting versus conservative management for fetal lower urinary tract obstruction (PLUTO): a randomised trial. *Lancet.* 2013; 382(9903):1496–1506.
159. Matsell DG, Tarantal AF. Experimental models of fetal obstructive nephropathy. *Pediatr Nephrol.* 2002;17(7):470–476.
160. Beck AD. The effect of intra-uterine urinary obstruction upon the development of the fetal kidney. *J Urol.* 1971;105(6):784–789.
161. Harrison MR, Nakayama DK, Noall R, de Lorimier AA. Correction of congenital hydronephrosis in utero II. Decompression reverses the effects of obstruction on the fetal lung and urinary tract. *J Pediatr Surg.* 1982;17(6):965–974.
162. Josephson S, Robertson B, Rodensjo M. Effects of experimental obstructive hydronephrosis on the immature nephrons in newborn rats. *Urol Int.* 1989;44(2):61–65.
163. Trnka P, Hiatt MJ, Ivanova L, et al. Phenotypic transition of the collecting duct epithelium in congenital urinary tract obstruction. *J Biomed Biotechnol.* 2010;2010:696034.
164. Trnka P, Ivanova L, Hiatt MJ, Matsell DG. Urinary biomarkers in obstructive nephropathy. *Clin J Am Soc Nephrol.* 2012;7(10):1567–1575.
165. Fern RJ, Yesko CM, Thornhill BA, et al. Reduced angiotensinogen expression attenuates renal interstitial fibrosis in obstructive nephropathy in mice. *J Clin Invest.* 1999;103(1):39–46.
166. Grandaliano G, Gesualdo L, Bartoli F, et al. MCP-1 and EGF renal expression and urine excretion in human congenital obstructive nephropathy. *Kidney Int.* 2000;58(1):182–192.
167. Chevalier RL. Obstructive nephropathy: towards biomarker discovery and gene therapy. *Nat Clin Pract Nephrol.* 2006;2(3):157–168.
168. Shappell SB, Mendoza LH, Gurpinar T, et al. Expression of adhesion molecules in kidney with experimental chronic obstructive uropathy: the pathogenic role of ICAM-1 and VCAM-1. *Nephron.* 2000;85(2):156–166.
169. Furness PD 3rd, Maizels M, Han SW, et al. Elevated bladder urine concentration of transforming growth factor-beta1 correlates with upper urinary tract obstruction in children. *J Urol.* 1999;162(3 Pt 2):1033–1036.
170. El-Sherbiny MT, Mousa OM, Shokeir AA, Ghoneim MA. Role of urinary transforming growth factor-beta1 concentration in the diagnosis of upper urinary tract obstruction in children. *J Urol.* 2002;168(4 Pt 2):1798–1800.
171. Palmer LS, Maizels M, Kaplan WE, et al. Urine levels of transforming growth factor-beta 1 in children with ureteropelvic junction obstruction. *Urology.* 1997;50(5):769–773.
172. MacRae Dell K, Hoffman BB, Leonard MB, et al. Increased urinary transforming growth factor-beta(1) excretion in children with posterior urethral valves. *Urology.* 2000;56(2):311–314.
173. Klein J, Lacroix C, Caubet C, et al. Fetal urinary peptides to predict postnatal outcome of renal disease in fetuses with posterior urethral valves (PUV). *Sci Transl Med.* 2013;5(198):198ra106.
174. Charlton JR, Norwood VF, Kiley SC, et al. Evolution of the urinary proteome during human renal development and maturation: variations with gestational and postnatal age. *Pediatr Res.* 2012;72(2): 179–185.
175. Clark TJ, Martin WL, Divakaran TG, et al. Prenatal bladder drainage in the management of fetal lower urinary tract obstruction: a systematic review and meta-analysis. *Obstet Gynecol.* 2003; 102(2):367–382.
176. Holmes N, Harrison MR, Baskin LS. Fetal surgery for posterior urethral valves: long-term postnatal outcomes. *Pediatrics.* 2001;108(1):E7.
177. Biard JM, Johnson MP, Carr MC, et al. Long-term outcomes in children treated by prenatal vesicoamniotic shunting for lower urinary tract obstruction. *Obstet Gynecol.* 2005;106(3):503–508.
178. Morris RK, Daniels J, Deeks J, et al. The challenges of interventional trials in fetal therapy. *Arch Dis Child Fetal Neonatal Ed.* 2014;99(6):F448–F450.

21

Index

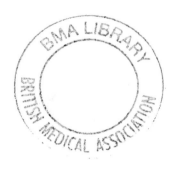